S0-BPZ-684

ULTRASONOGRAPHY OF DIGESTIVE DISEASES

ULTRASONOGRAPHY OF DIGESTIVE DISEASES

Francis S. Weill, M.D.

Head, Department of Diagnostic Radiology
University Hospital
Professor of Radiology
University of Besançon School of Medicine
Besançon, France

with 1336 *illustrations*

The C. V. Mosby Company

Saint Louis 1978

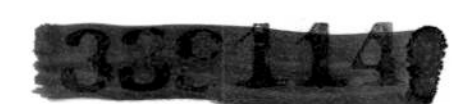

Printed in the United States of America

Distributed in Great Britain by Henry Kimpton, London

The C. V. Mosby Company
11830 Westline Industrial Drive, St. Louis, Missouri 63141

Library of Congress Cataloging in Publication Data

Weill, Francis Samuel, 1933-
Ultrasonography of digestive diseases.

Bibliography: p.
Includes index.
1. Diagnosis, Ultrasonic. 2. Digestive organs—Diseases—Diagnosis. I. Title. [DNLM: 1. Gastrointestinal diseases—Diagnosis. 2. Ultrasonics—Diagnostic use. WI141 W422u]
RC804.U4W44 616.3′6′0754 77-13046
ISBN 0-8016-5374-6

CB/CB/B 9 8 7 6 5 4 3 2 1

To my everloving wife,
who said that,
if I ever dared to write another book,
she would fly to Honolulu.
That was a mistake:
I will.

Preface

This book reflects ten years of ultrasonographic experience combining the techniques of real-time and contact scanning.

During the process of accumulating illustrations for this book, two important technical advances took place: first, gray scale imaging by scan converter became available in Europe in mid-1975; second, the greatly improved gray scale imaging of the contact machines of the third generation became available in France in March, 1977, at the very time this manuscript was completed. These changes are responsible for a rather large variability in the quality of images. Unusual cases that were encountered before 1975 and cannot be readily duplicated are shown in bistable imaging. A few demonstratively normal bistable images were also retained: in fact, the bistable image is a caricature of sectional anatomy and, as such, is a striking way of demonstrating typical acoustic interfaces.

I wish to supplement the information of new ultrasonographers, whose training, by apprenticeship, is long and without any assurance that in a limited time they will encounter a sufficient variety of pathological conditions. I also wish to familiarize radiologists, internists, surgeons, and other specialists with ultrasonographic images; without having practiced ultrasonography themselves, they should be able to understand and use information derived by this method. Finally, I believe that the large number of ultrasonographers now entering the domain of real-time and gray scale techniques will find this work to be a guide to a new methodology for ultrasonic symptomatology. Many of the ultrasonic signs described in this book should also be displayed by x-ray–computed axial tomography. Thus this study of ultrasonic imaging in digestive pathology may constitute a link between the recent, sophisticated method of CT scanning, which, in my opinion, should remain closely associated with ultrasonography, and the work of the pioneers in the field of ultrasonic diagnosis. To those pioneers, Dr. Joseph Holmes of Denver and Dr. Ian Donald of Glasgow, Scotland, I wish to express a respectful tribute.

Francis S. Weill

Acknowledgments

I want to thank Dr. Eisenscher, my former assistant, who contributed several personal ultrasonograms and collaborated in writing Chapter 22 and part of Chapter 10; Dr. Roussille and Dr. Duquesnel, from Lyons; Dr. Triller, from Bern; Mr. Planiol and Mr. Feil, from Tours; and Dr. Mauleon, from Rouen, who also contributed personal cases. Special thanks go to Mrs. M. T. Wackenheim and Mr. Rudolf Leonard, whose help was of great value in translating the text from French to English. I am particularly grateful to Dr. Fred Winsberg, from Montreal, who spent a long time reviewing the "Frenglish" version of this book and whose contribution of multiple scans helped to update the illustrations. Finally, I want to thank Miss Cheval, my secretary; Miss Chapuis; Miss Nussbaum; Mrs. Devèze; and Mr. Bernard, photographer, and Mr. Pellissioli, artist, for their technical help.

Francis S. Weill

Contents

PART II
THE LIVER

PART I

TECHNOLOGY: imaging, echopatterns, and echoanatomical introduction

CHAPTER 1

PRINCIPLES OF ULTRASONOGRAPHY AND TYPES OF ULTRASONOGRAPHIC IMAGES

To understand ultrasonography it is necessary to appreciate salami. Normally one cuts a salami in transverse slices (Fig. 1-1, *A*). This is the procedure of the ultrasonographer when confronted by an abdomen. One may also cut salami in longitudinal slices (Fig. 1-1, *B*) or in oblique slices (Fig. 1-1, *C*). When one is capable of cutting in all directions and can recognize all the details of the slice (Figs. 1-2 and 1-3), one has become a good ultrasonographer, member of the "salami club," so called by my friend George Leopold, of San Diego.

For those who do not like salami and are opposed to this gastronomical approach to digestive ultrasonography, there is another approach to ultrasonography: sadomasochism (Fig. 1-4).

PRINCIPLES OF ULTRASONIC LAMINAGRAPHY

The technique illustrated in Fig. 1-4 leaves one open to malpractice suits. One must therefore find something else. It is useful to recall certain principles of ultrasonographic scanning.

The basic tool is the transducer. It emits pulsating ultrasound, the emission of which lasts approximately a microsecond, with a millisecond interval. These intervals permit the use of the transducer as both an emitter and a receptor. When a transducer is placed in contact with the abdomen and emits its ultrasonic beam through the visceral organs, a certain number of echoes return from the interface zone (Fig. 1-5). These echoes are then visualized on a cathode-ray tube, either in the form of deflections, A mode (Fig. 1-5, *B*), or in the form of bright spots, B mode (Fig. 1-5, *C*).

If the transducer is displaced along the surface of the abdomen, at each new position a series of bright spots representing the interface zones will appear (Fig. 1-6). If one records the echoes from an infinite number of successive positions, the summation will construct an image of a transverse section of the abdomen (Figs. 1-7 and 1-8). Thus the construction of an ultrasonographic scan demands the following:

- Displacement of the transducer along a fixed plane
- Display of the echoes on a scope, in the form of bright spots
- Summation of these spots

The different modes of displacement and summation have led to the development of different types of imaging systems. These are, on the one hand, contact scanning, with bistable imaging and gray scale display, and, on the other hand, real time.

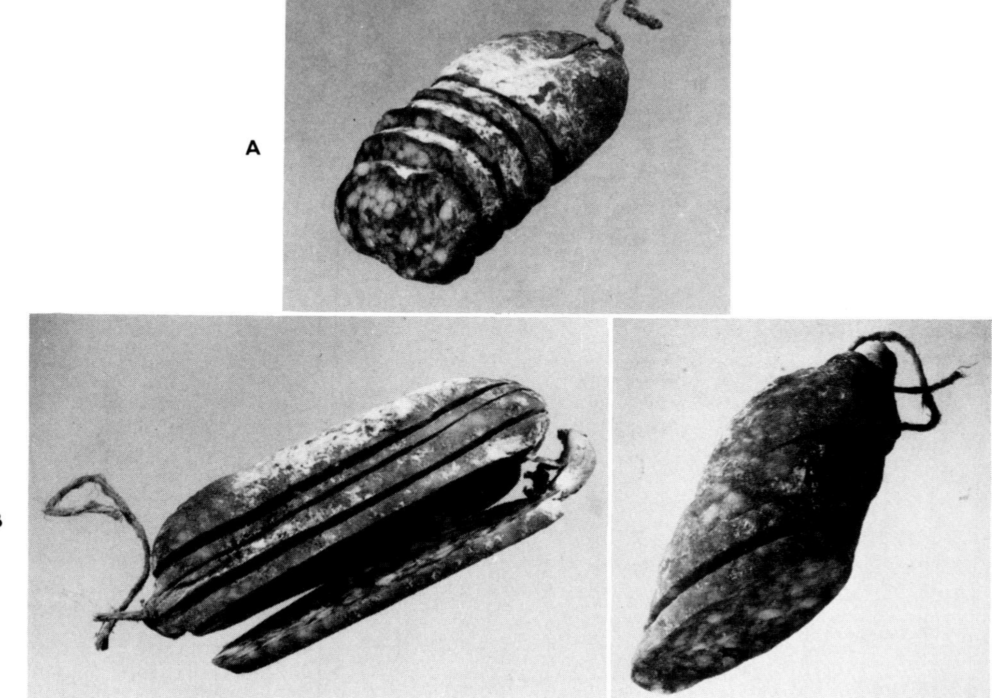

Fig. 1-1. Gastronomic approach to digestive ultrasonography. **A,** Transverse slices of French salami. **B,** Longitudinal slices. **C,** Oblique slices.

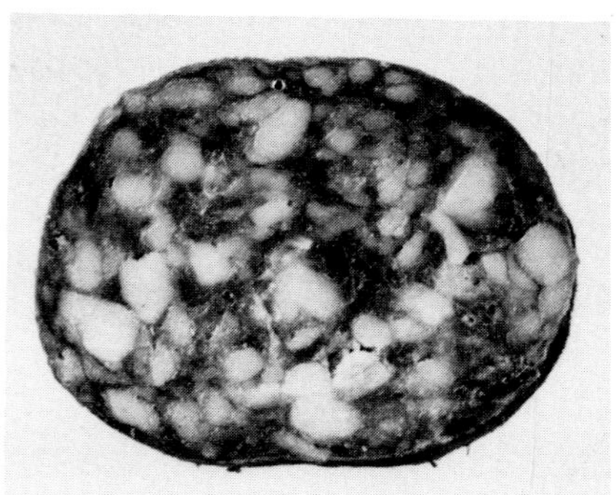

Fig. 1-2. Salami slice in close-up.

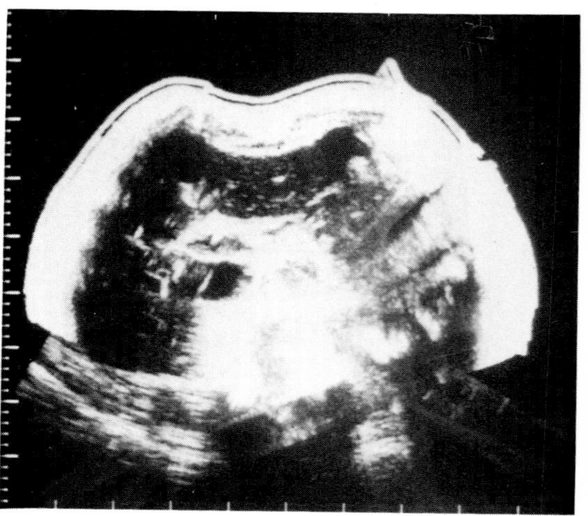

Fig. 1-3. Abdomen slice—same technique.

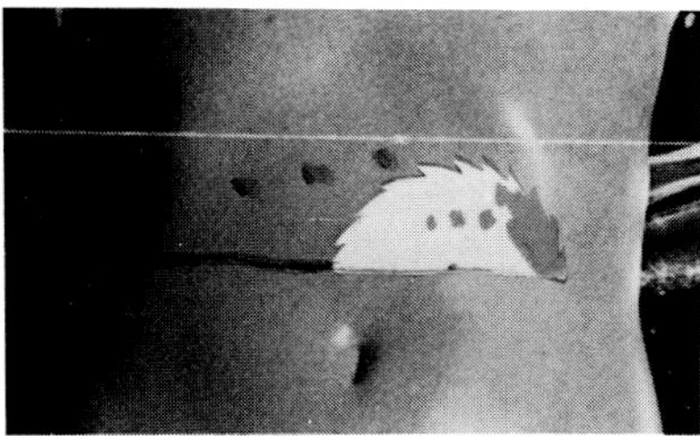

Fig. 1-4. Sadistic approach to digestive ultrasonography.

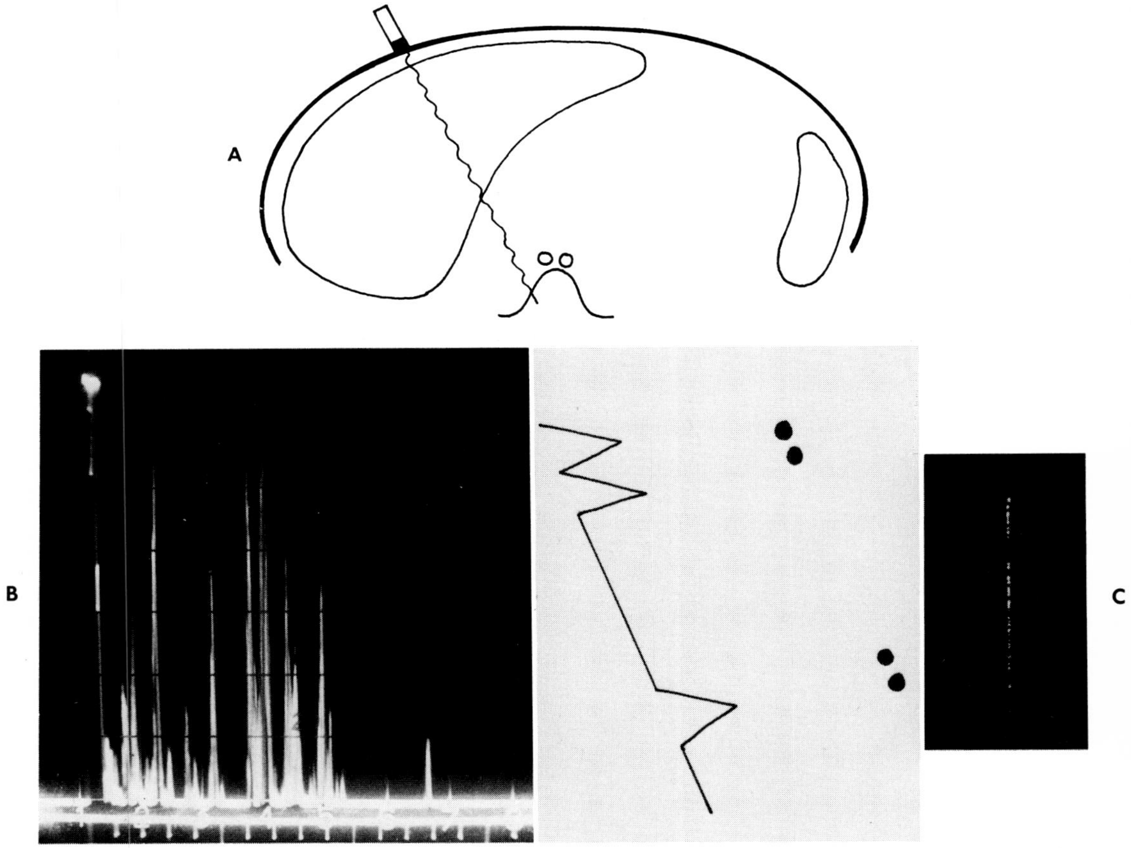

A

B

C

Fig. 1-5. A, Progression of ultrasonic beam across a liver displayed in transverse section. **B,** Deflections of A-mode display. **C,** B-mode display in which the deflections are replaced by bright spots.

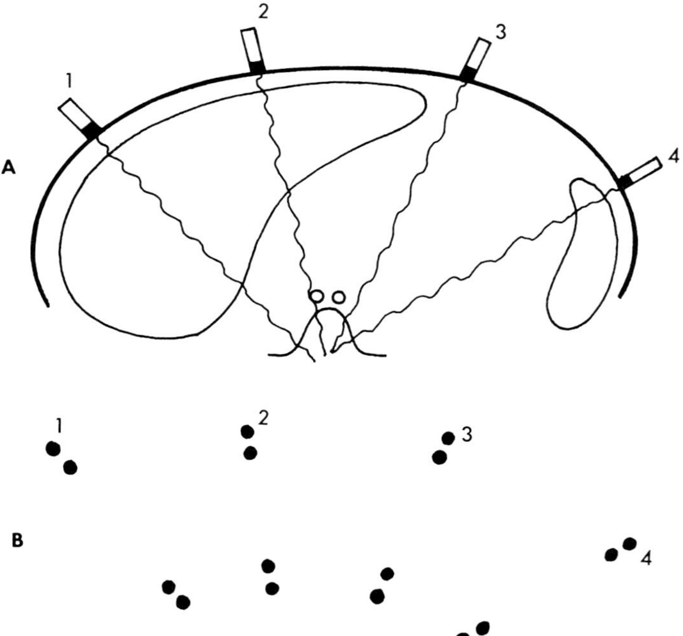

Fig. 1-6. A, Successive positions of transducer during transverse scan of abdomen. **B,** Connected bright spots.

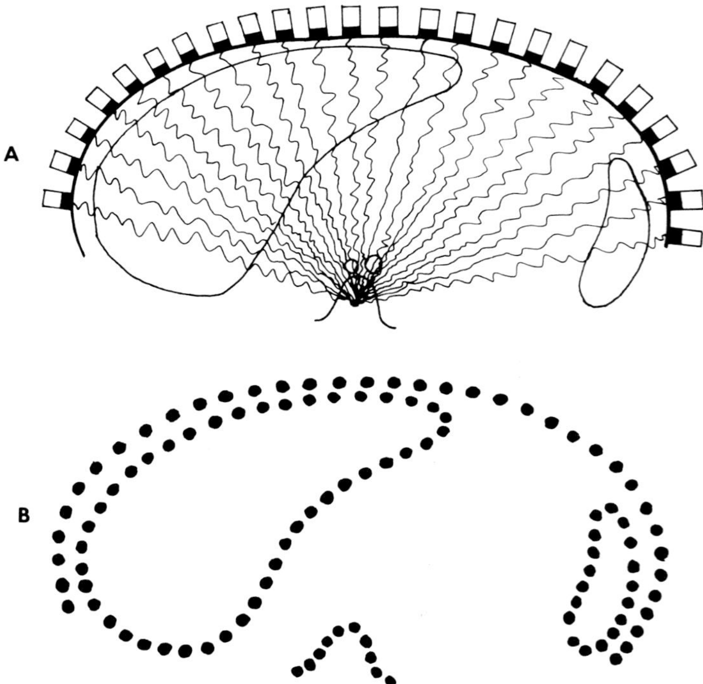

Fig. 1-7. A, Much closer successive positions of transducer during transverse scanning of abdomen. **B,** Summation of multiple bright spots belonging to successive positions of transducer. This summation builds up sectional image of different organs through which ultrasonic beam has passed.

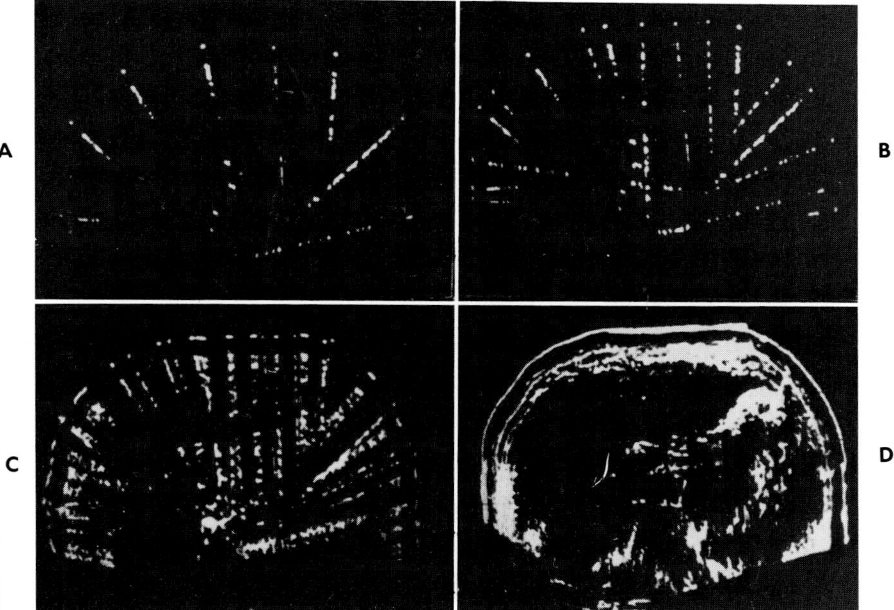

Fig. 1-8. Practical example of principle of B-mode ultrasonography: transverse section of abdomen. **A,** Bright spots displayed on storage tube by eight successive positions of transducer. **B,** Bright spots displayed through seventeen successive positions of transducer. **C,** Scanning is now almost continuous. **D,** Continuous scanning. Images of liver and spleen are now outlined.

CONTACT SCANNING

In the first type of ultrasonic system, the transducer of the machine is manually displaced along the surface of the region to be explored (Fig. 1-7). A contact gel, without which intervening air would reduce transmission to no more than 0.1%, is used. Obtaining a global tomographic section demands that the displacement be made along a single plane (Fig. 1-9). The transducer then is animated along its course, the explored region, by successive pendular movements, thus producing a compound scan (Fig. 1-10). The summation of the bright points is accomplished by means of a storage tube. The image produced by conventional contact scanning has the following properties:

1. The image is constructed progressively in several (approximately 1 to 5) seconds. Therefore this construction is rather slow and risks blurring of the image. For many anatomical regions, it is, however, possible to use a rapid (less than a second) passage of the transducer, either linear or sectorial, and thus reduce the blur. This is called a *single-sweep scan.*

2. The direct manipulation of the transducer by hand introduces a human factor, with associated hazards, which are drastically reduced with the single-sweep scanning technique. On the other hand, with the compound scanning technique it is possible to circumscribe the region completely with the transducer, resulting in global anatomical slices. These techniques may be usefully combined.

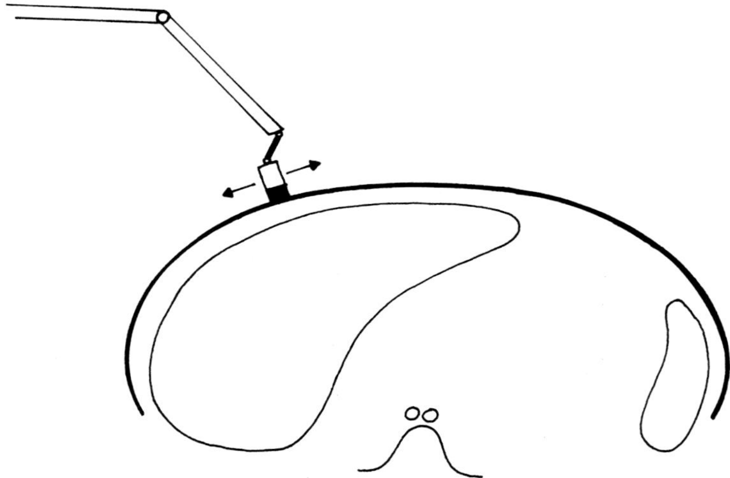

Fig. 1-9. Pantographic device assuring geometrical reliability of the section, which must be made in one plane only.

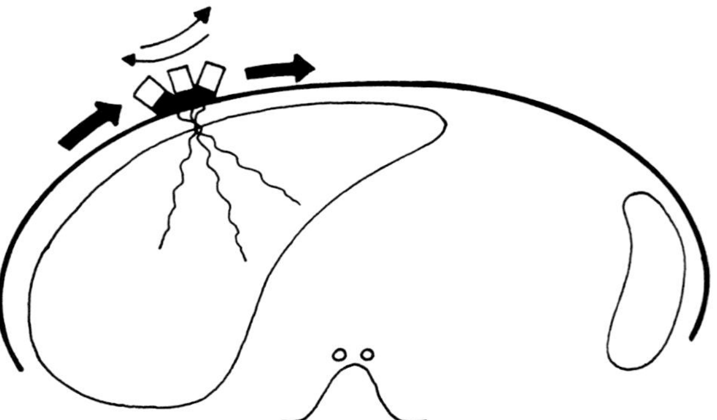

Fig. 1-10. Principle of compound scanning. To basic linear sweeping movement of transducer around body are added successive pendular movements. With recent machines, such pendular movements are less necessary.

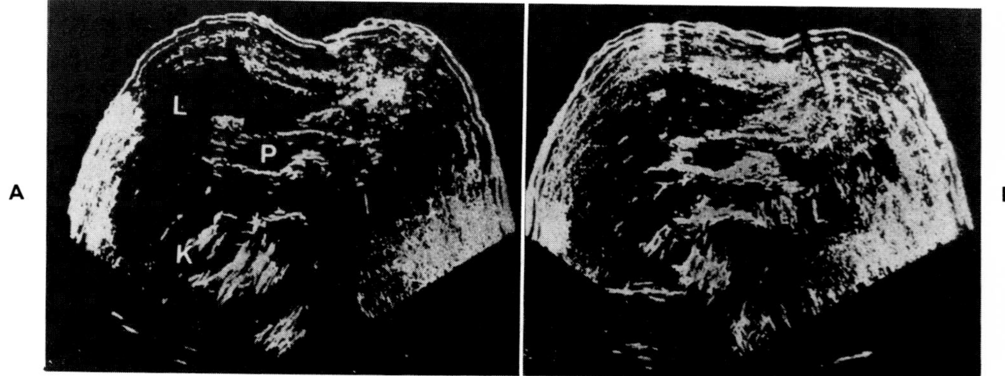

Fig. 1-11. Transverse section of upper abdomen in bistable imaging, with low sensitivity, **A,** and with higher sensitivity, **B.** Scattered echoes appear inside liver tissue *(L).* Certain areas remain echo-free; others tend to be saturated. *K,* kidney; *P,* pancreas.

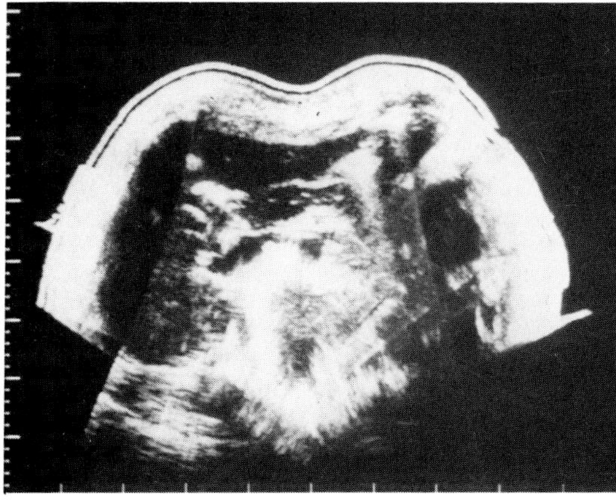

Fig. 1-12. Transverse scan of upper abdomen in gray scale imaging.

3. The mode of response of the storage tube is limited; it functions according to the principle of all or nothing. Below a certain intensity of the reflected beam the bright spots do not appear; above this minimal intensity they do appear. Whatever the intensity that is greater than the threshold, however, the bright spots remain the same, even for elevated intensities (Fig. 1-11). This all-or-nothing image is called *bistable.*

A more reliable and adaptive response is available with the scan converter. The storage tube is then replaced by a series of capacitors that reconstitute the intensity of the reflection: the bright spots are thus rendered proportional to the intensity of the reflected beam. This is gray scale display (Fig. 1-12). Gray scale resolution and rapid writing rate have been dramatically improved in machines of the last generation, many of which now have computer assistance. With such machines, rapid single-sweep scanning is used as often as possible. Kinetic blur can thus be avoided. For example, consider sectorial single-sweep scanning over 5 cm of skin for half a second. At a depth of 10 cm the ultrasonic beam will sweep across about 15 cm of tissue. If 150 mm of tissue are explored in half a second (500 msec), cutting across an anatomical structure 3 mm wide will take only 10 msec.

Two points are still to be emphasized in regard to contact scanning:

1. Since the transducer is easily accessible, it can be adapted to the region under examination or suited to the corpulence of the patient (by changes in the diameter, focus, or frequency of emission).

2. Finally, in contact scanning the scans are realized one by one, *discontinuously,* following a predetermined orientation—a time-consuming procedure.

DYNAMIC IMAGING (REAL TIME)

In this method the sound source also must move and the reflections be summated. *In first-generation machines* the movement of the transducer takes place at a distance from the skin, in distilled water (to avoid cavitation). This movement is far more rapid than that in manual scanning; it is repetitive and cyclical. The bright spots appear on a cathode-ray tube. One complete cycle of the transducer

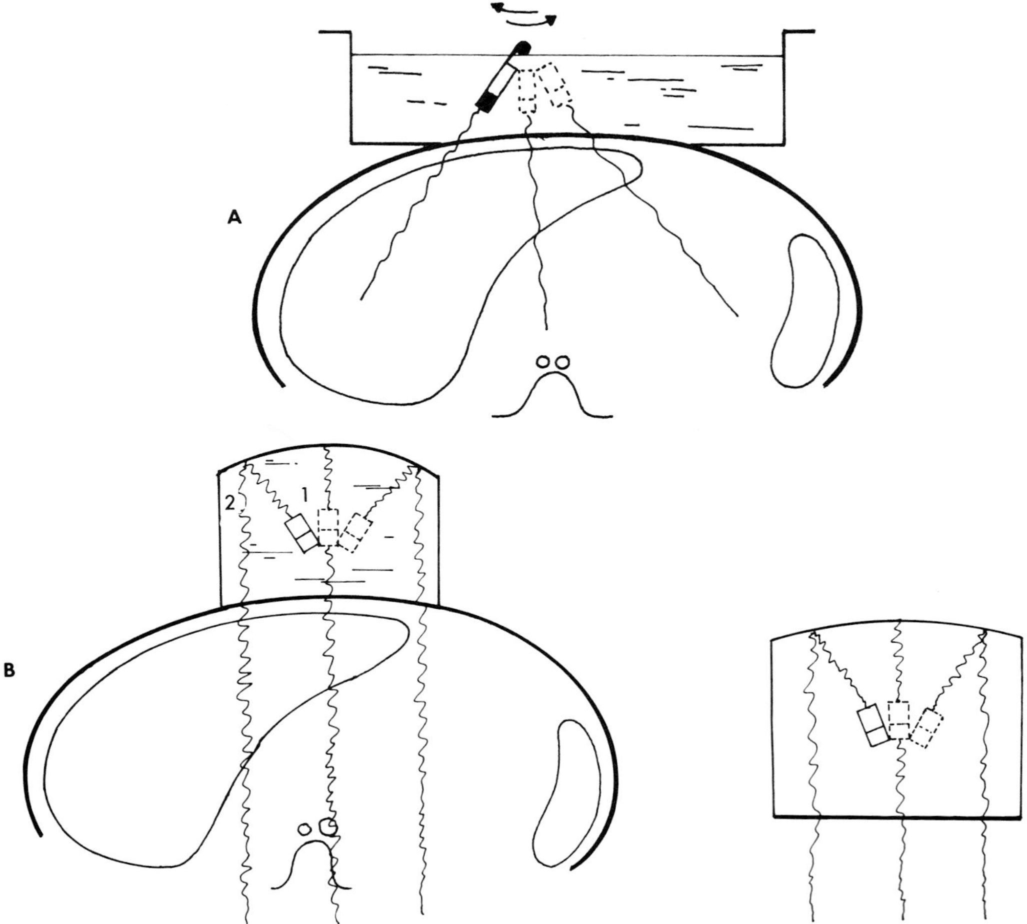

Fig. 1-13. Principle of transducer movement in real-time machines of first generation: the transducer moves in an enclosure filled with distilled water and placed on the region to be examined. **A,** Anterograde emission toward examined region with sector scanning. **B,** Retrograde emission toward parabolic mirror. Ultrasonic beam reflected toward examined region is therefore not sectorial, but parallel. All real-time images illustrated in this book are built with this type of real-time machine.

produces on the screen a fleeting image of the section. A succession of cycles produces a succession of images. The frequency of the transducer's movement and therefore the frequency of the successive images is sufficiently high to be perceived as a permanent image. Liberated from the storage tube, a real-time ultrasonic machine does not require an image converter to display an intensity-modulated representation of the echoes: gray scale display is intrinsically natural to real-time imaging.

The mechanical devices of first-generation dynamic machines are of different types. In some devices, the transducer revolves in contact with the skin, giving rise to a sector scan. In other machines the circular movement of the transducer takes place in an enclosure of distilled water. The enclosure is placed in contact with

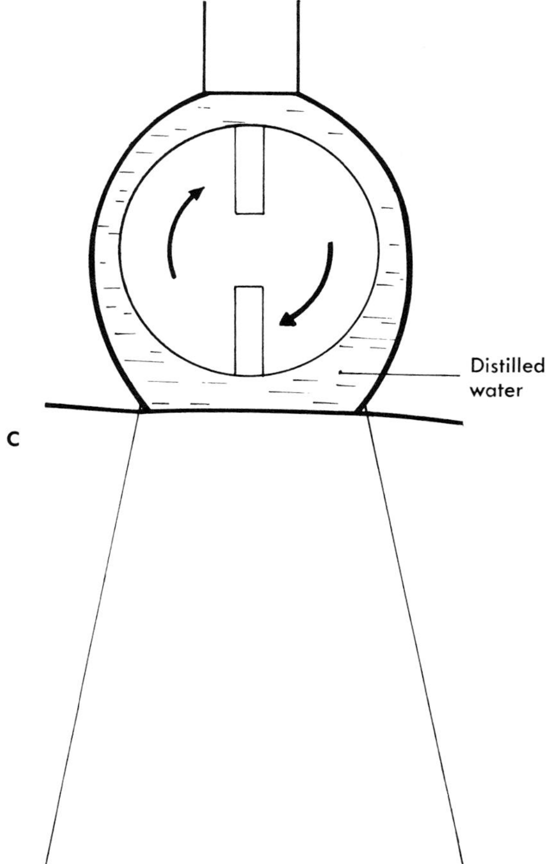

Fig. 1-13, cont'd. C, Smaller real-time head with sectorial scanning.

the skin, through a flexible membrane. The ultrasound emission is directed either straight toward the object (Fig. 1-13, *A* and *C*) or backward, toward a parabolic mirror (Fig. 1-13, *B*). In the latter case the ultrasonic beam, once reflected toward the object, propagates according to parallel lines. In such first-generation machines the frequency of rotation and therefore the frequency of the image are rather low, approximately 16 to 30 per second. A certain degree of flickering of the image is thus inevitable. The transducer can be of excellent quality, focused, with a relatively high frequency (2 or 3 MHz), which assures a bidimensional image of good quality. However, because it is situated inside an enclosure filled with water, the transducer cannot be changed.

In the dynamic machines of the second generation the mechanical displacement of the transducer is replaced by electronic means; a large number of transducers (thirty to sixty) are aligned in an array (Somer, 1969; Wagai, 1973). They emit one after the other, from the first to the last, or in groups, in successive phases (Fig. 1-14). The frequency of the image is much higher; therefore the image is stable, without flickering. Electronically switched arrays of different sizes and frequencies

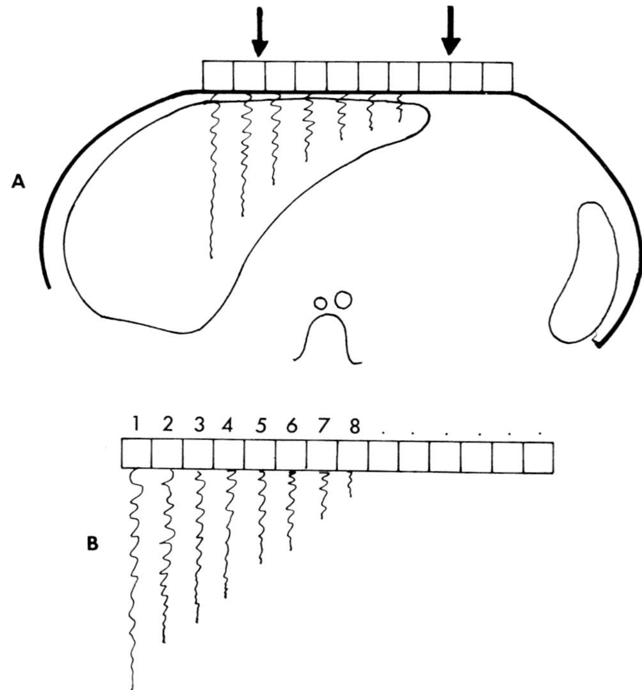

Fig. 1-14. Schematic drawing of switched array. **A,** Switched array *(arrows)* is applied to epigastrium. **B,** Successive triggering of different transducers.

are at the disposal of the user. In a switched array the transducers are necessarily very small in size. For this reason, the geometrical characteristics of the ultrasonic beam are of poorer quality than with the focused transducer of the first-generation machines. However, this disadvantage is minimized by firing the array of transducers in groups. Although contours and tubular (vascular for instance) images are of excellent quality with switched-array devices, parenchymal patterns are, in my experience, of poorer quality than with first-generation machines. However, the technology is changing rapidly. I used to call such a dynamic emitter, either electronic or mechanical, an *ultrasonic real-time head* (RTH).

In general, the properties of the image in real time are as follows:

1. The image is dynamic and persistent, permitting the observation of physiological movements. It can be photographed with a short exposure, which eliminates blurring, or recorded on movie film or videotape.

2. The anatomical field explored is limited by the size of the RTH. In the abdomen, for example, only one particular area is explored at a time. The image for a given location of the RTH never displays the global anatomical character of a compound scanning section, but such is also the case with contact single-sweep scanning.

3. Because of the persistence of the image, it is possible to displace the RTH along the surface of the examined region, displaying an almost infinite number of close parallel sections. This compensates for the limited size of the explored region

and enables one to construct *three-dimensional* visual impressions. The persistence of the images also permits instant change of orientation of scans and immediate adaptation to the direction of the anatomical structure under examination. For instance, if one searches for the image of the portal vein in contact scanning, one is obliged to carry out a series of oblique scans of the right upper quadrant, along a plane parallel to the presumed direction of the portal vein. If the orientation of the vessel does not coincide with that of the scan, a new series of scans must be made. The angle of correction can only be determined laboriously, by trial and error. On the other hand, with real time, movement of the RTH along the surface of the right upper quadrant permits immediate identification of the portal vein and its direction, enabling an instant adaptation of the scanning plane to the axis of the vein. The anatomical exploration is therefore more rapid and precise.

4. Also, remember that, because of its construction on a nonstore cathode tube, the image of real time is a gray scale image.

5. Unfortunately, at present the resolution of real-time imaging is greatly inferior to that of last-generation contact scanning imaging. This should not long be the case, since basic technological improvements, due to new tubes, are expected in the field of real time.

The majority of abdominal ultrasonographers are radiologists. For them, it will be easy to compare real-time imaging to x-ray fluoroscopy and contact scanning to radiography. Similarly, as the field in real time is more limited than that of compound scanning, the fluoroscopic field is reduced in relation to that of radiography because of the size of the image amplifier. At present, a real-time image, on a photograph, is less pleasing to the eye than a contact scanning image. However, it is a static representation of a dynamic phenomenon; it is well known that the frame-to-frame image of a radiocinematographic film or a videotape recording is of poorer quality than the dynamic sequence itself. Also, the detail in fluoroscopy is known to be inferior to that in radiography. Two final radiological analogies can be made: that of the bistable image (now commonly replaced by a black-and-white high-contrast gray scale image) with high-contrast radiography and that of an image in gray scale with radiography in low contrast.

Now is the moment to introduce to you two respectable gentlemen: Hillel and Schammai. Hillel and Schammai lived in the first century B.C. They were the most learned of their world, and what they did not know of the science of their time would largely have found a place on the surface of a Polaroid film. However, when Hillel considered something to be black, Schammai and his numerous disciples would prove, by many wise demonstrations, that in reality this thing was white; when Schammai showed that something was white, Hillel and his followers would, by reasoning just as clever, show that in reality this thing was black. The more they demonstrated, the more these gentlemen gathered disciples. Well, the schools of Schammai and Hillel seem to have survived through the generations, and the students of one or the other continue, more than ever, to oppose each other in the medical domain.

Those belonging to the school of Schammai maintain that the only valuable technique in ultrasonography is that of contact scanning. They thus obtain, after long and detailed explorations, excellent anatomical images that are not always free

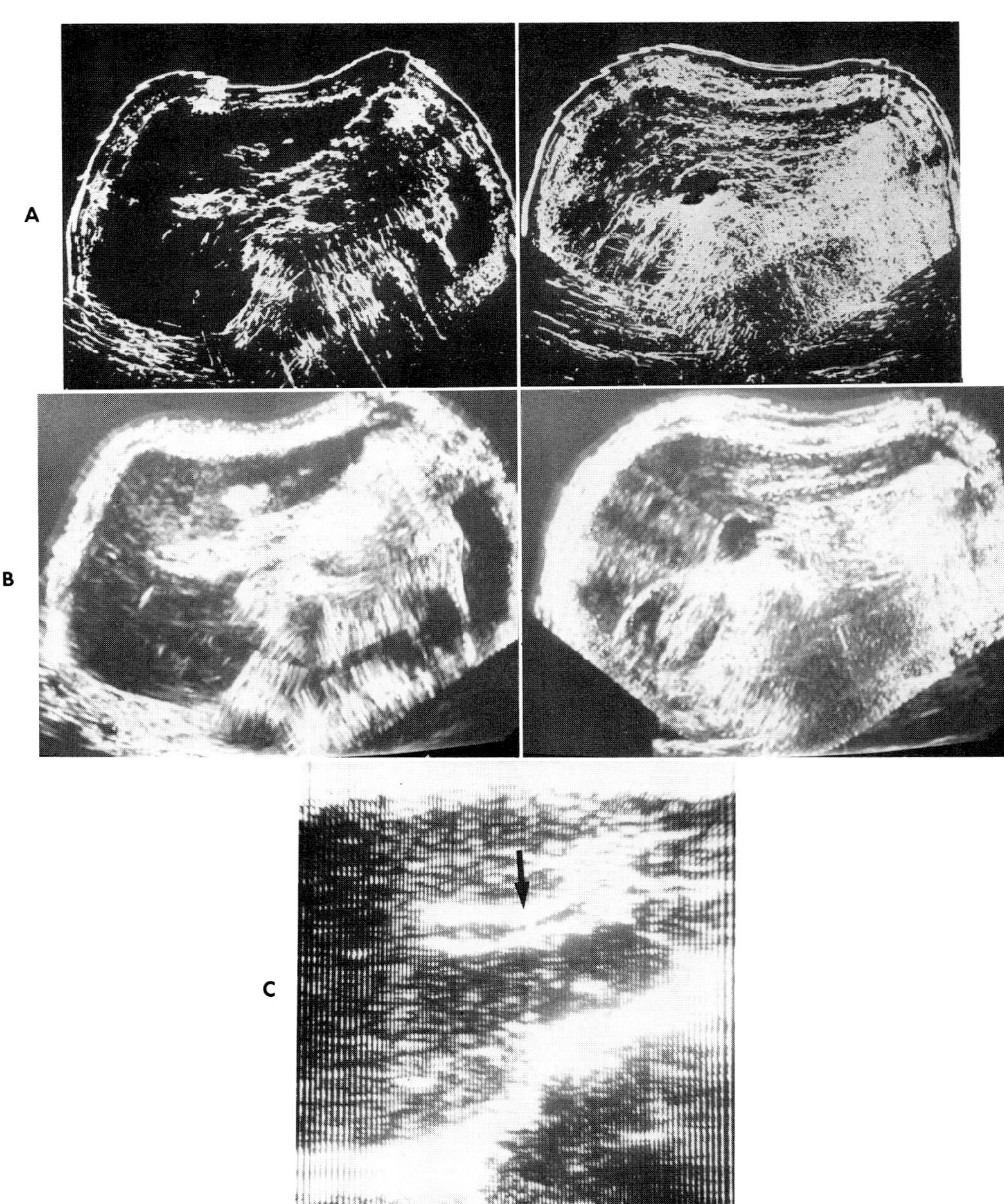

Fig. 1-15. Transverse scans of liver. **A,** Contact scanning in bistable imaging. **B,** Contact scanning with gray scale display. **C,** Real time—gray scale display *(arrow):* portal division.

of artifacts caused by the operator. For a long time, certain vascular elements completely escaped them because of blurring. The school of Hillel, on the contrary, maintains that the only valuable technique in ultrasonography is real time. Thus they rapidly obtain anatomical images that are often detailed, although difficult for the uninitiated to recognize. However, certain regions covered by the ribs or intestinal gas escape them. Doubtless the school of Hillel would opt for fluoroscopy as the only conventional radiology and that of Schammai for radiography as the only one; but everyone knows that, to disclose an ulcer on the posterior surface of the lesser gastric curvature, it is necessary to rotate the patient under fluoroscopic control. Only then does one take films. It is also known that, to appreciate the flexibility of a gastric or esophageal wall, it is necessary to use fluoroscopy; but the finest detail of the mucosal pattern is best shown by radiography. Exactly as in conventional radiology, in ultrasonography it is important to use the two techniques synergistically: static and dynamic (Fig. 1-15). A particular example of the utility of this association is shown in Fig. 1-16. In this case, metastases on the hepatic anterior surface are best shown in real time, since in contact scanning the superficial planes are often poorly distinguished.* Conversely, when an enlargement of the left hepatic lobe is hidden in real time by the lower ribs, the thin transducer of the contact scanning device is able to slide along the anterior intercostal spaces, thus displaying the abnormal area. The constant interdependence of real-time and contact scanning imaging will be frequently illustrated

*This is probably due to the presence of a water bag coupling in the RTH, so that the acoustic mismatch is only 10% of that with a direct transducer coupling.

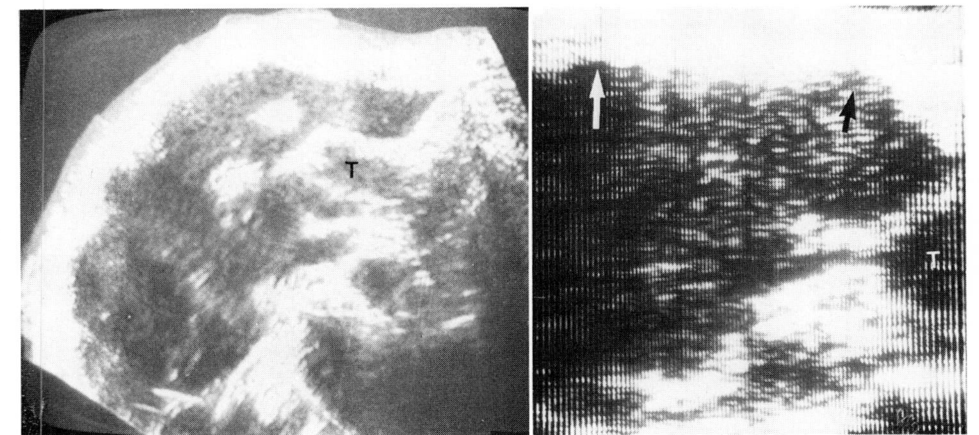

Fig. 1-16. Complementarity of contact scanning and real-time imaging. This patient has pancreatic tumor *(T),* which is displayed by both techniques. With both, abnormalities of hepatic tissue architecture are shown. **A,** In contact scanning, anterior aspect possesses quite regular outline. **B,** In real time, however, several elevations *(arrows)* are displayed. Such elevations indicate metastatic deposits ("hump sign"). Contact scanning image is more satisfying as anatomical section. Real-time image displays smaller field but may better demonstrate particular details of tissue echopattern or liver contours.

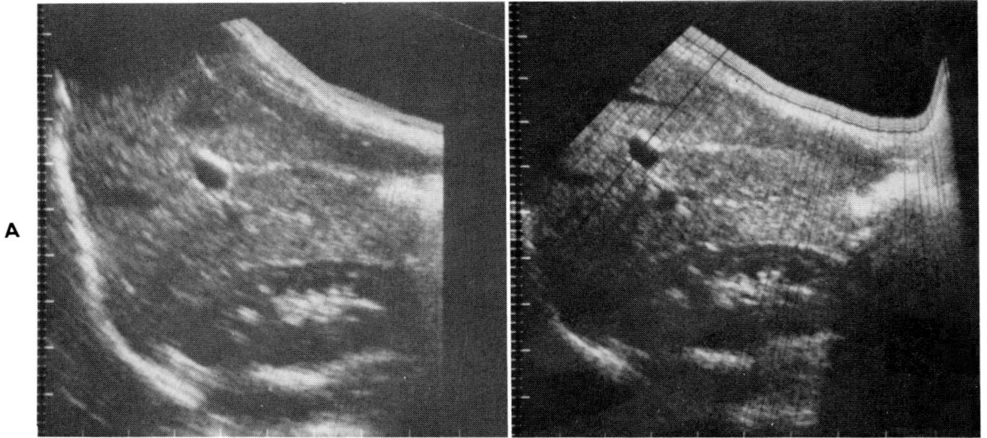

Fig. 1-17. The part played in ultrasonic imaging by the frequency and quality of the transducer: sagittal scans of right upper quadrant. **A,** Images of liver and kidney are built with focused transducer of 2.25 MHz. Note sharpness of diaphragm and kidney contours and of vascular sections. **B,** Previous transducer has been replaced by transducer of 3.5 MHz. With same setting of sensitivity, contour sharpness and tissue details are improved, but penetration is reduced.

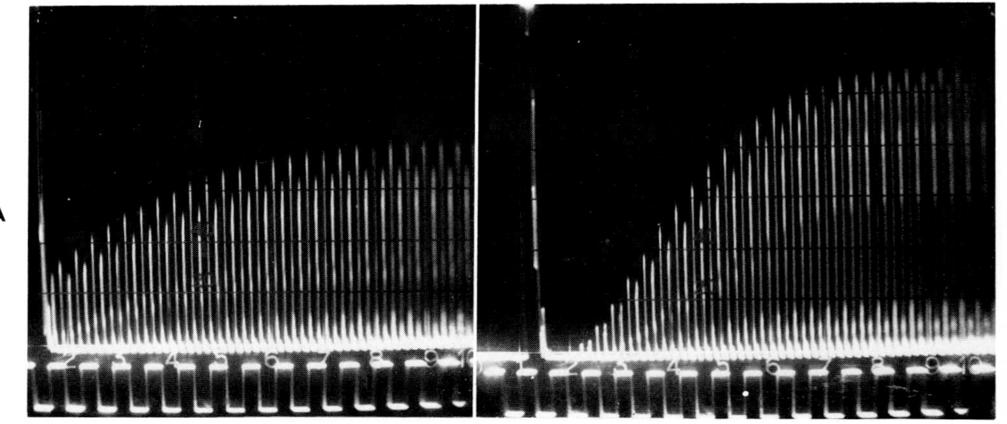

Fig. 1-18. Swept-gain curves (x-axis: depth in centimeters; y-axis: intensity). **A,** There is only small difference in gain between superficial and deep areas. This type of curve may be used to examine the abdomen of a child. **B,** There is now marked difference between superficial and deep amplification. This type of curve is generally used for abdominal examinations in adults. The ramp is lowered for thin patients and increased for stout ones.

in the following chapters on clinical applications of ultrasonography. The respective roles of real-time and contact scanning in ultrasonic examinations will perhaps change when the new high-resolution real-time equipment is available. Fully automatic contact scanning (Kossoff, 1976) is another element to be considered in relation to the future of ultrasonic techniques.

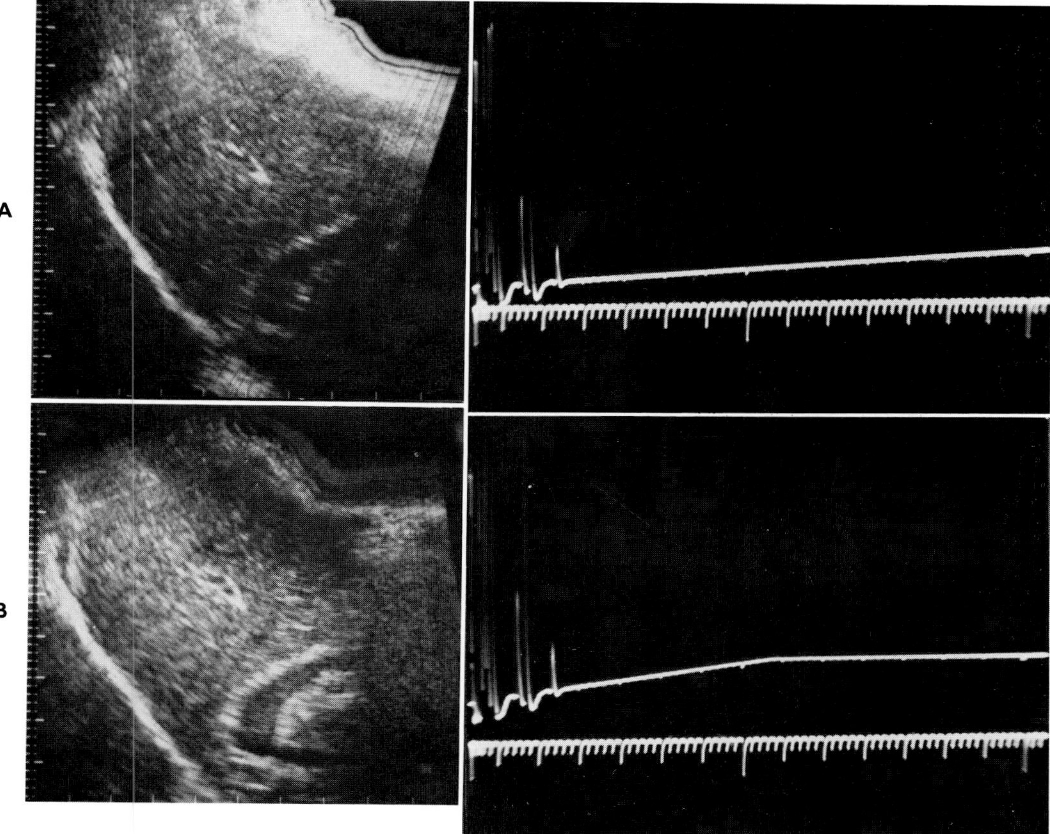

Fig. 1-19. The part played by swept gain: sagittal scans of abdomen through liver and kidney. **A,** Deep amplification is insufficient, since the time gain compensation (TGC) was too low (2.2 dB/cm). **B,** There is now too much deep amplification. Deep layers of tissue are displayed without information in superficial part of liver (TGC: 6.5 dB/cm).

OTHER TECHNICAL POINTS

The quality of the ultrasonographic image is improved as the *frequency* of the ultrasonic beam is elevated, and thus the wavelength is shortened (Fig. 1-17). However, as the frequency is increased, so is the attenuation in depth. Eventually one reaches the extreme, at which point the ultrasonic beam does not penetrate beyond the first few centimeters of tissue. In abdominal exploration of adults, one uses between 2.25 to 3.5 MHz. Referring back to the radiological comparison, one can compare the role of frequency to that of kilovolts, but with the inverse relation, since the penetration diminishes with the wavelength.

The quality of the image also depends on the *geometry* of the beam. The use of the focused transducer is now fairly widespread, replacing that of the old transducer, the beam of which was more dispersed. A number of parameters must still be considered.

Because of depth attenuation, it is necessary to subject the echoes returning

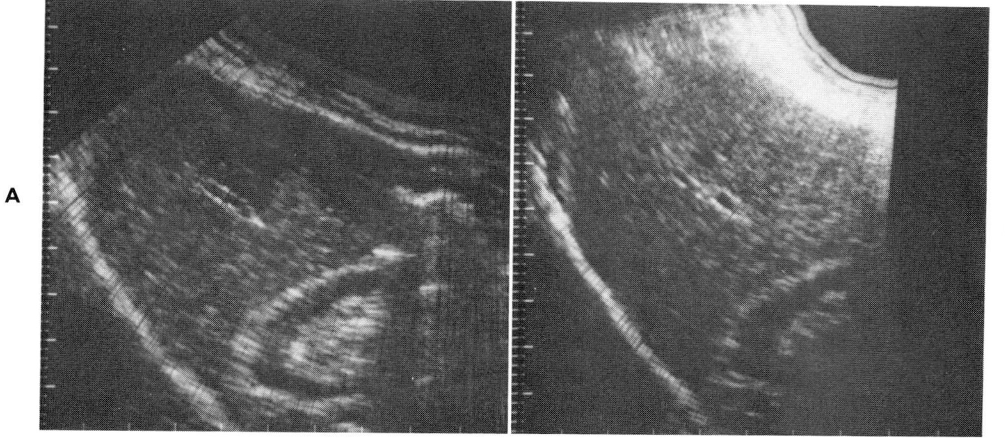

Fig. 1-20. The part played by the sensitivity (total gain). **A,** Low sensitivity. **B,** High sensitivity. In this case, swept gain is not ideally set. There is superficial saturation, whereas deep layers of tissue are poorly displayed.

from deep structures to an electronic amplification far greater than that to which the superficial echoes are subjected. All machines possess such a system of regulation of depth compensation—*swept gain* or TGC (Figs. 1-18 and 1-19). It is also possible to eliminate the less intense echoes *(threshold suppression)* or, on the contrary, to reduce the most intense pikes *(compression).*

Of particular importance is the ability to vary, in a global sense, the intensity of all the signals—*total gain* or *sensitivity* (Fig. 1-20). This control is usually an attenuation circuit. When attenuation is reduced, the overall sensitivity is increased. Returning to the domain of radiology, one can compare the total gain to the milliampere-second (mas). The *power of emission,* expressed in W/cm^2, is limited because of biological reasons but is considered to be well within safe limits in commercially available equipment.

All these adjustments may seem difficult to master. In reality, with most available machines and in most abdominal explorations, it is possible to adopt a routine average adjustment for almost all the parameters and to vary only that of sensitivity. Exceptionally, when the patient is very stocky, it will be necessary to set up a steeper swept-gain curve or to use a lower frequency or, on the contrary, to flatten the swept-gain curve for children.

Once gathered, the morphological information has to be interpreted; as in radiology, this step involves a certain degree of subjectivity. This is why different research teams have proposed a quantitative approach to ultrasonic data. One of the elements of such an analysis is the intensity, in decibels, at which certain images appear or disappear (Kobayashi, 1973). At the present time, we do not use this type of quantitative analysis in our study of ultrasonic images.

I have grouped in the following list the different parameters relating to the quality of the ultrasonographic image.

Qualities relative to the transducer
- Frequency, Diameter, Focusing — Beam profile
- Sensitivity of crystal

Settings
- Power*
- Suppression*
- Near gain
- Swept gain (dB/cm)
- Sensitivity (dB)
- Image contrast and brilliance

---

*Not available on all machines—fortunately.

REFERENCES

Barnett, E., and Morley, P.: Abdominal echography, Borough Green, England, 1974, Butterworth & Co. (Publishers), Ltd.

Bock, K., and Egermann, L.: Ultrasonographia medica, Proceedings of the World Federation of Ultrasound in Medicine and Biology First Congress, Vienna, 1972, Verlag der Wiener Medizinischer Akademie.

Goldberg, B. B., Kotler, M. N., Ziskin, M. C., and Waxham, R. D.: Diagnostic uses of ultrasound, New York, 1975, Grune & Stratton, Inc.

Gordon, D.: Ultrasound, Edinburgh, 1964, Churchill Livingstone.

Hassani, N.: Ultrasonography of the abdomen, Heidelberg, Germany, 1976, Springer-Verlag.

Holm, H. H., Kristensen, J. K., Rasmussen, S. N., Pedersen, J. F., and Hancke, S.: Abdominal ultrasound, Copenhagen, 1976, Munksgaard, International Booksellers & Publishers, Ltd.

Hussey, M.: Diagnostic ultrasound, Glasgow, Scotland, 1975, Blackie & Son, Ltd.

Kazner, E., de Vlieger, M., Muller, H. R., and McCready, V. R.: Ultrasonics in medicine, Proceedings of the World Federation of Ultrasound in Medicine and Biology Second European Congress, Amsterdam, 1975, Excerpta Medica Foundation.

Kossoff, G.: Classification of soft tissues by grey scale echography, Abstract No. 589, World Federation of Ultrasound in Medicine and Biology, San Francisco, 1976, American Institute for Ultrasound in Medicine.

Kobayashi, T.: Clinical evaluation of ultrasound techniques in breast tumors and malignant abdominal tumors, Proceedings of the World Federation of Ultrasound in Medicine and Biology Second Congress, Rotterdam, Holland, 1973, Excerpta Medica Foundation.

Leopold, G. R., and Asher, W. M.: Fundamentals of abdominal and pelvic ultrasonography, Philadelphia, 1975, W. B. Saunders Co.

Pourcelot, L., Pottier, J. M., Berson, M., and Planiol, T.: A fast ultrasonic imaging system. Usabel. Ultrasonics in medicine, Second European Congress, Amsterdam, 1975, Excerpta Medica Foundation.

Somer, J. C.: Electronic sector scanning with ultrasonic beams. Ultrasonographia medica, Proceedings of the World Federation of Ultrasound in Medicine and Biology First Congress, Vienna, 1972.

de Vlieger, M., White, D. N., and McCready, V. R.: Ultrasonics in medicine, Proceedings of the World Federation of Ultrasound in Medicine and Biology, Amsterdam, 1974, Excerpta Medica Foundation.

Wagai, T.: Advances in ultrasonography and its clinical evaluation, Proceedings of the World Federation of Ultrasound in Medicine and Biology Second Congress, Amsterdam, 1973, Excerpta Medica Foundation.

Weill, F., Becker, J. C., Kraehenbuhl, J. R., Heriot, G., and Walter, J. P.: Clinical atlas of ultrasonic radiography, Paris, 1973, Masson & Cie., Editeurs.

Wells, P. N. T.: Physical principles of ultrasonic diagnosis, London, 1969, Academic Press, Inc.

Wells, P. N. T.: Ultrasonics in clinical diagnosis, Edinburgh, 1972, Churchill Livingstone.

World Federation of Ultrasound in Medicine and Biology: Volume of abstracts, Third Meeting, San Francisco, 1976.

CHAPTER 2

DIFFERENT TYPES OF ECHOPATTERNS

Whatever type of image is used, ultrasonography is employed to display organ or lesion contours, as well as internal tissue images. These pathological anatomical elements can be reduced to a small number of fundamental image types.

CONTOUR IMAGES

A continuous, unindividualized line separating two areas between which there is a marked difference in acoustic impedance, for example, the border between a solid and a liquid area (Fig. 2-1), is called an *interface image*. Such images can also be found between certain visceral organs.

Images of *separation* make up the boundary between two liquid collections that are distinct (Fig. 2-2).

A marginated individual line separating two neighboring areas is designated as a *wall image*. The bladder (Fig. 2-1) and vascular walls (Figs. 2-3, *A*, 2-7, and 2-9) are representative of such wall images. It is also an image of this type that one would see between the liver and the kidney (Fig. 2-4).

The analysis of contour images is the first step in sonographic diagnosis: the sharpness, the regularity, and the continuity of the contours are all evaluated.

TISSUE IMAGES—SOLID, SEMISOLID, AND LIQUID AREAS

Liquid collections are very characteristic: they present themselves in the form of transparent areas, preserving the same pattern after several passes of the transducer or with higher gain (Fig. 2-2). There is usually reinforcement of the posterior interface of a liquid collection, with a zone of dense echoes behind it.

Solid tissues, on the contrary, are characterized by the presence of scattered echoes. Regularly dispersed echoes, of similar intensity, represent the *solid homogeneous echopattern* (Figs. 2-3 and 2-4) characteristic of normal parenchyma. At a given sensitivity the degree of reflection of the different tissues is variable. Thus the spleen is far less reflective than the liver; it appears as a translucent zone, whereas the hepatic tissue obviously possesses the character of solid tissue (Fig. 2-4). The solid character of weakly reflective tissues such as the spleen is manifest only with higher-gain settings. As previously mentioned, the gain required to produce reflections may serve as a quantitative approach to the morphological analysis of parenchyma. The presence of islands of unequal reflection, either extended or regularly dispersed, constitutes the *echopattern of a heterogeneous solid type.* This pattern is found in many pathological processes (Fig. 2-5). Different types of heterogeneous echopatterns may be distinguished:

- The nodular heterogeneous echopattern (macronodular and micronodular, with reflecting or sonolucent nodules)

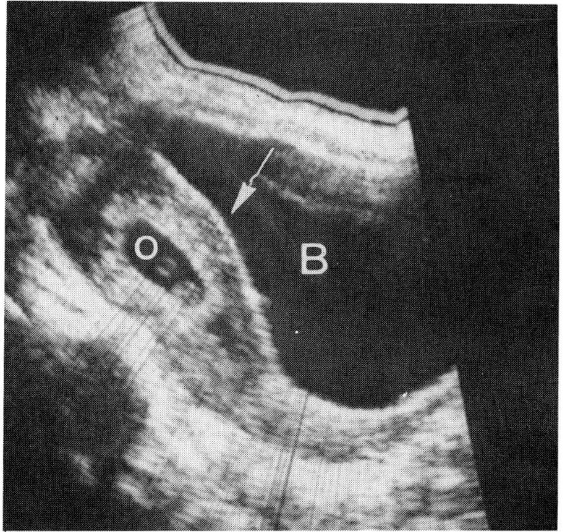

Fig. 2-1. Fundamental images displayed on sagittal scan of pelvis in pregnant woman (7-week pregnancy). Interface image delineates limit between ovular sac *(O)* and uterine muscle. Bladder *(B)* possesses typical liquid pattern. It is echo-free and well marginated by wall image *(arrow)*. One might wonder why an obstetrical image is displayed in a book dealing with digestive diseases: this is, of course, because the woman complained of vomiting.

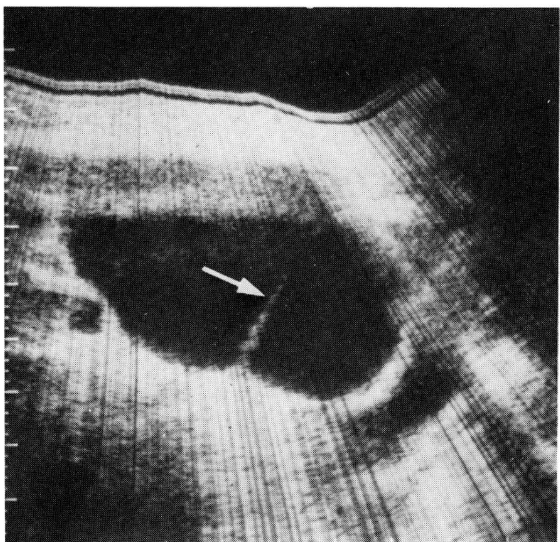

Fig. 2-2. Sagittal scan of abdomen in a case of septate ovarian cyst. Here again are typical liquid echopatterns, remaining echo-free even with high sensitivity setting and well delineated by interface images. Between two neighboring collections, separation image *(arrow)* is displayed.

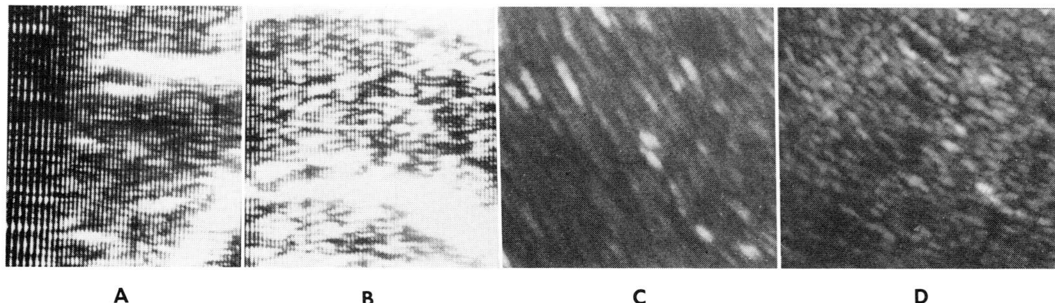

Fig. 2-3. Solid homogeneous echopatterns. **A** and **B,** Liver—real time. **C** and **D,** Liver—contact scanning gray scale display. In **A,** two parallel lines of reflection, displayed in upper part of figure, belong to branch of portal vein.

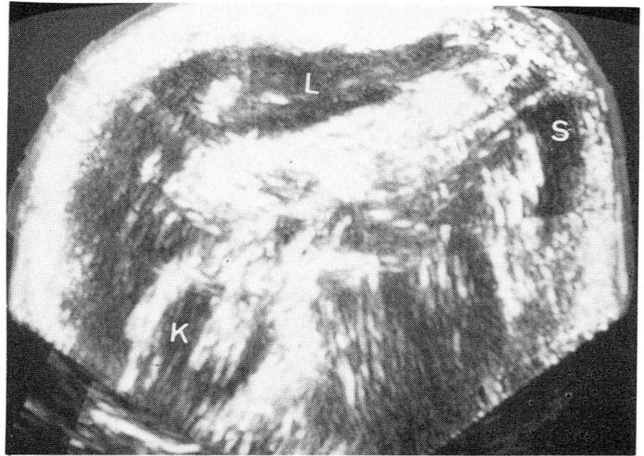

Fig. 2-4. Three examples of solid homogeneous echopattern: liver tissue *(L),* splenic tissue *(S),* and renal cortex *(K).*

- The heterogeneous echopattern in fields, with larger areas of abnormal reflection
- The infiltrative heterogeneous echopattern

An important element to be considered in solid tissues is attenuation. In certain pathological parenchyma, attenuation in depth is much greater than that found in normal tissue, even if the localized echopattern itself is barely changed (Rettenmaier, 1973a).

There exists another type of echopattern that is more difficult to categorize. It is characterized by apparently echo-free areas, which fill up very slightly when the sensitivity is set at a higher level and lack posterior reinforcement. Does such an echopattern belong to solid tissue or to fluid? As a matter of fact, the answer to that question often remains in doubt. This type of image, in agreement with the school of Hillel, is called a *semisolid echopattern.* (See Fig. 2-6.) (Evidently the school of Schammai called it *semiliquid.*) In a solid tissue, it indicates the presence of edema or of a necrotizing process; in liquid, the existence of a thick, lumpy

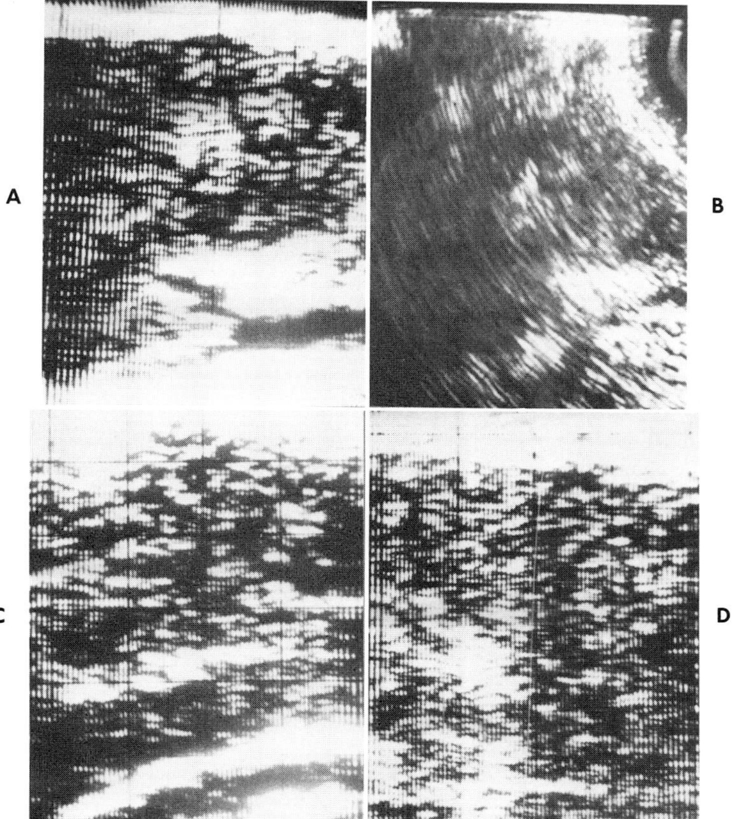

Fig. 2-5. Solid heterogeneous echopattern. **A** and **B,** Macronodular type. **C,** Micronodular type. **D,** In fields and infiltrative type.

collection, containing debris. This type of echopattern is often called *complex.* However, since a heterogeneous solid pattern is undoubtedly complex and there are so many other complex situations in ultrasonography, I prefer the designation *semisolid.*

The existence of this semisolid echopattern shows that the differentiation between solid tissues and liquid collections can present a difficult problem—all the more difficult since certain rather sonotranslucent solid tissues can possess a well-marked posterior interface. If the tissue echopattern is not immediately obvious, it is advisable to reconstruct the images several times with increasing sensitivity. Comparison between real-time and contact scanning images can be useful: the nature of the tissue is often easier to identify in real time. It is classic to advise an exploration at high frequency. In theory a solid sonotranslucent tissue quickly attenuates an ultrasonic beam of high frequency (greater than 4 MHz). Conversely, a high-frequency ultrasonic beam is able to penetrate a liquid collection as far as its posterior interface. A complementary help may be offered by the comparative method, which consists of using a known liquid image, such as the urinary bladder, gallbladder, or aorta, as a standard. The reference to such a typical image of liquid

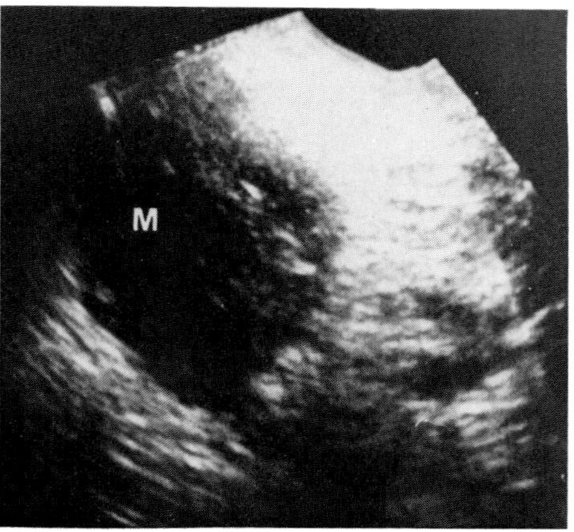

Fig. 2-6. Semisolid echopattern. Sagittal scan of left upper quadrant shows, in suprarenal area, well-marginated mass *(M)* with few echoes and without posterior reinforcement. At higher level of sensitivity and after multiple passes of transducer, echopattern remained poor. This type of echopattern belongs to either necrotic tumor, edematous tissue, or thick liquid with blood clots, necrotic debris, or pus. In this case the mass was a carcinoma of upper pole of kidney.

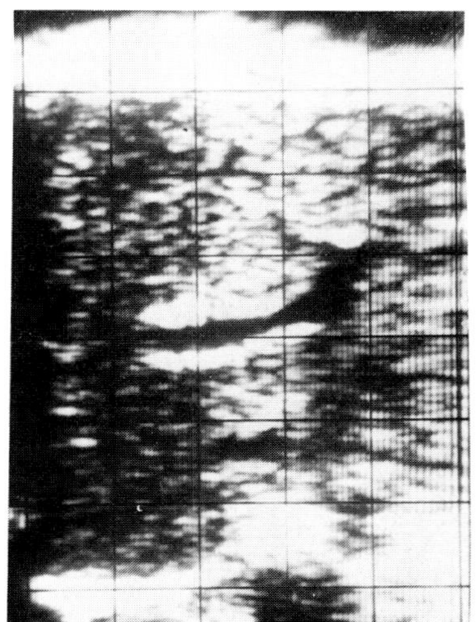

Fig. 2-7. Tubular structure. The duct displayed in this scan belongs to hilar portal network. Portal venous branches possess well-demarcated wall images.

collection is usually decisive. If any doubt persists, the echopattern must be considered undetermined; its nature can be ascertained only by an ultrasonically guided biopsy. Research in the field of tissular quantitative analysis (Hill and co-workers, 1976; Kobayashi, 1973; Levi and Keuwez, 1977; Rettenmaier, 1973b; Wagai, 1973) should eventually obviate such interpretational difficulties.

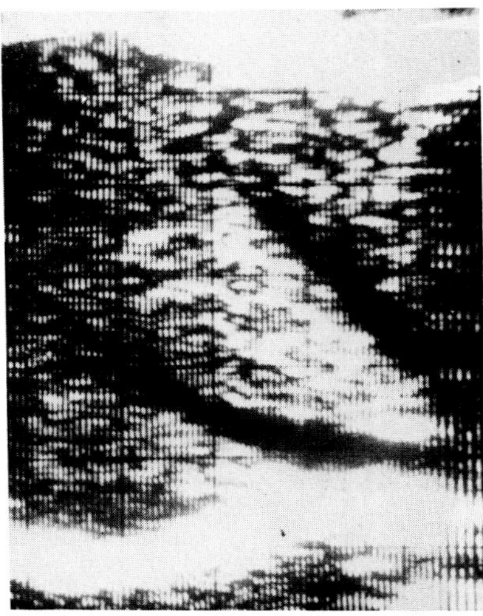

Fig. 2-8. Another tubular intrahepatic network. In this case, wall images are not well delineated. These tubular elements belong to network of hepatic veins.

TUBULAR IMAGES

There are many tubular structures, such as blood vessels and biliary ducts. Whether extraparenchymal or intraparenchymal, these structures appear with their echo-free lumen and their walls. These walls may appear as either proper, delineated wall images (Fig. 2-7) or simple tissue limits (Fig. 2-8). The delineation of a wall image, of course, is related to the thickness of the tubular wall, but it also depends on the angle at which the ultrasonic beam approaches the tubular element, as will be seen in dealing with the hepatic veins (Chapters 4 and 6).

The shape of the tubular element as it appears on an ultrasonic section is related to the geometrical orientation of the scanning plane—sagittal, transverse, or oblique sections (Fig. 2-9).

ACOUSTIC SHADOWS

The abundant juxtaposition of elements found in an ultrasonographic section is related to the gradient of impedance between various tissues, both normal and pathological. As long as the ultrasonic beam is capable of propagation, even though attenuated, it continues to produce reflections. However, if the ultrasonic beam reaches totally reflective (or attenuating) structures, no image is formed beyond that point. The absence of image behind a reflective structure is called an *acoustic shadow*. This phenomenon occurs when the ultrasonic beam encounters bone (or other calcified tissues) or air. The ribs (Fig. 2-10) produce acoustic shadows, but an image is formed at the level of the intercostal spaces. The vertebral body also interrupts the ultrasonic beam, but, if the latter passes through the intervertebral space, an image of the vertebral canal can be produced (Fig. 2-11). Gallstones and the calcified walls of chronic abscesses or cysts can also play a masking role. When an ultrasonic beam passes from a solid or liquid to a gas, its

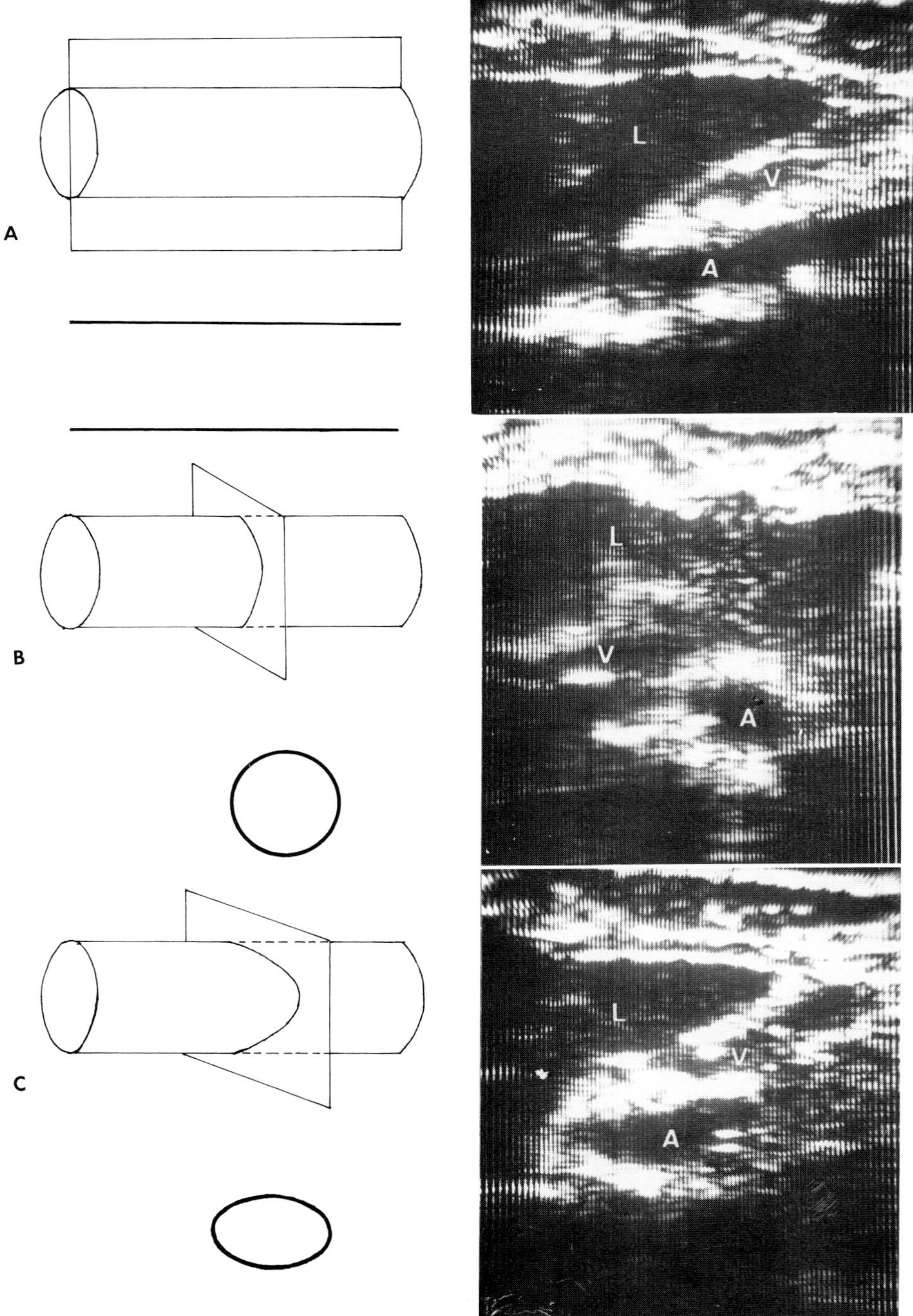

Fig. 2-9. Formation of tubular images. **A,** Sagittal section of tubular element. Schematic representation of section image and real-time example. Aorta *(A)* is cut sagitally. *V,* venous mesenteric-portal junction; *L,* liver. **B,** Transverse section of tubular element. Schematic representation of section image and real-time example. Aorta *(A)* is cut transversely; splenoportal venous axis *(V)* is cut sagittally. **C,** Oblique section of tubular element. Schematic representation of section image and real-time example. In this oblique scan of epigastrium, aorta is displayed in oblique section; therefore its section image is oval. Note mesenteric-portal junction.

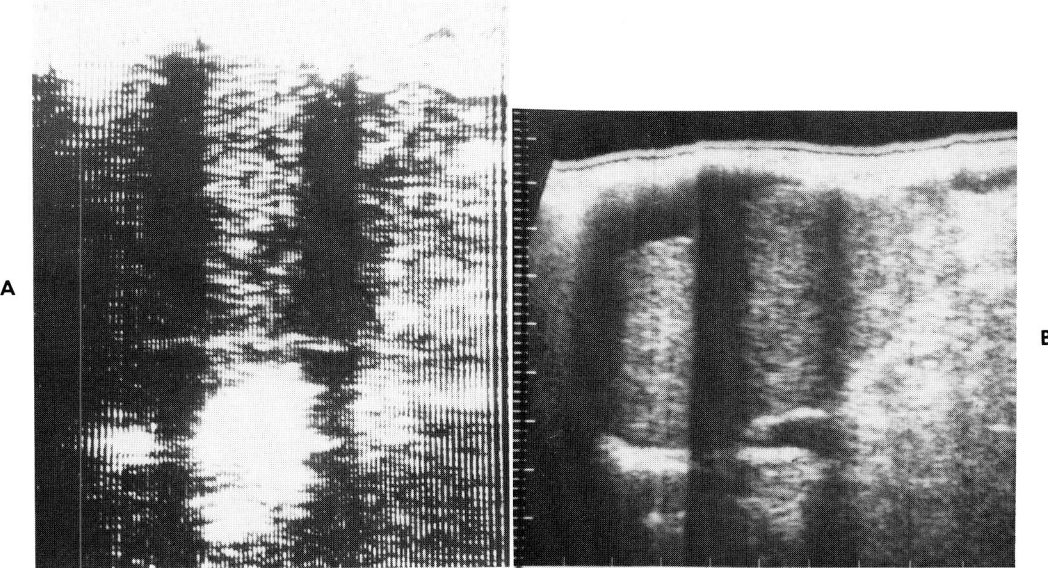

Fig. 2-10. Bone acoustic shadows (ribs). **A,** Sagittal lateral real-time scan of liver. Behind each rib, there is acoustic shadow. Liver tissue is displayed only between these shadow areas. **B,** Sagittal contact scan of spleen. Acoustic shadows of ribs are also displayed. They would be less sharply delineated on compound, instead of single-sweep, scan.

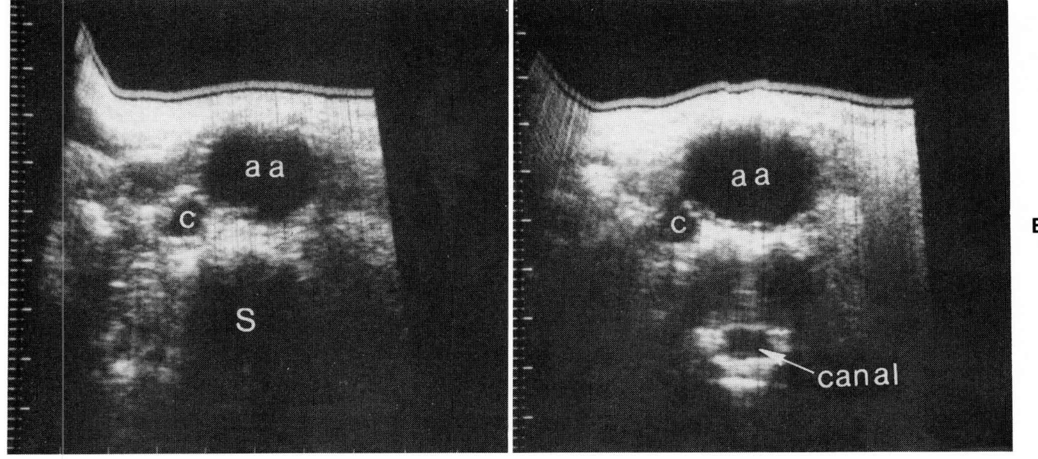

Fig. 2-11. Bone acoustic shadow (vertebral body) displayed on scans of patient with aortic aneurysm. **A,** Transverse scan at level of L-1 displaying acoustic shadow(s) behind anterior aspect of vertebral body. **B,** Parallel, more caudal scan at level of intervertebral space. Ultrasonic beam passes through intervertebral disc and displays outline of spinal canal. *aa,* aortic aneurysm; *c,* cava.

attenuation reaches 99.9%, producing an acoustic shadow. This is a common appearance behind duodenal or colic gas (Fig. 2-12). For the same reason, no image can be constructed above the diaphragm in normal circumstances (Fig. 1-20), whereas, if there is a pleural effusion, a liquid pattern appears above the diaphragm (Chapter 14). In that case, since the ultrasonic beam is now able to proceed, pulmonary elements may even be displayed.

The *fundamental images* previously discussed have been grouped as follows.

2:1 FUNDAMENTAL IMAGES

I. Contours
  A. Interface image
  B. Separation image
  C. Wall image
II. Tissues
  A. Liquid echopattern (transparent)
  B. Semisolid echopattern
  C. Solid echopattern
    1. Homogeneous
    2. Heterogeneous
      a. Macronodular } Translucent (transonic)
      b. Micronodular } or reflective
      c. In fields
      d. Infiltrative

Images should be analyzed as follows.

2:2 IMAGE ANALYSIS

Contours	*Tissue*
Sharpness	Type of echopattern
Regularity	Attenuation
Continuity	

Since I am now beginning to deal with methodology, one last principle of importance in interpreting ultrasonograms must be pointed out. According to an international convention, the sections are always presented with an identical orientation: for a sagittal scan the cephalic extremity of the patient is located to the left of the observer (Fig. 2-13, *A*). For a transverse scan the right of the patient appears to the left of the observer, as though the section were looked at from below (Fig. 2-13, *B*).

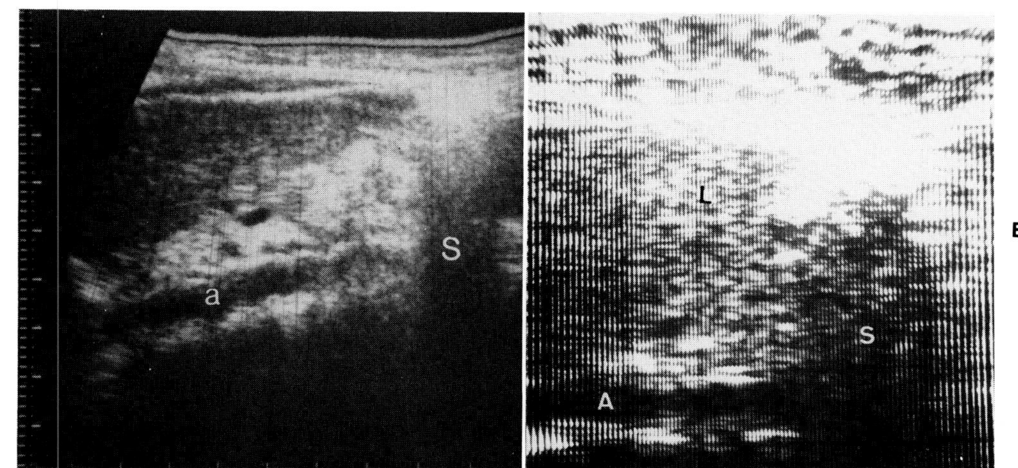

Fig. 2-12. Acoustic shadow of intestinal gas. These sagittal scans of abdomen display aorta *(A)* behind the liver *(L)*. Aortic image disappears below inferior edge of liver, since ultrasonic beam is interrupted by colonic gas, which gives rise to acoustic shadow *(S)*. **A,** Contact scan. *a,* aorta. **B,** Real-time scan.

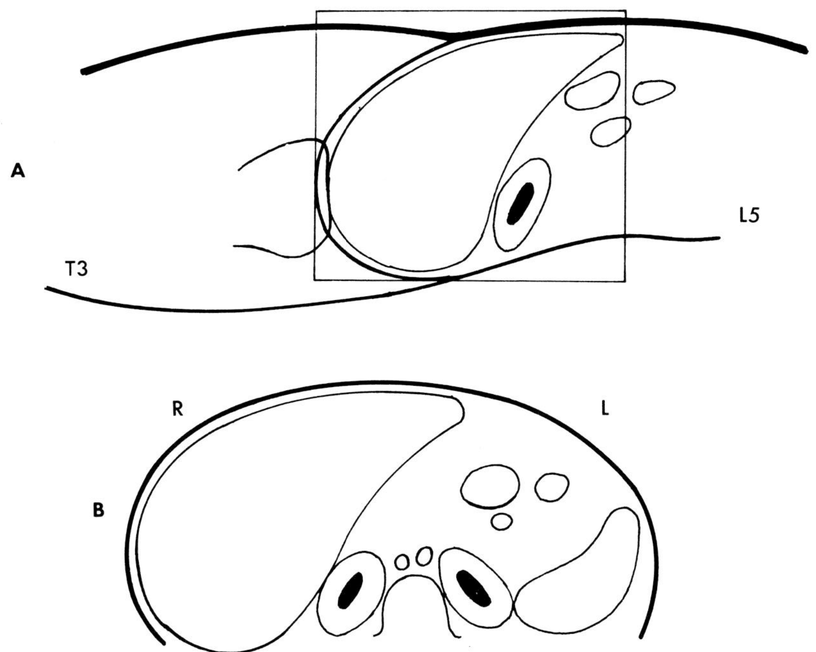

Fig. 2-13. The orientation of ultrasonic sections that is accepted international convention. **A,** Sagittal scan. **B,** Transverse scan.

REFERENCES

Hill, C. R., Nicholas, D., and Bamber, J. C.: Practical approaches to quantitative tissue characterization, Abstract No. 1120, World Federation of Ultrasound in Medicine and Biology, San Francisco, 1976, American Institute for Ultrasound in Medicine.

Kobayashi, T.: Clinical evaluation of ultrasound techniques in breast tumors and malignant abdominal tumors, Proceedings of the World Federation of Ultrasound in Medicine and Biology Second Congress, Amsterdam, 1973, Excerpta Medica Foundation.

Kossoff, G.: Classification of soft tissues by grey scale echography, Abstract No. 589, World Federation of Ultrasound in Medicine and Biology, San Francisco, 1976, American Institute for Ultrasound in Medicine.

Levi, S., and Keuwez, J.: An attempt to find a differential attenuation coefficient for ultrasonic diagnosis of pelvic tumors in vivo. In White, D. N., and Brown, R. E., editors: Ultrasound in medicine, vol. 3B, New York, 1977, Plenum Publishing Corporation.

Rettenmaier, G.: Echographic diagnosis and differential diagnosis of diffuse liver diseases. Start of quantitative evaluation and results, Verh. Dtsch. Ges. Inn. Med. **79:**962-964, 1973a.

Rettenmaier, G.: Quantitative criteria of intrahepatic echo patterns correlated with structural alteration. Ultrasonics in medicine, Second World Congress, Amsterdam, 1973b, Excerpta Medica Foundation.

Wagai, T.: Advances in ultrasonography and its clinical evaluation, Proceedings of the World Federation of Ultrasound in Medicine and Biology Second Congress, Amsterdam, 1973, Excerpta Medica Foundation.

Weill, F., Ricatte, J. P., Bonneville, J. F., and Prevotat, N.: Systématisation élémentaire de l'image tomo-échographique: applications cliniques, J. Radiol. Electrol. Med. Nucl. **5:**389-398, 1970.

CHAPTER 3

EXAMINATION METHODS AND POSITIONING

In the chapters dealing with the different upper abdominal organs, I shall describe in detail special positions of the patient and particular views. However, in general, the procedure for examining the upper abdomen is rather stereotyped.

POSITIONS AND SCANNING PLANES

1. *The examination begins with the real-time technique.* The patient is supine, and the RTH is placed along the midsagittal line for *sagittal scanning.* When the aorta has been displayed, the RTH is moved to the left side of the patient, then from the left to the right side, and then again from the right to the left side. This continuous sweeping permits the construction, in a few seconds, of an entire succession of sagittal sections. (See Fig. 3-1.) Next, the RTH is rotated 90 degrees to the tranvserse plane and placed over the xiphoid process. It is then moved toward the umbilicus or lower and back to the xiphoid process. Use of this maneuver produces multiple *transverse sections.* (See Fig. 3-2.) Then, the patient is placed on the left side, in a more or less oblique position. The fundamental subcostal *oblique recurrent* view is then produced by the following method. The RTH is placed on the abdominal wall just below the costal margin. (See Fig. 3-3, *A* and *B*.) It is then rocked in the axis that is parallel to the costal margin, in a craniocaudal direction, and then caudocranially, back and forth (Fig. 3-3, *C* to *F*). This rocking movement permits visualization of a succession of retrocostal sections. The next step in this real-time examination is *intercostal scanning.* The patient remains in the same position (left posterior oblique decubitus). The RTH is then placed on the lateral thoracic wall. (See Fig. 3-4.) The orientation of the intercostal spaces is determined by palpation and echoscopic monitoring. A series of intercostal scans is then obtained by an RTH displacement in a craniocaudal direction. This entire succession of scans is performed during normal respiration, as well as in *suspended deep inspiration.* As necessary, complementary oblique scans, specifically oriented for such anatomical elements as the gallbladder and the portal vein (Fig. 3-5), can be obtained. This first phase of the examination, performed in real time, permits a complete exploration of the two upper quadrants of the abdomen in approximately 2 to 3 minutes.

2. *The exploration is completed by contact sagittal and transverse scans* (Fig. 3-6). Other scanning planes are used as in real time (oblique, lateral, intercostal, or posterior cuts). After a few global compound scans are made, most others are performed by the single-sweep technique.

ADJUSTMENTS

In *real time* the different scans are made with a level of sensitivity capable of showing both the organ contours and the tissue texture. This is also the case in

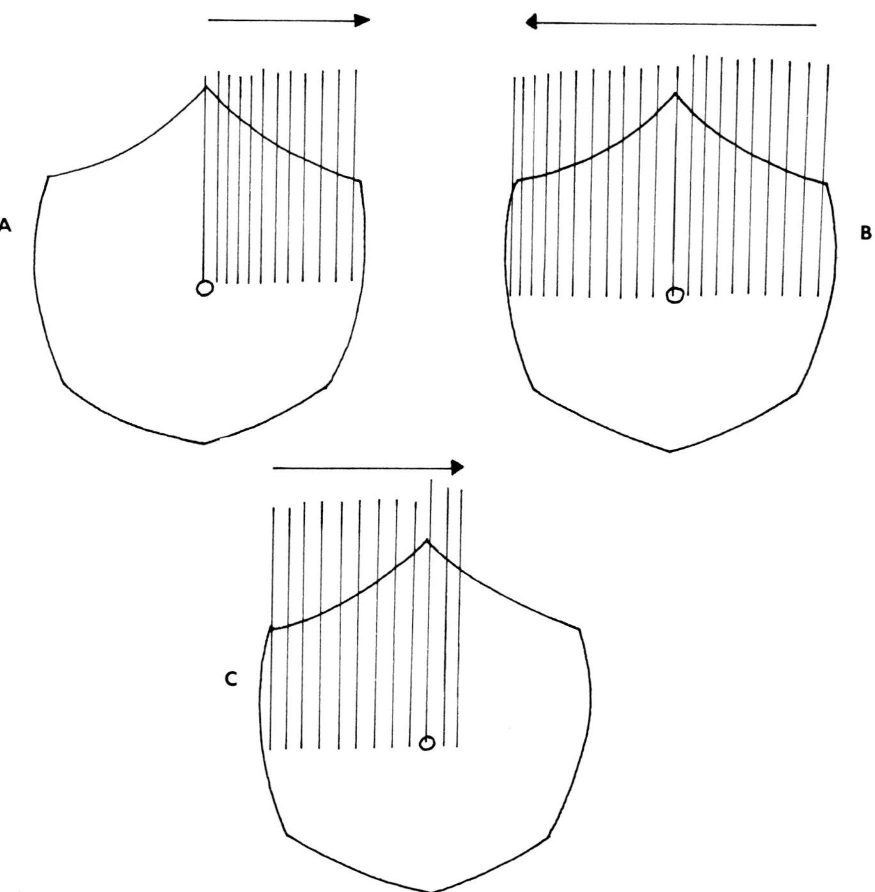

Fig. 3-1. Real-time sagittal scanning of upper abdomen. RTH is placed over midline. **A,** It is then displaced, with sweeping movement, from midline to left, then, **B,** from left to right, and then again, **C,** from right to left.

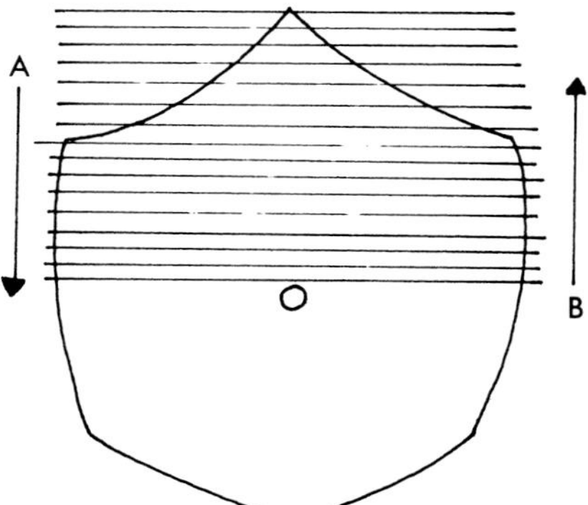

Fig. 3-2. Real-time transverse scanning of upper abdomen. RTH is placed transversely at level of xiphoid process. It is then moved downward from xiphoid process to umbilicus *(A)* and then back to xiphoid *(B)*.

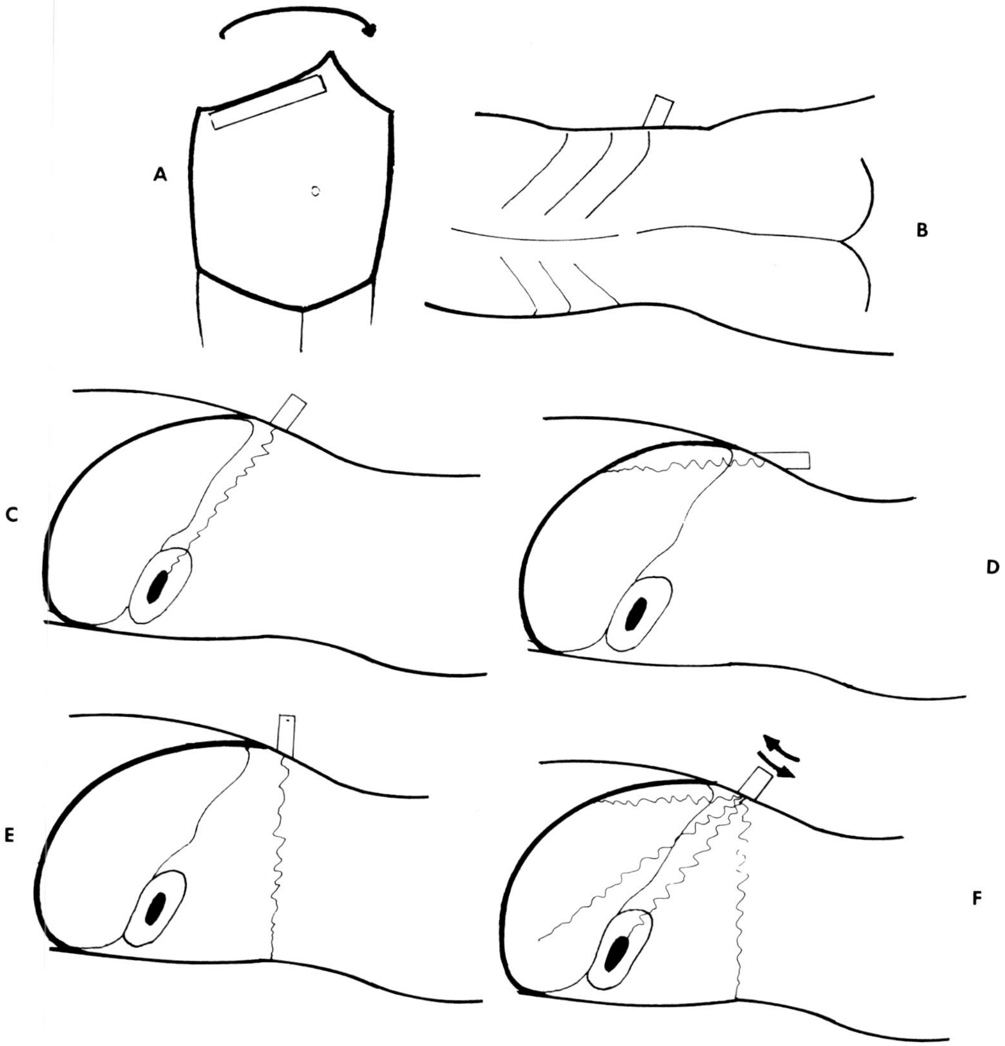

Fig. 3-3. Oblique recurrent subcostal scanning. **A** and **B,** Patient is placed in left posterior oblique position with RTH immediately under right costal edge. **C** to **F,** Rocking movement of RTH assures complete scanning of liver area, with caudal, medial, and cranial sections.

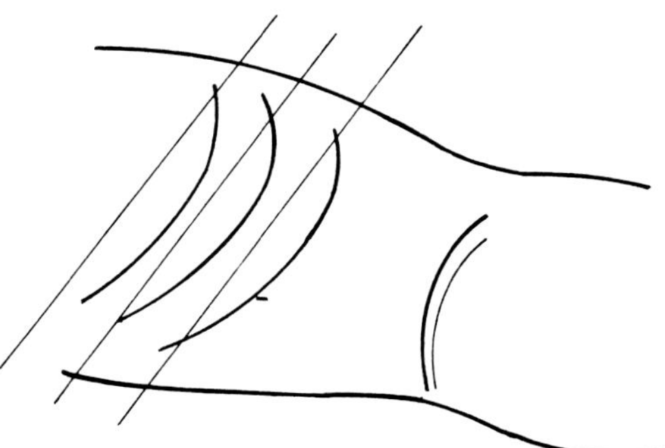

Fig. 3-4. Real-time intercostal scanning. RTH is oriented to direction of intercostal spaces and is then displaced from seventh to eleventh intercostal space.

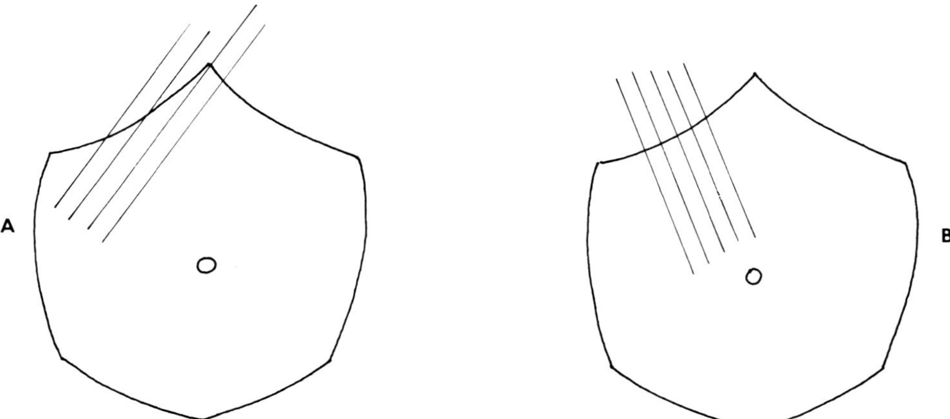

Fig. 3-5. Complementary scans in real time. RTH is oriented in other directions suited to axis of different anatomical elements. **A,** Gallbladder. **B,** Portal vein and common bile duct.

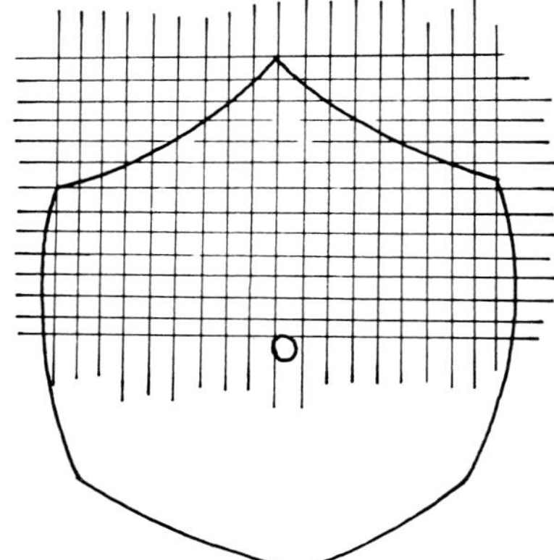

Fig. 3-6. Transverse and sagittal contact scanning.

contact gray scale scanning. The use of low sensitivity or high-contrast adjustment, instead of the old bistable imaging, may prove useful for analyzing organ contours.

ULTRASONICALLY GUIDED BIOPSY

Puncture can be done either with contact scanning or in real time (Hancke and co-workers, 1975; Holm and co-workers, 1975; Rasmussen and co-workers, 1972; Smith and co-workers, 1974). In contact scanning it is aided by the use of a special transducer (Fig. 3-7) containing a central canal. The operator first constructs the images of the organ to be punctured and then evaluates the depth of the lesion and the direction required for insertion of the puncture needle, since the direction of the ultrasonic beam can be displayed on the scope (Fig. 3-8). The needle is then introduced into the tissues, through the special transducer, according to the coordinates of the lesion. In real time the needle is guided by a comple-

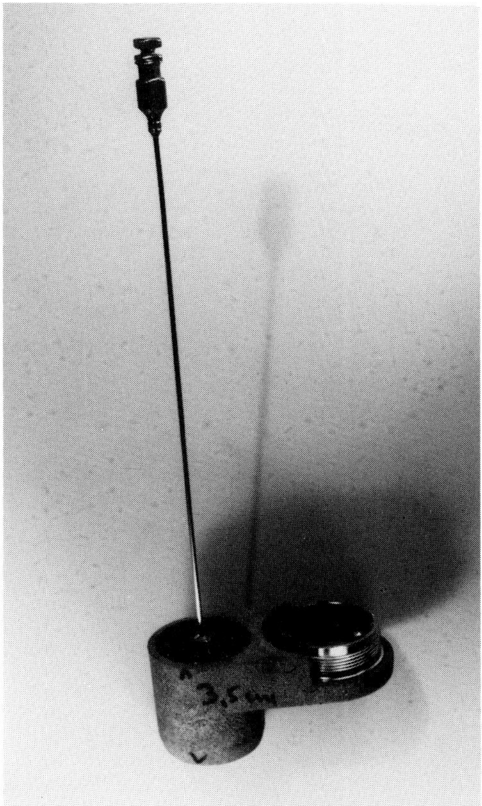

Fig. 3-7. Special transducer for ultrasonically guided puncture. Puncture needle is pushed through central canal.

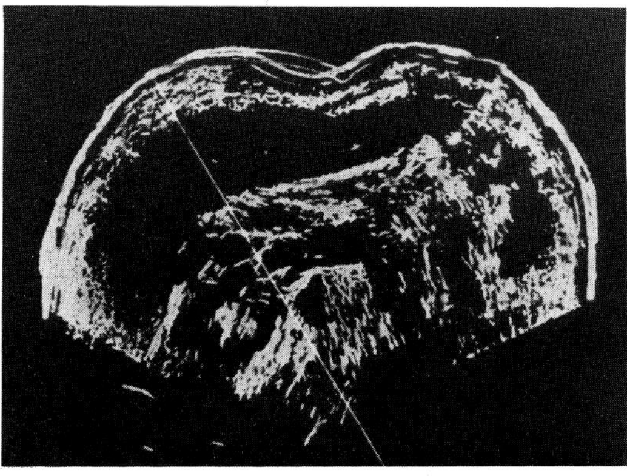

Fig. 3-8. Direction of transducer and therefore of puncture needle is displayed on storage tube screen. Since height of transducer and depth of lesion are known, it is possible to direct needle precisely to biopsy area.

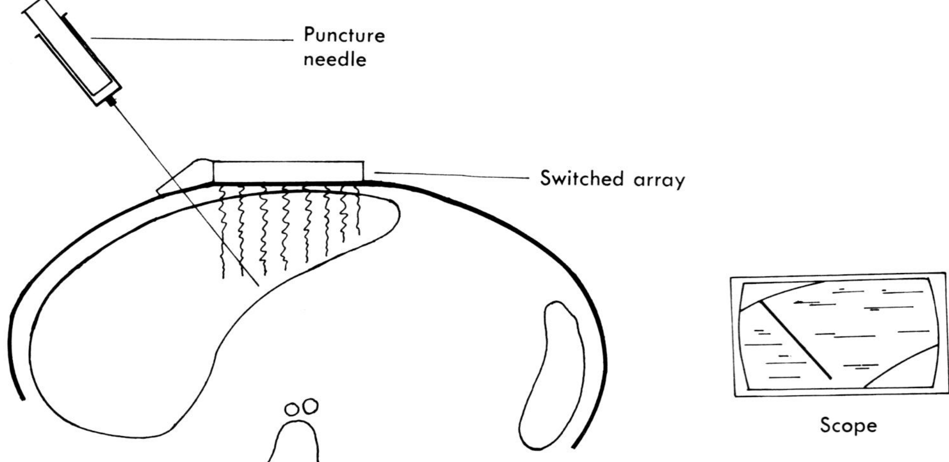

Fig. 3-9. Adaptation of ultrasonic RTH to ultrasonically guided biopsy (Holm, 1975). Lateral device guides puncture needle, progression of which is directly monitored on echoscopic screen.

mentary device that permits the orientation of the needle toward the structure that is to be punctured (Fig. 3-9). The progression of the needle is directly followed under echoscopic monitoring.

We now know *how* to perform ultrasonographic scans. It is still necessary to try to answer two questions: with which *machine* should these scans be done and by *whom?*

SELECTION OF AN ULTRASONIC MACHINE

Selection of an ultrasonic machine will be examined in more detail in Chapter 29. A *contact scanning machine* should be simple to operate, with a rigid arm, precise geometrical references, a gray scale display of quality and excellent resolution, and a rapid writing rate. Its gray scale display must include a wide range of shades: this can be judged in liver imaging; another criterion is the capability of differentiating pancreatic tissue from the stomach on a transverse scan of the epigastrium (Chapter 25). Image resolution is a fundamental element in choice. An excellent resolution test is display of the intrahepatic vascular network; another test is the capability of outlining Wirsung's duct in the pancreas (Chapter 19). The image should be easily reproducible, with equal quality from one patient and one operator to the next, with as little modification of the controls as possible. The transducers should be focused and of sufficiently high frequency (2.25 to 5 MHz). A real-time module of good quality should be coupled with contact scanning. *Good quality* is understood to mean an apparatus having a field of exploration that is sufficient in width, as well as depth, and of satisfactory resolution. This can also be easily judged by the quality of the vascular images that will be described in the next chapter and by the texture of the hepatic tissue echopattern. The synergistic use of the two types of techniques, as already mentioned, is *indispensable.*

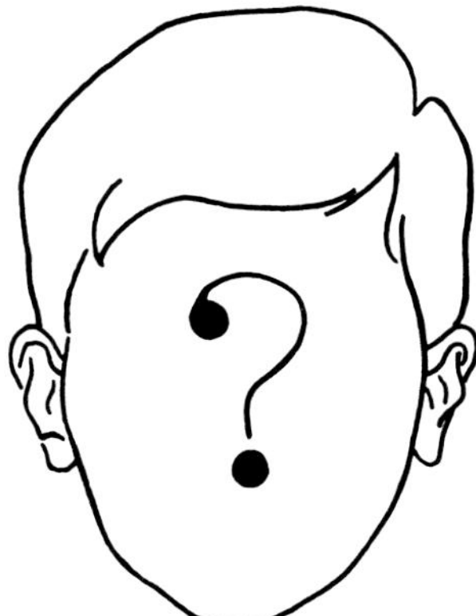

Fig. 3-10. Who should perform ultrasonography?

WHO SHOULD PERFORM ULTRASONOGRAPHY? (Fig. 3-10)

The school of Hillel says that ultrasonographers should be radiologists. The school of Schammai says that they should be technicians. I say that the choice should be those who know how to produce images of good quality but are also able to make a diagnosis on the spot—the diagnosis of a simple anatomical anomaly, as well as a lesion. An ultrasonographer should be able to follow clinical reasoning, leading to the examination of another organ or area if the first step of the examination is negative, exactly as is done in other types of gastrointestinal (GI) radiology, such as GI series, barium enemas, and celiac trunk angiography. The performance of real-time ultrasonography demands more medical knowledge than does the making of routine, repetitive single-sweep contact scans. In my department, trained radiologists themselves used to perform ultrasonography for most abdominal examinations. At the least, a close collaboration between technician and radiologist is necessary.

REFERENCES

Barnett, E., and Morley, P.: Abdominal echography, Borough Green, England, 1974, Butterworth & Co. (Publishers), Ltd.

Goldberg, B. B., Kotler, M. N., Ziskin, M. C., and Waxham, R. D.: Diagnostic uses of ultrasound, New York, 1975, Grune & Stratton, Inc.

Hancke, S., Holm, H. H., and Koch, F.: Ultrasonically guided percutaneous fine needle biopsy of the pancreas, Surg. Gynecol. Obstet. **140:**361-364, 1975.

Hassani, N.: Ultrasonography of the abdomen, Heidelberg, Germany, 1976, Springer-Verlag.

Holm, H. H., Kristensen, J. K., Rasmussen, S. N., Pedersen, J. F., and Hancke, S.: Abdominal ultrasound, Copenhagen, 1976, Munksgaard, International Booksellers & Publishers, Ltd.

Holm, H. H., Pedersen, J. F., Kristensen, J. K., Rasmussen, S. N., Hancke, S., and Jensen, F.: Ultrasonically guided percutaneous puncture, Radiol. Clin. North Am. **13:**493-503, 1975.

Leopold, G. R., and Asher, W. M.: Fundamentals of abdominal and pelvic ultrasonography, Philadelphia, 1975, W. B. Saunders Co.

Rasmussen, S. N., Holm, H. H., Kristensen, J. K., and Barlebott: Ultrasonically-guided liver biopsy, Br. Med. J. **2:**500-502, 1972.

Smith, E. H., Bartrum, R. J., Jr., and Chang, Y. C.: Ultrasonically guided percutaneous aspiration biopsy of the pancreas, Radiology **112:**737-738, 1974.

Weill, F., Becker, J. C., Kraehenbuhl, J. R., Heriot, G., and Walter, J. P.: Clinical atlas of ultrasonic radiography, Paris, 1973, Masson & Cie., Editeurs.

Wells, P. N. T.: Ultrasonics in clinical diagnosis, Edinburgh, 1972, Churchill Livingstone.

CHAPTER 4

ANATOMICAL GUIDE TO ULTRASONIC EXPLORATION OF UPPER ABDOMEN: echoangiography

THE AORTA AND ITS BRANCHES

As indicated in the preceding chapter, the aorta is the first anatomical element to be identified during an ultrasonic exploration of the upper abdomen. The first approach is by *sagittal midline scans* performed on the supine patient. The aorta appears as a tubular structure. (See Figs. 4-1 and 4-2.) Its pulsations are clearly apparent in real time. The diameter of the aorta diminishes regularly from its entry into the abdomen to the bifurcation (Fig. 4-1), that is, from T-12 to L-4. It is practically impossible to distinguish the posterior aortic wall from the vertebrae on which it rests (Figs. 4-1 and 4-2). As the aorta proceeds caudally, it becomes superficial, so that in a thin patient at the level of the bifurcation it may be found 2 to 3 cm beneath the skin (Fig. 4-2, *B* and *C*) or even closer if the skin is depressed by palpation. Since the superficial character of the vessel is accentuated by atheromatosis, it is not surprising that the clinician who is feeling intense pulsations during an abdominal examination may misdiagnose an aneurysm. The superior subdiaphragmatic segment of the abdominal aorta tends to be masked by the acoustic shadow of the xiphoid process. Therefore it is easier to visualize this segment of the aorta with contact scanning than in real time, since the transducer can be angled cephalad under the xiphoid process. (See Fig. 4-3.) Caudal to the liver the

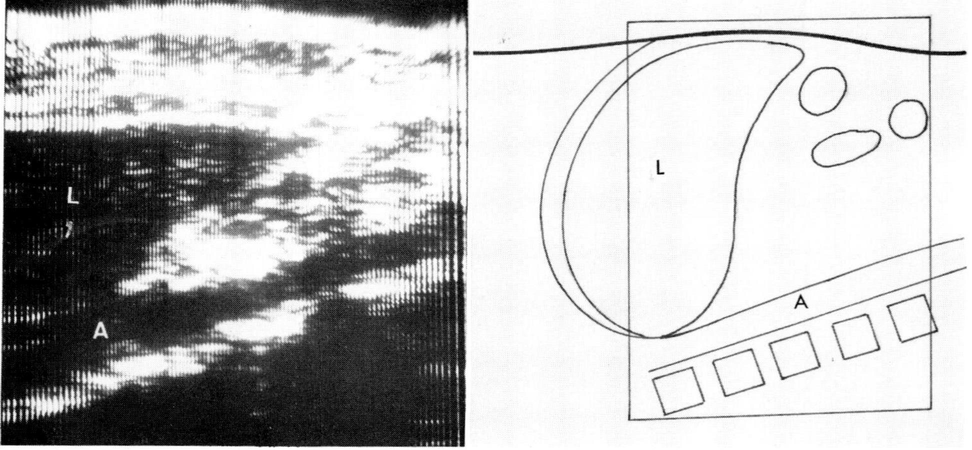

Fig. 4-1. Real-time sagittal abdominal scan and schematic drawing displaying aorta *(A)* in sagittal section, behind liver *(L)*.

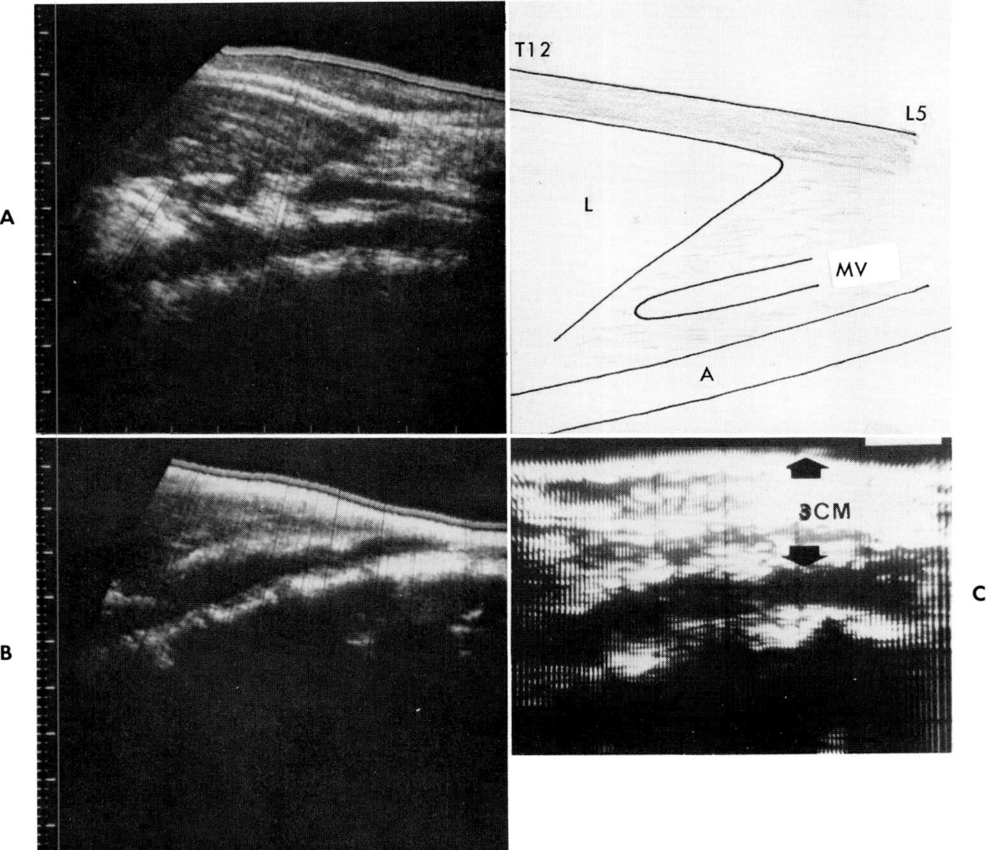

Fig. 4-2. Other examples of sagittal scans and schematic representation of aorta. **A,** Contact scan and schematic drawing. Note sagittal section of mesenteric vein *(MV)*. *A*, aorta; *L*, liver. **B,** Sagittal scan of aorta in lean and aged patient. Vessel is very superficial in its distal part. Its anterior wall lies at distance of 2 cm from skin. **C,** Real-time sagittal scan of aorta in another aged patient. Only 3 cm separates skin from anterior vascular wall.

aorta can be masked by colic gas, particularly in a patient whose left hepatic lobe is small. This inconvenience can be circumvented by two means: the use of suspended deep inspiration or changing the position of the patient. Deep inspiration displaces the liver and the transverse colon caudally. Standing displaces the liver caudally and gas cranially, toward the colic flexures. In decubitus, the rotation of the trunk into an oblique position also effects a migration of the gas from the transverse colon toward the colic flexures. Finally, in certain patients a lateral, transhepatic approach may permit good visualization of the aorta (Fig. 4-4); a left transrenal approach is also possible. In some elderly patients it is difficult to show the abdominal aorta in a single cut, since the vessel is tortuous. It is then necessary to select the different oblique orientations of the RTH that display the different segments of the aorta successively. (See Fig. 4-5.)

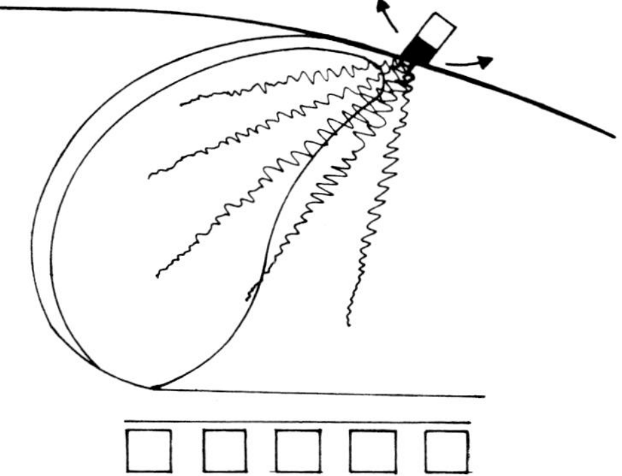

Fig. 4-3. Scan of retrohepatic portion of aorta. Upper segment of vessel is displayed on sector scan, with transducer applied on skin immediately below xiphoid process.

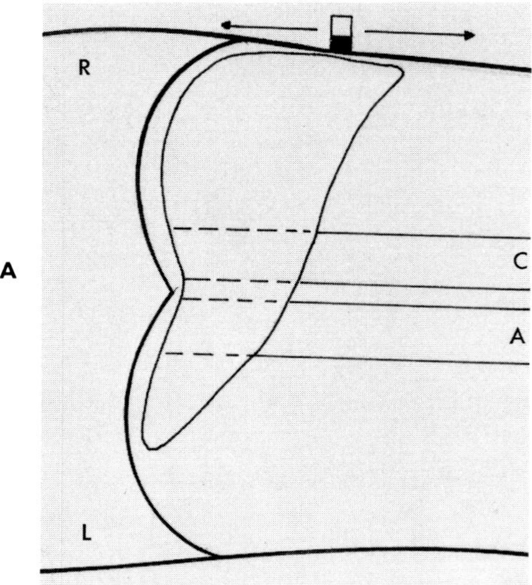

Fig. 4-4. Aorta and vena cava in frontal display. These images were obtained by lateral sagittal scanning with patient lying in left lateral decubitus position. **A,** Schematic representation of scanning plane. *C,* vena cava; *A,* aorta. **B,** Section itself. Ultrasonic beam has crossed liver *(L)* and shows frontal sections of vena cava and aorta side by side. **C,** Another example of sagittal lateral transhepatic vascular section. *Arrows* point to hepatic vein, merging with vena cava. Aorta is seen more internally.

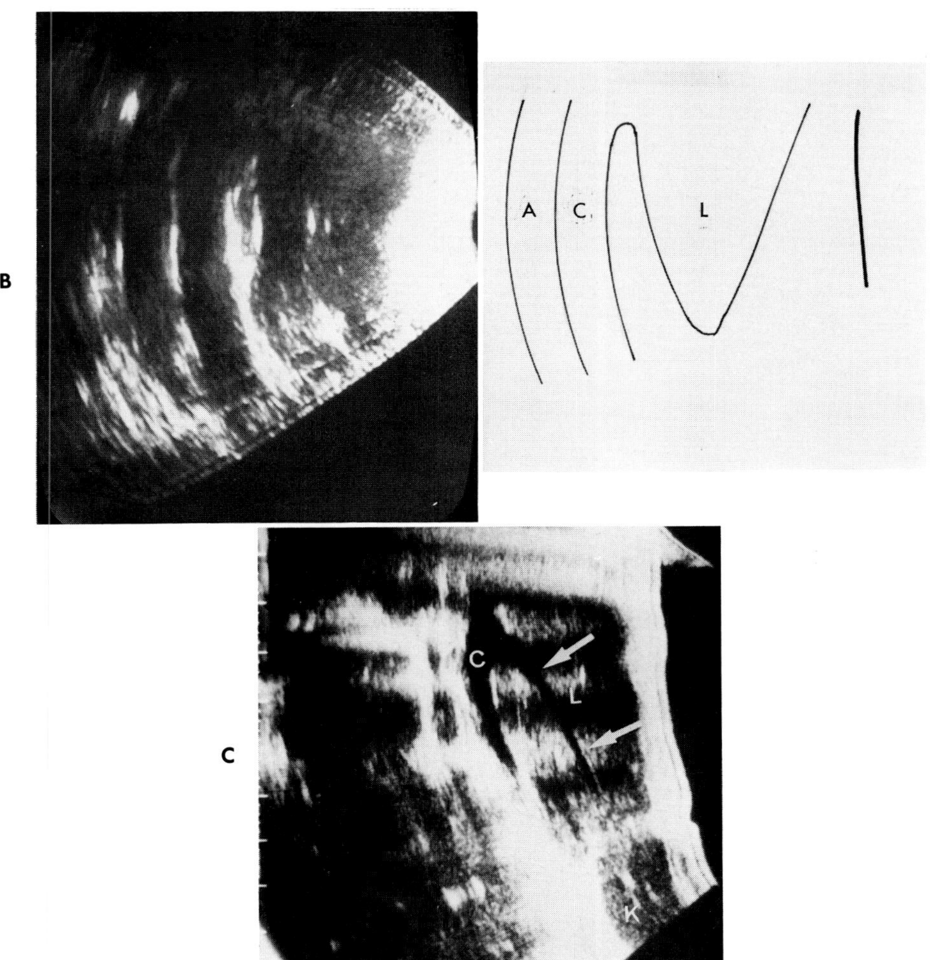

Fig. 4-4, cont'd. For legend see opposite page.

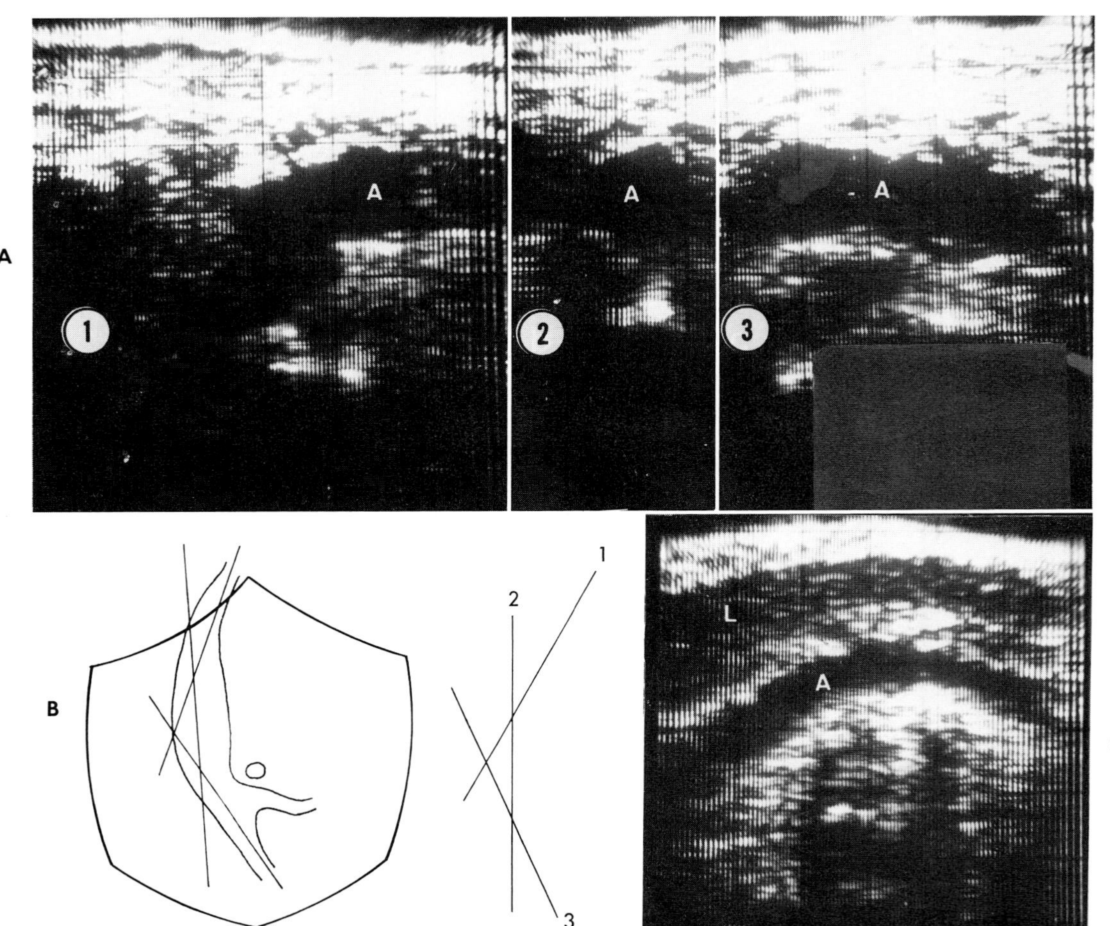

Fig. 4-5. A, Section of tortuous aorta *(A)*. In this elderly patient, it was not possible to display entire sagittal section with single scanning plane. Different scanning planes, adapted to direction of different vascular segments, were necessary. Summation of vascular sections, as displayed by each scan, permitted construction of image of entire aorta. **B,** Schematic drawing of angles used to obtain section in **A. C,** Another sinuous aorta, this time with anterior curvature. *L,* liver.

The image of the iliac arteries is often difficult to visualize because of intestinal gas in the pelvis, but the visceral branches of the aorta are more readily accessible, as will be discussed subsequently.

In *transverse scans* the aorta appears in front of the anterior edge of the vertebra and to the left of the section of the vena cava, in the form of a circle, or ring. Successive sagittal scans show its succesive sections in the fashion of the sliced sausage in Fig. 1-1. (See Fig. 4-6.) It is important to have first constructed an image of the aorta in sagittal scans: if the tortuosity of the vessel is not appreciated, one risks mistaking an oblique section for an aneurysm (Fig. 4-7).

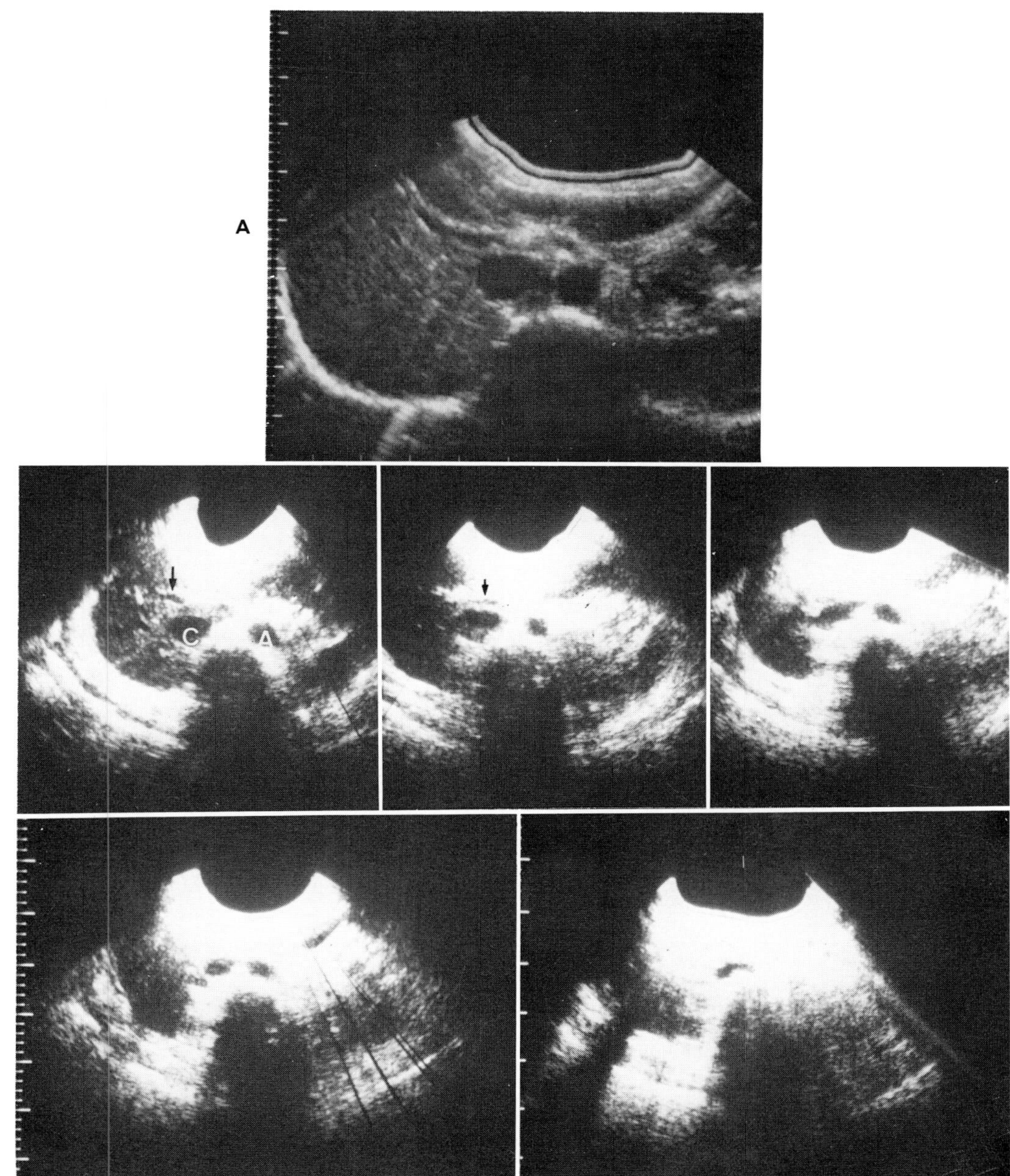

Fig. 4-6. A, Transverse section of aorta and vena cava in suspended respiration. **B,** Parallel transverse scans of aorta *(A)* and vena cava *(C)* from L-1 to L-4 (aortic division). In first two scans, note portal vein *(arrows)* in front of vena cava. Portal division is also displayed in **A.**

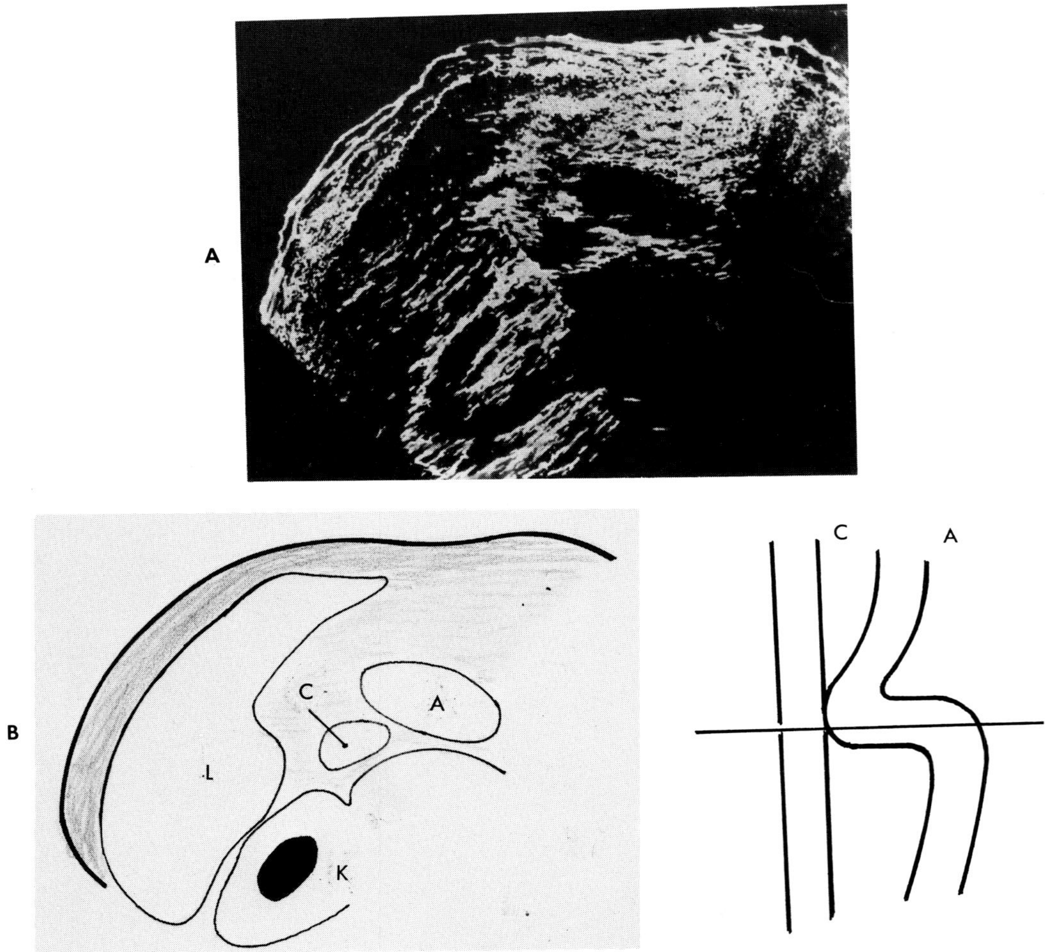

Fig. 4-7. A, Transverse section of aorta in elderly patient. Scan passes through bend in vessel, as shown in schematic drawing at right, so that aortic section is not rounded, but oval. **B,** Schematic drawings of **A.** Right, scanning plane. *A,* aorta; *C,* vena cava; *K,* right kidney; *L,* liver.

Aortic branches

The visceral branch of the aorta that is easiest to show on sagittal scans is the superior mesenteric artery (SMA), which is often preaortic over several centimeters (Figs. 4-8, 4-9, and 4-19). The celiac trunk can also be recognized (Fig. 4-8) on sagittal scans, as well as some of its branches, such as the hepatic artery, the splenic artery, and the gastric (coronary) artery (Fig. 4-10). (See also Fig. 15-23.) The inferior mesenteric artery is thin and only rarely seen on ultrasonographic scans (Fig. 4-8, *D*). The descending posterior orientation of the renal arteries makes them difficult to identify with regularity in transverse cuts (Fig. 4-11).

VENA CAVA

Parallel sagittal cuts just to the right of the aorta demonstrate the vena cava. The image of the inferior vena cava (IVC) is quite different from that of the aorta. The vena cava tends to run along the anterolateral aspect of the vertebral column, whereas the aorta is frankly prevertebral. Thus the IVC maintains a depth that is almost constant from its origin until it reaches the liver. (See Fig. 4-12.) The aorta, on the other hand, ascends from T-12 to L-4. Behind the liver the vena cava describes a curve slightly concave to the anterior (Fig. 4-12). Rarely, the vena cava may lie frankly lateral to the vertebral body, so that it is surrounded by liver tissue even posteriorly (Fig. 4-12, *D*), instead of lying on the paravertebral muscles (Fig. 4-12, *A* to *C*). The IVC is much flatter than the aorta. As a matter of fact, its diameter is constantly changing, as is readily evident in real-time scanning (Weill and associates, 1973a; Weill and associates, 1973b). This caval motion

Text continued on p. 50.

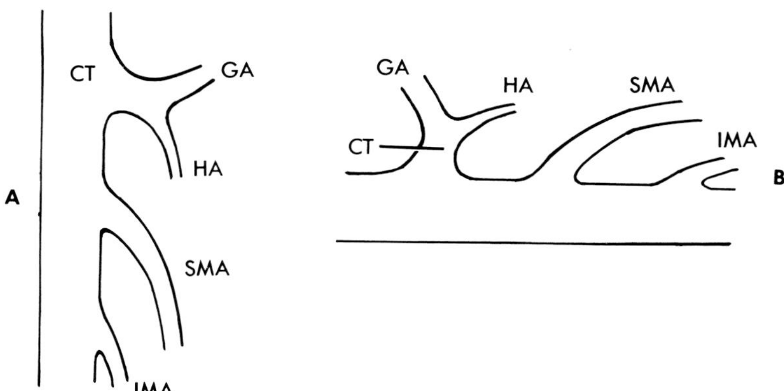

Fig. 4-8. Sagittal sections of digestive branches of aorta. **A,** Schematic representation of anatomy of different branches. *CT,* celiac trunk; *HA,* hepatic artery; *SMA,* superior mesenteric artery; *IMA,* inferior mesenteric artery; *GA,* gastric (coronary) artery. **B,** Same scheme presented with ultrasonographic orientation. **C,** Gray scale sagittal midline scan displaying aorta, celiac trunk, gastric artery, hepatic artery, and superior mesenteric artery. *L,* liver. **D,** Real-time display of celiac trunk, superior mesenteric artery, and inferior mesenteric artery. **E,** Branch of celiac trunk with superior mesenteric artery. *PV,* portal vein. *Continued.*

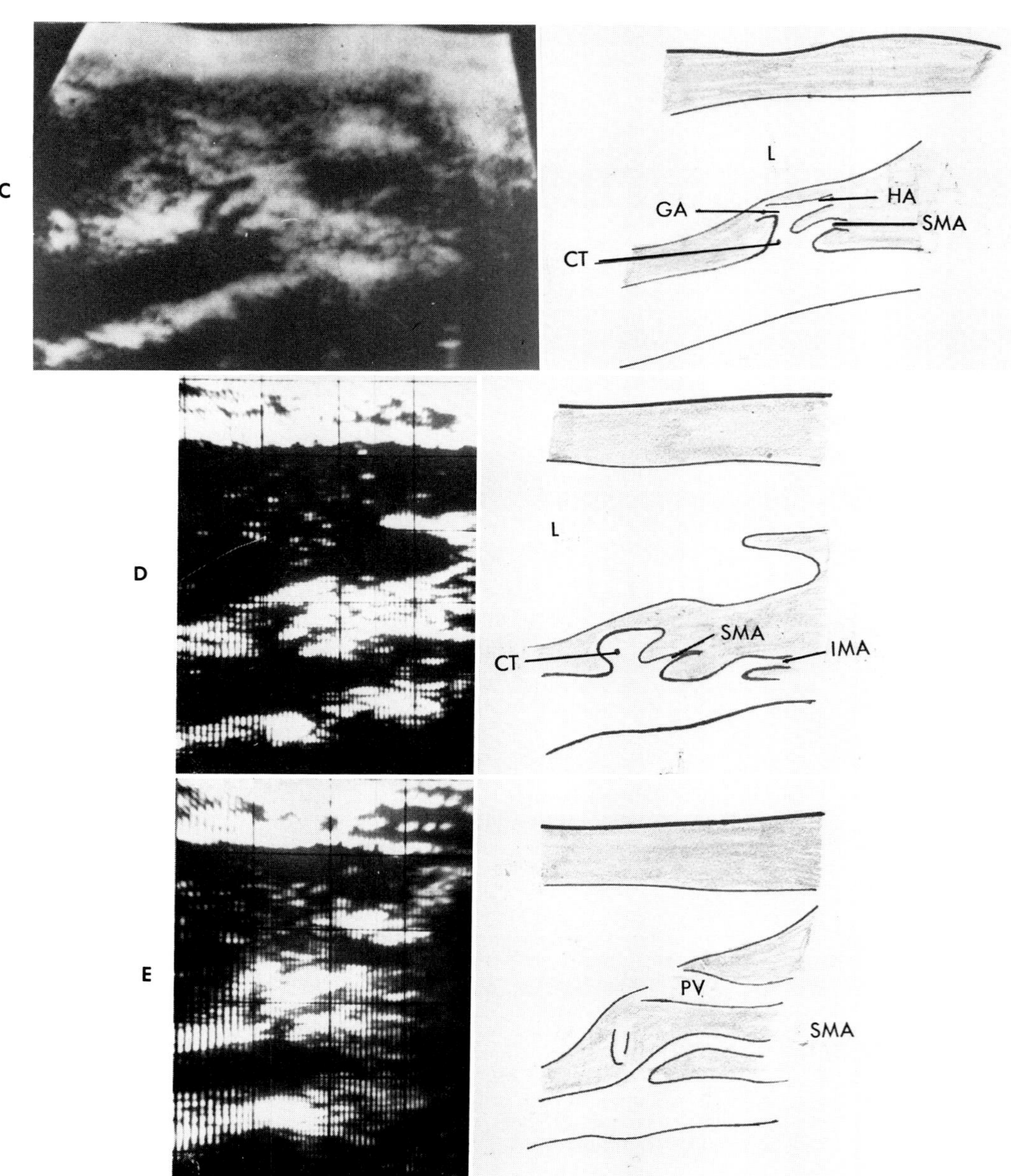

Fig. 4-8, cont'd. For legend see p. 45.

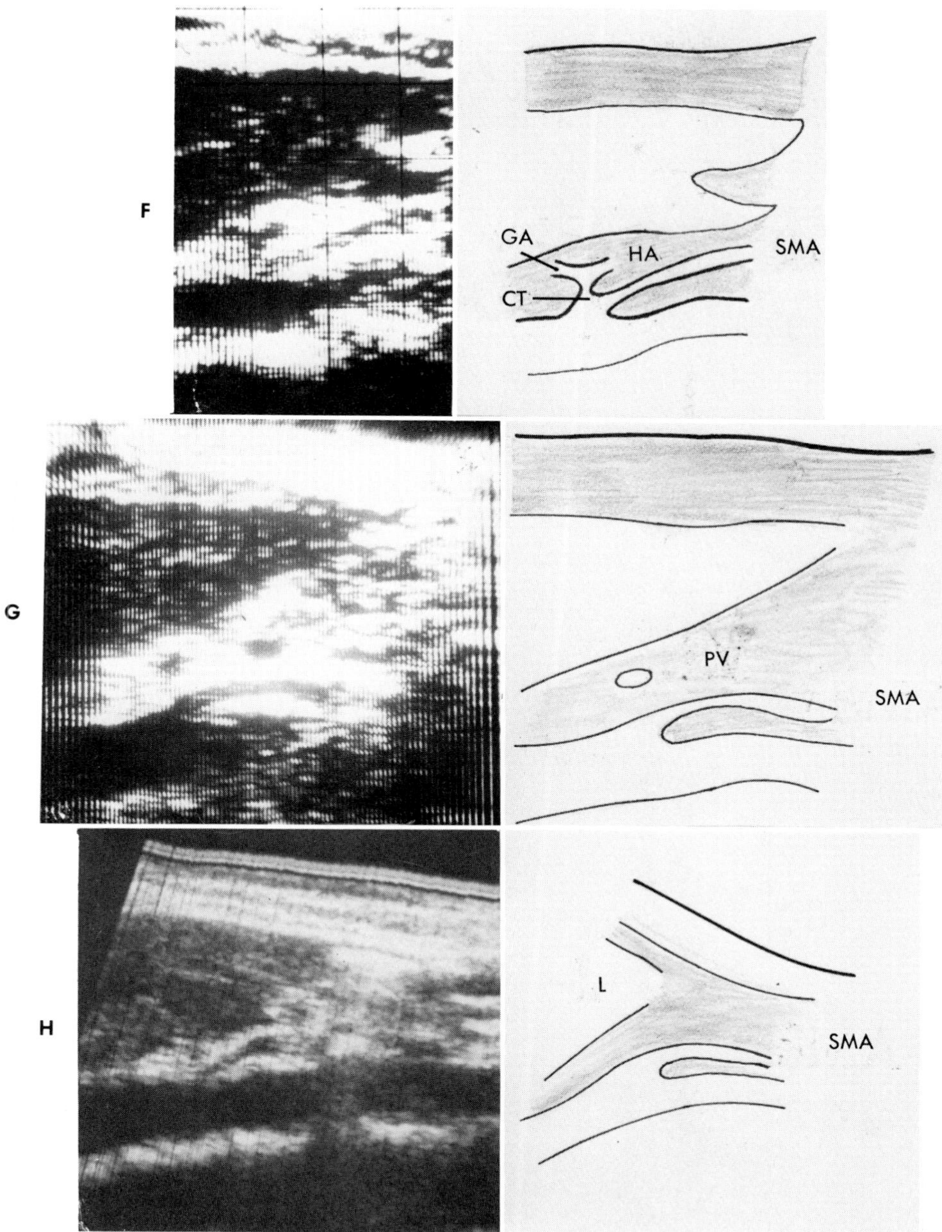

Fig. 4-8, cont'd. F, Celiac trunk with its branches and superior mesenteric artery. **G,** Superior mesenteric artery. *PV,* portal vein in sagittal section. **H,** Gray scale image of superior mesenteric artery.

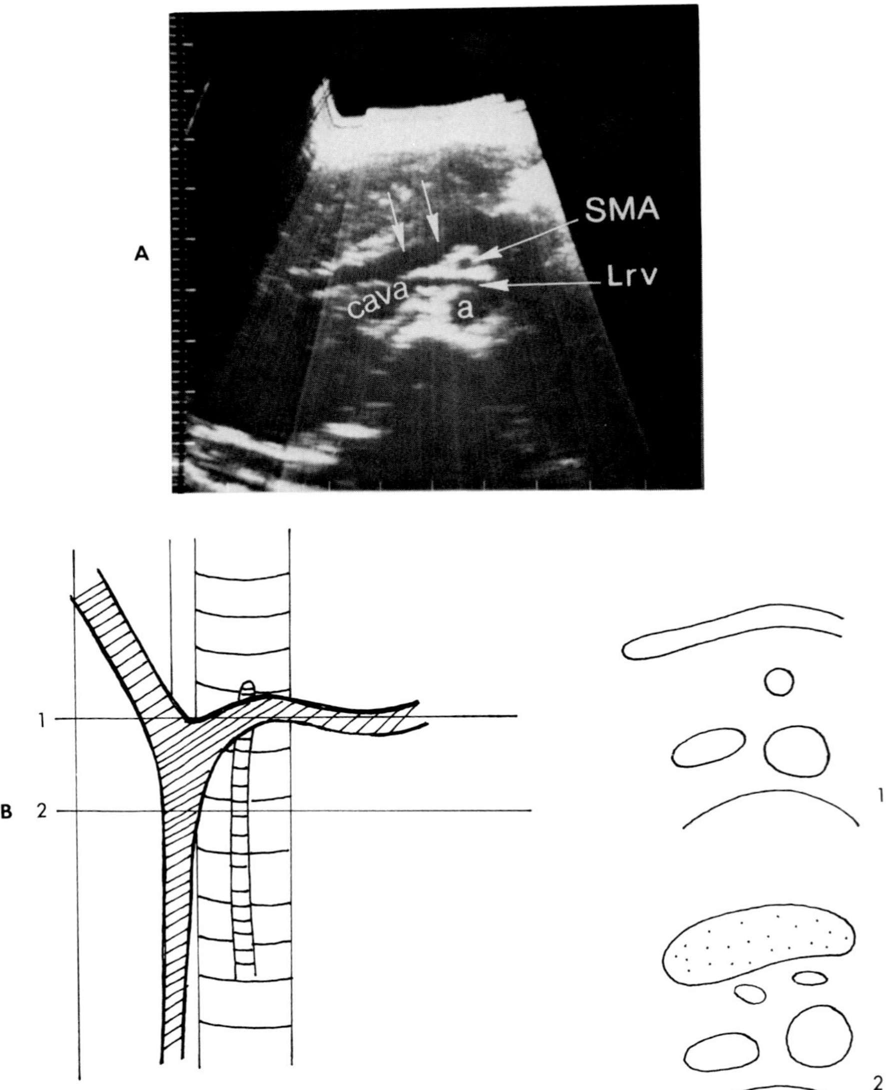

Fig. 4-9. A, Different arterial and venous elements. **A,** Transverse scan of upper abdomen showing aorta *(a)* and vena cava with left renal vein *(Lrv)*. In front of aorta and left renal vein, small sonolucent rounded area belonging to superior mesenteric artery *(SMA)* is displayed. Between superior mesenteric artery and left lobe of liver, splenic vein *(arrows)* is outlined. Thus, from front to back, between liver and vertebral body, splenic vein is displayed in its course toward portal vein and then mesenteric artery, left renal vein, and aorta. Splenoportal junction lies in front of cava. **B,** Schematic frontal representation of abdominal vessels. Scan in **A** was made along scanning plane *1,* which passes through splenic vein and shows only mesenteric artery, but not mesenteric vein. Parallel, more caudal scan along plane *2* would display both mesenteric artery and vein behind pancreas.

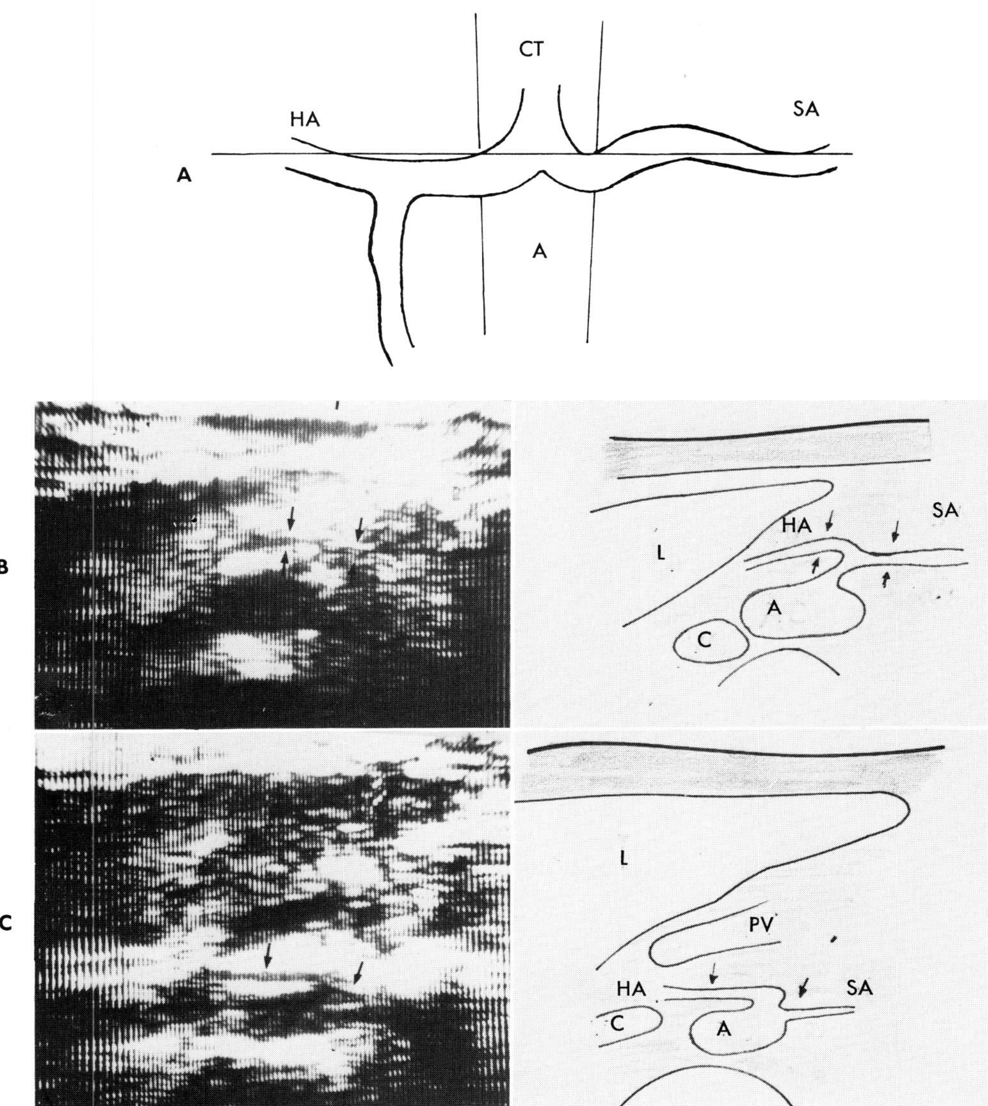

Fig. 4-10. Transverse section of celiac trunk branches. **A,** Scanning plane. *CT,* celiac trunk; *HA,* hepatic artery; *SA,* splenic artery; *A,* aorta. **B,** Real-time display of celiac trunk, hepatic artery *(HA, arrows),* and splenic artery *(SA, arrows). C,* vena cava; *L,* liver. **C,** Another example of transverse scan of both hepatic and splenic artery. In front of hepatic artery, note another tubular element, portal vein *(PV).* *Continued.*

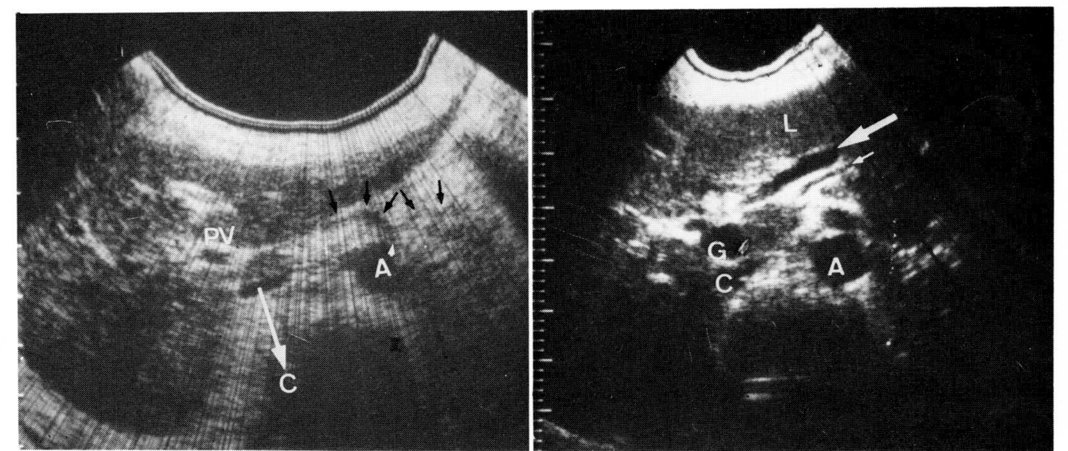

Fig. 4-10, cont'd. D, Another example of transverse section of celiac trunk *(white arrowhead)* and hepatic and splenic arteries *(black arrows). C,* vena cava; *A,* aorta; *PV,* portal vein. **E,** Splenic artery *(small arrow),* running along splenic vein *(large arrow). G,* gallbladder.

is surprising to one used to the large diameter of the cava in x-ray cavography, even though it is a well-known physiological phenomenon.

Thus the vena cava expands when intrathoracic pressure is increased after inspiration, and it flattens markedly after expiration. (See Fig. 4-12.) With shallow respiratory movements, in the majority of subjects the anteroposterior diameter does not exceed a few millimeters. The discrepancy between the ultrasonographic image and the radiographic appearance is due to the fact that cavography is carried out in suspended respiration. This procedure, similar to the Valsalva maneuver, also dilates the vena cava in ultrasonography. Thus suspended respiration is a good method of displaying a flat IVC. (See Fig. 4-13.) In sagittal contact scanning it is the only way to display the cava without respiratory blurring. In addition to respiratory caval movements, there are, in the retrohepatic segment of the vessel, pulsations that are synchronous with the cardiac cycle (Fig. 4-13, *A*). In my opinion, they correspond to cardiac pulsations transmitted directly from the right atrium.*

The respiratory movement of the vena cava is an important criterion of hemodynamic normality. In certain normal subjects, the vena cava may appear to be rather large and display only slight respiratory change; but with ample respiratory movements in normal subjects the variations in the retrohepatic venous diameter are evident, since it is reduced at least 50% after expiration. A vena cava that remains distended and akinetic is indicative of venous hypertension. (See Fig. 4-13.) (This will be discussed further in Chapter 7.)

Text continued on p. 55.

*In fact, these pulsations likely correspond to those classically described in the jugular venous pulse, including the a, v, and c waves. This triphasic pulsation is occasionally observed under exceptionally favorable conditions (Winsberg, 1977).

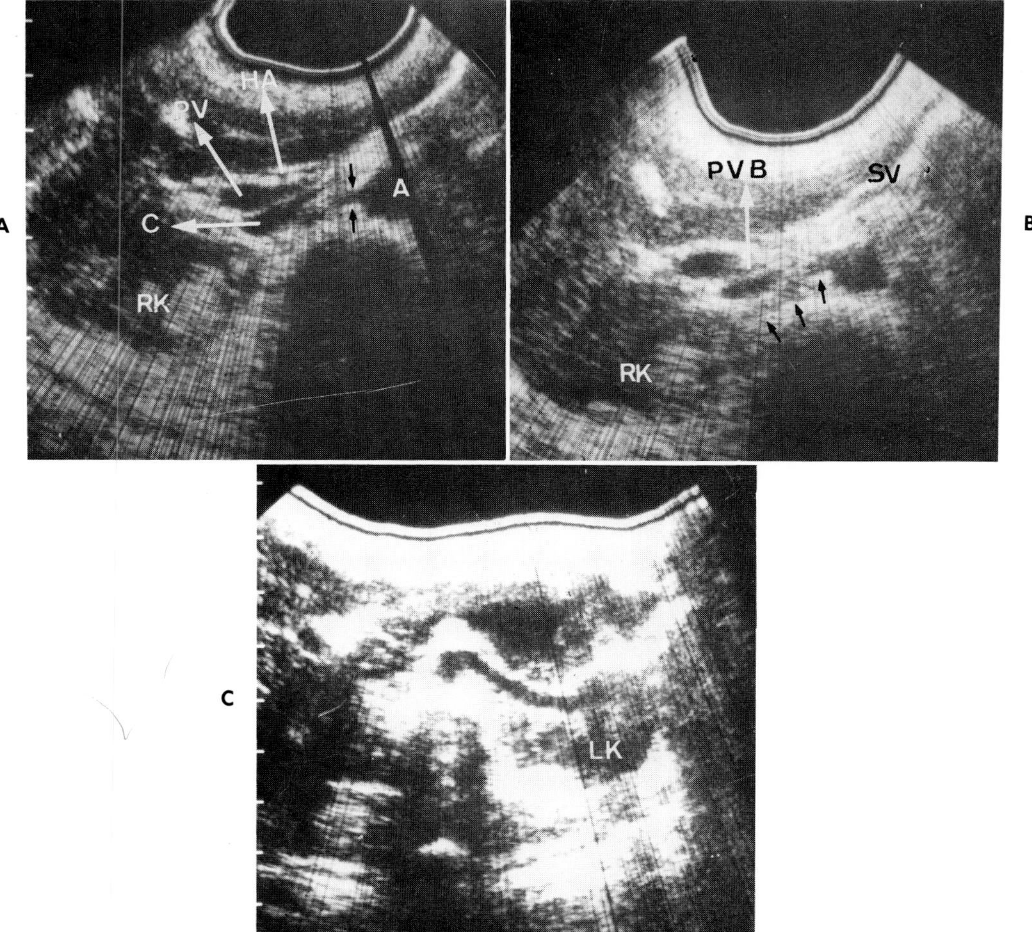

Fig. 4-11. Renal arteries. **A** and **B,** Right renal artery. Two parallel transverse scans show origin and course of vessel *(black arrows).* Note also hepatic artery *(HA),* portal vein *(PV),* splenic vein *(SV),* portal vein branch *(PVB)* (duodenal vein?), and vena cava and origin of left renal vein *(C). RK,* right kidney; *A,* aorta. **C,** Left renal artery outlined from origin to renal hilus. *LK,* left kidney.

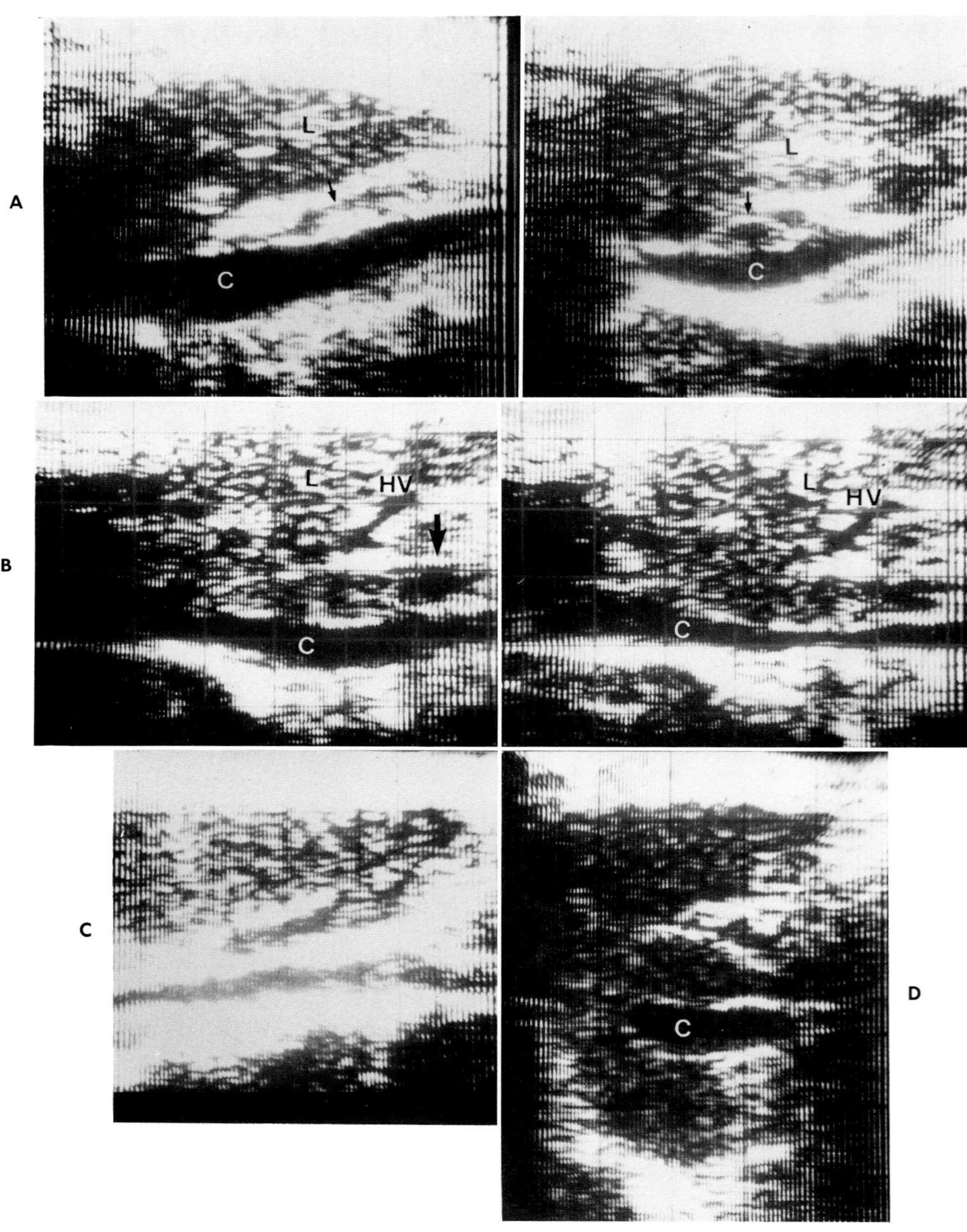

Fig. 4-12. For legend see opposite page.

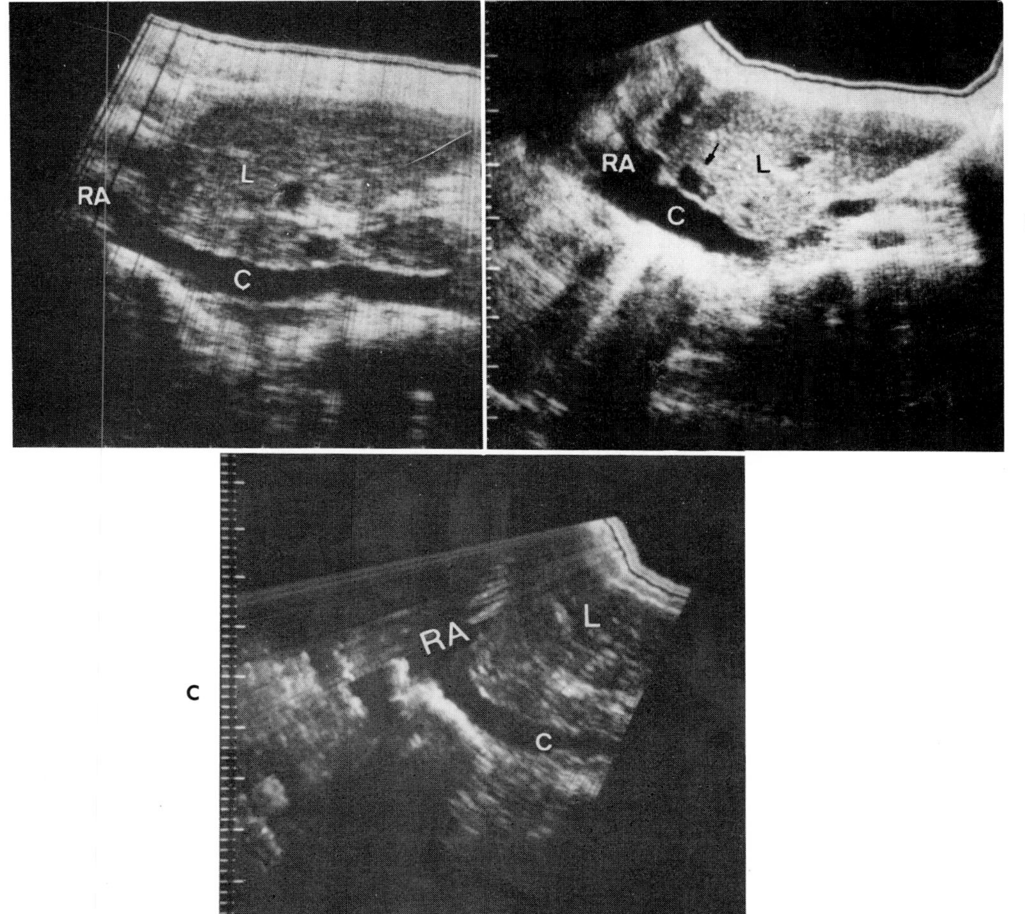

Fig. 4-13. Sagittal scan of vena cava. **A,** This scan was made during suspended inspiration. Subxiphoid sector scan displays junction between vena cava *(C)* and right atrium *(RA)*. Cardiac movements blur right atrium. Note undulated pattern of anterior wall of vein. It corresponds to systolic-diastolic pulsations of vessel, persisting even when respiratory movements were blocked; such pulsations are registered if transducer is moved slowly. *L,* liver. **B,** Identical scan in patient having cardiac insufficiency. Even without suspended respiration, vena cava is dilated. Junction between vessel and right atrium is evident. **C,** In this slowly performed scan with lower gain, pulsation of right atrial wall can be seen.

Fig. 4-12. Sagittal scans (real-time study) of vena cava showing respiratory changes. **A,** Vena cava *(C)* outlined behind liver *(L),* on left during inspiration and on right during expiration. Expiratory collapse of vena cava is accompanied by changes in position of mesenteric-portal venous axis: mesenteric-portal image *(arrow)* is quite different on left and on right. These changes are only positional. There are no respiratory changes in diameter of portal system. **B,** Another example of respiratory changes of vena cava, on left during inspiration and on right during expiration. *HV,* section of hepatic vein; *arrow,* section of portal vein. **C,** Caval lumen is almost virtually behind liver. Portal vein is outlined between liver and IVC. **D,** Sagittal section of vena cava lying more laterally. There is now liver tissue behind vessel, instead of paravertebral muscles.

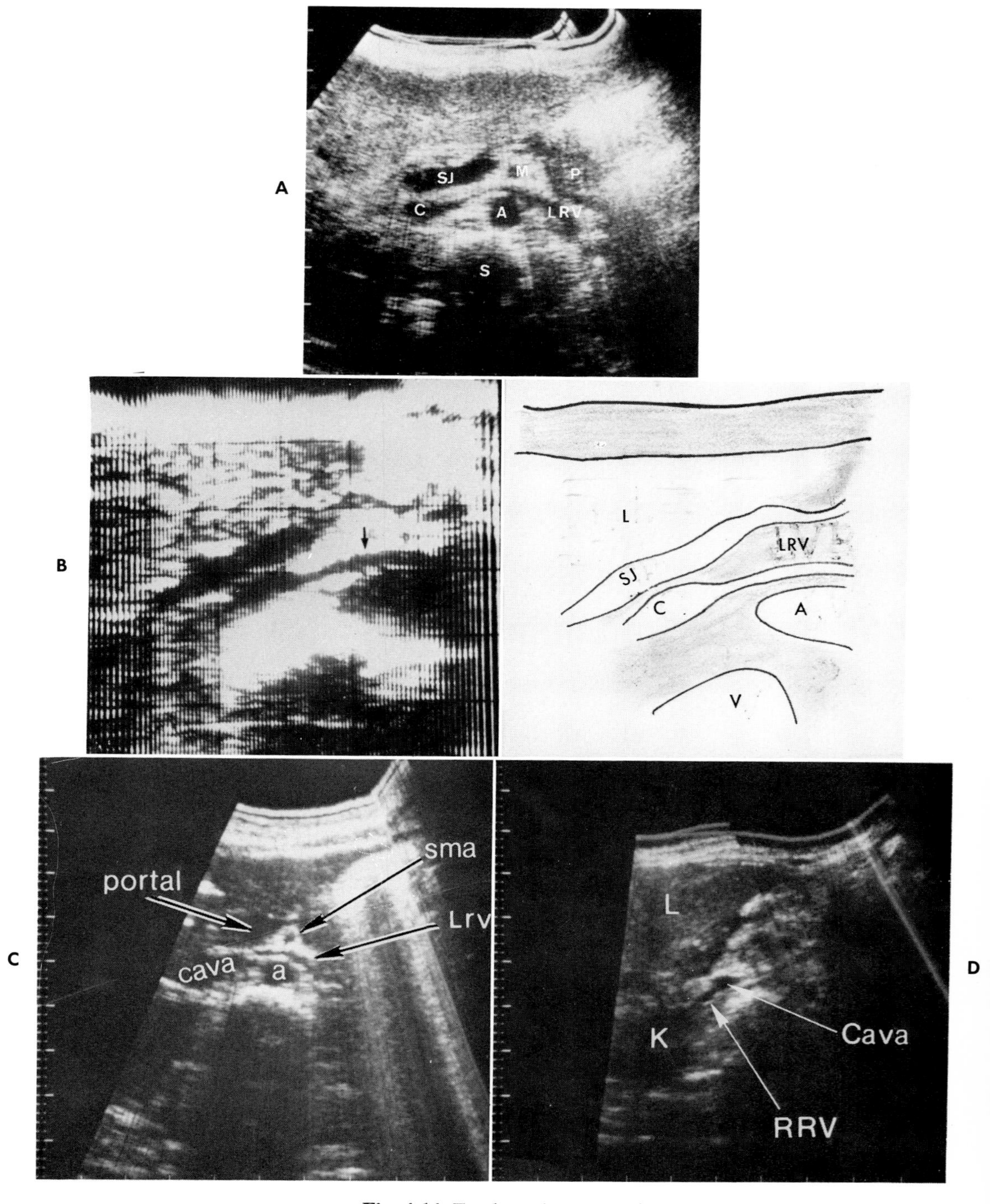

Fig. 4-14. For legend see opposite page.

The IVC is in close relation to the portal vein (Fig. 4-12); that relation will be studied in more detail later. The vena cava can be seen on lateral transhepatic scans (Fig. 4-4). Its image is then identical to that of a frontal cavogram, and no movement is visible.

The termination of the vena cava in the right atrium can be readily shown with a rapid sagittal contact sector scan (Fig. 4-13). This image of the junction is even more evident when there is venous stasis (Fig. 4-13, *B*).

On transverse scans the image of the IVC appears oval or flattened to the right of the aorta, from L-4 to L-2. At the level of L-1 and T-12 the vessel becomes more anterior in its retrohepatic enclave (Fig. 4-6).

Branches of vena cava

The image of certain branches of the IVC can be demonstrated: the left renal vein appears readily on close serial parallel transverse scans (Leopold, 1975; Meire, 1976). It crosses over the anterior wall of the aorta behind the SMA. (See Fig. 4-14.) One may speculate why the renal vein is more often displayed than the renal artery. The venous phase of renal angiography shows very well that the renal vein has a more horizontal course than does the artery. The image of the right renal vein can also be obtained (Fig. 4-14, *D*).

The *hepatic veins* appear in approximately half of normal subjects on hepatic recurrent oblique subcostal real-time scans performed with machines of the first generation and still more often when real-time equipment of the second generation is used. Such recurrent scans usually display the whole venous network, since the major branches are all in the same plane. (See Fig. 4-15, *A* to *I*.) This section clearly shows their harmonious convergence toward the IVC (Weill and associates, 1975b; Weill and Eisencher, 1976). In most subjects the diameter of the hepatic veins is no larger than 4 to 5 mm at a distance of 2 cm from the junction. When the hepatic veins are narrower, they can be only momentarily visualized as the RTH is rocked rapidly. In some normal subjects the diameter of the hepatic veins is somewhat larger, up to 1 cm. Rarely, changes in diameter with respiration may parallel those which occur in the IVC (Fig. 4-15, *J* and *K*), at least in the distal segment of the hepatic veins. These veins, embedded in the homogeneous hepatic parenchyma, show a typical branching pattern, often without distinct wall images, a point that will be examined in Chapter 6.

Fig. 4-14. Renal veins. **A,** Transverse scan of upper abdomen, displaying left renal vein *(LRV)* running in front of aorta *(A)*, to merge with IVC *(C)*. *S,* spine; *SJ,* splenoportal junction; *M,* SMA; *P,* pancreas. **B,** Oblique real-time scan and schematic representation displaying left renal vein running in front of aorta to enter vena cava *(C)*. In front of vena cava, in close contact with liver *(L)*, is splenoportal junction. *V,* vertebral body. **C,** Another image, on transverse scan, of left renal vein *(Lrv)*. Portal vein *(arrow)* and superior mesenteric artery *(sma)* are displayed between liver and left renal vein. *a,* aorta. **D,** Right renal vein. This transverse scan, slightly more caudal than previous ones, passes through right kidney *(K)*. Right renal vein *(RRV)* is displayed from renal hilus to its junction with vena cava.

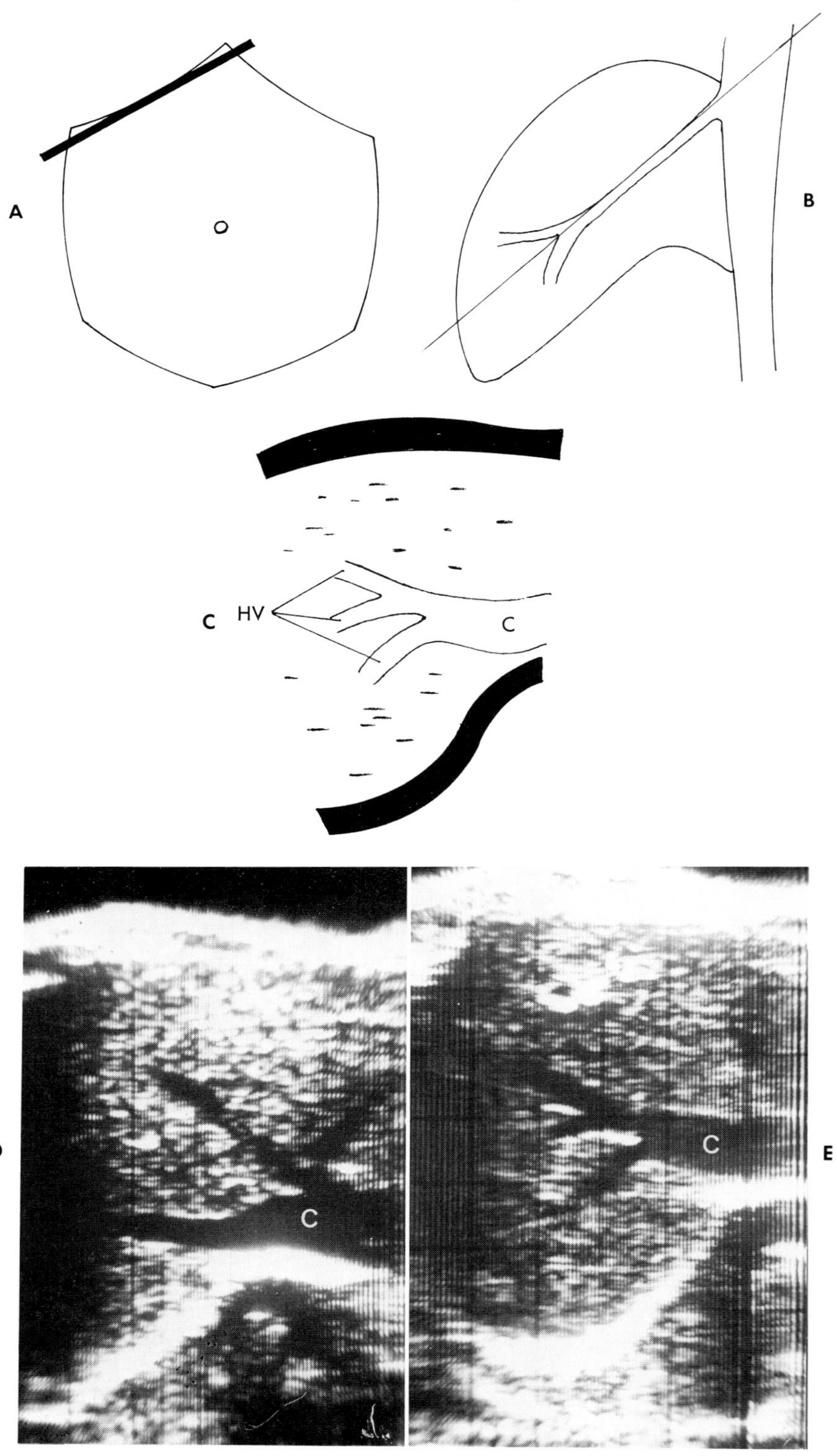

Fig. 4-15. For legend see opposite page.

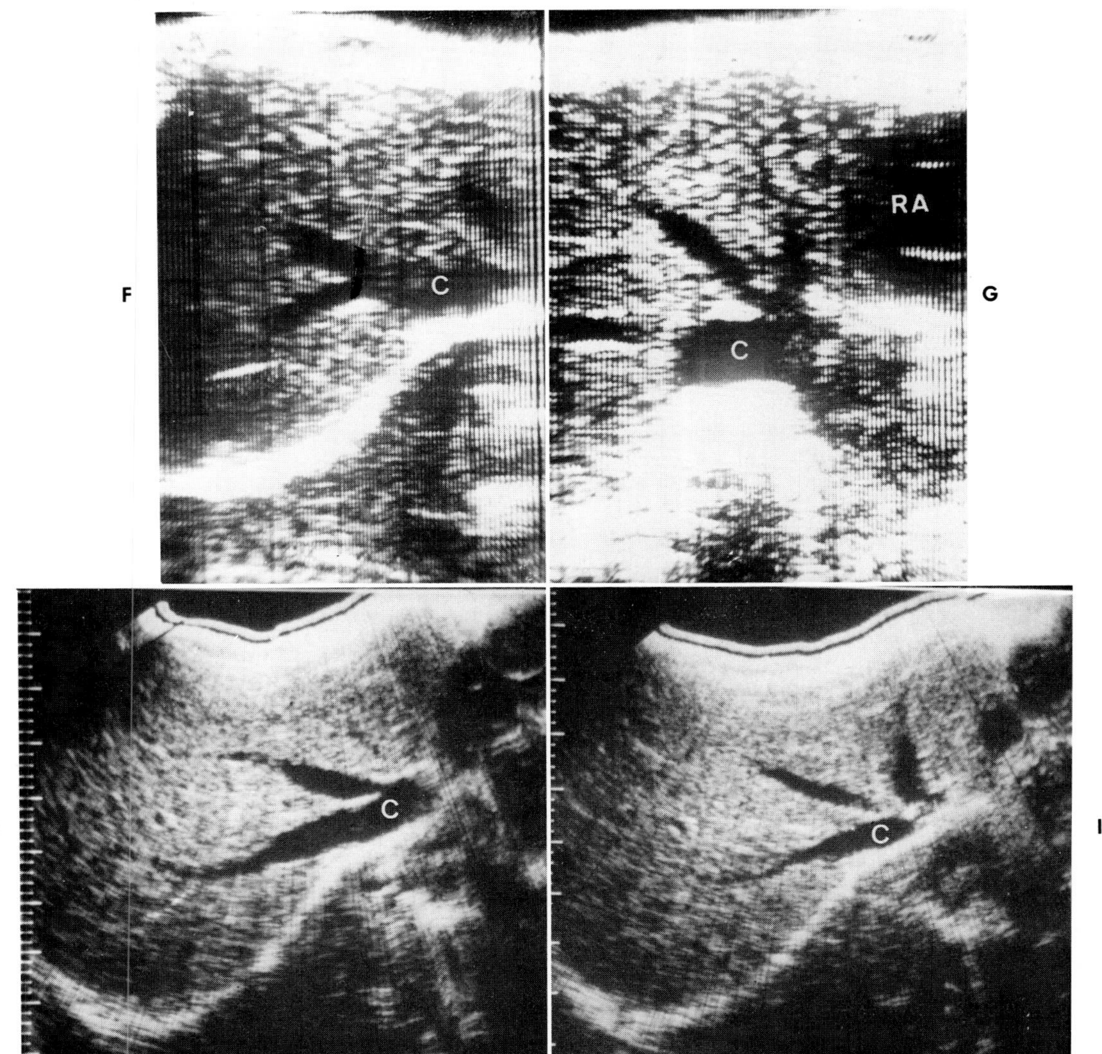

Fig. 4-15. Hepatic veins displayed through oblique recurrent subcostal scans. **A,** Orientation of RTH under costal edge. **B,** Scanning plane through hepatic veins. **C,** Schematic representation of hepatic vein network and its junction with vena cava *(C)*. *HV,* hepatic vein. **D** to **G,** Real-time examples of hepatic venous branching and junction with vena cava. In **G,** recurrent scan is so oblique that it shows heart *(RA)*. **H** and **I,** Contact scans. Note that wall image of hepatic vein is not always well displayed. *Continued.*

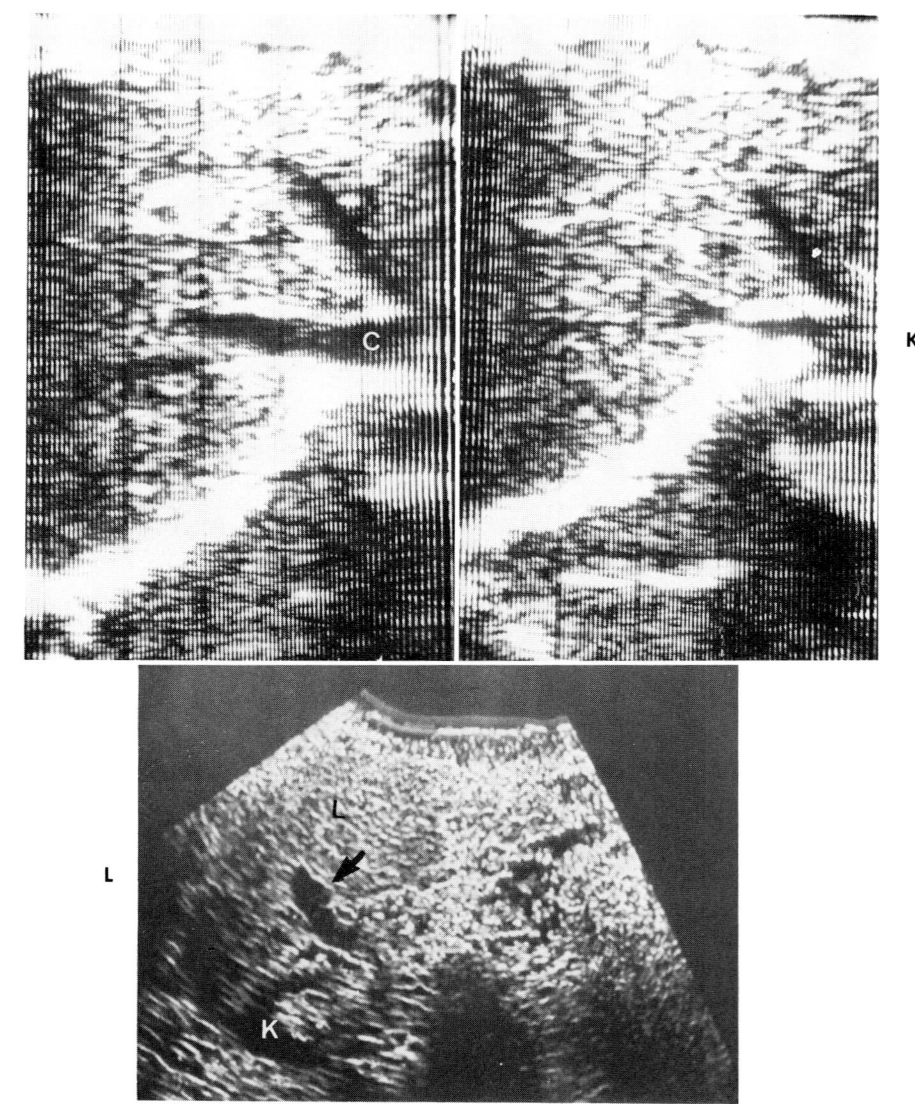

Fig. 4-15, cont'd. J and **K,** Changes in diameter of hepatic vein during respiration. **J,** Inspiration, and **K,** expiration. **L,** Abnormally low hepatic vein *(arrow)* merging with IVC at same level as right renal vein. *K,* kidney; *L,* liver.

The fanlike configuration of the hepatic veins, as it appears in Fig. 4-15, explains why the veins are so much more difficult to display as a whole in sagittal scans. It is only possible to show the median vein in axial sections of the vena cava, and even that branch is not visible unless the cut is in precisely the right plane (Fig. 4-16, *A* to *E*). As in all vascular ultrasonic examinations, the image of the hepatic veins in sagittal section is more readily shown in real time, but the anastomosis of the hepatic vein and the IVC is often masked by the xiphoid process because of the parallelism of the ultrasonic beam. Contact sector scanning with the

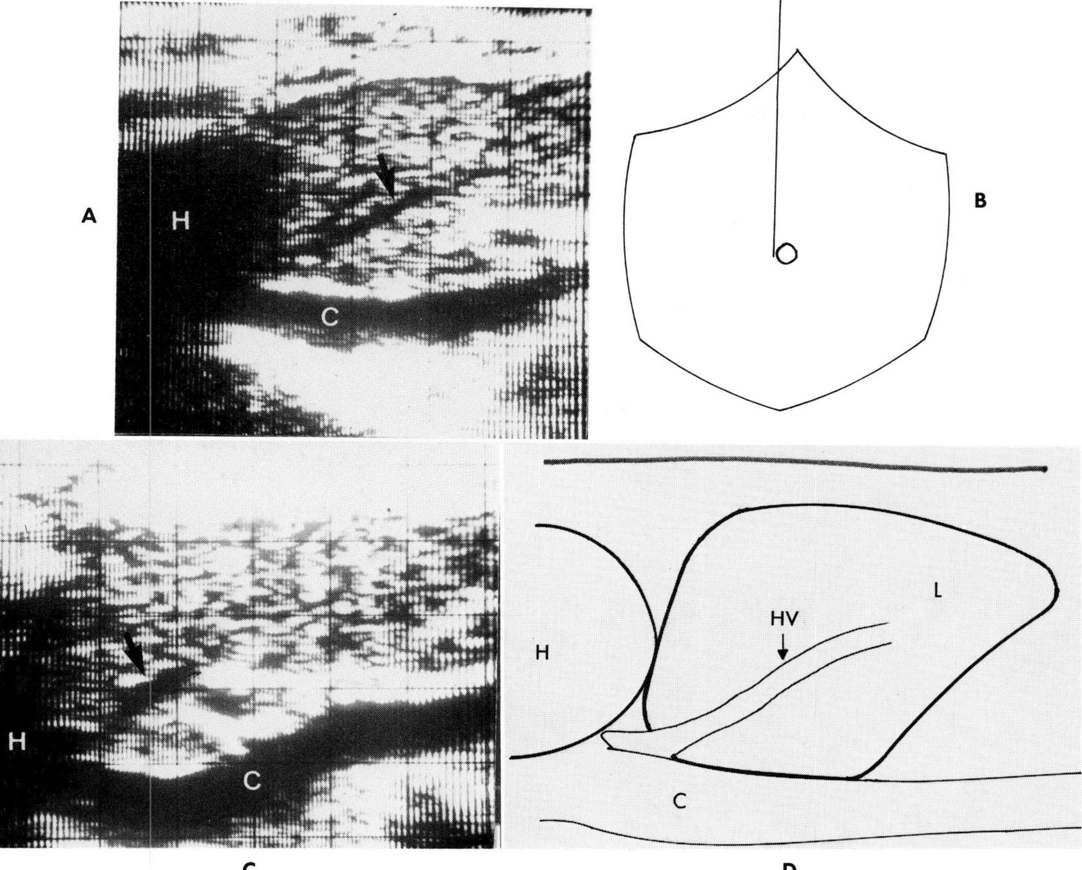

Fig. 4-16. **A** and **C,** Sagittal sections of hepatic veins. **B,** Scanning plane. **D,** Schematic representation. *H,* heart; *C,* vena cava; *L,* liver; *HV,* hepatic veins.

Continued.

transducer in the subxiphoid region is thus better able to show this zone of anastomosis. (See Fig. 4-16, *F* and *G.*)

PORTAL SYSTEM

The different structures of the portal system are regularly displayed by an ultrasonic investigation of the upper abdomen. Sagittal sections of the aorta always show the superior mesenteric vein (SMV). (See Figs. 4-2, *A,* and 4-17.) This vessel is usually found anterior to the right side of the aorta (Fig. 4-17). Study of the venous phase of a mesenteric angiogram shows that the relation of the SMV to the aorta is variable and the SMV is sometimes frankly to the right of the aorta or even somewhat to the left. The same variability is evident in ultrasonic studies. The SMV is best displayed in real-time sagittal scans of the epigastric region. The vein is identified as a tubular structure, and its differentiation from the mesenteric artery is straightforward, since it is completely independent of the aorta. Whereas

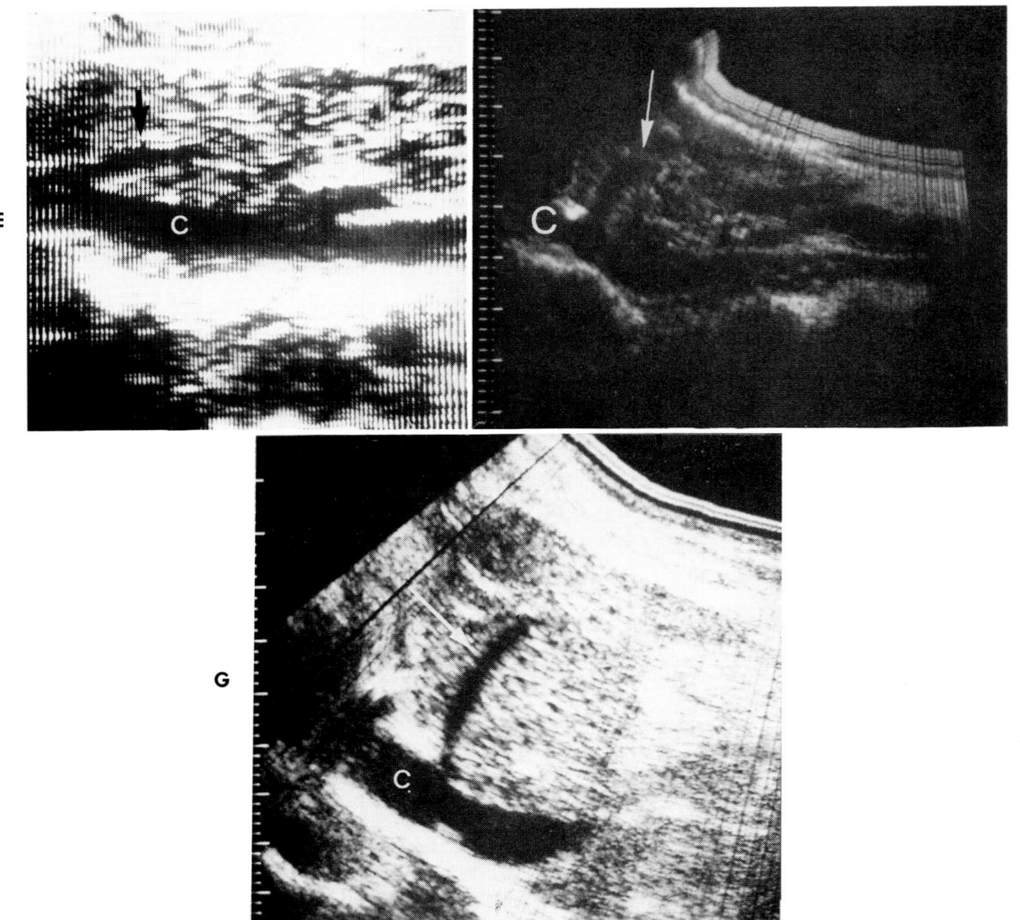

Fig. 4-16, cont'd. E to **G,** Examples of sagittal sections of hepatic veins *(arrows).* All scans were made during deep suspended inspiration.

the SMA joins the aorta, the SMV continues into the portal vein (Fig. 4-18), which prolongs the mesenteric venous axis anteriorly to the level of the vena cava.

In transverse scans the section of the SMV appears to the side of the homologous image of the SMA. These two structures resemble a pair of glasses. (See Fig. 4-19.) They lie just under the neck of the pancreas, for which they constitute an essential echoanatomical landmark (Chapter 19).

The *portal vein* appears on sagittal scans of the vena cava, which it crosses at a variable angle (Fig. 4-20) (Burcharth and Rasmussen, 1974; Leopold, 1975; Weill and co-workers, 1973a; Weill and co-workers, 1973b). If the orientation of the portal vein is close to the vertical, its infrahilar segment appears along several centimeters in a true sagittal scan (Fig. 4-20, *A*). If the portal vein is closer to the horizontal, a sagittal scan of the IVC shows it as a more or less round image (Fig. 4-20, *B*). A good way to approach the hilar segment of the vessel is by intercostal scans (Fig. 4-20, *C*). The branching of the vessel can then be followed over

Text continued on p. 65.

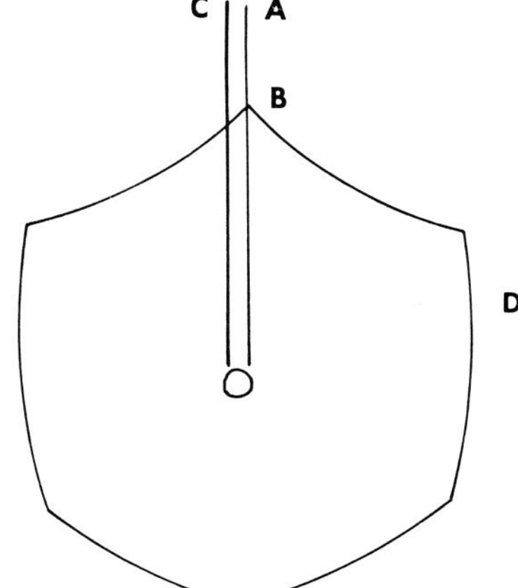

Fig. 4-17. Mesenteric vein displayed on real-time sagittal scans. **A,** Mesenteric vein (*MV* and *arrow*) is displayed between liver *(L)* and aorta *(A)*. Since vessel is slightly oblique, only short segment of it is displayed on this sagittal scan. **B,** Longer segment of more sagittal venous axis is displayed on this section, belonging to another patient. Vein again lies in front of aorta. **C,** Mesenteric vein appears in front of vena cava *(C)* in this patient. **D,** Scanning planes of three sections.

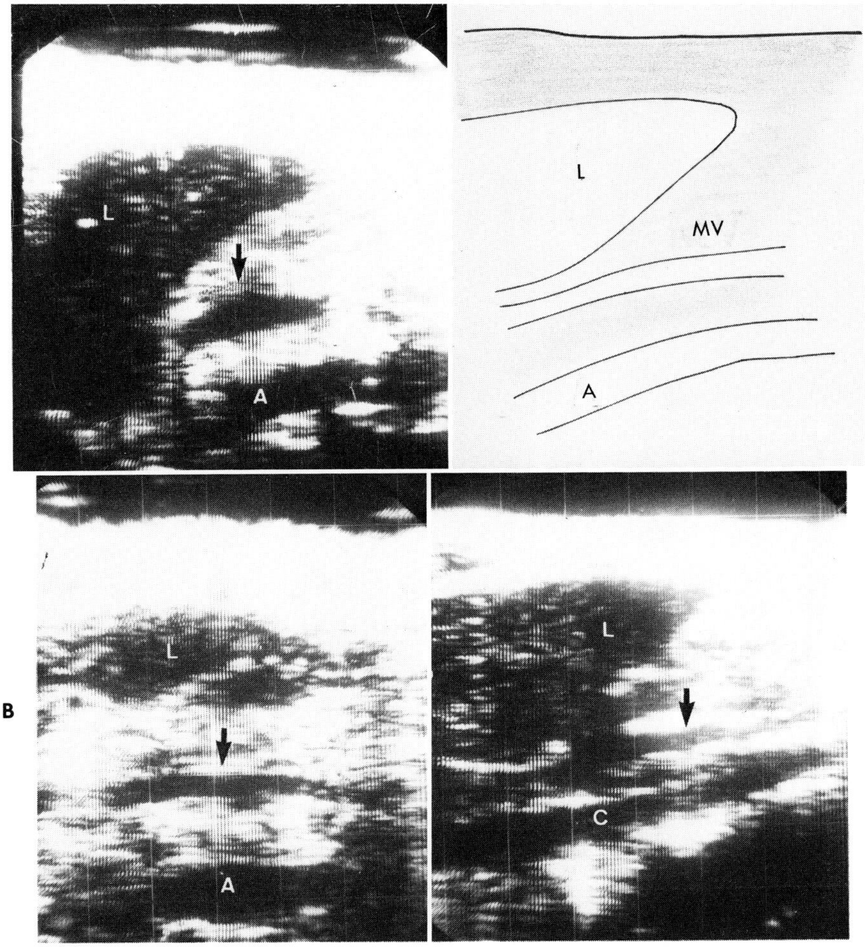

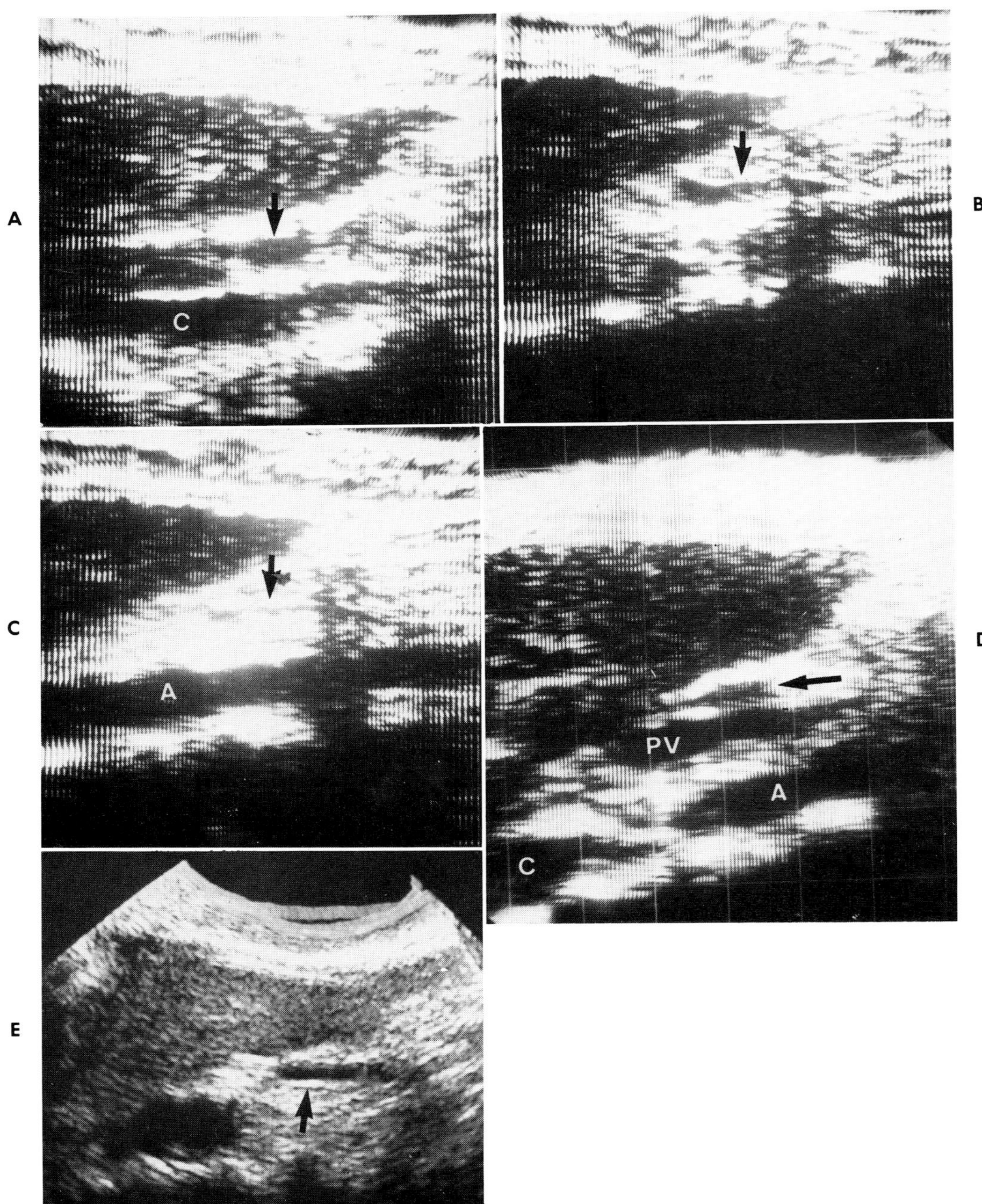

Fig. 4-18. Mesenteric vein and mesenteric-portal junction on sagittal scans. **A,** This scan displays junction *(arrow)* in front of vena cava *(C)*. **B,** Second scan was made 1 cm to left. It passes between vena cava and aorta and shows mesenteric vein alone *(arrow)*. **C,** Another parallel scan made 1 cm farther left. It passes through aorta *(A)*. Narrow tubular element running parallel to aorta *(arrow)* belongs to mesenteric artery. **D,** Direction of scan is now oblique. Therefore sections of aorta and vena cava are oval. Mesenteric-portal junction and portal vein *(PV)* appear in sagittal section. Immediately in front of portal vein, another tubular element is displayed *(arrow)*. This is common hepatic duct. **E,** Previous images were in real time. This is contact sagittal scan of mesenteric vein, along same plane of section as that in **D.**

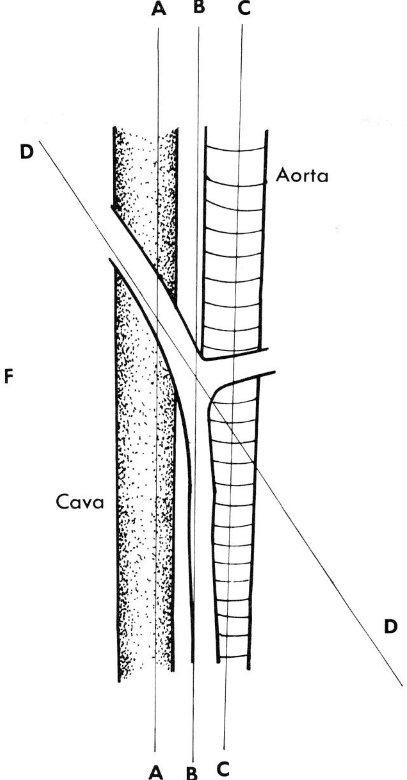

Fig. 4-18, cont'd. F, Scanning planes in **A** to **D.**

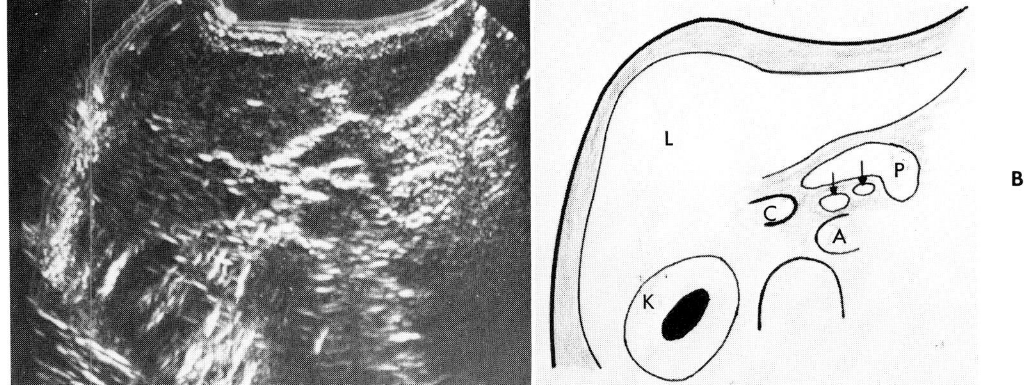

Fig. 4-19. Mesenteric vessels in transverse sections. **A,** Contact scan of upper abdomen outlining twin sections of mesenteric artery and vein between great vessels and pancreas. **B,** Schematic representation. *Arrows,* mesenteric artery and vein; *C,* vena cava; *A,* aorta; *P,* pancreas; *L,* liver; *K,* kidney.

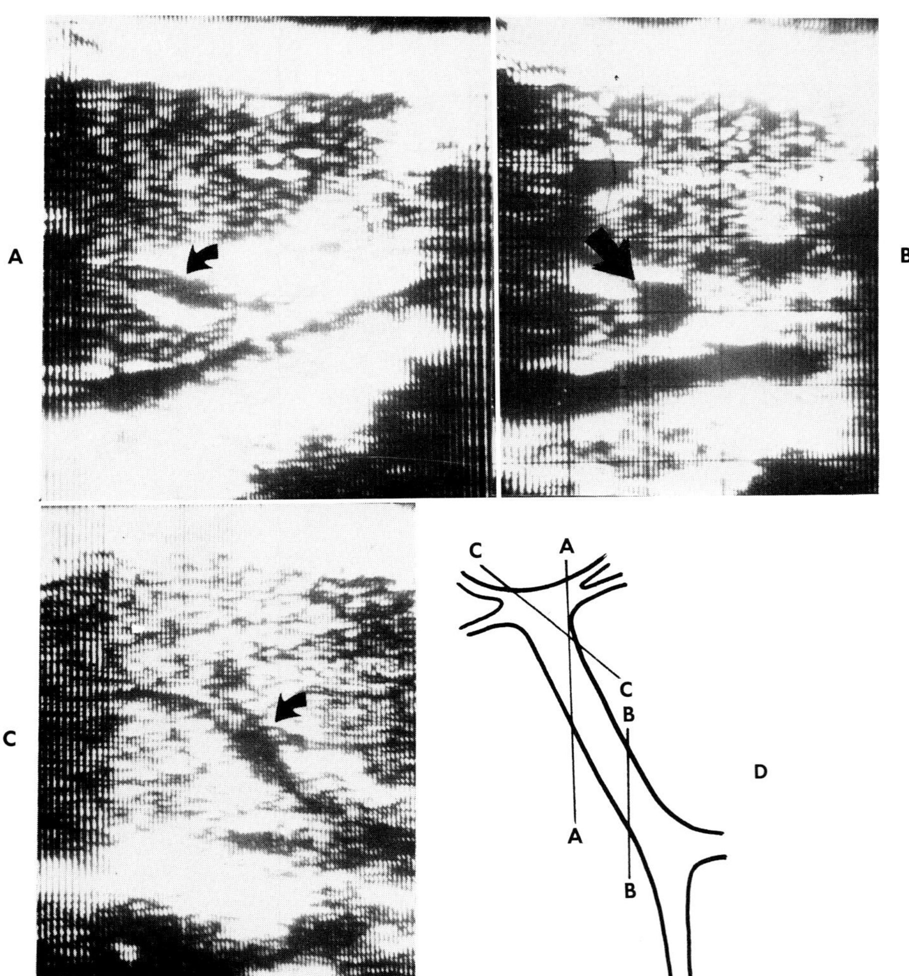

Fig. 4-20. Different types of real-time sections of portal vein *(arrows)*. **A,** Sagittal scan passing through vena cava displays upper segment of portal trunk in sagittal scan. If such a long segment of portal vein appears on sagittal scan, direction of portal vein is almost vertical. **B,** Another sagittal scan of upper abdomen passing through vena cava displays portal vein as rounded element. This means that portal vein direction is almost horizontal. **C,** Intercostal scan displaying terminal segment of portal vein and its branching. **D,** Different scanning planes.

several centimeters. However, the easiest approach to the portal vein is by oblique scans of the right upper quadrant. If the orientation of the real-time ultrasonic head is adapted to the orientation of the vessel, the latter appears in its entirety, along its sagittal axis, from its origin at the splenic mesenteric-portal junction up to the hilus. (See Figs. 4-21 and 4-22.) Often, on scans made in the plane of the portal vein the common hepatic duct can be seen along the anterior aspect (Figs. 4-21, *A,* and 4-22, *B*) of the vein. The anteroposterior diameter of the portal vein varies from approximately 8 to about 15 mm. Since the axis of the portal vein is oblique in relation to that of the aorta and the vena cava, a sagittal scan of the portal vein displays the two large vessels in an oblique section, and they appear oval in shape (Fig. 4-21). Although the portal vein does not change in diameter with respiration, its position, of course, does change with the respiratory cycle (Fig. 4-23).*

Transverse scans of the upper abdomen also show the *splenic vein* and the splenoportal anastomosis (Figs. 4-10, *E,* and 4-24 to 4-27) (Leopold, 1975; Weill and associates, 1973b; Weill and associates, 1975b). The splenic vein, which curls around in front of the great vessels, can be relatively straight, in which case it appears on a section as a tubular structure several centimeters in length (Figs. 4-25, *B,* to 4-27). However, it may be tortuous, so that one transverse scan shows only a short segment (Figs. 4-25, *A,* and 4-27, *B*) and one must sweep the real-time

*The portal division presents a constant hilar pattern on oblique recurrent subcostal liver scans. It will be studied in Chapters 6, 15, and 26. (See Figs. 6-9, 15-25, *C,* and 26-19, *A.*)

Text continued on p. 72.

A

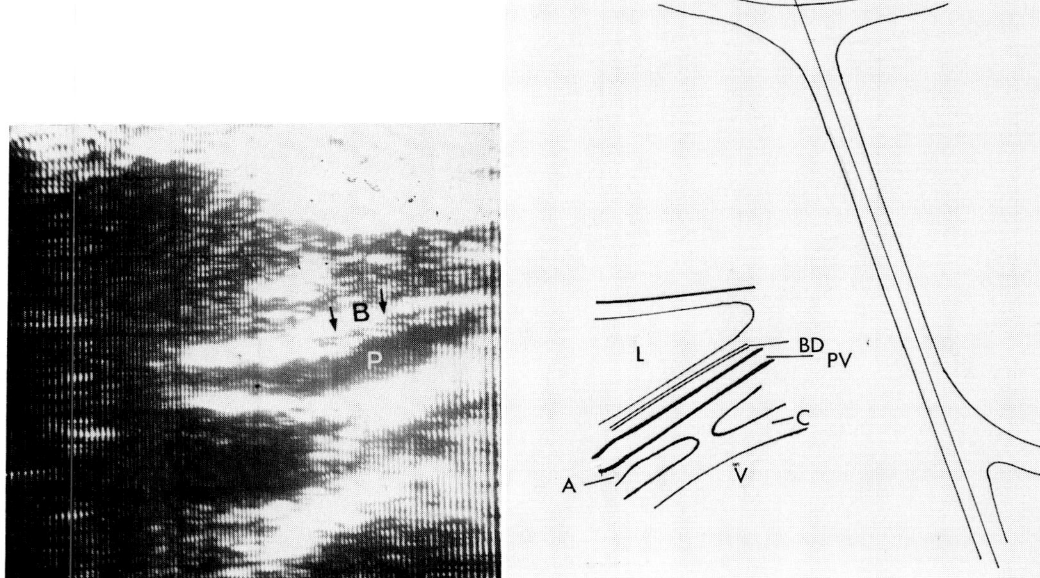

Fig. 4-21. A, Narrow tubular element *(arrows)* displayed in front of portal vein *(P)* belongs to common hepatic duct *(B).* Center, schematic drawing. Right, scanning plane. *A,* aorta; *C,* vena cava; *L,* liver; *BD,* common hepatic duct; *PV,* portal vein; *V,* vertebral body.

Continued.

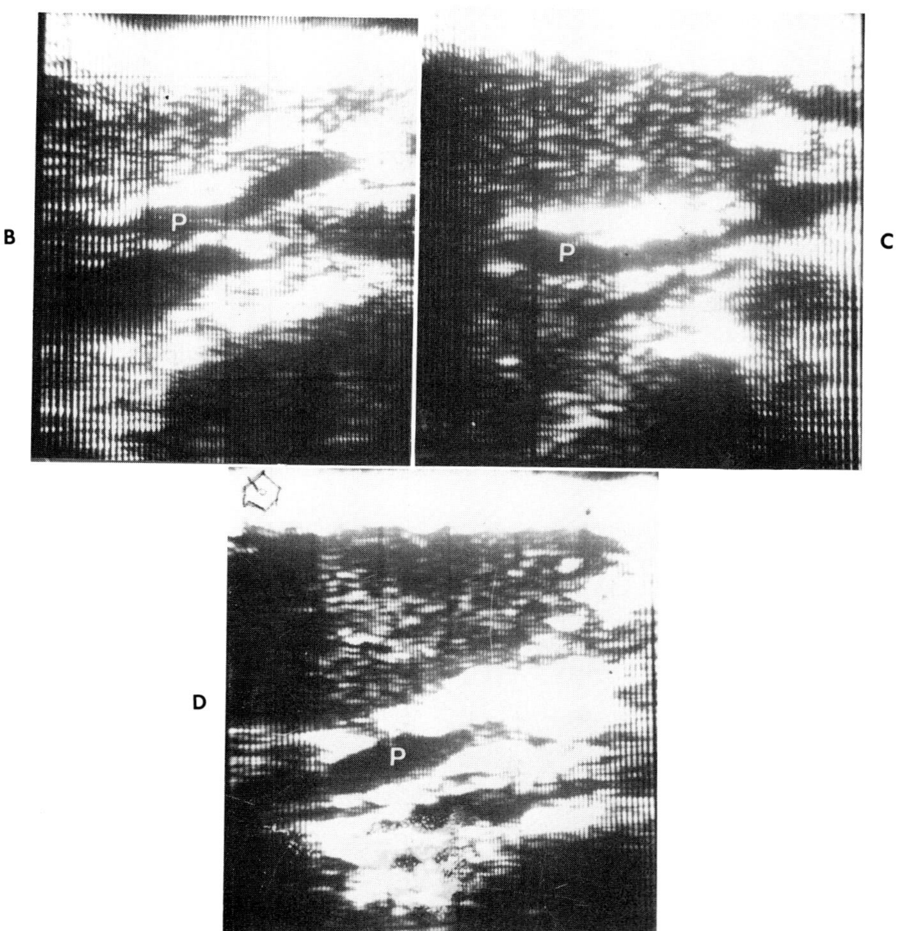

Fig. 4-21, cont'd. B to **D,** More examples of sagittal sections of portal vein shown on real-time oblique scans of right upper quadrant. Since portal vein is cut sagittally, section images of vena cava and aorta are oval. In **C,** note left renal vein behind portal vein.

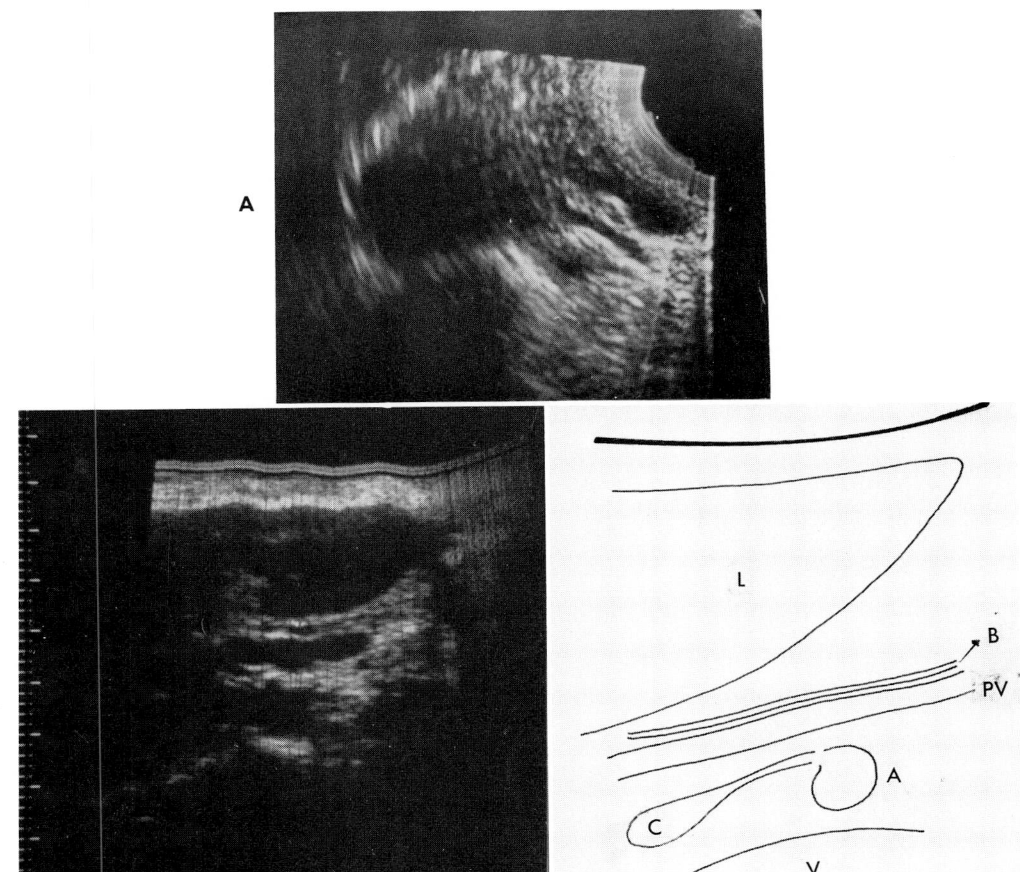

Fig. 4-22. Portal vein. **A,** Sagittal contact gray scale scan of right upper quadrant showing upper segment of portal vein. **B,** Oblique scan of right upper quadrant showing portal vein *(PV)* in sagittal section. Between liver *(L)* and portal vein, main bile duct *(B)* (common hepatic duct plus short segment of common bile duct) is outlined. *A,* aorta; *C,* vena cava; *V,* vertebral body.

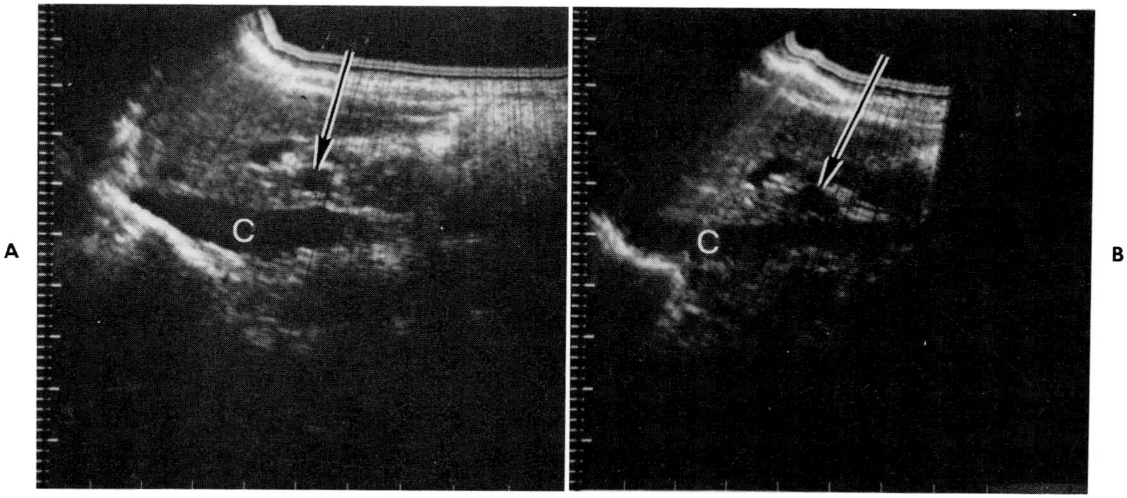

Fig. 4-23. Positional respiratory changes of portal vein. **A,** Sagittal portal vein *(arrow)* displayed from its origin up to hilus, between liver and large vena cava *(C)*. This scan was performed during deep suspended inspiration. **B,** Second scan made after partial expiration. Vena cava is now narrower. Portal vein *(arrow)* has moved, and its shape is somewhat different.

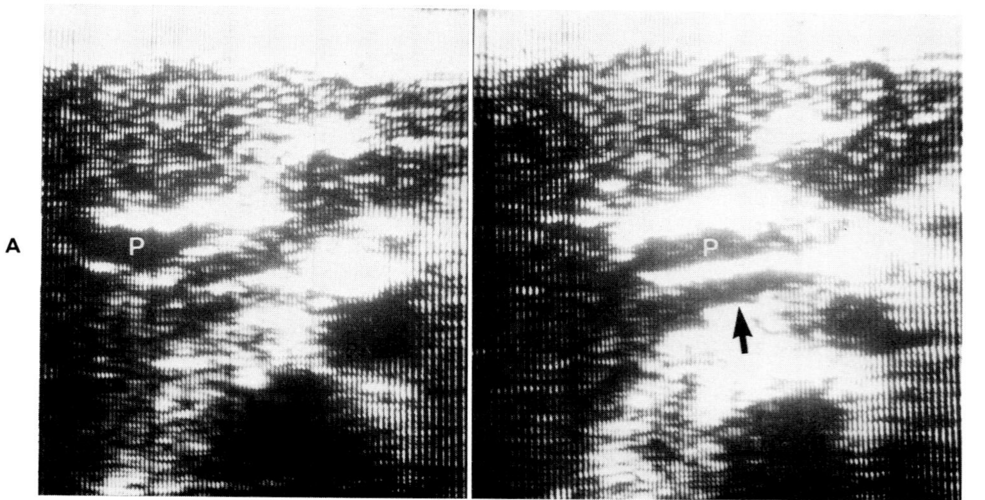

Fig. 4-24. For legend see opposite page.

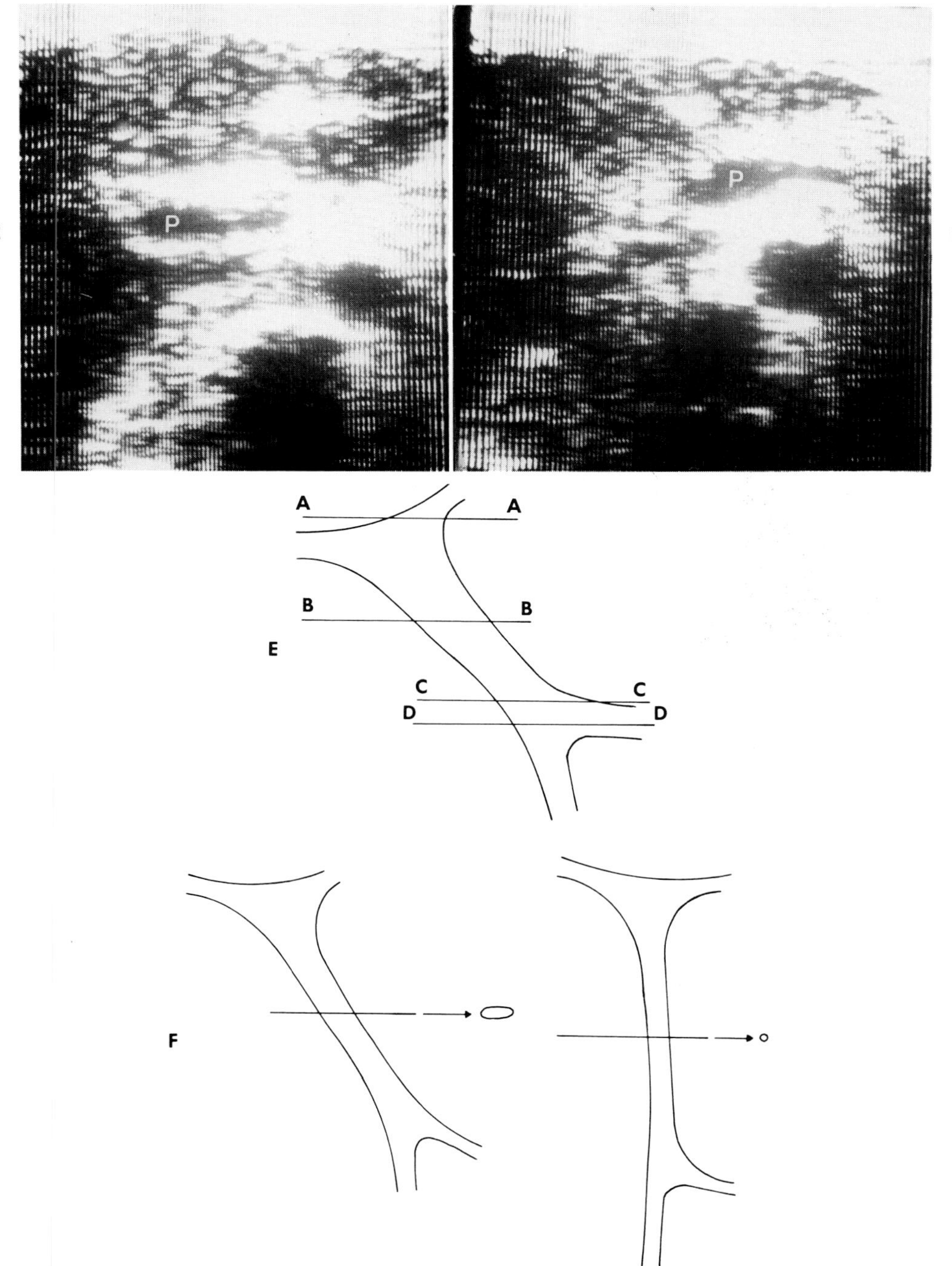

Fig. 4-24. Parallel transverse scans of portal vein *(P)* in real time. **A,** Transverse scan of hilar segment of portal system. **B,** More caudal scan through splenoportal junction at level of left renal vein *(arrow).* **C** and **D,** Parallel, more caudal scans displaying splenoportal junction and splenic vein. **E,** Different scanning planes. **F,** Different patterns of portal vein section according to direction of vessel. If portal vein is horizontal, transverse section displays tubular or oval section. If portal vein is more sagittal, transverse scan displays rounded section. Such a section will be found in Figs. 4-11, *B,* and 4-27, *A*.

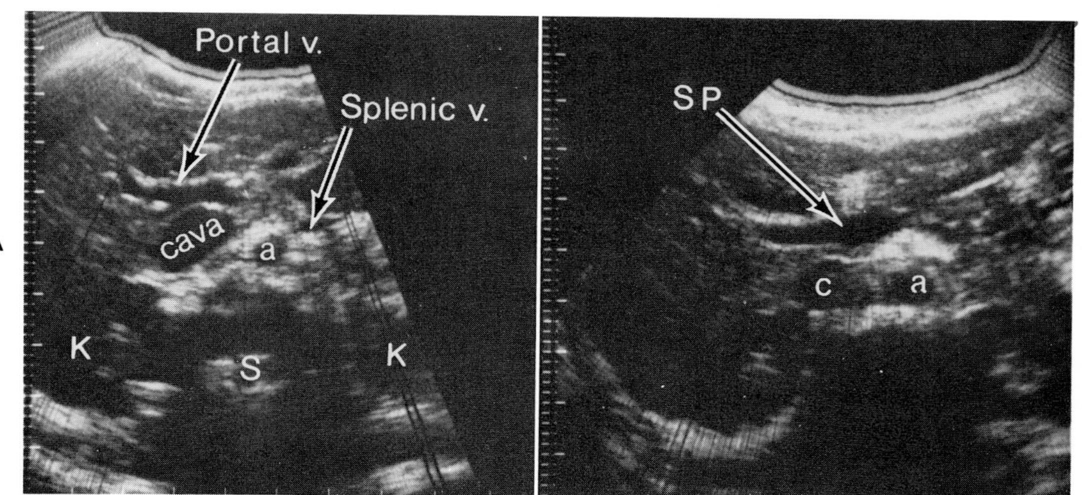

Fig. 4-25. Portal and splenic veins. **A,** Transverse section of upper abdomen showing liver and portal vein. Part of splenic vein is displayed on left in front of aorta *(a)*. Small segment of right renal artery is seen between cava and spine. *K*, kidney; *S*, spine. **B,** Parallel, more caudal scan passes through splenoportal junction *(SP)*. Splenic vein runs in front of aorta and mesenteric artery to its portal junction. *C*, vena cava.

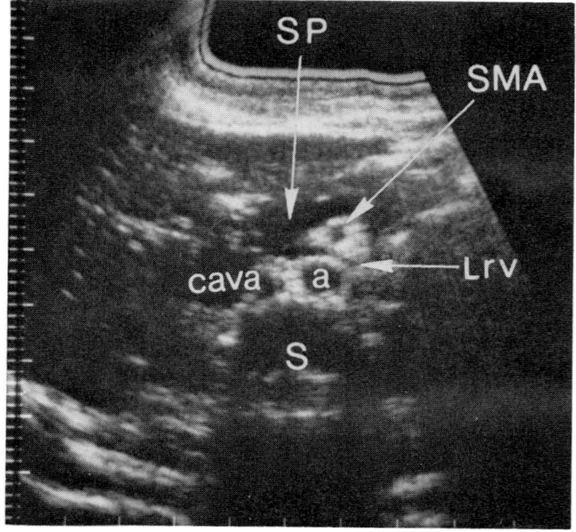

Fig. 4-26. Different vascular elements on transverse scan of upper abdomen: in front of vertebral body *(S)*, transverse sections of aorta *(a)* and vena cava are displayed. Between aorta and superior mesenteric artery *(SMA)*, left renal vein *(Lrv)* is shown. Splenoportal *(SP)* junction lies below liver. (Same plane as that in Fig. 4-9, *A*.)

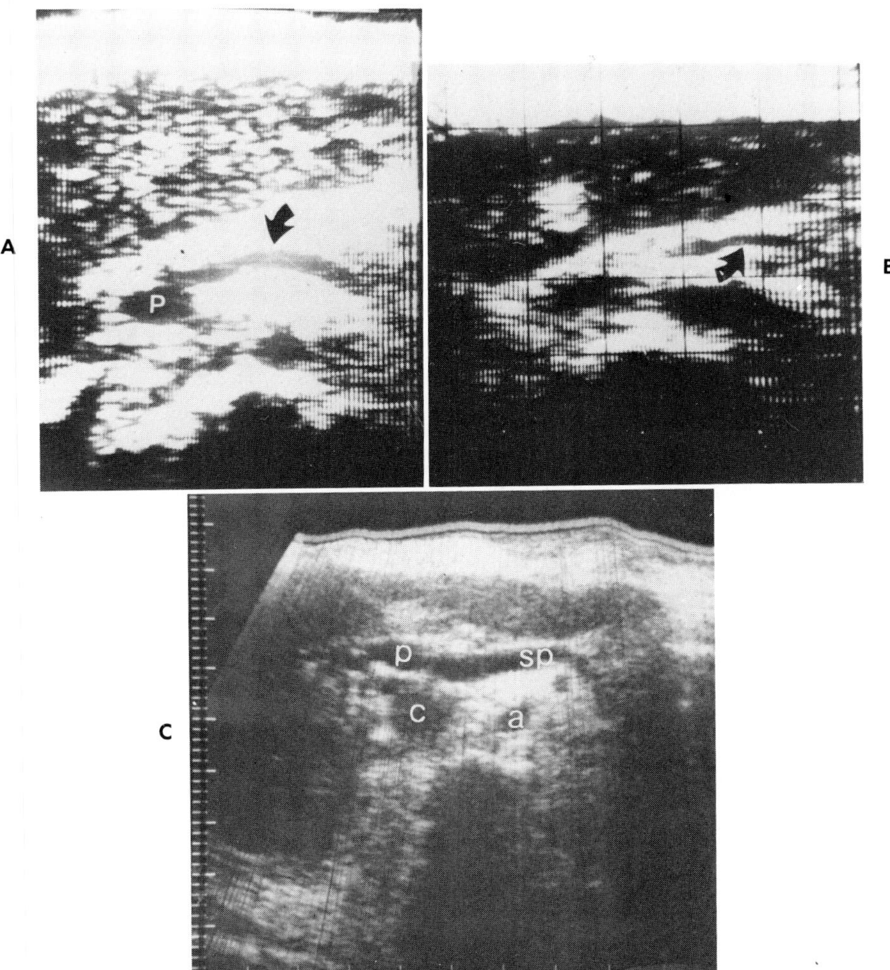

Fig. 4-27. Splenic veins in sagittal section, by transverse scans of upper abdomen. **A,** Exceptional pattern of splenic vein *(arrow)*. Vessel is linear and therefore appears entirely on same section, from splenic hilum up to portal junction *(p)*. **B,** Common pattern of splenic vein. Since vessel is sinuous, only short venous segment *(arrow)* is displayed on one transverse section. **C,** Gray scale example of exceptional pattern as in **A.** *sp,* splenic vein; *c,* vena cava; *a,* aorta.

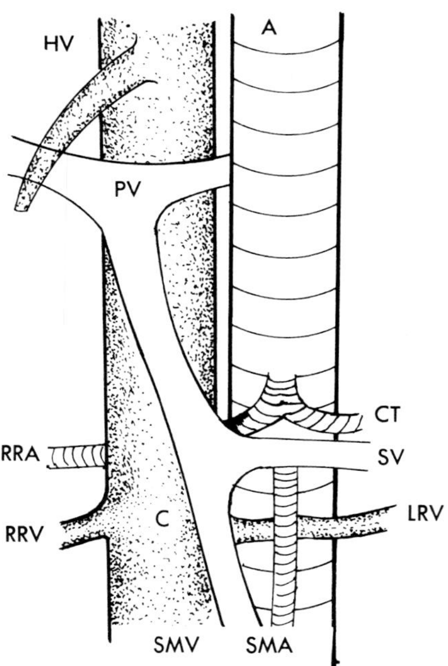

Fig. 4-28. Schematic representation of different vessels that transverse, sagittal, or oblique scans of upper abdomen can display. *A,* aorta; *C,* vena cava; *CT,* celiac trunk; *SMA,* superior mesenteric artery; *RRA,* right renal artery; *LRV,* left renal vein; *RRV,* right renal vein; *HV,* hepatic vein; *PV,* portal vein; *SV,* splenic vein; *SMV,* superior mesenteric vein.

scanner over the epigastric region, from above to below and below to above, to visualize the entire course of the vessel.

In Fig. 4-28 the different vessels that can be demonstrated by ultrasonography are summarized. For those who recall the proximity of the mesenteric vessels and splenic vein to the pancreas, as well as the close relation of the portal axis to the biliary tree, and of the aorta, the vena cava, and their branches to other elements of the retroperitoneal region, the interest of this echoangioanatomical study is immediately apparent. It is possible to obtain the images of these elements by single-sweep scanning with gray scale (Leopold, 1975), but only the rapid repetition rate of real-time scans permits the analysis of vascular anastomosis and branching. This is why many of my illustrations are real-time images, even though their quality is sometimes less pleasing to the eye than that of contact scans. Why struggle for several minutes to see what appears in a few seconds and with greater precision on an echoscopic screen? You now know that I am not only a glutton (Fig. 1-1) and a sadomasochist (Fig. 1-4) but also rather lazy.

REFERENCES

Burcharth, F., and Rasmussen, S. N.: Localization of the porta hepatis by ultrasonic scanning prior to percutaneous transhepatic portography, Br. J. Radiol. **47:**598-600, 1974.

Goldberg, B. B., Ostrum, B. J., and Isard, H.: Ultrasonic aortography, J.A.M.A. **124:**119-124, 1966.

Leopold, G. R.: Gray scale ultrasonic angiography of the upper abdomen, Radiology **117:**665-671, 1975.

Meire, H. B.: Upper abdominal vascular anatomy demonstrated by gray scale ultrasound, World Federation of Ultrasound in Medicine and Biology, San Francisco, 1976, Abstract No. 519.

Rettenmaier, G.: Ultrasonic angiography, Deutsche Arbeitsgemeinschaft für ultraschall Diagnostik (D.A.U.D.), Hannover, Germany, May 16-18, 1974.

Saunders, R. C.: Correlation of the ultrasonic appearance of the portal vein with abdominal arteriography, J. Clin. Ultrasound **3:**263-266, 1975.

Weill, F., Aucant, D., Bourgoin, A., Eisenscher, A., and Gallinet, D.: Ultrasonic visualization of abdominal veins: vena mesenterica, vena splenica, vena portae, hepatic veins, vena cava, Second European Congress, Munich, Germany, 1975a, Abstract No. 103.

Weill, F., Becker, J. C., Kraehenbuhl, J. R., Heriot, G., and Walter, J. P.: Clinical atlas of ultrasonic radiography, Paris, 1973a, Masson & Cie., Editeurs.

Weill, F., and Eisenscher, A.: Echo-angiostructure hépatique: étude écho-anatomique des structures canalaires intraparenchymateuses, J. Radiol. Electrol. Med. Nucl. **57:**311-319, 1976.

Weill, F., Eisenscher, A., Aucant, D., Bourgoin, A., and Gallinet, D.: Ultrasonic study of venous patterns in the right hypochondrium, J. Clin. Ultrasound **3:**23-28, 1975b.

Weill, F., Kraehenbuhl, J. R., Aucant, D., and Maurat, J. P.: Etude échotomographique des gros troncs veineux abdominaux, Coeur Méd. Interne **12:**431-439, 1973b.

Winsberg, F.: Personal communication, 1977.

PART II

THE LIVER

CHAPTER 5

TECHNIQUES OF EXAMINATION

In the normal subject the liver is in large part covered by the ribs, so that it is only directly accessible in the epigastric region except during deep inspiration or in the upright position. Extension of the liver beyond the limits of the thoracic cage is a pathological sign, which will be discussed later. The first step in the examination is to determine the relationship of the liver to the costal margin during normal breathing with the patient in the supine position. After that first step, it is helpful to ask the patient to hold a deep breath, so that the liver clears the costal margin and becomes more accessible. For the same reason one should always use the left lateral decubitus, or rather a left posterior oblique position, as one of the phases of the examination. A gravitational displacement of the liver is thus added to the respiratory displacement. Finally, it may be necessary to accentuate this gravitational displacement occasionally by examining the patient in the standing position, a maneuver that is difficult with contact scanning but relatively easy with real-time equipment.

I shall describe a rather large number of views for the hepatic examination. Since ultrasonography proceeds by successive slicing, only a large number of sections realized with different views assures one that the entire hepatic volume has been explored. The smaller the number of sections carried out and the fewer angles used, the greater the risk that a lesion has been overlooked.

CHOICE OF TECHNIQUE: REAL-TIME OR CONTACT SCANNING

The considerations discussed in the first chapter concerning the combination of real-time and contact scanning techniques can be applied to the hepatic examination. A large number of sections are mandatory: the rapid, extensive, and repeated sweeping movement of the RTH over the hepatic region satisfies that requirement. It is necessary to produce these sections with diverse positions: the flexibility of the RTH also meets this requirement. Assessment of the general morphology of the organ is better done by contact scanning, since that method is able to display the general contours of the liver, including the left hepatic lobe, which can be visualized with contact scanning even if partly hidden behind the ribs. The small contact scanning transducer is better able to show the image of the diaphragmatic dome in sagittal section than the larger RTH. An analysis of the hepatic tissue texture is also necessary: here both methods are useful, but the rich tubular pattern of the liver is well studied with the flexibility of real time. On the other hand, the outstanding resolution of last-generation contact scanners is at present irreplaceable both for displaying the intrahepatic vessels and for tissue analysis.

Finally, if one has identified a lesion successively by two different methods, one's confidence in the diagnosis is increased. These multiple arguments point to the need for both methods in a complete examination of the liver.

We begin the examination with real time and then proceed with contact scanning. The successive steps of this procedure will be described in the following paragraphs. As a matter of fact, an isolated description of the hepatic examination is somewhat artificial: any ultrasonic examination in this area is in practice an exploration of the entire upper abdomen. The images of the vascular system, the biliary tree, the liver, the pancreas, and the spleen are all produced at the same time. These are different elements of a whole and are, of course, simultaneously displayed on a single section. The global character of the ultrasonic examination will again be considered as other viscera are discussed. Another problem must be considered when dealing with the technique of ultrasonic examination of the liver: the place of ultrasonography among other radiological procedures. It is not illegal to glance at a plain film of the abdomen or GI series before beginning the ultrasonic scanning.

VIEWS AND POSITIONING

In real-time ultrasonography. The patient is first placed in decubitus. With the RTH machine the anterior aspect of the abdomen is explored by successive sagittal and horizontal scans (Figs. 5-1 and 5-2), during normal respiration and then in deep suspended inspiration. The patient is then placed in a left posterior oblique position for the subcostal oblique recurrent view already described in Chapter 3. The RTH is placed below the right costal edge. During suspended deep inspiration the RTH is rocked in a caudocranial and craniocaudal sectoring movement, which results in an exploration of the entire hepatic volume (Fig. 5-3). Finally, the RTH is placed over the right lateral rib cage, with its orientation in the direction of the intercostal spaces, so as to minimize acoustic shadowing. Deep inspiration is not necessary during intercostal scanning. The RTH is then moved successively down along the last four intercostal spaces (Fig. 5-4). Usually only the last three interspaces permit visualization of the liver. Above that level the lung intervenes. A small liver is often accessible only through intercostal scanning.

In contact scanning. The patient is again supine. Sagittal scans in neutral apnea show the situation of the hepatic margin in relation to the costal edge. Then the patient is asked to hold a deep breath, and successive parallel scans are performed from the right to the left ("sagittal salami scans"). (See Fig. 5-5.) When the transducer reaches the costal margin, it is angled up toward the diaphragm (Fig. 5-5, *A* and *B*). Finally, transverse parallel scans are carried out, from the xiphoid process to the umbilicus, producing "horizontal salami scans" (Fig. 5-6). Sector scans made perpendicular to the right costal edge with the patient in left lateral decubitus may prove useful when the liver is small or in a high position. So also are intercostal scans, as already noted. Intercostal scans may also be made to verify lateral abnormalities discovered in real time. These scans are performed in the lateral decubitus or left posterior oblique position. If the left lobe is large, left subcostal oblique scans can be carried out as well (Fig. 5-7). Liver scans must, of course, be performed with gray scale, but study of the liver size and shape can be carried out with high contrast.

In infants, we use only the real-time technique. Since the patient is small, the limited field is no handicap, and, in addition, there is no risk of blurring due to motion of the child.

Text continued on p. 85.

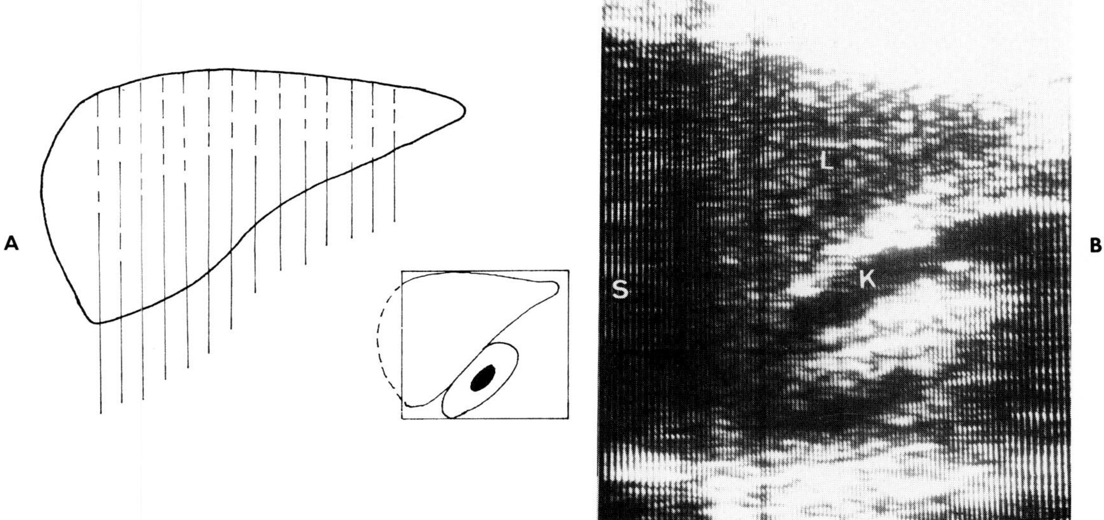

Fig. 5-1. Sagittal real-time scanning. **A,** Successive scans made with sweeping movement of RTH, sagittally positioned, along surface of hepatic region. Even with deep suspended inspiration, ribs hide upper part of liver. **B,** Sagittal scan displaying right kidney *(K)* behind liver *(L)* and acoustic shadow *(S)* of ribs.

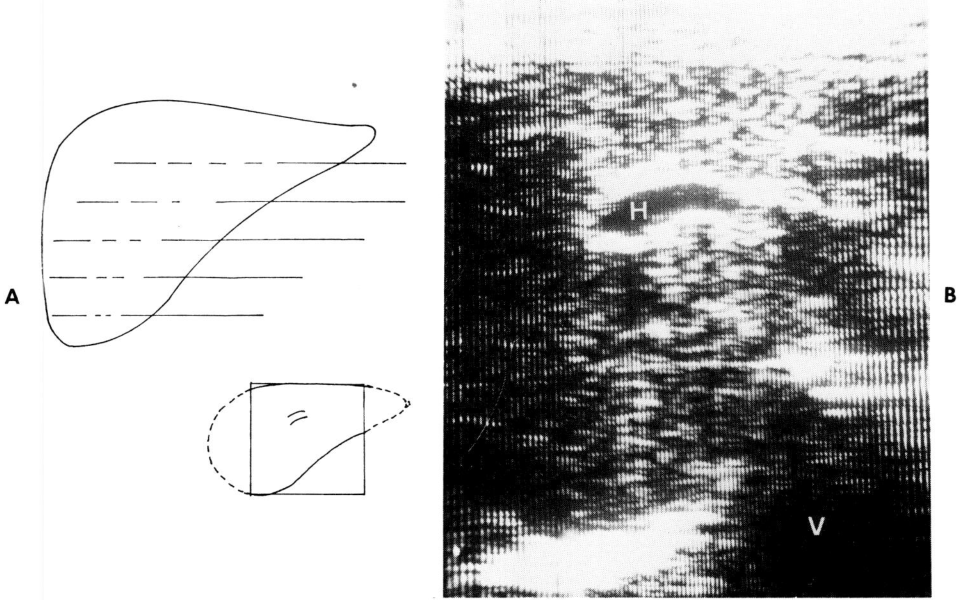

Fig. 5-2. Real-time transverse scanning. **A,** Successive scans made during sweeping movement of RTH, horizontally positioned, along surface of hepatic region. Rib shadows are lateral. **B,** Transverse real-time scan of liver. Tubular structure *(H)* belongs to portal hilar division. *V,* vertebral body.

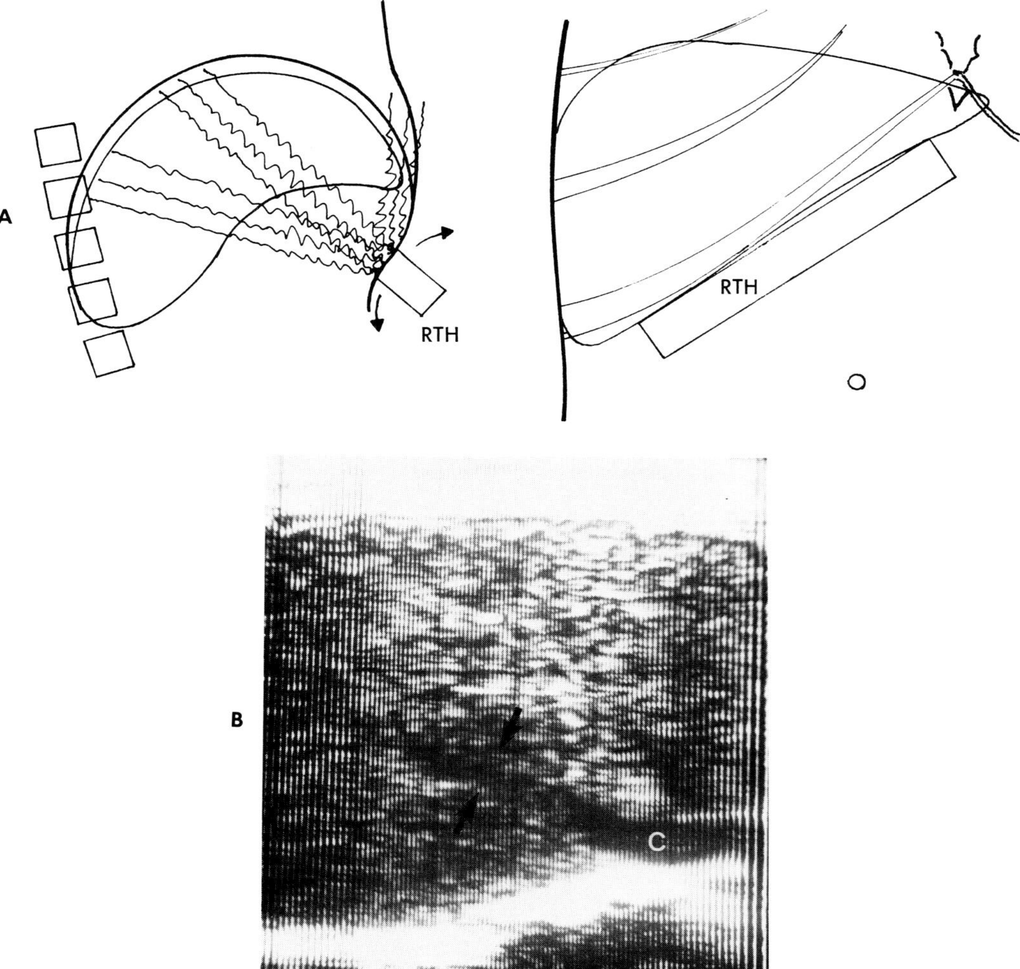

Fig. 5-3. Real-time oblique recurrent subcostal view. **A,** Patient is placed in left lateral decubitus (left oblique posterior) position. RTH is applied on skin immediately below right anterior costal edge. With help of rocking movement of RTH, every part of liver tissue is successively cut. **B,** Real-time oblique recurrent subcostal liver scan passing through vena cava *(C)* and right hepatic vein *(arrows)*.

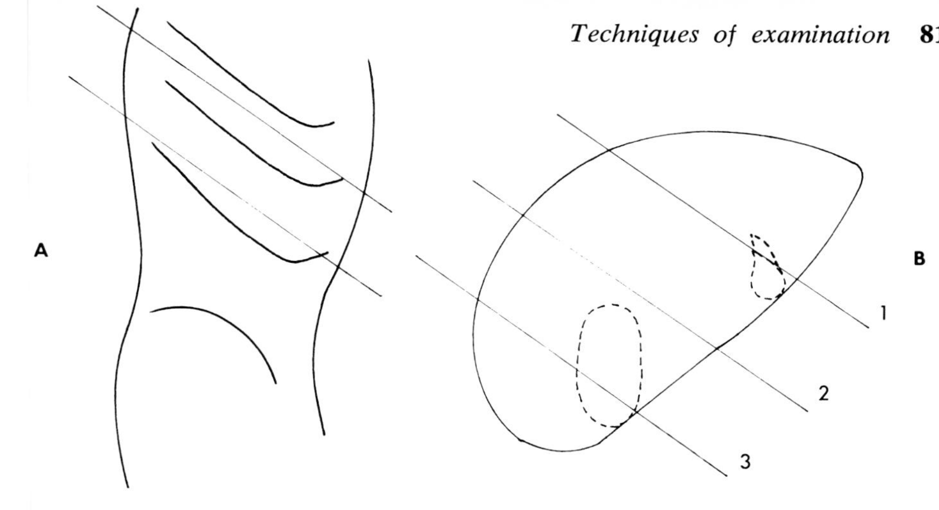

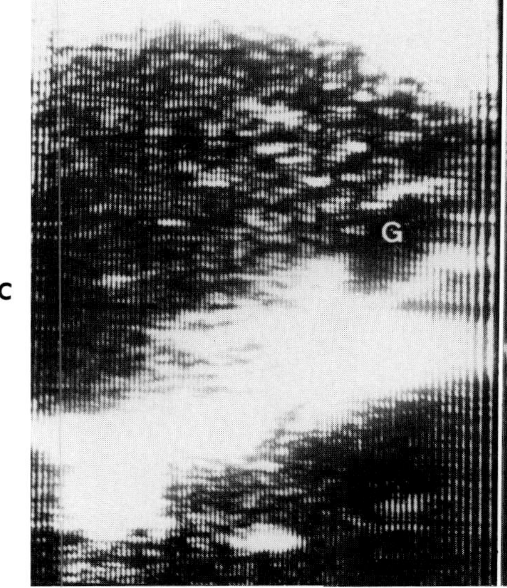

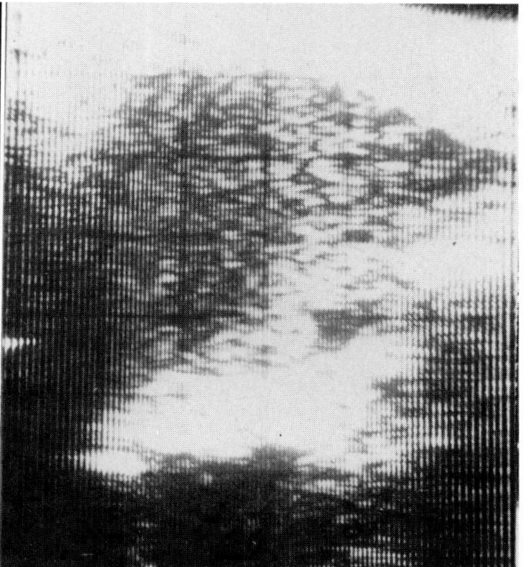

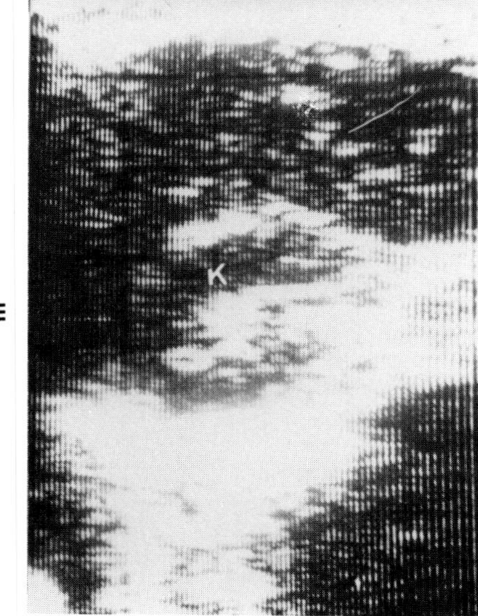

Fig. 5-4. Real-time intercostal scanning. **A,** Patient remains in same left lateral decubitus position. Orientation of RTH is adapted to direction of intercostal spaces. **B,** Successive scans, from above to below, cut liver and gallbladder *(1),* liver *(2),* and liver and right kidney *(3).* **C,** Intercostal section of liver and gallbladder *(G)* (plane *1* of **B**). **D,** Hepatic intercostal section (plane *2* of **B**). **E,** Intercostal section of liver and right kidney *(K)* (plane *3* of **B**).

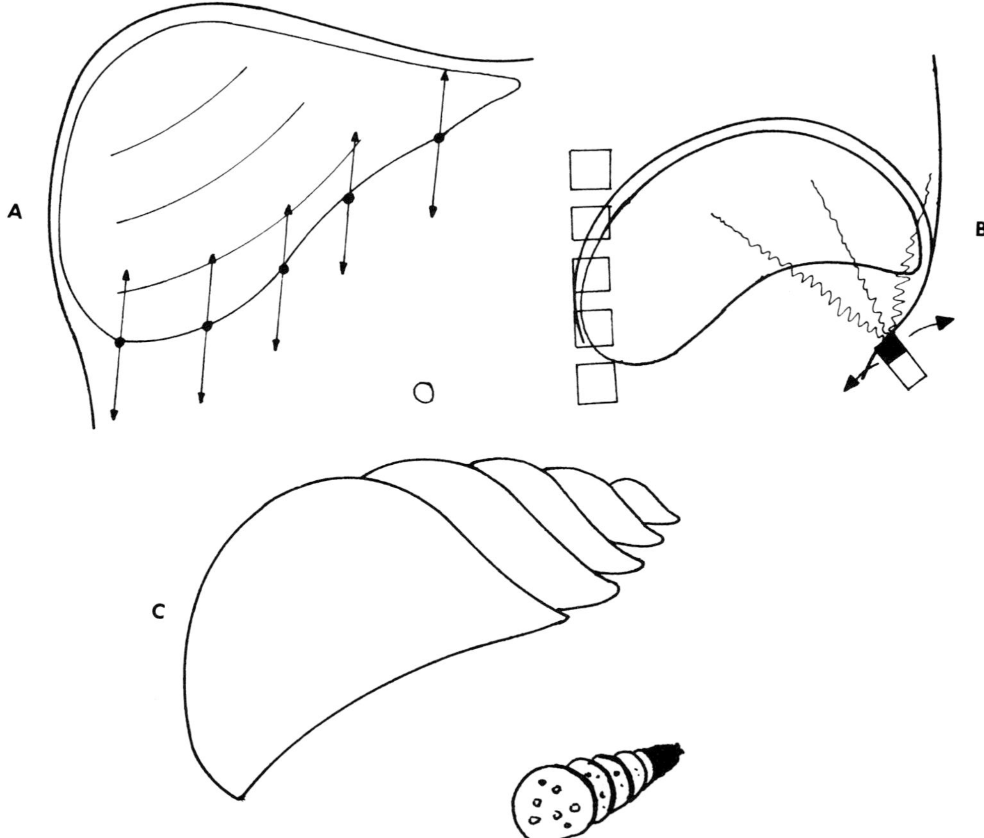

Fig. 5-5. Sagittal sector contact scanning. **A,** Successive positions of transducer applied to skin immediately below right anterior costal edge (frontal view). **B,** Sectoring movement of transducer applied under costal margin (lateral view). **C,** Schematic representation of successive hepatic sections ("salami scans").

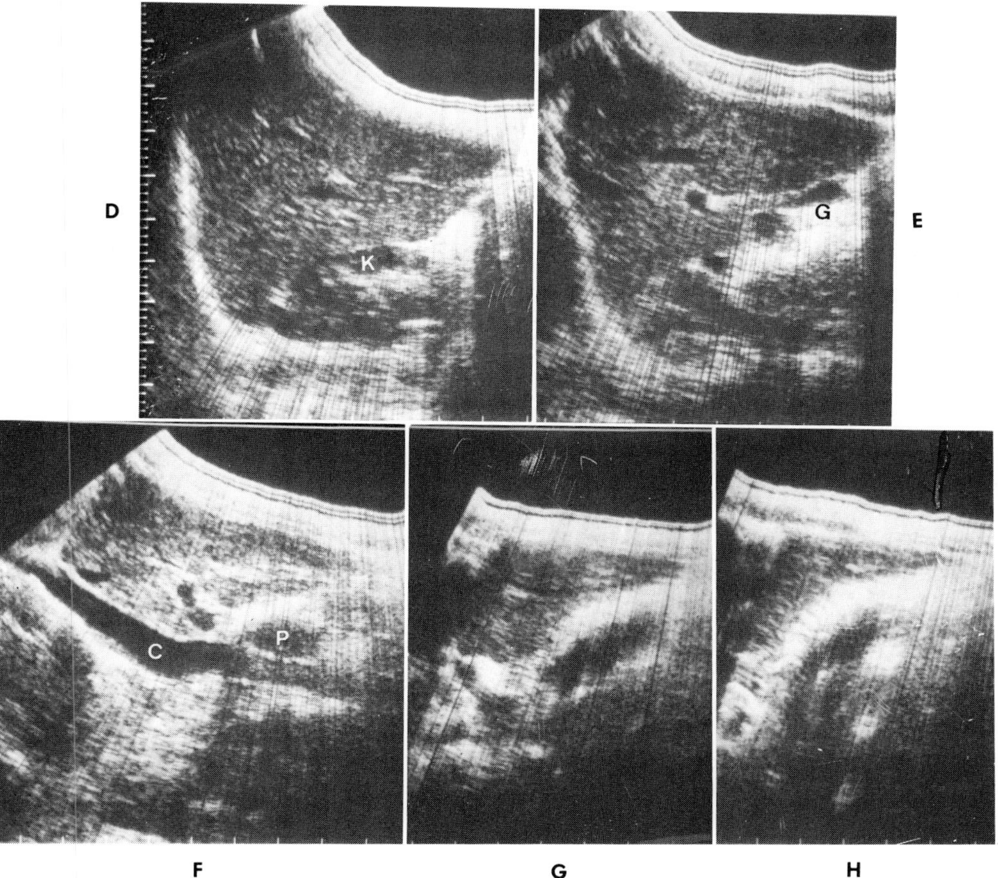

Fig. 5-5, cont'd. Successive liver sections. **D,** Through right kidney *(K).* **E,** Through gallbladder *(G).* **F,** Through vena cava *(C),* portal vein, and head of pancreas *(P).* **G** and **H,** Through left lobe of liver.

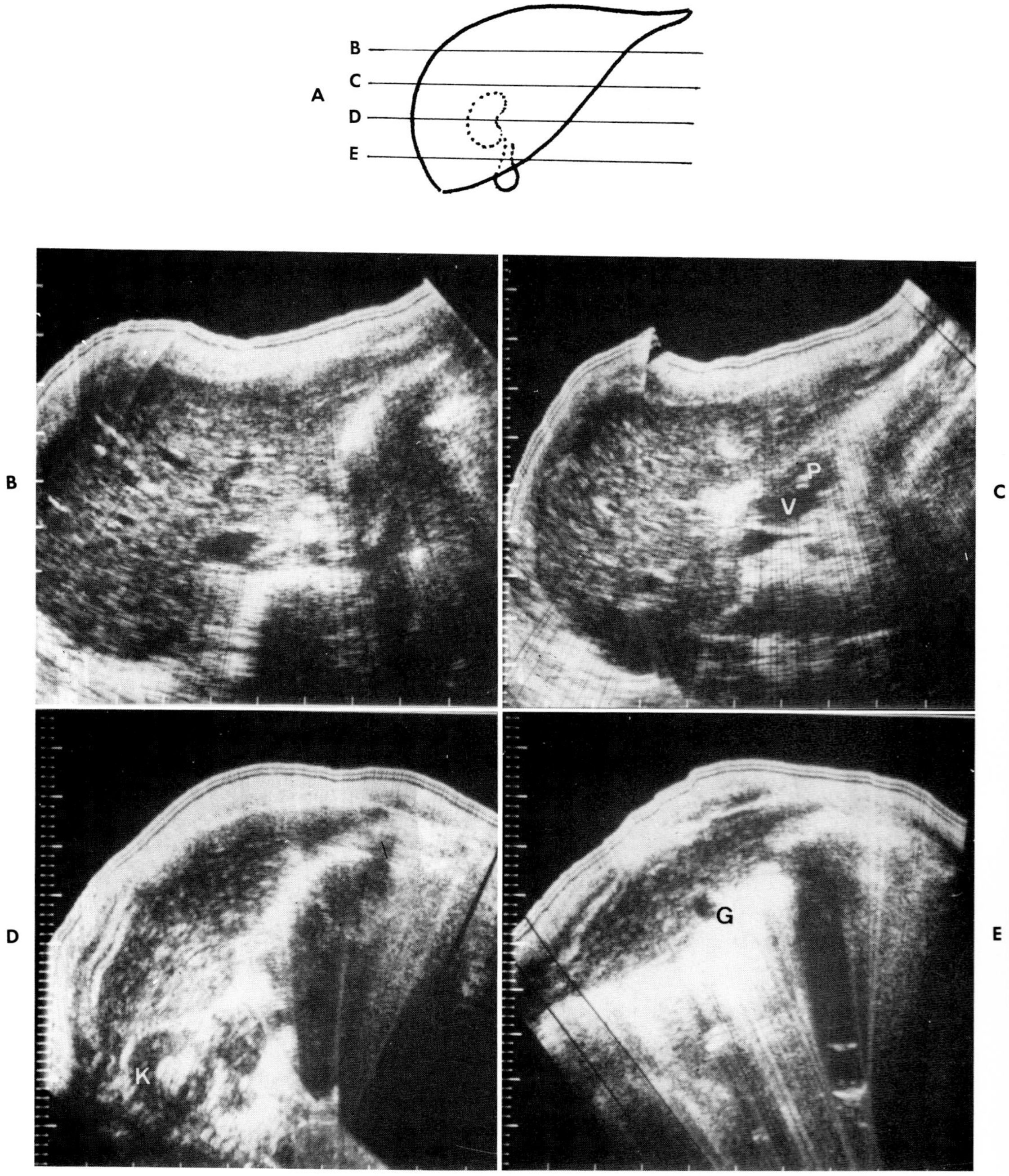

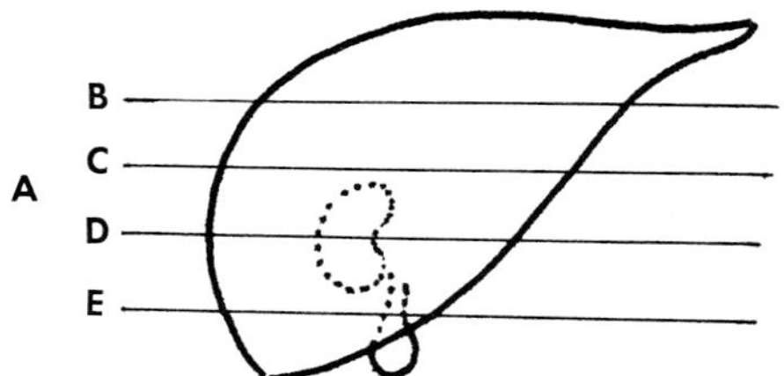

Fig. 5-6. Horizontal contact scanning of liver. **A,** Different scanning planes. **B** to **E,** Successive parallel scans from top to bottom (horizontal salami scans). **B,** Through liver. **C,** Through liver, pancreatic head *(P),* and portal vein *(V).* **D,** Through right kidney. **E,** Through gallbladder *(G).*

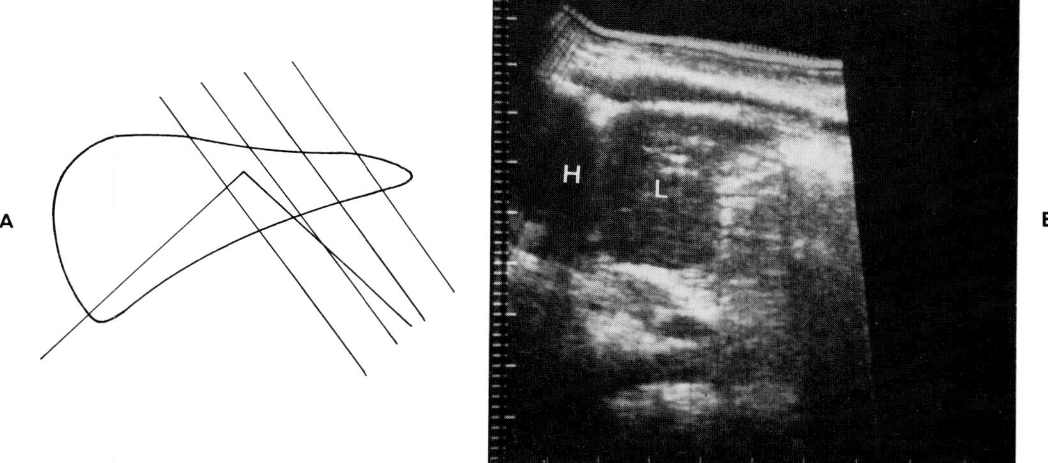

Fig. 5-7. Oblique scanning of left hepatic lobe parallel to left costal edge. **A,** Scanning planes. **B,** Example of resulting section, which also cuts heart *(H),* mesenteric vein, and aorta. Posterior bulge of liver *(L)* is not pathological (Chapter 6).

Table 5-1. Different steps in ultrasonic exploration of the liver

Real time	*Contact scanning*
In normal respiration and then deep inspiration	In neutral apnea, but mainly in deep inspiration
Sagittal scans	Sagittal scans
Horizontal scans	Horizontal scans
Subcostal recurrent oblique view	Occasionally, subcostal oblique scans
In normal respiration and then expiration	In neutral apnea
Intercostal scans	Occasionally, intercostal scans

In children over 4 years of age, single-sweep scanning with good results is possible. This protocol, which is summarized in Table 5-1, may appear to be somewhat long and complicated. As a matter of fact, however, the real-time phase of the examination lasts less than 3 minutes. The rapidity of the gray scale contact scanning, after a first examination in real time, is such that the whole examination does not exceed 6 to 7 minutes for a normal subject. Of course, the discovery of a pathological process requires a verification by repeated and complementary scans, but the systemic character of this protocol permits a trained operator to work far faster than with contact scanning alone.

ULTRASONICALLY GUIDED BIOPSY

Biopsy, or puncture, can complete the morphological phase of ultrasonography; its different methods have been described in Chapter 3. Patients suffering from a liver disease are, of course, subject to disorders of blood coagulation. The enthusiasm that physicians may feel behind their needles, like matadors behind their swords, should not make them forget to check the prothrombin time before a puncture. Moreover, if there is the least possibility of a vascular tumor, it is advisable to perform angiography *before* the puncture, rather than *afterward*—when the object may be embolization, to control hemorrhage.

REFERENCES

Barnett, E., and Morley, P.: Abdominal echography, Borough Green, England, 1974, Butterworth & Co. (Publishers), Ltd.

Goldberg, B. B., Kotler, M. N., Ziskin, M. C., and Waxham, R. D.: Diagnostic uses of ultrasound, New York, 1975, Grune & Stratton, Inc.

Hassani, N.: Ultrasonography of the abdomen, Heidelberg, Germany, 1976, Springer-Verlag.

Holm, H. H., Kristensen, J. K., Rasmussen, S. N., Pedersen, J. F., and Hancke, S.: Abdominal ultrasound, Copenhagen, 1976, Munksgaard, International Booksellers & Publishers, Ltd.

Hussey, M.: Diagnostic ultrasound, Glasgow, Scotland, 1975, Blackie & Son, Ltd.

Leopold, G. R., and Asher, W. M.: Fundamentals of abdominal and pelvic ultrasonography, Philadelphia, 1975, W. B. Saunders Co.

Rasmussen, S. N., Holm, H. H., Kristensen, J. K., and Barlebott: Ultrasonically-guided liver biopsy, Br. Med. J. **2**:500-502, 1972.

Weill, F., Becker, J. C., Kraehenbuhl, J. R., Heriot, G., and Walter, J. P.: Clinical atlas of ultrasonic radiography, Paris, 1973, Masson & Cie., Editeurs.

Wells, P. N. T.: Ultrasonics in clinical diagnosis, Edinburgh, 1972, Churchill Livingstone.

CHAPTER 6

ECHOANATOMY

HEPATIC CONTOURS AND SIZE

Those who frequent the butcher's shop or the department of pathology are familiar with a slice of liver, which has regular, smooth, but sharply outlined, contours, sharply angulated margins, and, on the whole, a harmonious shape. Such are, as a matter of fact, the morphological features displayed by ultrasonographic scans of the liver, as already illustrated in the previous chapter (Figs. 5-5 and 5-6). The general character of the hepatic contours is best displayed by contact scans. However, real-time images often display more accurately, as shown in Chapter 1, the morphological details of the liver surface and margins, the latter probably because of the absence of operator manipulation. This is especially true for the anterior hepatic surface. The normal liver may clear the costal margin in the epigastric area, but it does not extend beyond the last rib on the axillary line.

The smoothness of the hepatic contour is interrupted in only a few places. One such zone is a hollow that is displayed on sagittal scans at the level of the hilus (Fig. 6-1, *A*).

There are *four convex areas* as follows:

1. A very discrete and inconstant elevation, the height of which does not exceed 3 to 4 mm, with a long radius of curvature. It is found at the point at which the

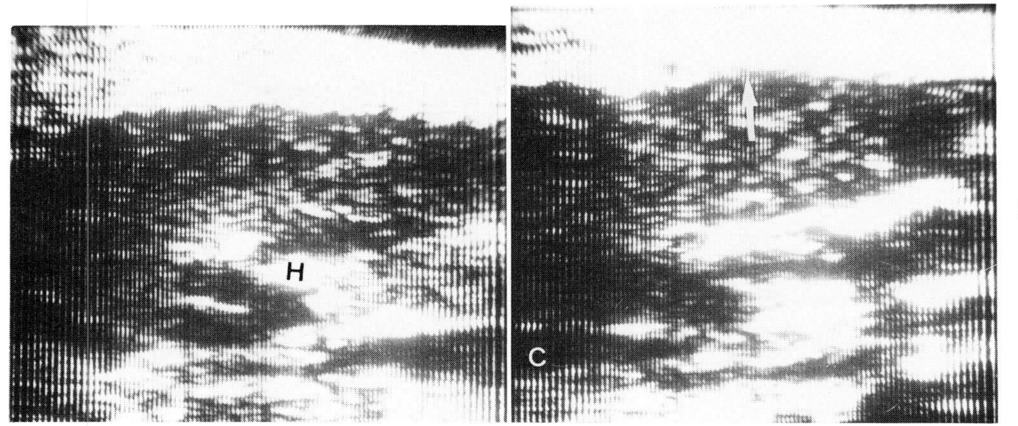

Fig. 6-1. A, Real-time intercostal hepatic section. Anterior hepatic contour is perfectly regular, without elevation. On posterior aspect of liver a relief is created by inner inflection toward hilus *(H)*. This relief will be encountered again when caudate lobe is discussed. **B,** Sagittal real-time scan passing through vena cava *(C)* in same patient. As it clears costal margin, anterior aspect of liver is slightly elevated *(arrow)*.

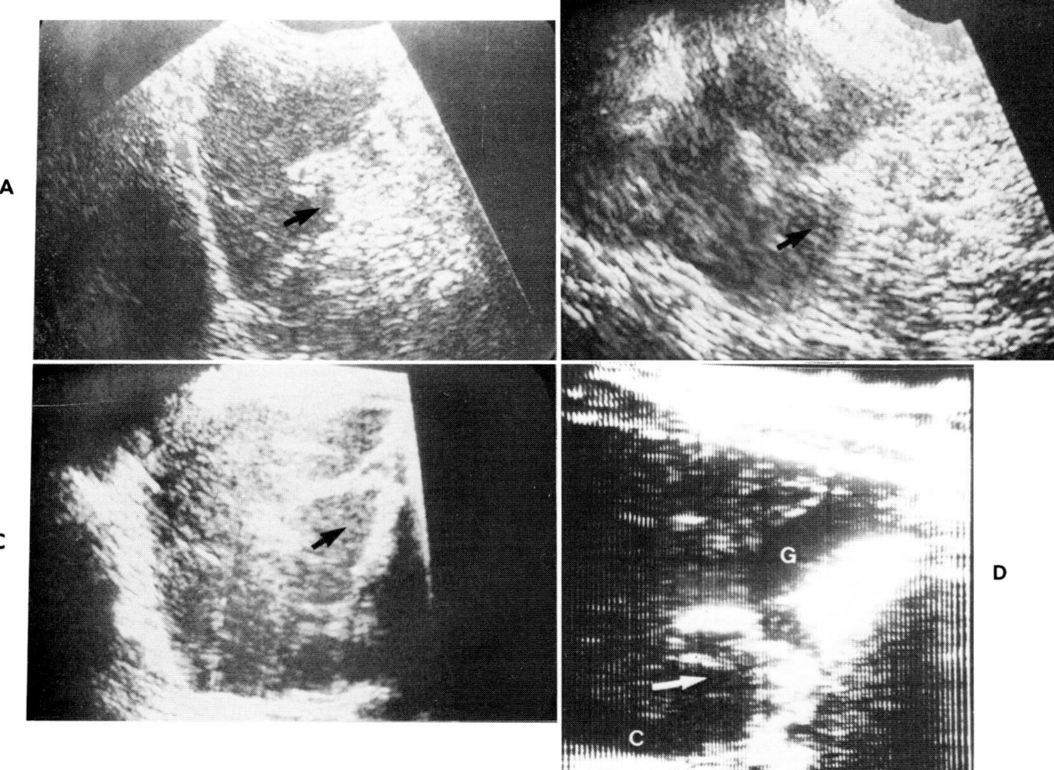

Fig. 6-2. Caudate lobe. **A** to **C,** Sagittal contact scans of liver displaying differently shaped caudate lobes *(arrows)*. **D** to **F,** Real-time sagittal scans also displaying different shapes of caudate lobe *(arrows)*. *G,* gallbladder; *C,* vena cava. In **F,** note abnormally rounded shape of inferior margin of liver (edge sign, explained in Chapter 8). **G,** Caudate lobe *(arrow)* shown in front of vena cava, on transverse scan of liver.

anterior hepatic surface clears the costal margin in the epigastric region (Fig. 6-1, *B*).

The three other normal elevations are posterior.

2. The caudate lobe. On sagittal scans, this lobe produces a rather marked convexity, which may be angular or rounded, lying just in front of the vena cava (Fig. 6-2, *A* and *F*). Its convexity may also be seen on transverse scans in less sharp relief, anterior to the transverse section of the vena cava.

3. A related, quite similar convexity is often visible on transverse scans in front of the aorta (Fig. 6-3).

4. Finally, on sagittal scans, the posterior aspect of the liver bulges above the lower pole of the kidney (Fig. 6-14, *B*).

Some of those normal elevations may be quite marked and should not be misinterpreted to be enlargements. The falciform ligament, which separates the right and left lobes of the liver, is seen only in the presence of ascites.

The *margins* of the liver are also an important element in the analysis of the

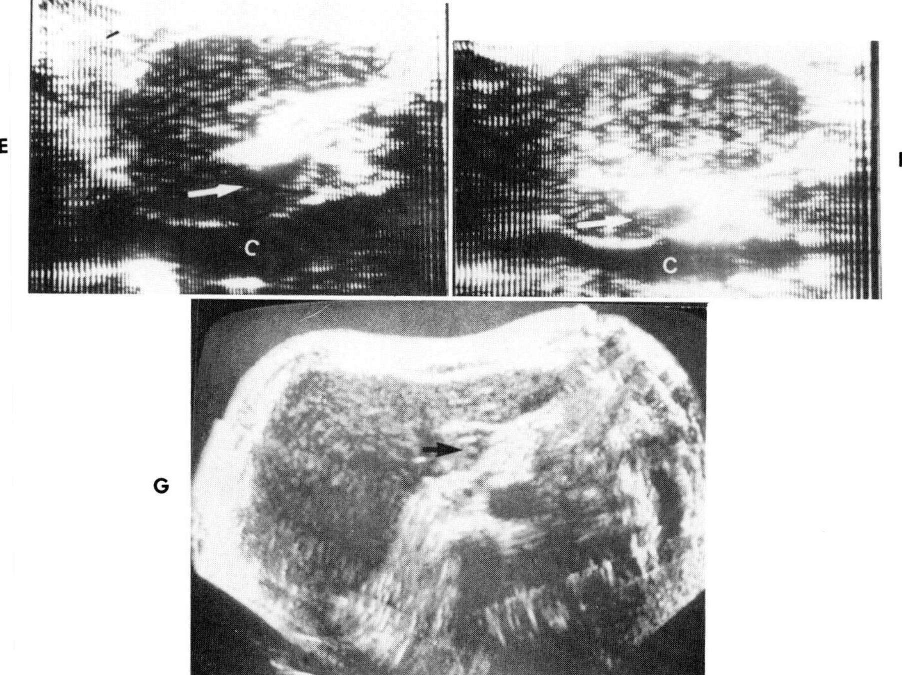

Fig. 6-2, cont'd. For legend see opposite page.

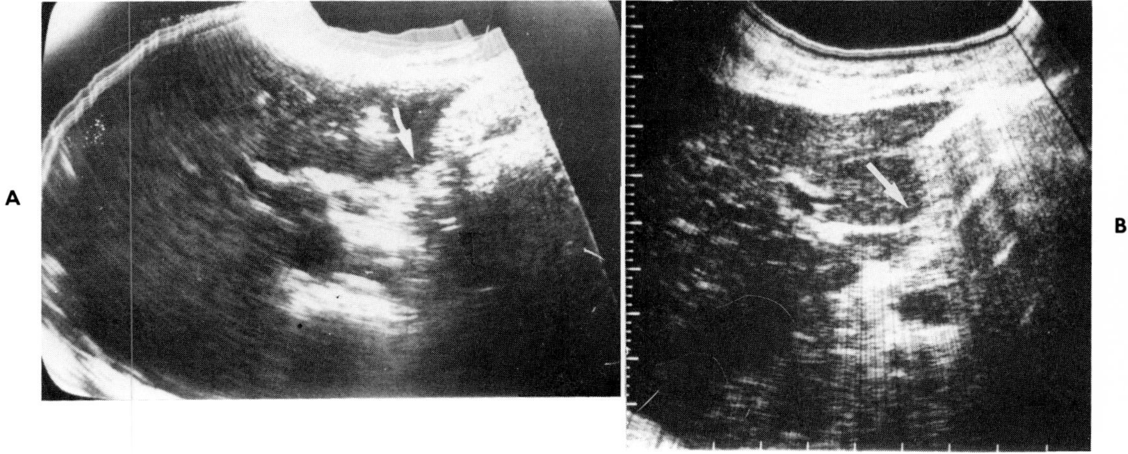

Fig. 6-3. A, Another type of normal contour convexity. There is a bulge of posterior aspect of left lobe of liver *(arrow),* this time in front of aorta (transverse scan). **B,** Rare caricatural pattern.

hepatic contours. On a section, these margins appear as well-delineated angles with two exceptions. One is the area of insertion of the falciform ligament, where the liver margin may be rounded. The other is the left margin: on transverse scans made at the level of the xiphoid process or lower, the liver margin has an angular shape. More cranial cuts do not pass through the external limit of the left lobe, but rather through the superior aspect of the liver. The left outline of such a liver section, as well as a section passing through the liver dome, would be convex or frankly rounded. Ultrasonic sections are seldom so cranial because of costal masking. CT scans can display very cranial liver sections. (The same part of the liver is accessible to ultrasound with sagittal scanning.) This is the reason that the left limit of the liver may look so different on CT scans and ultrasonograms. A rounded left margin shown on ultrasonograms is pathological if the level of transverse scanning was the xiphoid process or below.

Marginal angles can be measured (Fig. 6-4). The first marginal angle to be considered is the left lateral marginal angle, which in normal subjects does not exceed 45 degrees (Fig. 6-4, *A*). The others are the inferior marginal angles. The right inferior marginal angle many reach 75 degrees, whereas the left inferior marginal angle does not usually exceed 45 degrees (Fig. 6-4, *B* and *C*). There is only one exception to these normal values: when the left hepatic lobe is short,

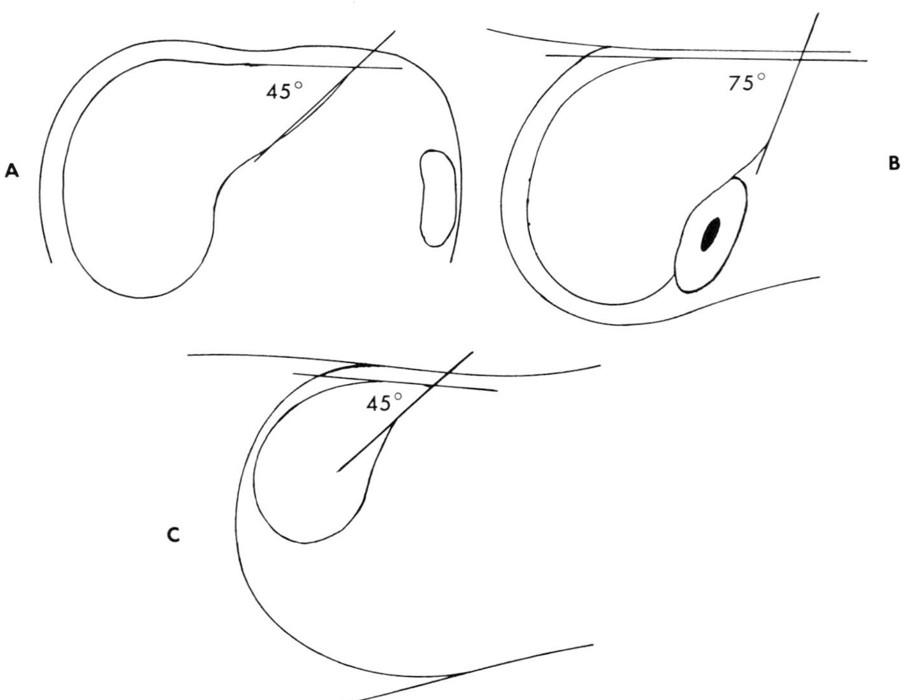

Fig. 6-4. Marginal angles. **A,** Left marginal angle, transverse cut. **B,** Right inferior marginal angle, sagittal cut. **C,** Left inferior marginal angle, sagittal cut.

the left lateral marginal angle may measure more than 45 degrees (Fig. 6-5, *D*). The configuration of the left lobe is variable (Fig. 6-5). When well developed, it may extend to the left and approach the spleen. In other subjects, it is almost absent. Therefore one does not rely on the transverse development of this part of the liver, but rather on its thickness, as a criterion of normality. The left lobe thickness is measured along a tangent to the left aspect of the vertebral body (Fig. 6-5, *A*). Along this line the liver tissue should not measure over 5 cm. This point will be discussed in Chapter 7, on hepatomegaly.

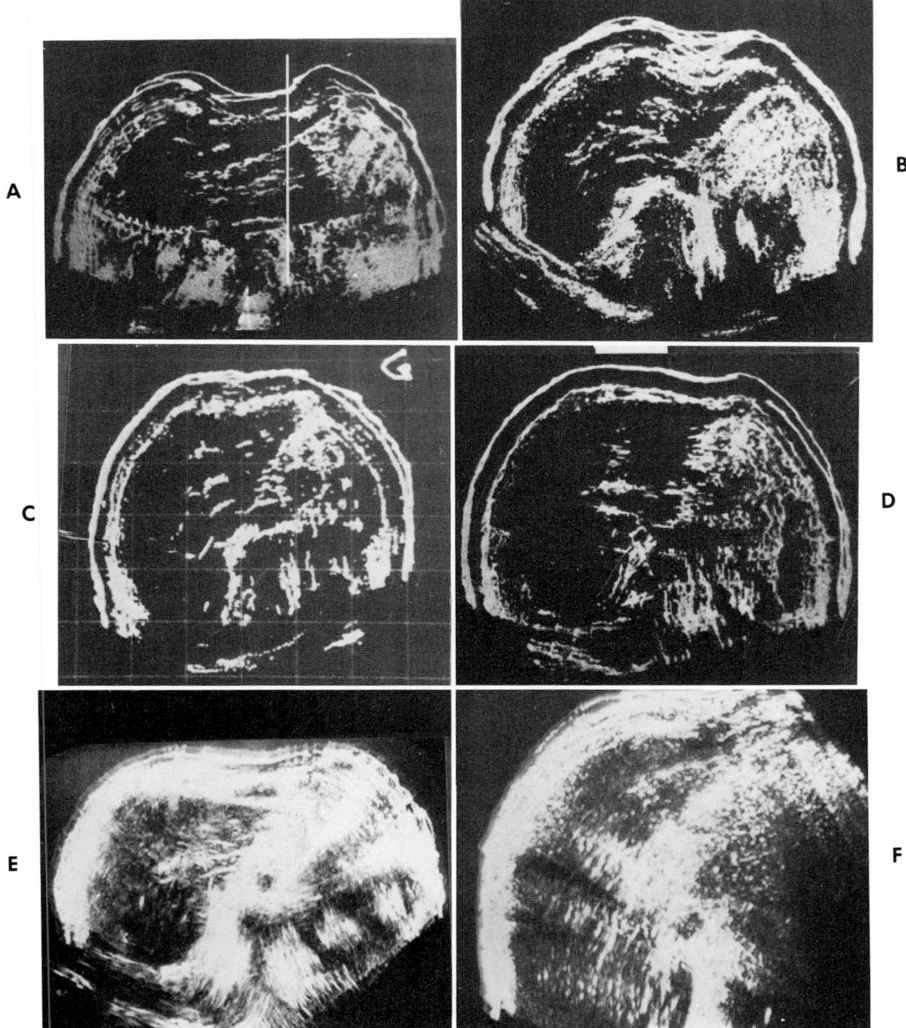

Fig. 6-5. Different shapes of left hepatic lobe, displayed on transverse sections. **A** and **B,** Slender left hepatic lobe. In **A,** tangent to left margin of vertebral body has been drawn. Along that line, left lobe of liver must not be thicker than 5 cm. **C** to **E,** Short left hepatic lobe. **F,** Hypoplastic left hepatic lobe. Short or hypoplastic left hepatic lobe may outline left marginal angles exceeding 45 degrees.

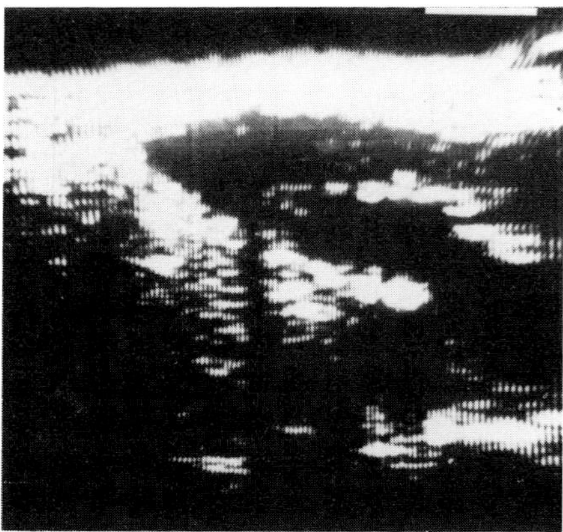

Fig. 6-6. Transverse scan of left hepatic lobe, with small field of real-time image, in a case of situs inversus.

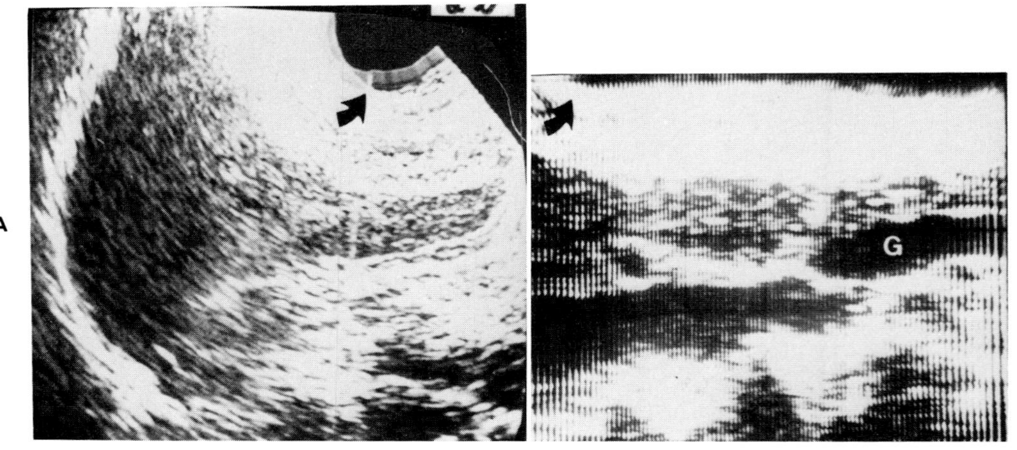

Fig. 6-7. Normal ptosed liver in aged woman. Narrow strip of liver tissue extends well below costal edge *(arrow)* without true hepatomegaly. **A,** Contact scan. **B,** Real-time scan. *G,* gallbladder.

More precise methods for measuring the *size* of the liver have been proposed. Rasmussen (1972) calculates the liver volume from serial scans with the help of a computer. Carr and colleagues (1976) propose a simpler geometrical method. In our opinion the criteria just described (marginal angles and left lobe thickness), available without complicated calculations, are adequate in most cases. Evaluation of liver volume by precise methods is, of course, necessary in a few particular clinical situations.

The right lobe has a less variable configuration. Situs inversus (Fig. 6-6) may prove temporarily puzzling when one observes the small field of a real-time machine. In some elderly and thin women the right lobe may appear thin and

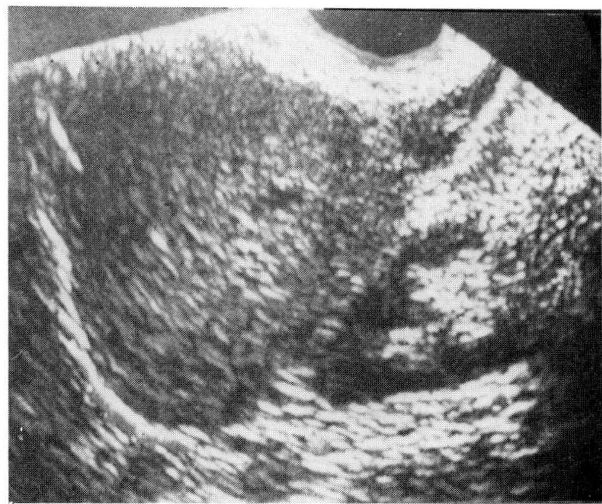

Fig. 6-8. Normal attenuation. On this sagittal scan of right lobe of liver, passing through right kidney, tissular echopattern is homogeneous. Intensity and number of echoes remains about the same from surface to depth, since, in this normal tissue, swept gain was able to balance attenuation.

elongated, extending far below the costal edge (Fig. 6-7). Precise evaluation of the liver volume, however, would show the absence of a true hepatomegaly. In any case, there is no sagittal enlargement on the liver sections, and the inferior marginal angle is well below its maximal value.

THE PARENCHYMA

The examples of homogeneous solid-type echopattern illustrated in Figs. 2-3 and 2-4 were of hepatic tissue. Even though a few echoes may be more intense than others, the intensity gradient remains small, and the more intense echoes are scattered so that the general appearance remains that of homogeneity (Rettenmaier, 1973a; Taylor and associates, 1973; Weill and associates, 1973) (Figs. 5-5, 5-6, 6-2, 6-7, and 6-8).

This general impression of homogeneity is strengthened by a good balance of the intensity of echoes in the superficial and deep areas of the liver tissue, owing to a normal attenuation. In a normal subject, it is thus possible to obtain, with an average sensitivity and a standard swept-gain curve, satisfactory images of the whole parenchyma, especially on oblique recurrent and sagittal scans (Figs. 6-8, 6-10, *B,* 6-13, and 6-14). When, in spite of identical technical conditions (excepting very obese patients), the ultrasonic beam is attenuated to such an extent that it is no longer possible to obtain an image of the deeper areas, one must increase the sensitivity, saturating the image of the superficial layers of tissue. Such a pattern is, of course, pathological, as will be seen in Chapter 10.

TUBULAR STRUCTURES

Branches of the portal vein are always displayed. In Chapter 4 the main portal branches in the hilar area were described (Figs. 4-20, *C,* and 4-24, *A*). Slow and

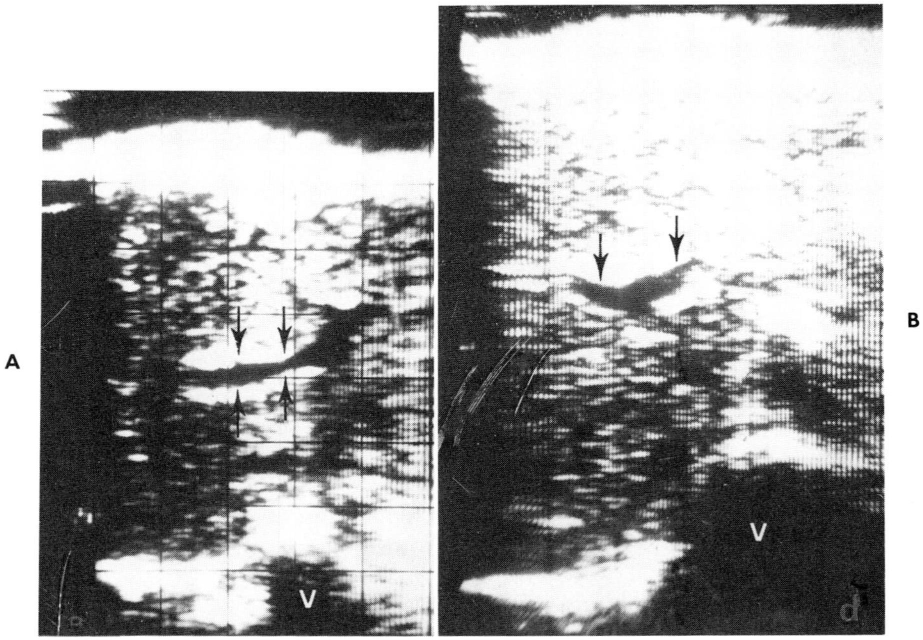

A

B

Fig. 6-9. Hilar division of portal vein *(arrows).* **A** and **B,** Oblique recurrent subcostal scans in two different patients. *V,* vertebral body.

progressive movements of the RTH allow one to follow the course of some of these branches and to outline their successive arborizations (Fig. 6-9). The image of the portal division may also be displayed with rapid single gray scale scans (Fig. 6-10, *B* and *C*). In bistable imaging the slow scan construction, with its kinetic blur, often led one to misinterpret these vascular echoes as pathological nodules (Fig. 6-11). This could still be the case with gray scale at too high a sensitivity, saturating the vascular lumen (Fig. 6-11, *C*). *Another pitfall* is a reflective strip often displayed on transverse scans, extending from the portal division to the posterior aspect of the liver (Fig. 6-12). This strip may be rather thick; if cut perpendicularly or obliquely, it may give rise to pseudonodular images. It likely belongs to connective tissue.

Bile ducts. The bile ducts are usually too narrow to be viewed except in the hilar region, where the biliary junction is usually displayed in front of the portal division (Chapter 15). The biliary network will be studied in more detail in the discussion of jaundice (Chapter 26), since in obstructive jaundice the dilated biliary ducts are readily visible.

Hepatic veins. The *hepatic veins* have already been dealt with (Chapter 4). According to Schammai's school, these veins are readily recognized on any type of scan, even if they are isolated or reduced to a short segment because they have no proper wall image. This is often true; but, as I reviewed my own collection of images of hepatic veins—kept in a combination-lock safe, in a bank in the Galápagos Islands—I found that, in about half the cases, there was a wall image, at least on some venous segments. As a matter of fact, the sharpness of the venous

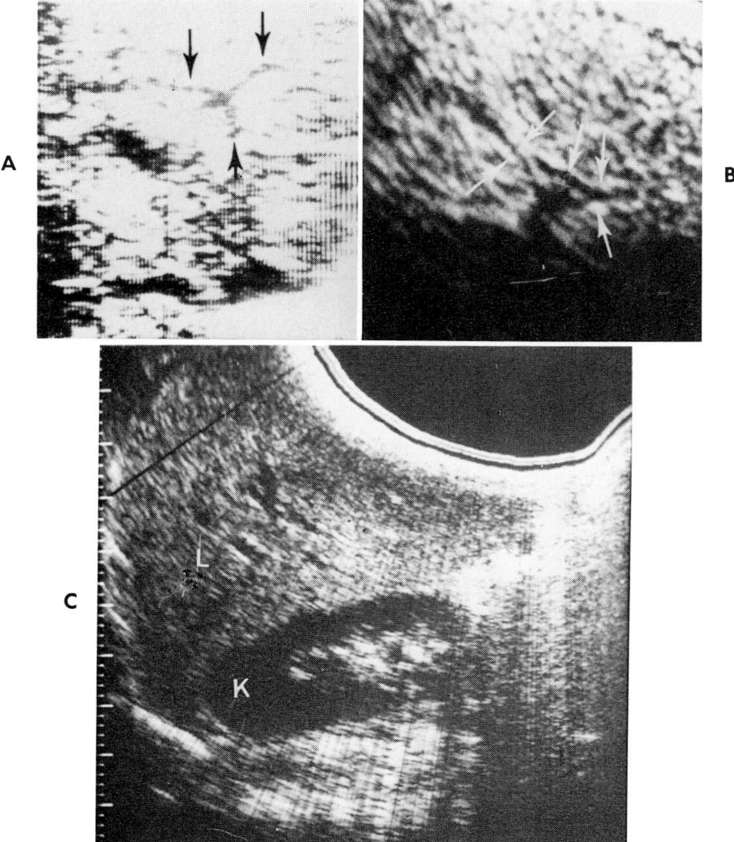

Fig. 6-10. Secondary portal branches *(arrows).* **A,** Real-time scan. **B** and **C,** Rapid single-contact scans.

wall image depends on the angle with which the ultrasonic beam approaches the hepatic veins. It is sharp and well marginated when this angle is close to 90 degrees and absent when the approach is tangential (Fig. 6-13). I do hope that Hillel's school will pick up this information and that an interesting discussion will arise. In my opinion, the real identification of the tubular structures, whether biliary or venous and portal or systemic, rests mainly on the study of their anatomical relations and their possible anastomosis with a dilated main bile duct, the portal vein, or the vena cava, displayed by the real-time technique.

ECHOANATOMICAL RELATIONS OF THE LIVER

Hepatic scans show the following, as well as the liver:

1. The gallbladder in fasting patients (Figs. 5-4 to 5-6, 6-2, *D,* and 6-7, *B*). This will be studied in more detail in Chapter 15.
2. The inferior vena cava, aorta, portal vein, and splenic vein.
3. The right kidney (Figs. 6-8 and 6-14). Part of the kidney margin may

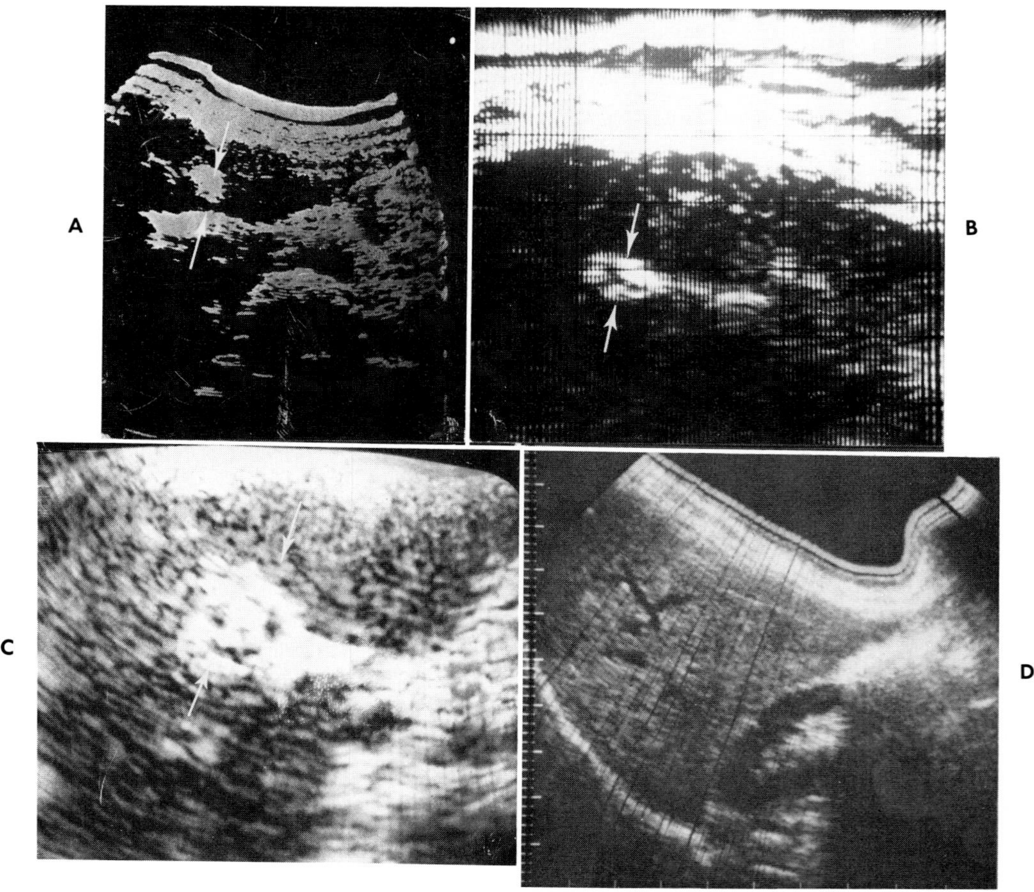

Fig. 6-11. Interpretation pitfall—portal branching. **A,** Contact scan bistable imaging. Several passes of transducer were necessary to build the image. Kinetic blur changes venous branching image into apparent reflective nodule *(arrows)*. **B,** Real-time scan displaying, at this level, T-shaped venous branching *(arrows)*. **C,** Venous branching displayed on almost saturated single-sweep contact scan. **D,** Evident branching on another single-sweep contact scan.

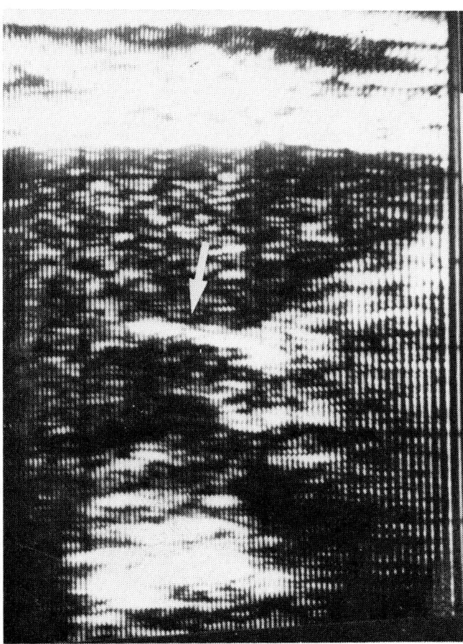

Fig. 6-12. Nonpathological linear image *(arrow)* often encountered between hilar region and posterior aspect of liver.

appear on liver scans. This must be kept in mind before diagnosing a pathological marginal deformity or sonolucency.

4. The pancreas, already shown in Figs. 4-19 and 5-6, *C,* which will be studied in Chapter 19; and the spleen, encountered in Figs. 6-2, *G,* and 6-5, which will be studied in Chapter 27.

5. The diaphragmatic dome (Figs. 6-2, 6-7, *A,* 6-8, and 6-14, *B*). In normal conditions the diaphragmatic dome cannot be distinguished from the superior aspect of the liver. Successive passages with the transducer in sagittal scanning without respiratory blockage show the mobility of the diaphragm (Fig. 6-15). When there is a subdiaphragmatic or interhepatodiaphragmatic liquid collection, the diaphragmatic image is separated from the liver parenchyma (Chapter 14). In normal subjects, no image of the thoracic content is obtained, since the ultrasonic beam is interrupted by the pulmonary air. The appearance of images above the diaphragm thus indicates consolidated lung or pleural fluid in the lower thorax. Colonic gas, in case of colonic interposition, may mask the diaphragm.

Following are the fundamental criteria of normality in the liver examination:

- Regular contours, without elevation, except for the subcostal elevation, caudate lobe, preaortic elevation, and infrarenal elevation
- Acute marginal angles (left marginal angle—45 degrees, inferior marginal angle—75 degrees, and left marginal angle—45 degrees)
- Thickness of the left hepatic lobe—5 cm maximum along the left tangent to the vertebral body
- Parenchyma—homogeneous, with balanced attenuation
- Tubular structures—portal and systemic networks regularly outlined, with

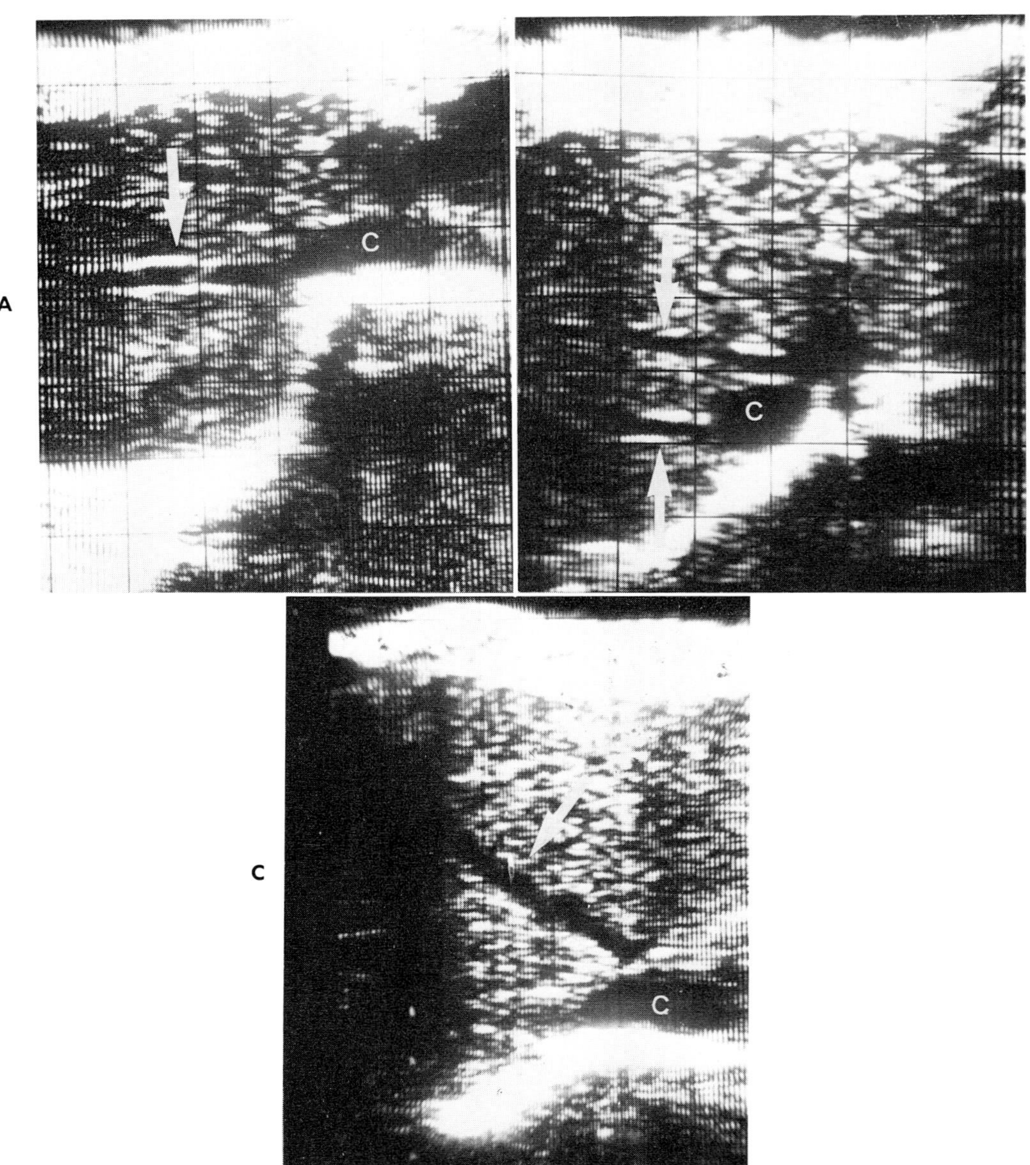

Fig. 6-13. Different examples of hepatic veins displayed on oblique recurrent subcostal real-time scans. *C,* vena cava. **A** and **B,** Hepatic veins have proper wall image *(arrows),* probably owing to the fact that ultrasonic beam was perpendicular to venous wall. **C,** Direction of hepatic vein is more oblique and wall image *(arrow)* now less sharply delineated.

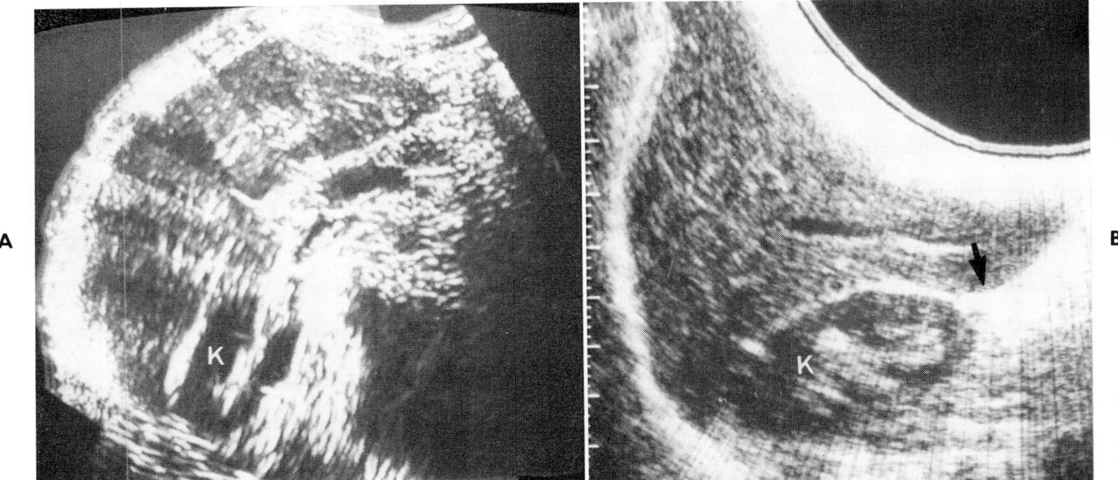

Fig. 6-14. Relation between liver and right kidney *(K)*. **A,** Horizontal scan displays difference in reflectivity between liver tissue and renal cortex. **B,** Sagittal scan. Note presence of a convexity of posterior aspect of liver *(arrow)* at the level of lower pole of right kidney. Such an elevation is not pathological. Also note proper wall image of venous branches.

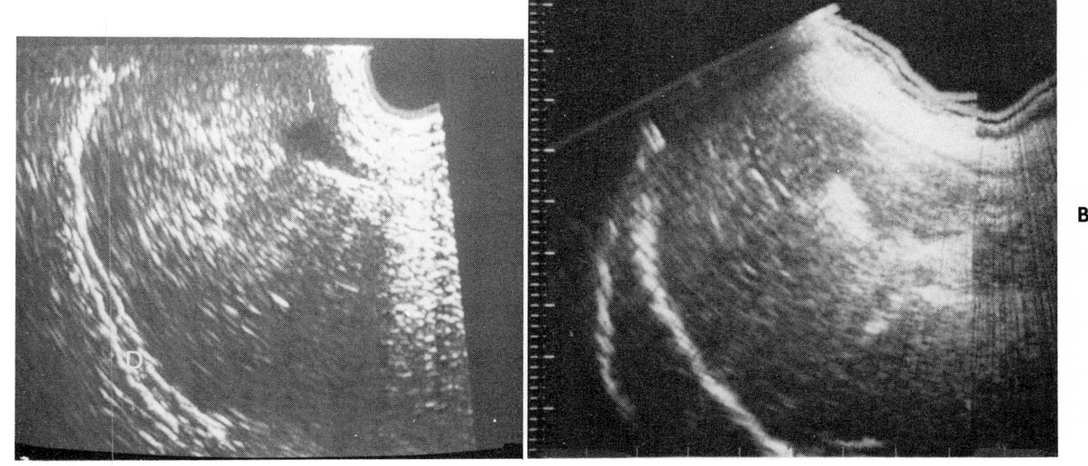

Fig. 6-15. Diaphragm. **A,** This sagittal scan of right hepatic lobe passes through gallbladder *(arrow)*. The image was built in two rapid contact passes. Since patient was breathing, there are two distinct diaphragmatic images *(D)*, indicating, as in conventional radiology, mobility of diaphragm. **B,** Another example of diaphragm mobility.

intrahepatic bile ducts not visible except for the junction of the right and left hepatic ducts.

REFERENCES

Barnett, E., and Morley, P.: Abdominal echography, Borough Green, England, 1974, Butterworth & Co. (Publishers), Ltd.

Carr, D., Duncan, J. G., Railton, R., and Smith, C. B.: Liver volume determination by ultrasound: a feasible study, Br. J. Radiol. **49:**776-778, 1976.

Goldberg, B. B., Kotler, M. N., Ziskin, M. C., and Waxham, R. D.: Diagnostic uses of ultrasound, New York, 1975, Grune & Stratton, Inc.

Haber, K., Asher, M., and Freimanis, A. K.: Echographic evaluation of diaphragmatic motion in intra-abdominal diseases, Radiology **114:**141-144, 1975.

Hassani, N.: Ultrasonography of the abdomen, Heidelberg, Germany, 1976, Springer-Verlag.

Holm, H. H., Kristensen, J. K., Rasmussen, S. N., Pedersen, J. F., and Hancke, S.: Abdominal ultrasound, Copenhagen, 1976, Munksgaard, International Booksellers & Publishers, Ltd.

Leopold, G. R., and Asher, W. M.: Fundamentals of abdominal and pelvic ultrasonography, Philadelphia, 1975, W. B. Saunders Co.

Rasmussen, S. N.: Liver volume by ultrasonic scanning, Br. J. Radiol. **45:**579-585, 1972.

Rettenmaier, G.: Echographic diagnosis and differential diagnosis of diffuse liver diseases. Start of quantitative evaluation and results, Verh. Dtsch. Ges. Inn. Med. **79:**962-964, 1973a.

Rettenmaier, G.: Quantitative criteria of intrahepatic echo patterns correlated with structural alteration. Ultrasonics in medicine, Second World Congress, Amsterdam, 1973b, Excerpta Medica Foundation, pp. 199-206.

Taylor, K. J., Carpenter, D. A., and McCready, V. R.: Grey scale echography in the diagnosis of intrahepatic disease, J. Clin. Ultrasound **1:**284-287, 1973.

Weill, F., Becker, J. C., Kraehenbuhl, J. R., Heriot, G., and Walter, J. P.: Clinical atlas of ultrasonic radiography, Paris, 1973, Masson & Cie., Editeurs.

CHAPTER 7

NONSPECIFIC HEPATOMEGALIES

CRITERIA OF HEPATOMEGALY

Referring to the list of criteria of normality in the liver examination (p. 97), one may readily deduce the criteria of hepatomegaly. Since an enlarged liver is so easily palpated, one might wonder why it is necessary to set up ultrasonic criteria of hepatomegaly. In fact, however, the liver is difficult to palpate in some obese patients, and some partial hepatomegalies, especially of the left lobe, escape detection by palpation.

The liver is enlarged when the following signs are observed:

1. When it extends below the costal margin at the right axillary line in a recumbent patient and in the absence of deep inspiration (Fig. 7-1, *A*). There is, as already mentioned, an exception: in some women the liver is ptosed and elongated anteriorly.

2. When the thickness of the gland is more than 5 cm along the tangent to the left aspect of the vertebral body (Figs. 7-1, *B,* to 7-3): this is what we call the *tangent sign.*

3. When the left marginal angle measures more than 45 degrees and the right and left inferior angles measure, respectively, more than 75 and 45 degrees: this was termed the *angle sign* (Figs. 7-4 and 7-5).

In many cases of hepatomegaly the tissue echopattern is not altered or displays only minor and nonspecific changes. In these cases, the hepatomegaly itself

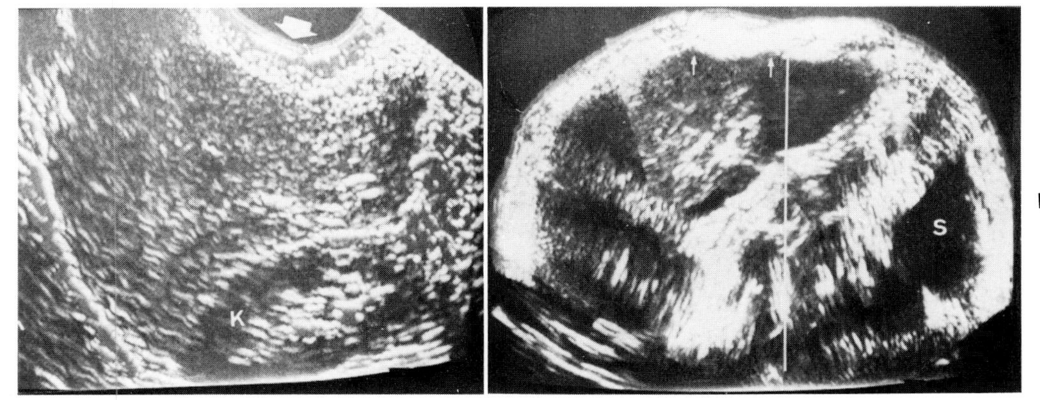

Fig. 7-1. Hepatomegaly. **A,** Sagittal scan. Liver clears costal margin *(arrow).* Normal convexity of posterior aspect of liver at the level of lower pole of right kidney *(K)* is exaggerated. **B,** Transverse scan. On anterior aspect of liver are several small elevations *(arrows)* at the level of intercostal spaces, toward which enlarged liver bulges. *S,* spleen.

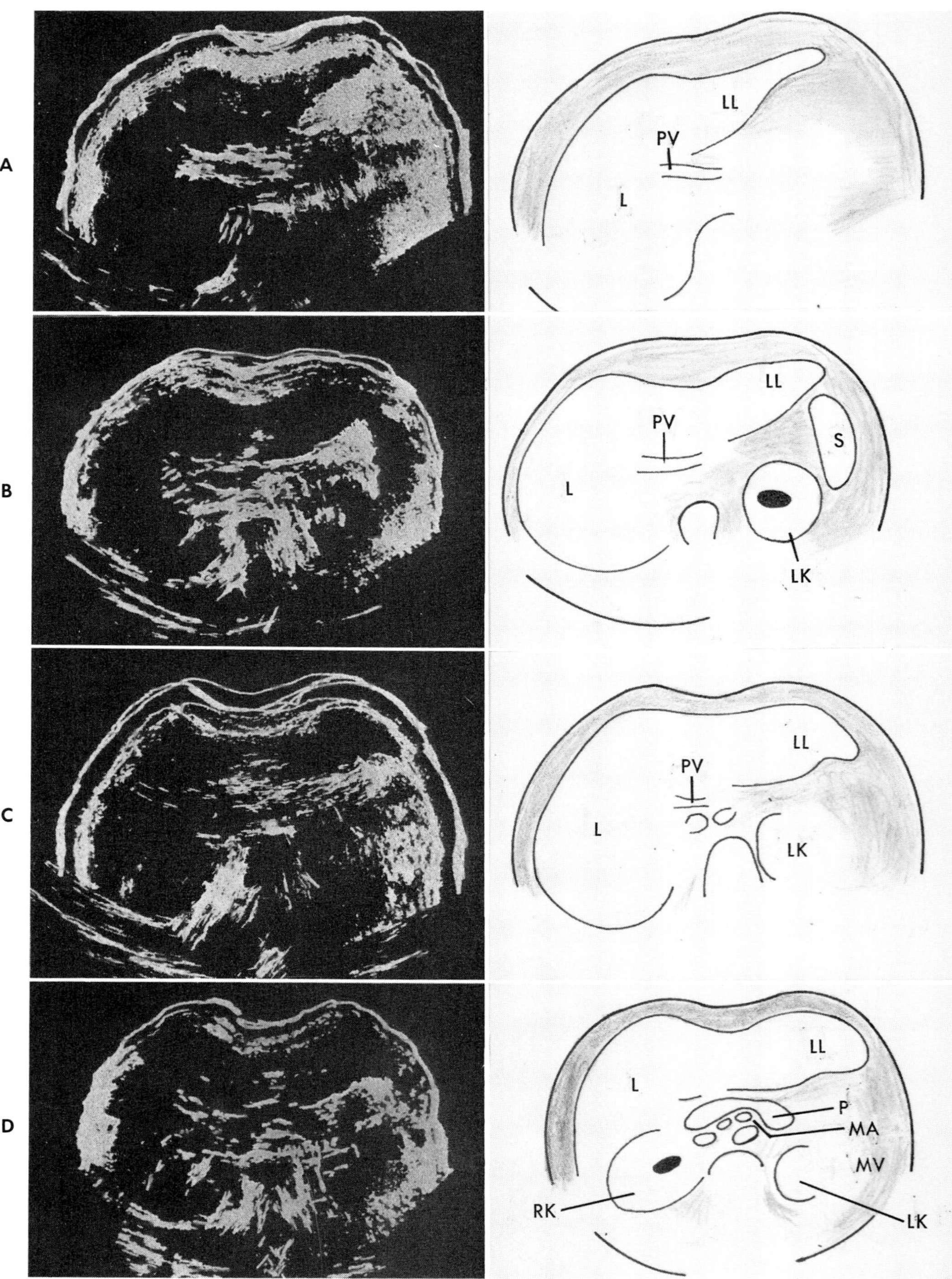

Fig. 7-2. Hepatomegaly: tangent sign displayed on three transverse scans and schematic representations. **A,** *Normal* liver *(L),* for comparison. **B** to **D,** Three examples of left hepatomegaly. Left hepatic lobe *(LL)* is thicker than 5 cm along tangent to left margin of vertebral body. *RK* and *LK,* right and left kidneys; *PV,* portal vein; *P,* pancreas; *MA* and *MV,* mesenteric artery and vein; *S,* spleen.

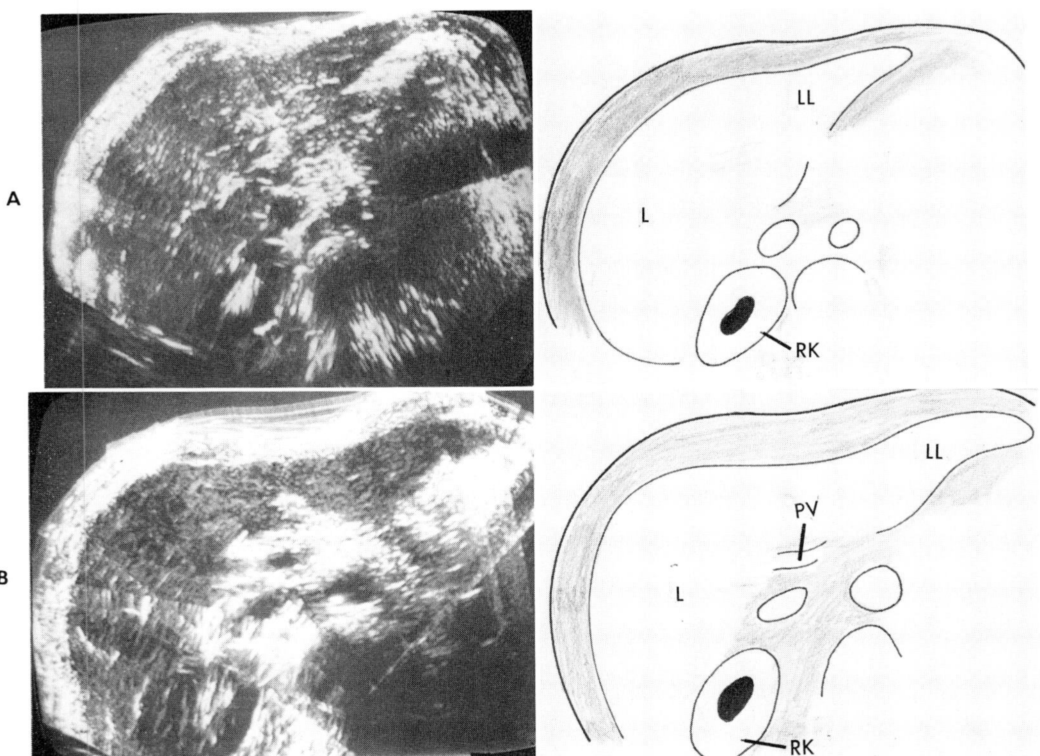

Fig. 7-3. Hepatomegaly: tangent sign. **A,** Normal left hepatic lobe. **B,** Positive tangent sign. Note that left hepatic margin remains angular despite hepatomegaly, as in Fig. 7-2. *L,* liver; *LL,* left lobe; *RK,* right kidney; *PV,* portal vein.

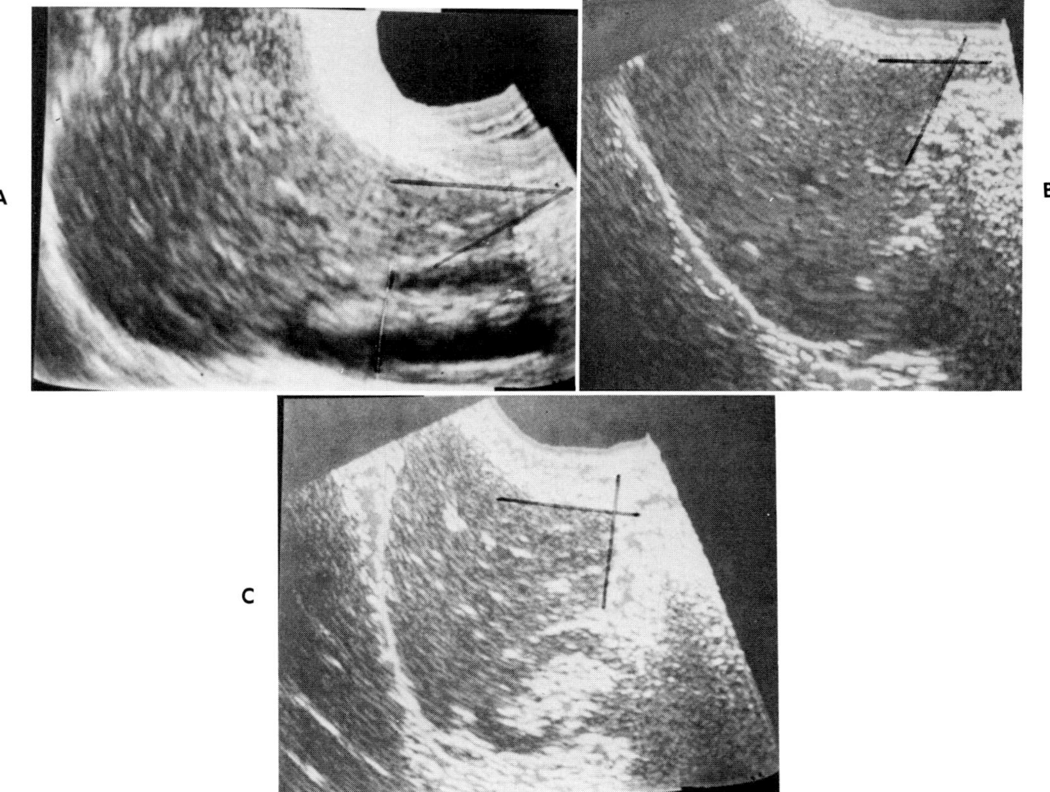

Fig. 7-4. Hepatomegaly: angle sign (inferior marginal angle). **A,** Liver tissue extends past the level of lower pole of right kidney. Right inferior marginal angle, however, remains less than 45 degrees. **B,** Right inferior marginal angle, here at 72 degrees, almost reaches its upper limit (75 degrees). **C,** Positive angle sign. Right inferior marginal angle here reaches almost 90 degrees.

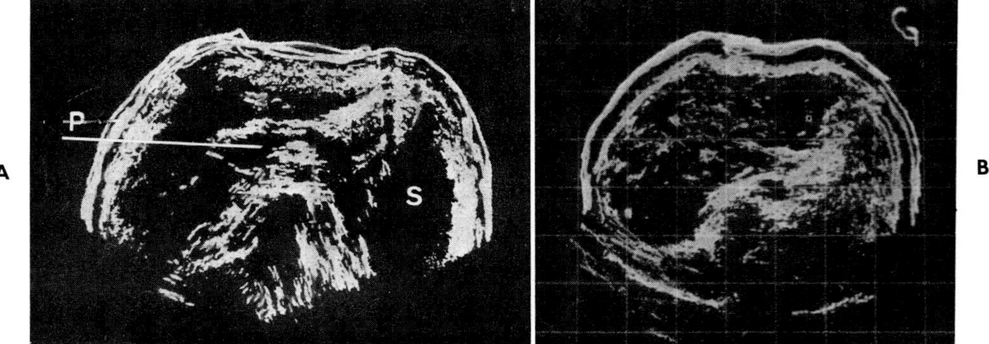

Fig. 7-5. Hepatomegaly: angle sign (left lateral marginal angle). **A,** Normal left hepatic lobe. Left lateral marginal angle is less than 45 degrees. *S,* spleen; *P,* pancreas. **B,** Enlarged left lobe of liver. Left lateral marginal angle is over 45 degrees.

represents the pathological element. Different examples of such "nonspecific" hepatomegalies will now be examined.

CARDIAC LIVER

In the cardiac liver there are usually no changes of the tissue echopattern. The liver tissue is easily traversed by the ultrasonic beam; tissue attenuation is diminished because of the stasis. It is then particularly easy to display the image of the vena cava, especially since the vessel shows evidence of increased venous pressure; in right cardiac insufficiency the inferior vena cava is congested *(vena cava sign)* (Figs. 7-6 to 7-9 and 7-11) (Weill and co-workers, 1973; Weill and Maurat, 1974). The vessel has lost any respiratory variability.* This is a reliable sign allow-

*There is often exaggerated systolic expansion of the anterior wall of the vena cava when the cardiac decompensation is due to or results in tricuspid regurgitation (Winsberg, 1977) (Fig. 7-8, *E*).

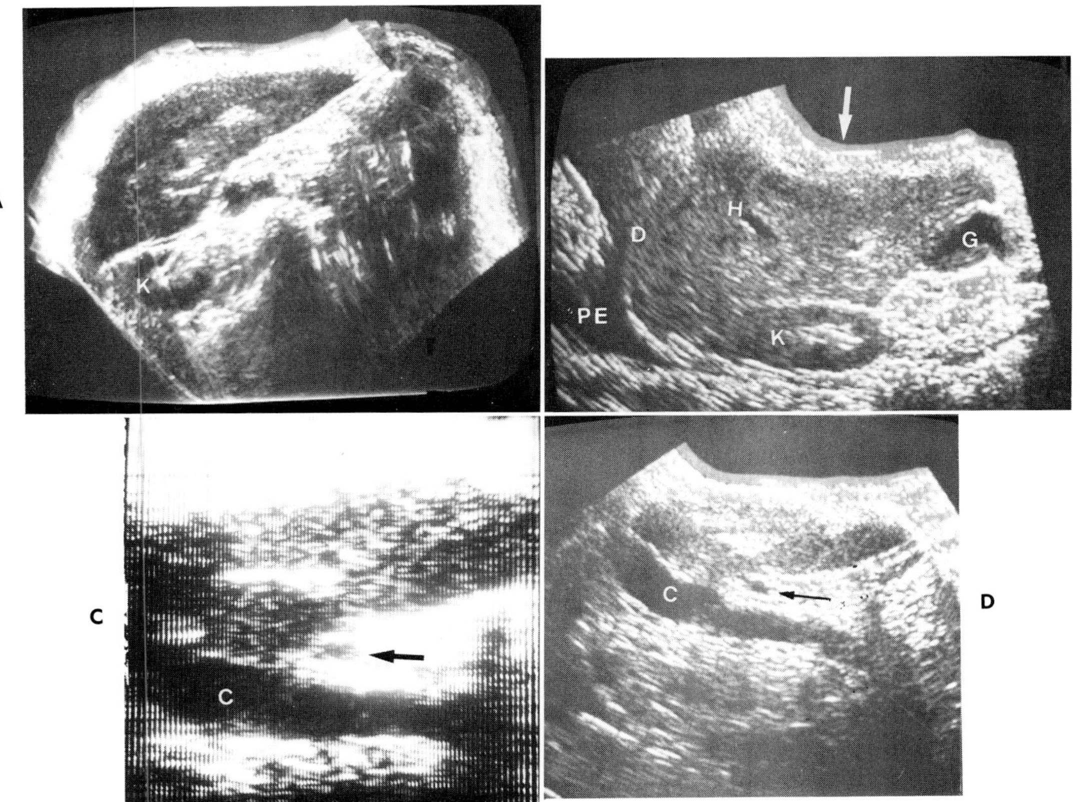

Fig. 7-6. Cardiac liver—direct and indirect signs. **A,** Horizontal section of liver showing normal tissue echopattern. On this rather caudal scan, liver enlargement is not evident. **B,** Sagittal liver scan displaying right kidney *(K)*, venous hilar elements *(H)*, and gallbladder *(G)*. Liver extends well below costal edge *(arrow)*. Typical associated sign—pleural effusion *(PE)*—is seen above diaphragm *(D)*. **C,** Sagittal scan in real time shows dilated cava *(C)*, which has lost its respiratory variability. *Arrow,* portal vein. **D,** Identical image in contact scanning.

A 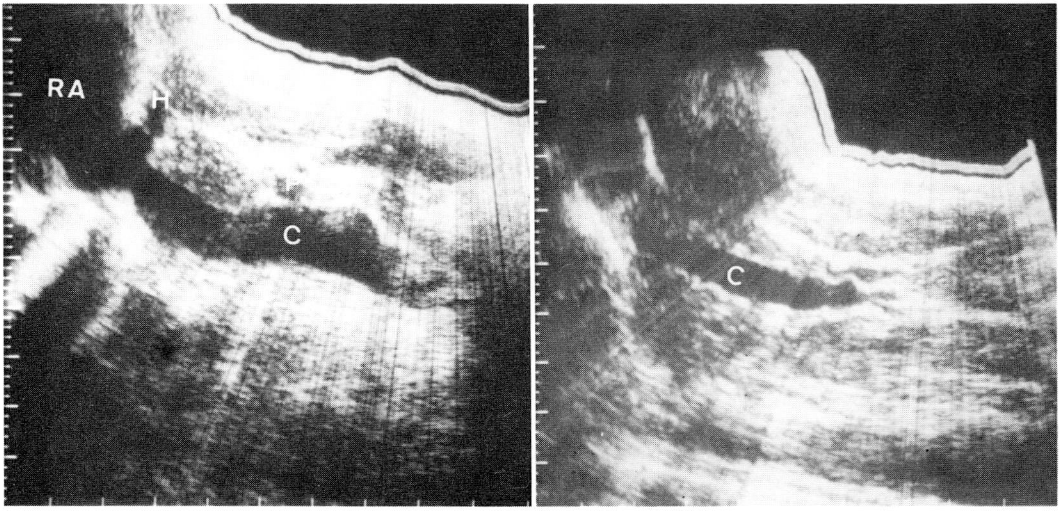 B

Fig. 7-7. Right cardiac insufficiency shown on sagittal scans of vena cava. **A,** Vena cava *(C)* is markedly dilated. Its junction with enlarged right atrium *(RA)* is displayed. *H,* hepatic vein; *P,* portal vein. **B,** In another case of caval dilatation, slow scanning brings about undulated aspect of vascular walls because of systolic pressure waves, which may be displayed even in normal subject, but less sharply.

ing one to recognize the cardiac origin of a hepatomegaly. The reappearance of a respiratory variability at subsequent examinations occurs with therapeutic improvement. Dilatation of the hepatic veins may be recorded at the same time (Fig. 7-8). Large hepatic veins with a diameter of less than 1 cm are, however, not sufficient evidence to conclude the presence of venous hypertension. In Chapter 4 the variability of the diameter of the hepatic veins was discussed. Contact sagittal scans of the vena cava often show the right atrium to be dilated (Fig. 7-7). This is a more reliable associated sign. The vena cava sign is pathognomonic for right cardiac insufficiency with one exception: Taylor and associates (1973) demonstrated that part, at least, of the inferior vena cava loses its respiratory variability in cases of thrombosis. This possibility should be considered when the clinical data include edema of the lower limbs. In fact, in cases of caval obstruction a solid echopattern is usually displayed in the vascular lumen, and dilated supplemental venous branches may be encountered. When a vena cava sign has been displayed, the RTH must be displaced toward the cardiac area in search of a *pericardial effusion.* Even contact scanning can display a pericardial effusion if abundant enough (Fig. 7-9).

Another abnormal image may be associated with a cardiac liver: the presence of a *pleural effusion.* This is displayed as an abnormal supradiaphragmatic image on a contact sectorial sagittal scan. Although in normal subjects the ultrasonic beam is completely interrupted above the diaphragm (Chapter 6), in cases of pleural effusion an evident liquid pattern is displayed at the thoracic level (Figs. 7-6 and 7-10). Examples of small pleural effusions visible on liver scans will be depicted in Chapter 14. The finding of ascites (Fig. 7-11) is exceptional. In the chronic cardiac liver a micronodular tissular pattern may appear (Fig. 7-12).

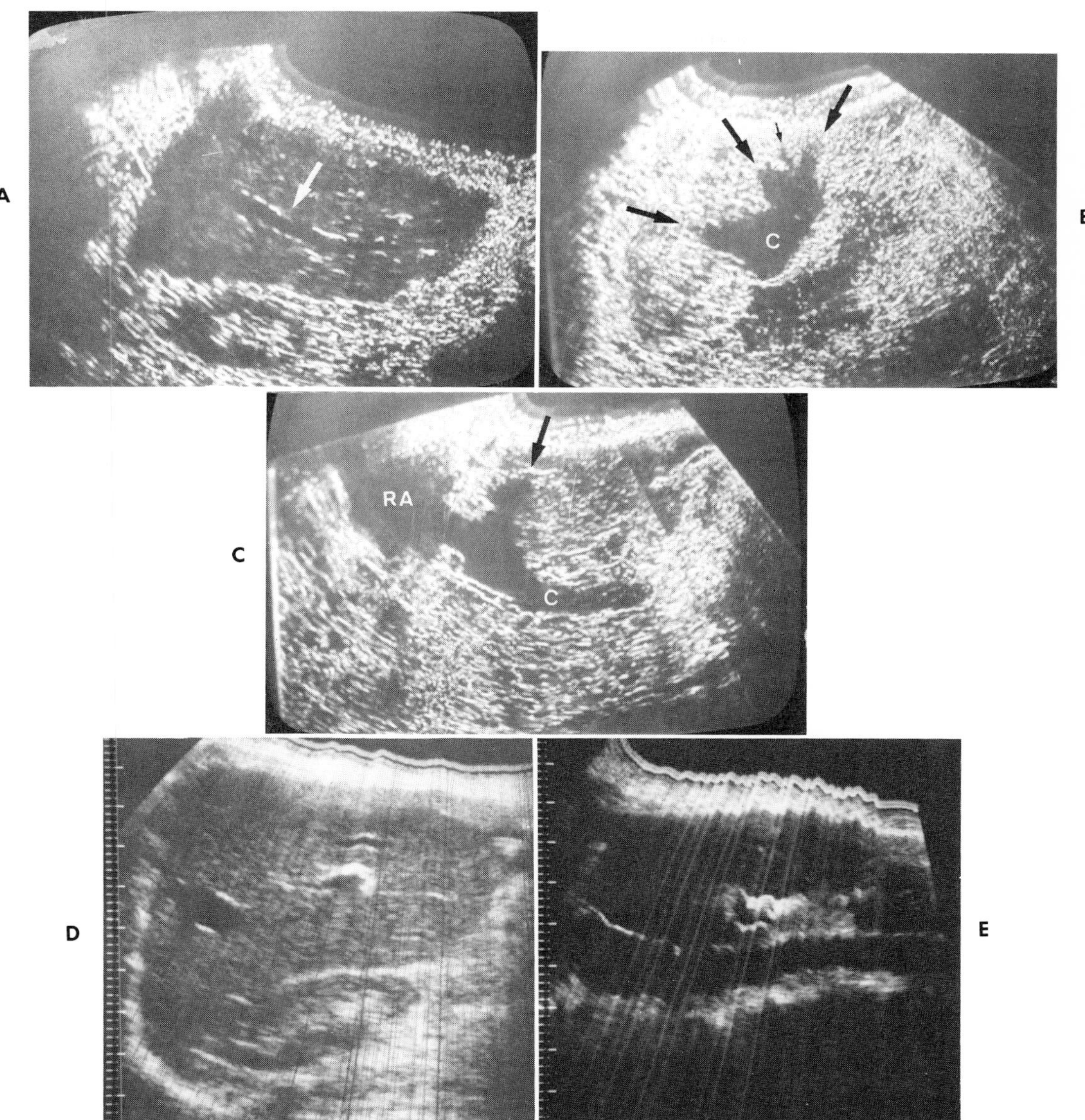

Fig. 7-8. Cardiac liver. **A,** Sagittal scan. Liver is massively enlarged, extending far below right kidney. There is dilated hepatic vein *(arrow)*. **B,** Oblique recurrent scan displays enlarged vena cava *(C)* and its junction with dilated hepatic veins *(arrows)*. **C,** Sagittal scan, more medial than that in **A,** passes through dilated vena cava and junction with hepatic veins *(arrow)*. Intrathoracic segment of vena cava, its junction with right atrium *(RA)*, and atrium itself, which is dilated, are clearly displayed. **D** and **E,** Enlarged liver with tricuspid regurgitation. Note pulsations of liver and dilated cava.

The different direct and indirect signs of cardiac liver are grouped below.

7:1 SIGNS OF CARDIAC LIVER

Hepatic sign: homogeneous hepatomegaly (with micronodulation in the chronic cardiac liver)

Extrahepatic signs
- Vena cava sign
- Dilatation of the hepatic veins and right atrium
- Possible pleural effusion
- Possible pericardial effusion

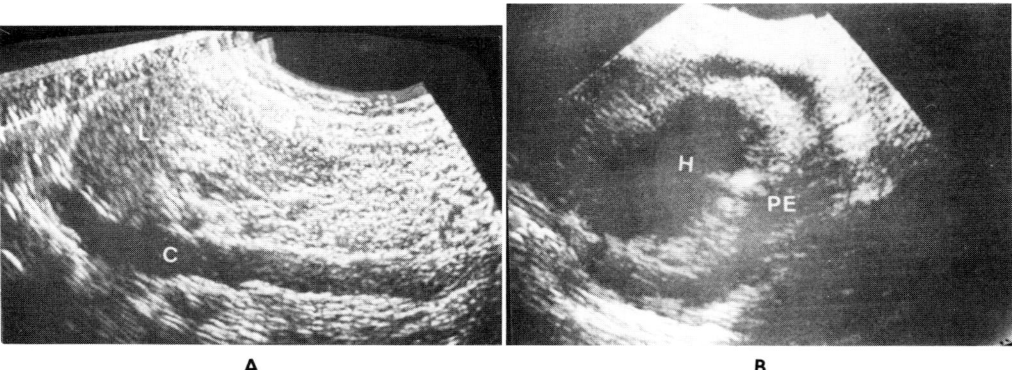

Fig. 7-9. Vena cava sign due to pericardial effusion. **A,** Sagittal display of enlarged vena cava *(C)*. **B,** Sagittal sector scan of heart *(H)* displays double wall image delineating pericardial effusion *(PE)*. Contact scanning display of pericardial effusion is possible only when effusion is very large. Usually it is much more easily and reliably displayed through real-time imaging. *L,* liver.

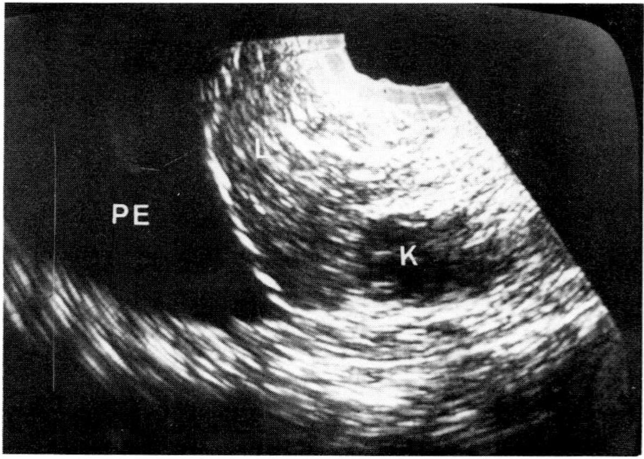

Fig. 7-10. Pleural effusion of cardiac origin. Liver clears the level of lower pole of right kidney *(K)*. Above diaphragm is typical liquid pattern of pleural effusion *(PE)*.

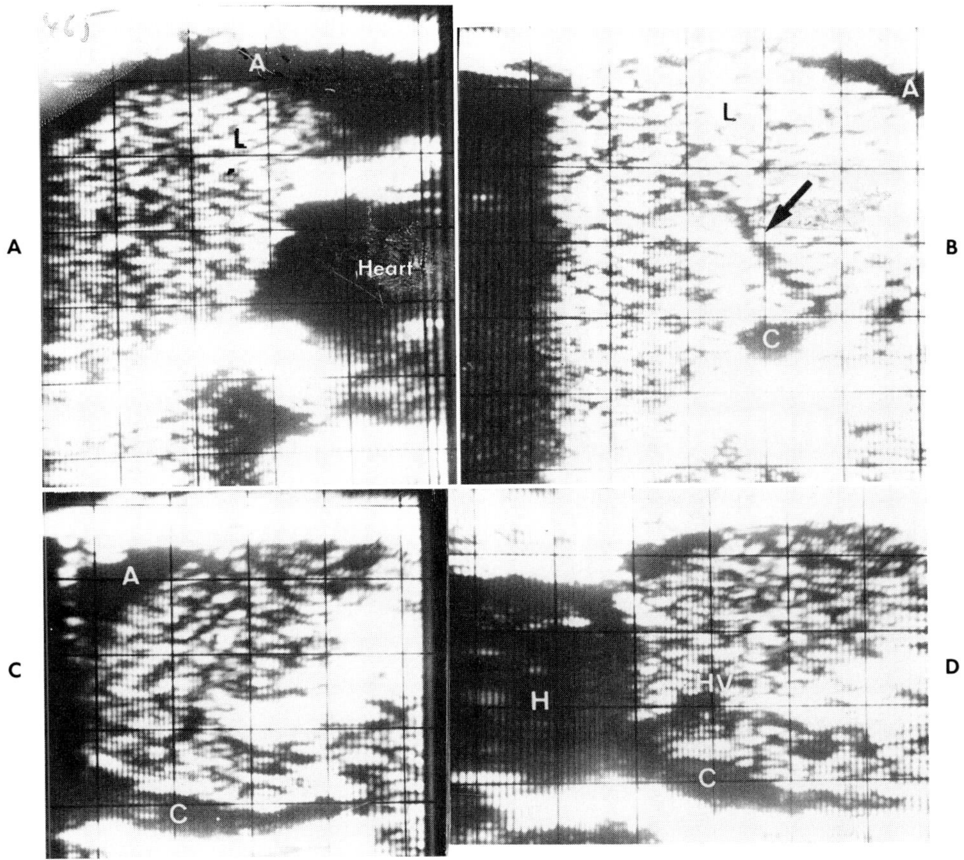

Fig. 7-11. Different scans performed on 8-year-old child, referred for abdominal examination because of edema in lower limbs. **A,** Oblique recurrent subcostal real-time scan of upper abdomen immediately shows sonolucent strip due to ascites *(A)* between liver *(L)* and anterior abdominal wall. This oblique recurrent scan passes through the heart. **B,** Another oblique recurrent scan showing ascitic fluid again between liver and anterior abdominal wall. This scan passes through vena cava *(C)* and hepatic vein *(arrow)*. **C,** Sagittal scan again showing ascitic fluid between liver and abdominal wall. Vena cava is dilated and has lost its respiratory variability. **D,** Another sagittal scan, displaying enlarged hepatic vein *(HV)*. Heart *(H)* is grossly enlarged. There is neither pleural nor pericardial effusion. The association of cardiomegaly, vena cava sign, and ascites is the expression of cardiac insufficiency, which had been overlooked in clinical examination.

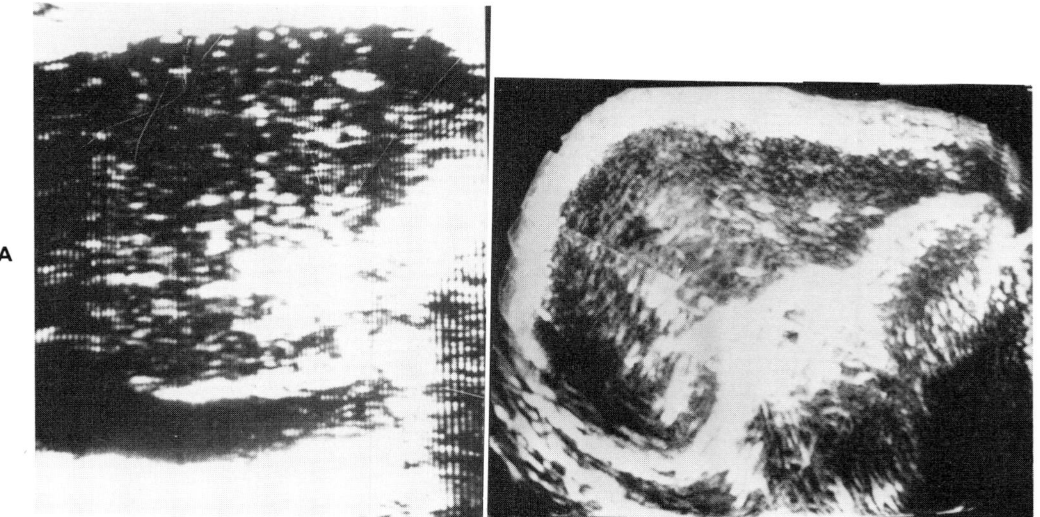

Fig. 7-12. Chronic cardiac liver. **A,** Sagittal scan of enlarged liver showing vena cava sign. Tissue echopattern is abnormal; it displays micronodular reflective pattern. Inferior edge of liver is biconvex, but not frankly rounded. **B,** Another example of chronic cardiac liver, on transverse scan, again with micronodular tissue echopattern. Note, on posterior aspect of liver, normal preaortic elevation.

HEPATITIS

In acute hepatitis there are no signs other than hepatomegaly (Fig. 7-13). The attenuation is normal. In chronic hepatitis there are increased attenuation and micronodulation (Fig. 7-14). Similar changes are encountered in cirrhosis (Chapter 10). These changes may occur very early. We had the opportunity to observe an example of an obviously increased attenuation, which had not existed previously, as early as the sixth week. Hepatitis will be discussed in Chapter 26, concerning jaundice, and in Chapter 19, about acute pancreatitis, since a transitory enlargement of the pancreas is not an uncommon feature during hepatitis. The nature of the histological changes in the pancreas during hepatitis is not known. Nonetheless, the pancreatic enlargement is an objective feature, and follow-up examinations show its rapid decrease. An inflammatory pancreatic enlargement may thus be considered an associated sign in acute hepatitis. This fact has also been reported by Rabsch and Rettenmaier (1975).

OTHER NONSPECIFIC HEPATOMEGALIES

I shall not enumerate all the causes of hepatomegaly, which a well-trained resident should know by heart. Nonspecific hepatomegaly will again be encountered in the early stage of cirrhosis (Chapter 10), as well as in some cases of lymphoma with abdominal involvement (Chapter 8). Since the origins of a nonspecific hepatomegaly are diverse, the search for associated signs is always important: not only caval enlargement or pericardial effusion but also splenomegaly, retroperito-

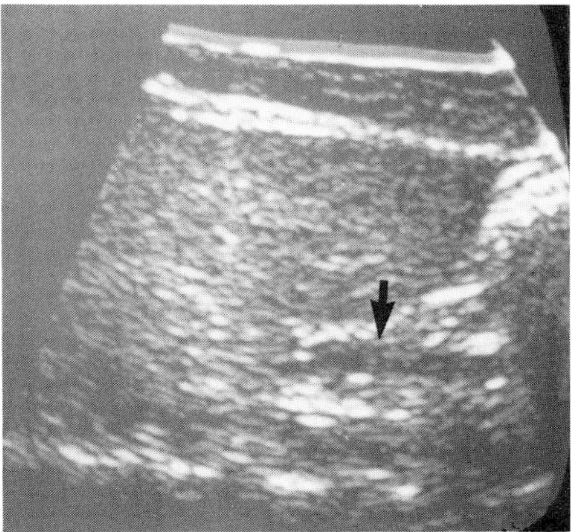

Fig. 7-13. Recent hepatitis: hepatomegaly. This sagittal scan passes through mesenteric-portal junction *(arrow)* and left margin of aorta. Inferior marginal angle is increased (80 degrees). Tissue echopattern is homogeneous.

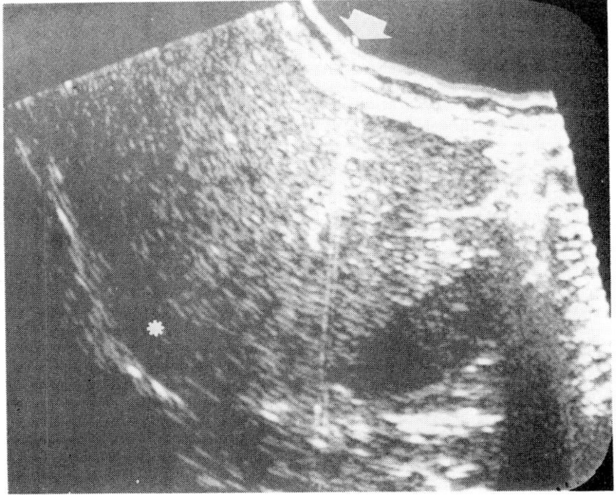

Fig. 7-14. Less recent hepatitis: persistent hepatomegaly (*arrow,* costal edge) a few months after acute phase. Attenuation is frankly increased in deeper part of liver (*). This indicates developing fibrosis. Rounded shape of inferior hepatic edge is due to contact scanning artifact.

A

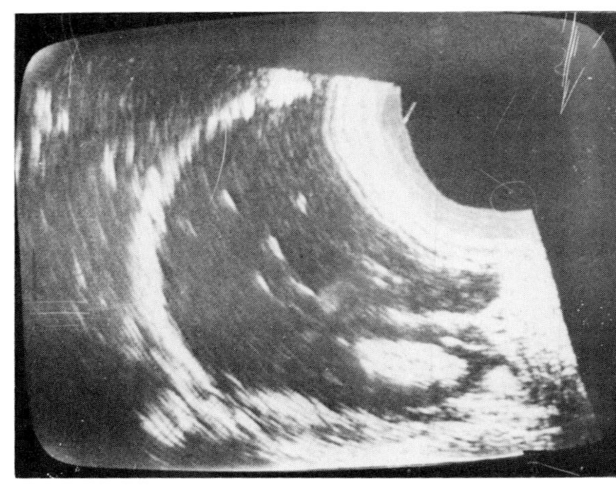

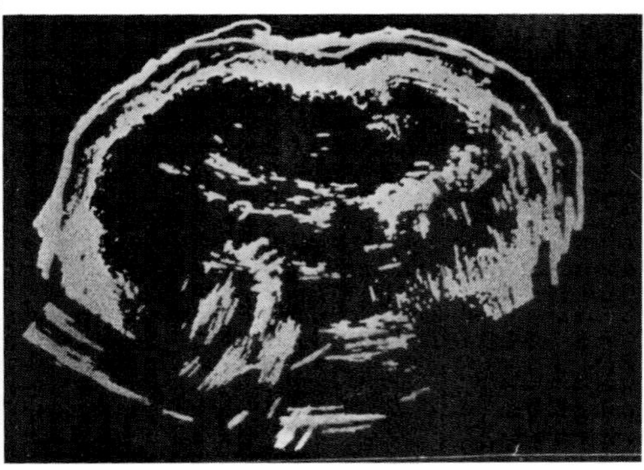

B

Fig. 7-15. Nonspecific hepatomegaly: amyloidosis due to chronic tuberculosis. **A,** Sagittal scan. Tissular echopattern remains homogeneous. **B,** Transverse scan displaying tangent sign at the level of left hepatic lobe.

neal lymph nodes, ascites, and other such symptoms. Fig. 7-15 shows an example of nonspecific hepatomegaly due to amyloidosis.

What is nonspecific for the radiologist is usually quite specific for the pathologist. In concluding this chapter, I should like to remind you of ultrasonically guided needle puncture.

REFERENCES

Barnett, E., and Morley, P.: Abdominal echography, Borough Green, England, 1974, Butterworth & Co. (Publishers), Ltd.

Goldberg, B. B., Kotler, M. N., Ziskin, M. C., and Waxham, R. D.: Diagnostic uses of ultrasound, New York, 1975, Grune & Stratton, Inc.

Hassani, N.: Ultrasonography of the abdomen, Heidelberg, Germany, 1976, Springer-Verlag.

Holm, H. H., Kristensen, J. K., Rasmussen, S. N., Pedersen, J. F., and Hancke, S.: Abdominal ultrasound, Copenhagen, 1976, Munksgaard, International Booksellers & Publishers, Ltd.

Leopold, G. R., and Asher, W. M.: Fundamentals of abdominal and pelvic ultrasonography, Philadelphia, 1975, W. B. Saunders Co.

Rabsch, U., and Rettenmaier, G.: Sonographically found asymptomatic enlargement of the pancreas in viral hepatitis and pneumonia, Second Congress of European Ultrasonics in Medicine, Munich, Germany, 1975, Abstract No. 100.

Taylor, K. J., Carpenter, D. A., and McCready, V. R.: Grey scale echography in the diagnosis of intrahepatic disease, J. Clin. Ultrasound **1:**284-287, 1973.

Weill, F., Becker, J. C., Kraehenbuhi, J. R., Heriot, G., and Walter, J. P.: Clinical atlas of ultrasonic radiography, Paris, 1973, Masson & Cie., Editeurs.

Weill, F., and Maurat, J. P.: The sign of the vena cava: echotomographic illustration of the right cardiac insufficiency, J. Clin. Ultrasound **2:**27-32, 1974.

Winsberg, F.: Personal communication, 1977.

CHAPTER 8

METASTASES

Although hepatic metastases are usually multinodular, solitary nodules also occur. Some multiple nodules may be so small that their juxtaposition produces an infiltrative pattern. Because of this proteiform morphological appearance, it is indispensable to have many hepatic scans at one's disposal and to analyze them carefully. The diagnosis of metastases is based on two kinds of pathological features, either contour abnormalities or textural tissue echo abnormalities.

FUNDAMENTAL SIGNS

Changes in contours

Hump sign. Superficial metastases produce small localized convex elevations on the surface of the liver and thus on sections of the hepatic contours (Fig. 8-1). Such "hump" images must be considered pathological, even if there is no obvious associated change in the tissue echopattern, except in the diaphragmatic area, where contour deformities may exist in a normal subject. Diaphragmatic humps must be considered only with associated tissue echopattern changes. When a hump sign is recorded, it is, of course, necessary to exclude anatomical humps,* which have already been discussed in Chapter 6.

Edge sign. The section of the inferior edge of the gland and the section of the lateral margin of the left lobe usually show an angular aspect (Chapter 6). In most benign hepatomegalies this angular aspect is not modified, whereas in metastatic hepatomegaly the hepatic edge may become rounded, convex (Fig. 8-2), and even polycyclic if humps are associated with the primary deformity (Fig. 8-3). To these signs, which are specific for metastatic deposits, may, of course, be added the signs described in Chapter 7, concerning hepatomegaly itself, that is, the angle and the tangent signs, since the liver is frequently enlarged.

Modifications of the echopattern

Sonolucent areas. Nodular metastases may appear as rounded translucent areas, which stand out clearly against the homogeneous and rich echopattern of the normal hepatic tissue (Fig. 8-4). This type of sonolucent change can be termed *sieve pattern* if nodules are scattered amid the hepatic parenchyma. Only rarely are liver metastases purely sonolucent. Some of these zones of diminished reflectivity may take on a frankly liquid (sonotransparent) pattern when there is necrosis of the metastatic tissue (Fig. 8-5, *A*), particularly after chemotherapy or radiotherapy.

Areas of increased reflection. Much more commonly the metastatic echopattern

*Subcostal elevation, caudate lobe, and suprarenal and preaortic elevations.

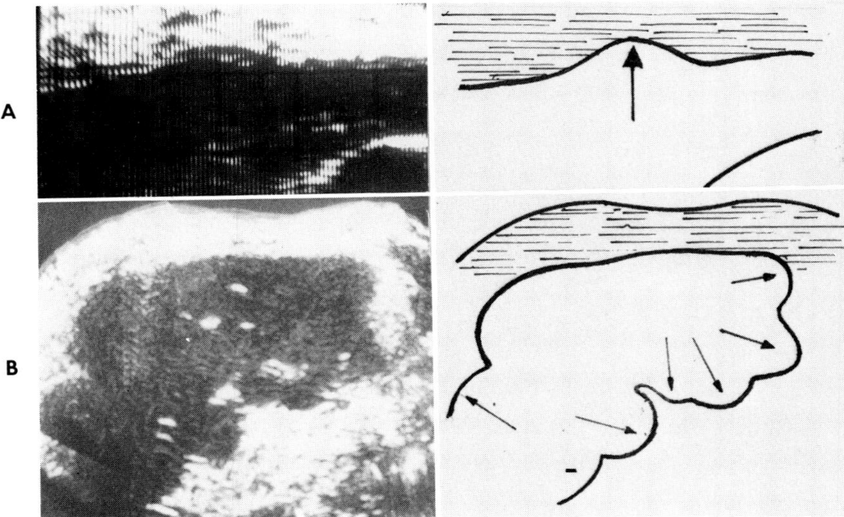

Fig. 8-1. Hump sign. **A,** Anterior hump *(arrow).* **B,** Posterior and lateral humps *(arrows).*

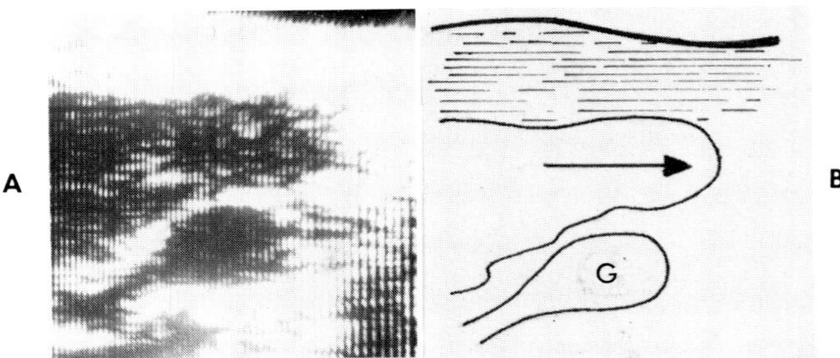

Fig. 8-2. Edge sign. **A,** Inferior margin is rounded and convex. **B,** Schematic representation of **A.** *Arrow,* inferior edge; *G,* gallbladder.

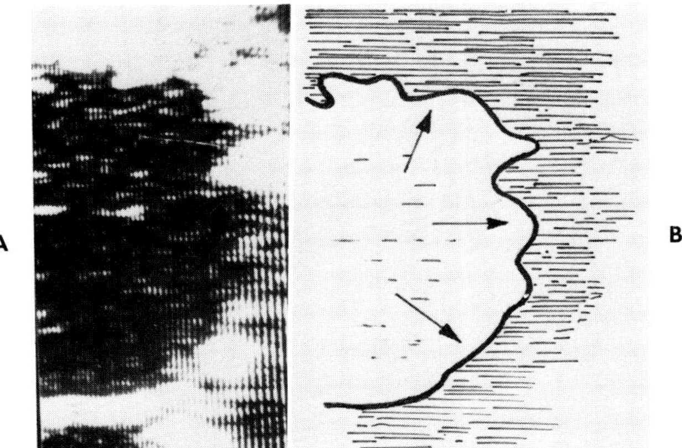

Fig. 8-3. Association of humps *(arrows)* with caricatural edge sign. **A,** Scan. **B,** Schematic drawing of **A.**

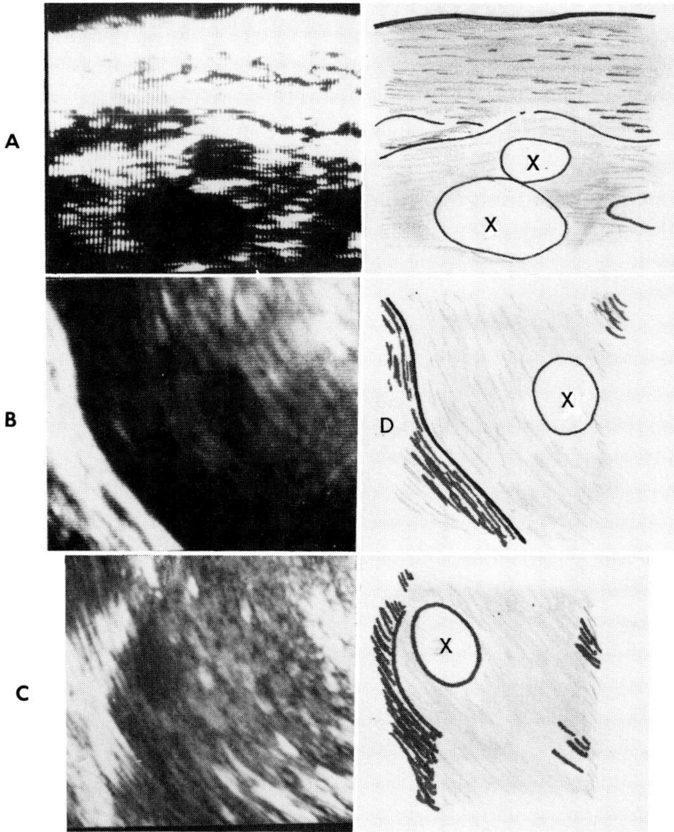

Fig. 8-4. Sonolucent nodules *(X).* **A,** Real-time display. **B** and **C,** Contact scanning gray scale display. In **C,** note convex deformation (associated hump sign) of diaphragm *(D).* Presence of multiple sonolucent areas of this type constitutes what is called *sieve pattern.*

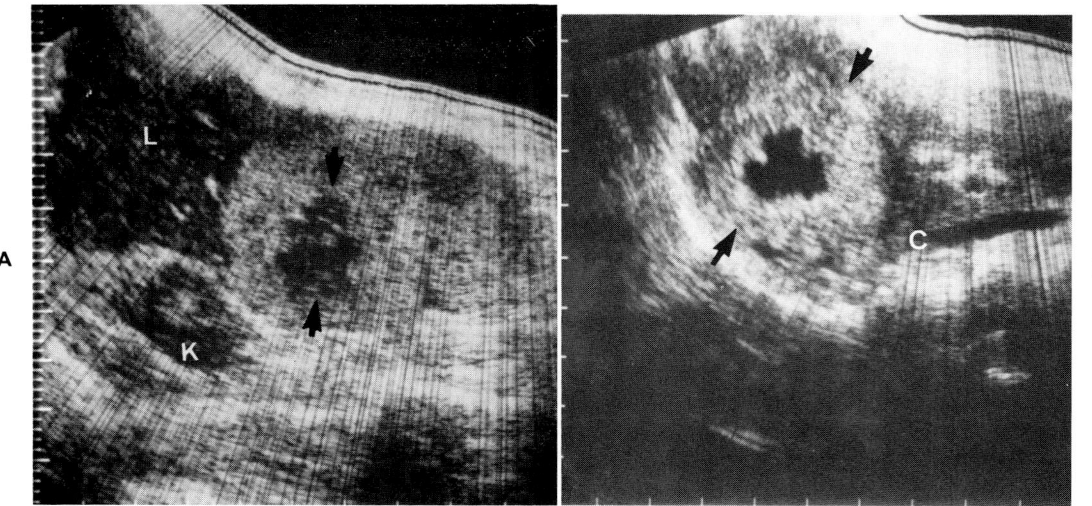

Fig. 8-5. Necrotized metastases. **A,** Sagittal scan of liver displaying transparent zone of necrosis *(arrows)* with debris amid reflective area. Note caudal field of diffuse increased reflectivity. *L,* liver; *K,* kidney. **B,** Sagittal scan of another patient showing rounded reflective nodule of large diameter *(arrows)* with central necrosis. In this case, necrotized area has almost liquid echopattern. Well-delineated, irregular limits and necrotized debris, as in **A,** are typical for necrosis. *C,* cava.

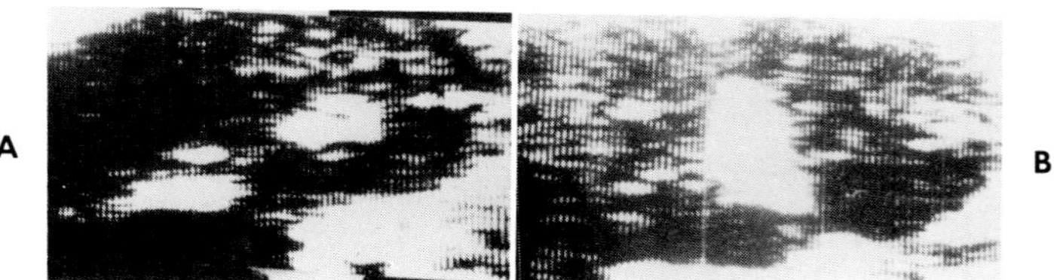

Fig. 8-6. Reflective nodules. Note presence in **A** of associated edge sign and in **B** of associated humps. Multiple reflective nodules of this type constitute what is called *hailstorm pattern.*

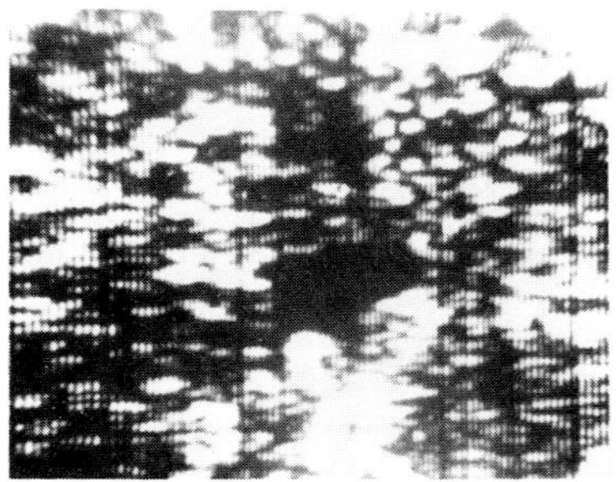

Fig. 8-7. Association of reflective nodules with sonolucent nodules, constituting mottled pattern.

is made up of nodular elements of increased reflectivity (Fig. 8-6). Such reflective nodules, if surrounded by sonolucent tissue, may give rise to a "bull's-eye pattern" (Fig. 8-12). The very heterogeneous pattern caused by multiple reflective nodules is called the *hailstorm pattern.* Another pattern is increased reflectivity in fields (Fig. 8-5, *A*).

Composite images. Areas of both increased and decreased reflection may be associated and form an extremely heterogeneous echopattern called a *mottled pattern* (Fig. 8-7).

Discussion

Hump sign. I call to your attention, once again, the normal elevations, that is, the subcostal elevation, caudate lobe, and suprarenal and preaortic elevations. A caudate lobe and subcostal and infrarenal elevations will again be seen in Figs. 8-8 to 8-10. Since diaphragmatic humps are not an uncommon feature on a chest film, humps in that area that are displayed on ultrasonograms are not, as previously stated, consistently pathological.

Edge sign. First, remember the area of insertion of the falciform ligament. Besides, a well-marked infrarenal elevation may bulge very close to the inferior hepatic edge and give rise to a localized false edge sign. Also, in some nonspecific hepatomegalies the surfaces of the liver may become slightly convex, giving the liver edge a somewhat less angular appearance (Fig. 10-2); but this type of edge deformity is quite different from the frankly rounded border produced by metastases.

Lucent and transparent areas. On some oblique recurrent sections, the gallbladder (Chapter 15), which is displayed as a rounded sonotransparent area, may seem to be situated within the hepatic parenchyma. As a matter of fact, this is an anatomical image that, as soon as it becomes familiar, cannot be confused with a

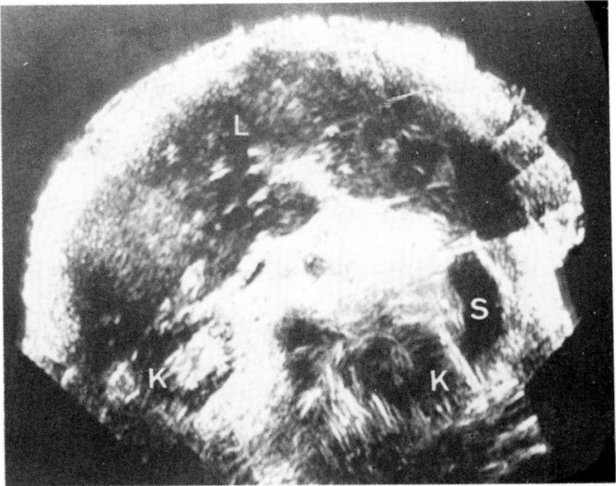

Fig. 8-8. Caricatural metastatic hepatomegaly. Left hepatic lobe is so enlarged that it extends laterally between anterior limit of spleen *(S)* and lateral abdominal wall. There is left edge sign associated with small humps. General echopattern is of hailstorm type. *L,* liver; *K,* kidneys.

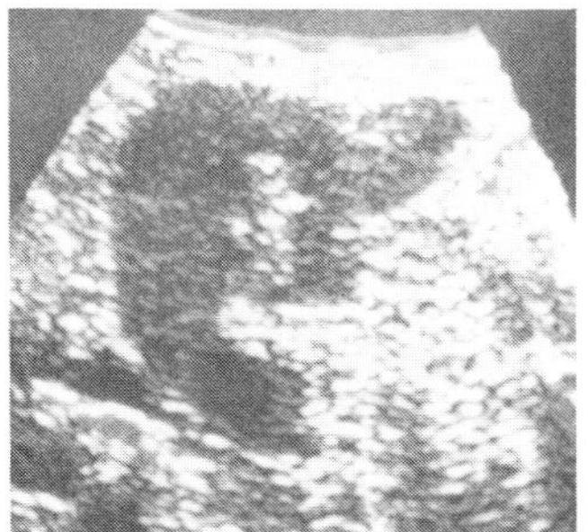

Fig. 8-9. Normal hump of caudate lobe.

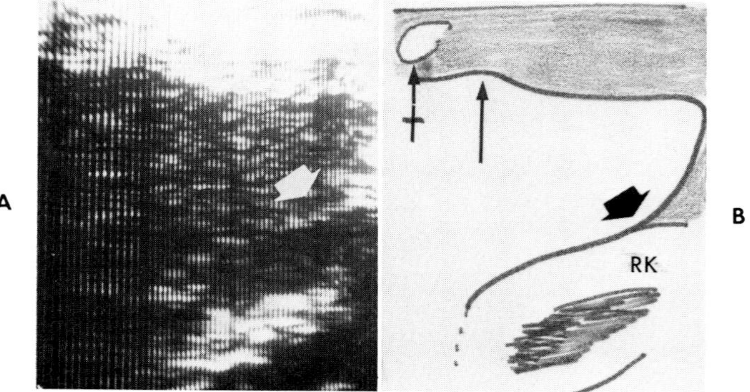

Fig. 8-10. Sagittal scan, **A,** and schematic representation, **B,** displaying two normal convexities: subcostal elevation *(arrow)* and posterior convexity *(broad arrows)* above lower pole of right kidney *(RK)*. *Arrowhead,* last rib.

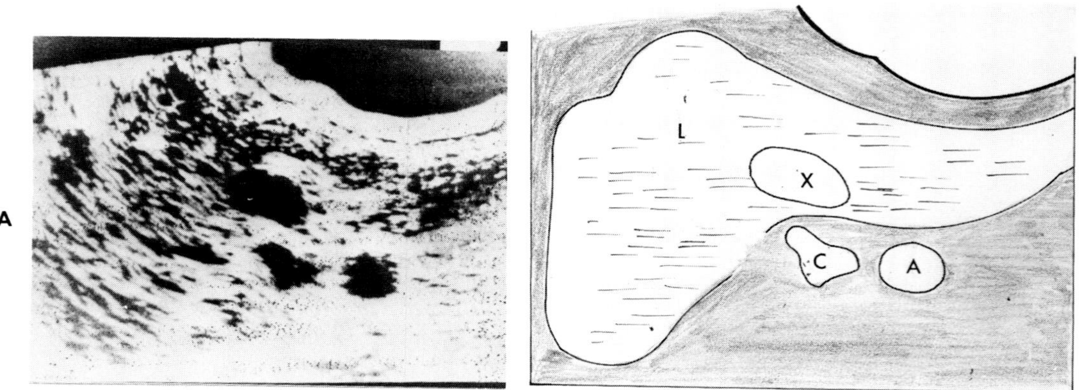

Fig. 8-11. Sonolucent nodule *(X)* in front of vena cava *(C)*. This image does not belong to gallbladder. It probably represents hepatic venous network. **A,** Scan. **B,** Schematic drawing of **A.** (See also Fig. 12-1.) *A,* aorta; *L,* liver.

pathological feature. If necessary, a contraction test will remove all doubts. Another image of about the same type may give rise to a problem. We have twice encountered within the hepatic parenchyma, in front of the vena cava, a well-delineated sonotransparent image (Fig. 8-11). This rounded structure moved with respiration and was evident on sagittal scans. There was no duplication of the vena cava, and the possibility of a simple gallbladder image had, of course, been ruled out. To clarify the nature of these images we undertook certain investigations (scintigraphic and angiographic), the results of which were all normal, and follow-

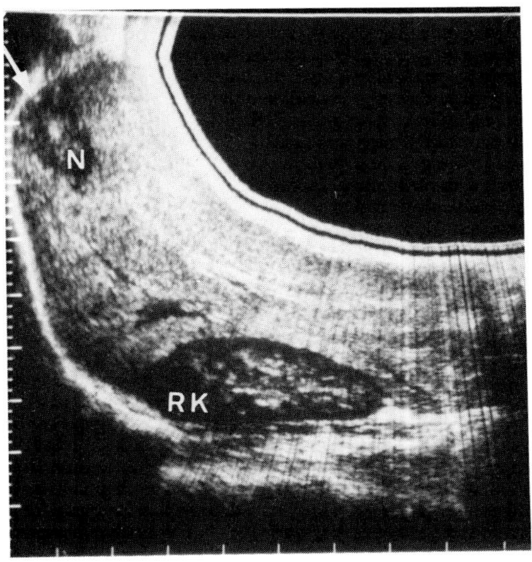

Fig. 8-12. Solitary bull's-eye nodule *(N)* displayed on sagittal scan. Nodule gives rise to diaphragmatic hump *(arrow)*. *RK*, right kidney.

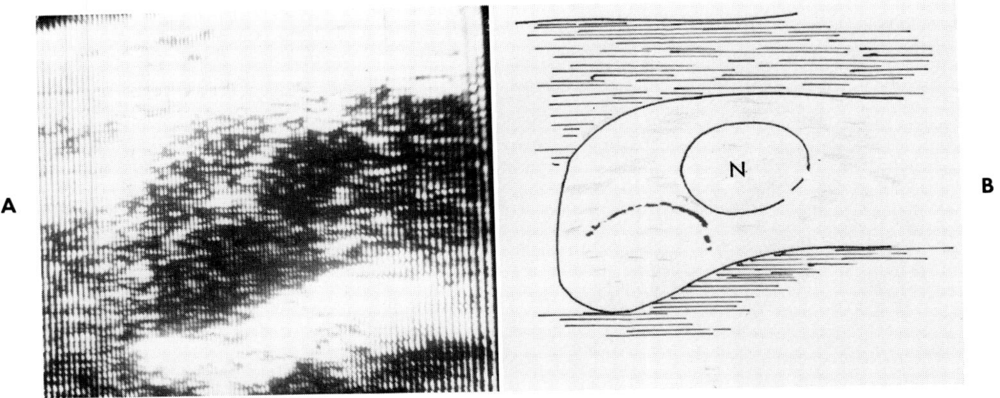

Fig. 8-13. Two localized solitary nodules *(N)* shown on intercostal scan, **A,** and schematic drawing, **B.**

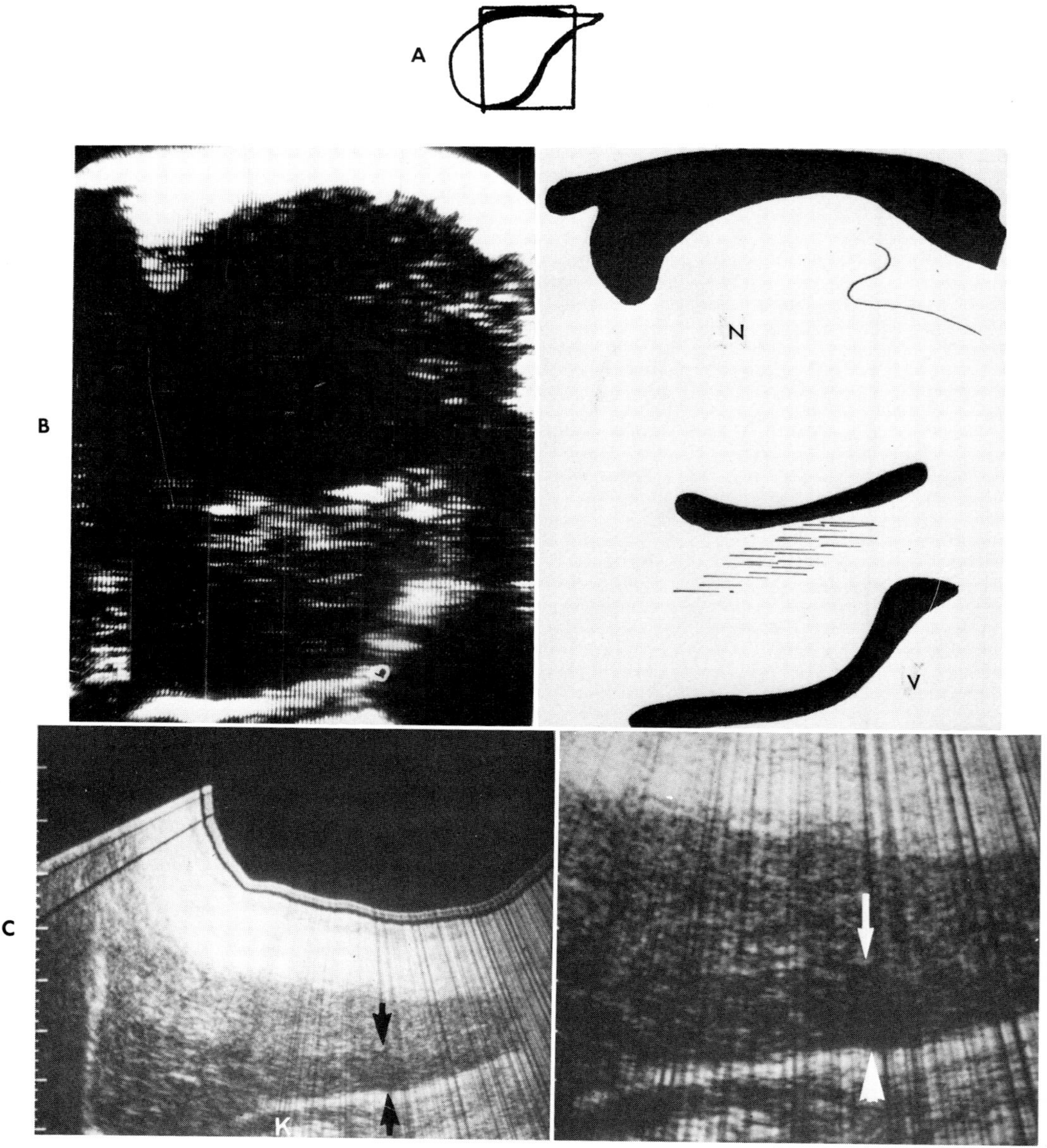

Fig. 8-14. A, Schematic drawing showing area of liver presented in **B. B,** Large solitary sonolucent anterior nodule *(N)* displayed on oblique recurrent subcostal real-time scan (left) and schematic representation (right). *V,* vertebral column. **C,** Enlarged liver with small, sonolucent solitary nodule *(arrows)*—metastatic deposit of breast cancer—displayed on sagittal scans. *K,* kidney.

up of the patients showed no change after two years. We believe that the most probable explanation is ectasis of the terminal segment of the hepatic veins before their junction with the vena cava.

Reflective areas

As already seen in Chapter 6, for lack of dynamic imaging, some vascular tubular structures may give rise to pseudonodular images: this hazard was a serious one only with bistable imaging. Bull's-eye nodules are rather specific.

DIFFERENT ULTRASONIC TYPES OF HEPATIC METASTASES

Solitary nodules

When solitary nodules are located superficially, they produce modifications of contours, such as a localized hump sign (Fig. 8-12) or a localized edge sign (Fig. 8-2). These solitary nodules produce chiefly localized changes in the echopattern, such as an isolated sonolucent area (Figs. 8-13 and 8-14), or, on the contrary, an isolated area of increased or modified reflectivity (Fig. 8-15).

Multiple nodules

In cases involving multiple nodules, humps, marginal deformations, and multiple alterations of the echopattern are associated with hepatomegaly (Figs. 8-8 and 8-16 to 8-23).

Text continued on p. 126.

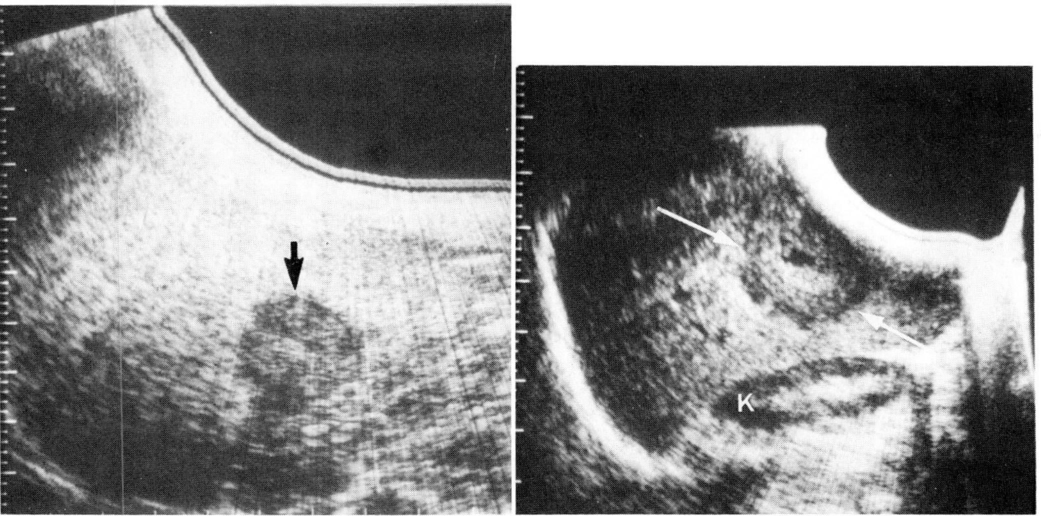

Fig. 8-15. A and **B,** Solitary nodules *(arrows)* of "bull's-eye" type seen in two different patients. *K,* kidney.

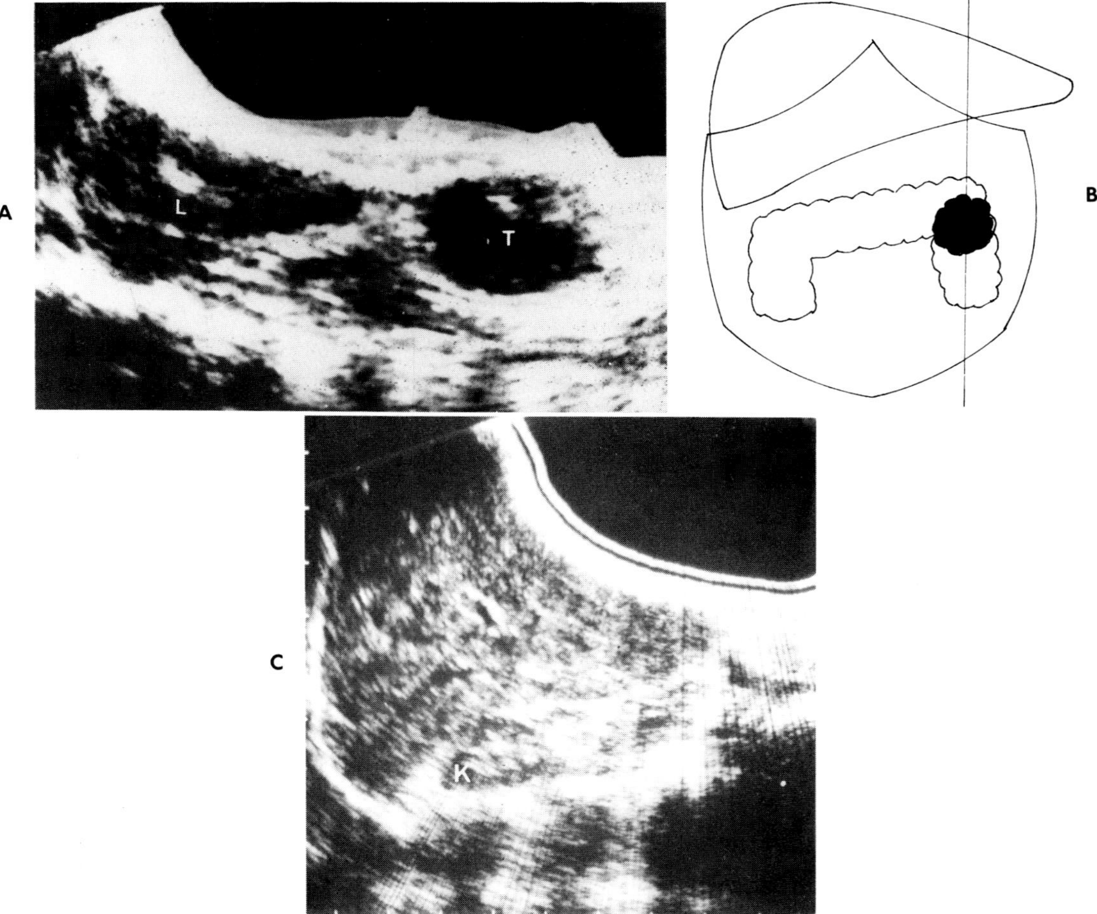

Fig. 8-16. Mottled pattern. **A,** Sagittal scan of left upper quadrant displaying enlarged left hepatic lobe *(L)* with mottled tissue echopattern. This section passes through primary tumor *(T)* of colonic origin. **B,** Scanning plane used in **A.** *Black area,* colonic tumor. **C,** Sagittal scan of another patient showing reflective bull's-eye and sonolucent nodules in right lobe of liver. *K,* right kidney.

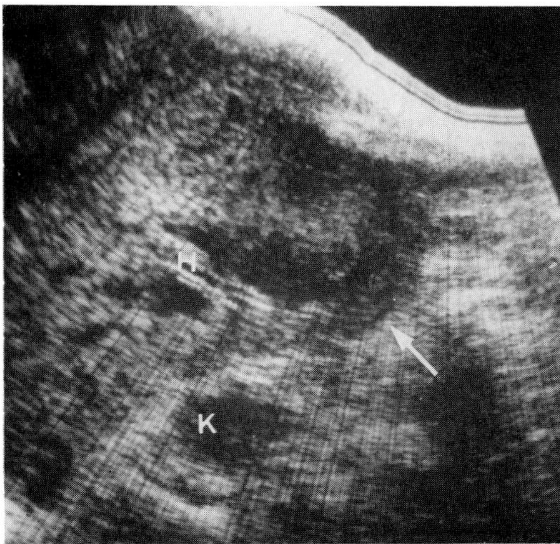

Fig. 8-17. Sagittal scan in a case of hepatomegaly accompanying gastric carcinoma. There is inferior angle sign, pathological posterior hump *(arrow)*, several sonolucent areas, and reflective area near hilus *(H)* constituting mottled pattern. *K*, kidney.

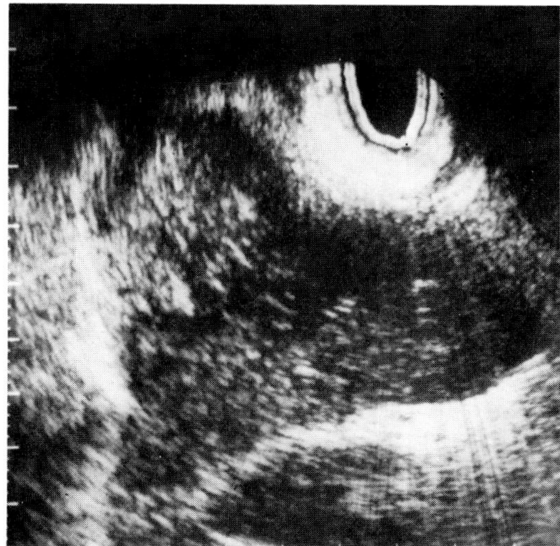

Fig. 8-18. Metastatic hepatomegaly. Sagittal scan of right hepatic lobe displays multiple reflective nodules constituting hailstorm pattern. There are diaphragmatic humps.

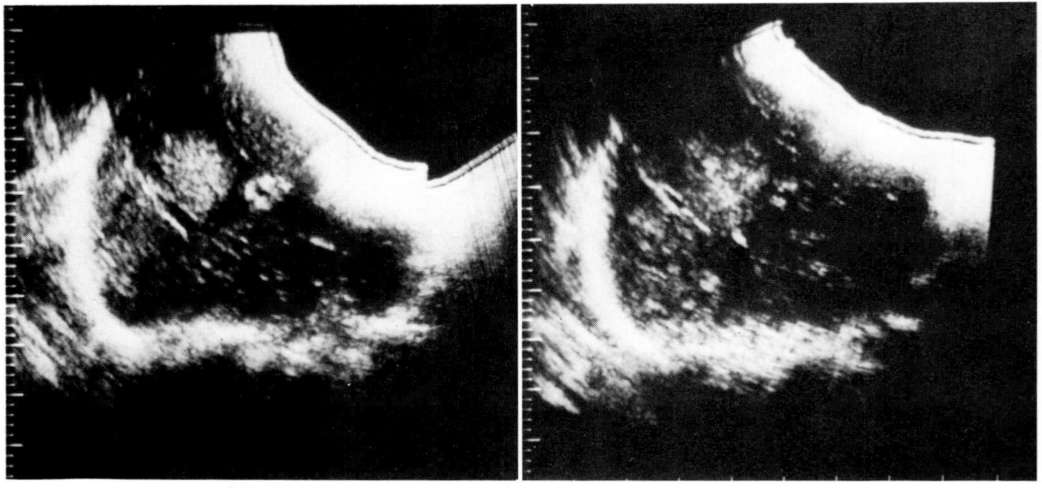

Fig. 8-19. Metastatic hepatomegaly. These two sagittal scans display reflective nodules of hailstorm pattern, inferior angle sign, edge sign, and humps.

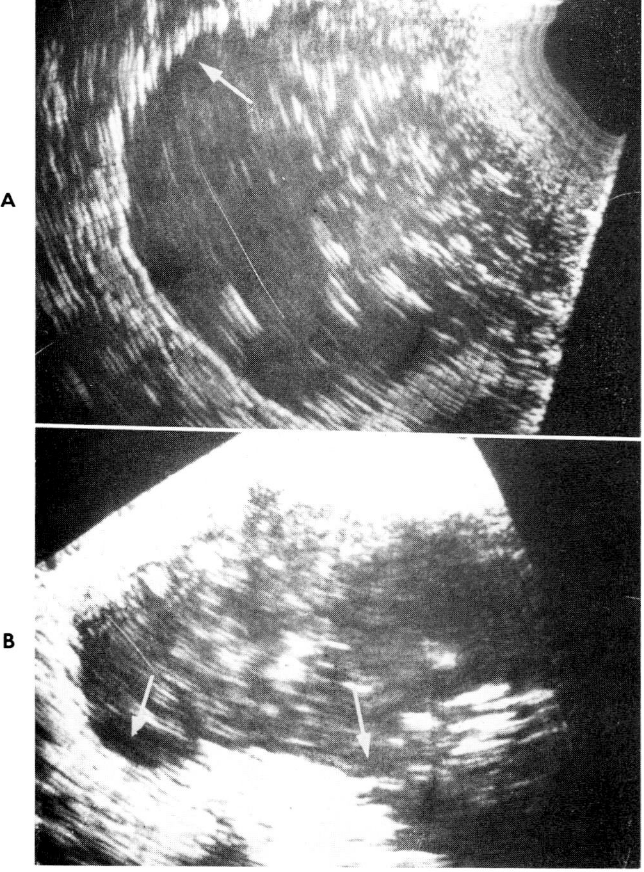

Fig. 8-20. Metastatic hepatomegaly. **A,** Sagittal scan displaying frank angle and edge signs. There are diaphragmatic humps *(arrow).* Echopattern is of hailstorm type. **B,** Intercostal scan also displaying frank humps *(arrows)* and hailstorm pattern.

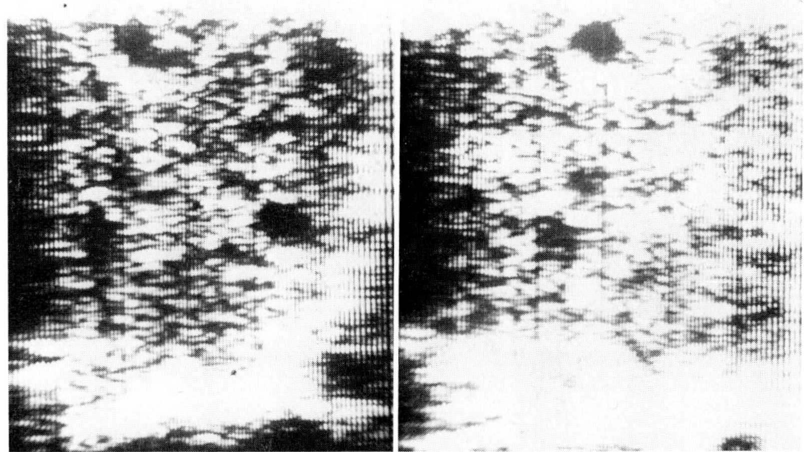

Fig. 8-21. Sieve pattern. These multiple sonolucent nodules belong to deposits of a melanosarcoma, rather typical in this type of tumor.

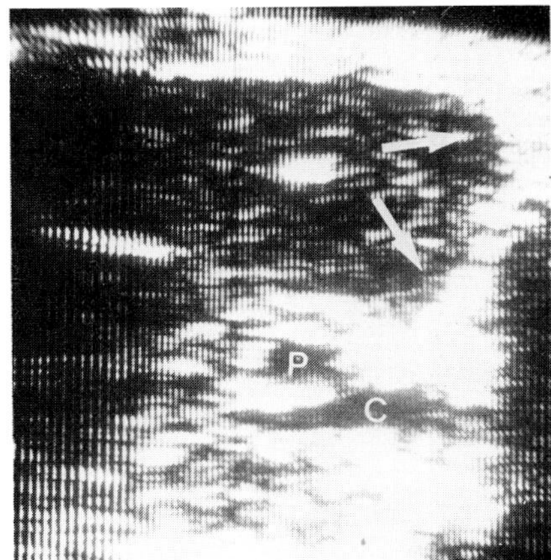

Fig. 8-22. Sagittal scan of right hepatic lobe, passing through vena cava *(C)* and portal vein *(P)*. Edge sign is associated with angle sign, humps *(arrows)*, and hailstorm pattern.

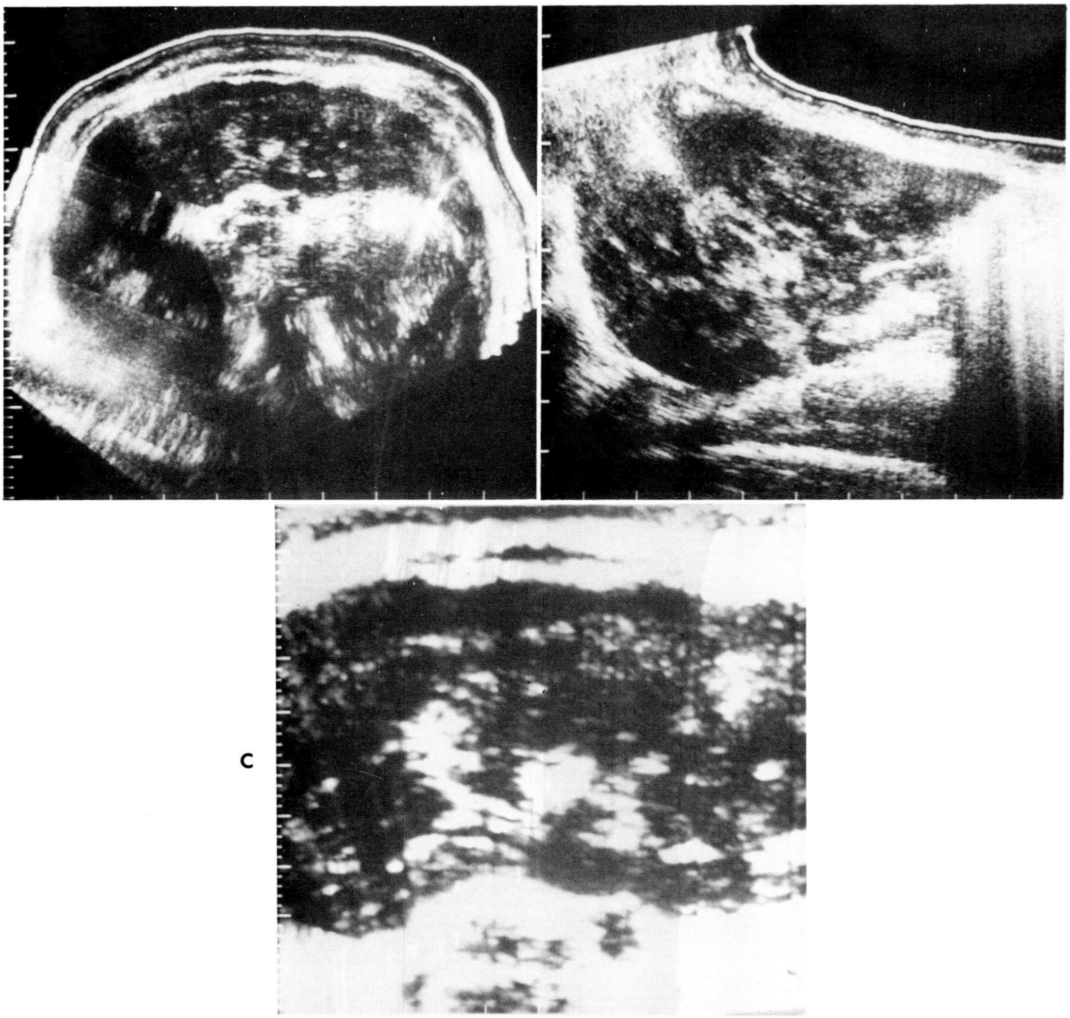

A

B

C

Fig. 8-23. Metastatic deposits of breast carcinoma, associating hepatomegaly, humps, and hailstorm pattern. **A,** Transverse scan. **B,** Sagittal scan. **C,** Magnification.

Infiltrative processes

Increased reflectivity in fields or very small nodules lead to very discrete modifications in the echopattern. The presence of a hump sign or of an edge sign may then constitute the only reliable indication (Figs. 8-24 to 8-26).

HISTOLOGICAL CORRELATION

It would be deceptive to try to make a histological diagnosis based on the morphological analysis of the tissue echopattern. The only consistent pattern we have observed is the multinodular and sonolucent pattern of the metastases in melanoma (Fig. 8-21). Metastases from renal or breast carcinomas are usually

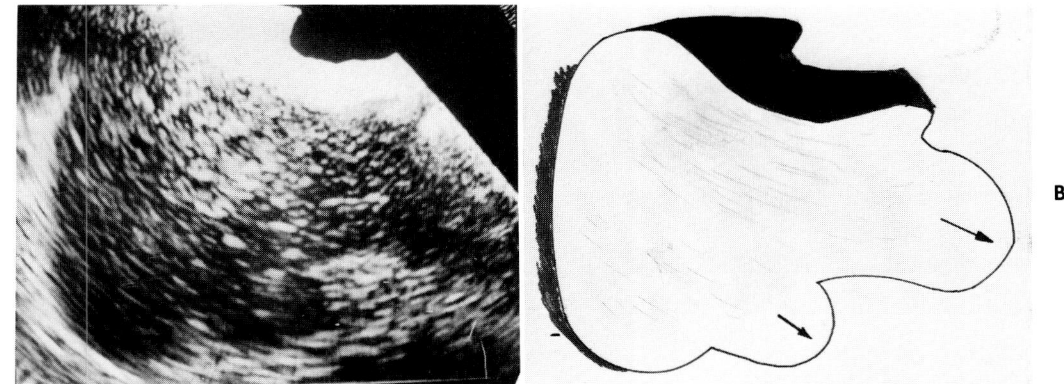

Fig. 8-24. Infiltrative pattern displayed on sagittal scan, **A,** and schematic drawing, **B.** There are only small micronodular and infiltrative changes. Posterior humps are obvious, however.

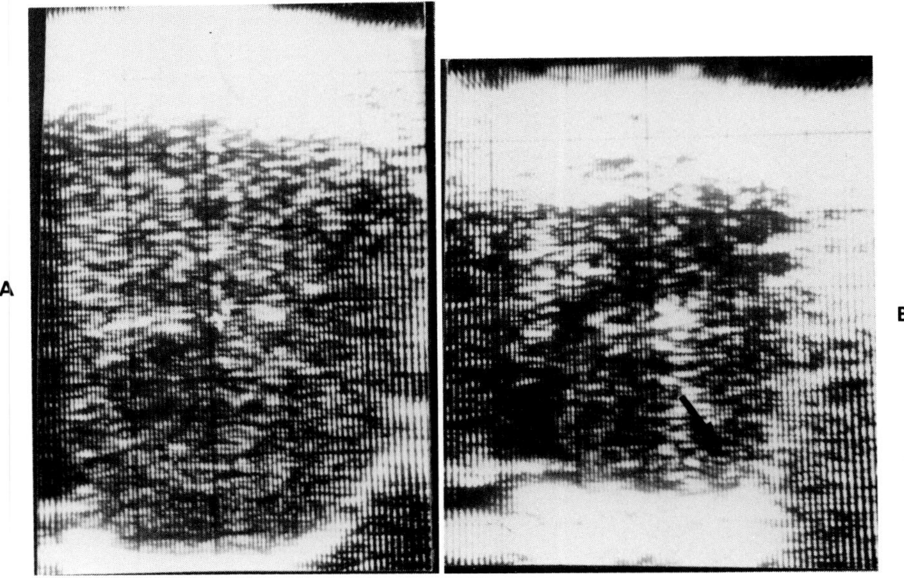

Fig. 8-25. Infiltrative pattern. **A,** Oblique subcostal recurrent scan displaying only micronodular changes. **B,** Sagittal scan of left hepatic lobe showing more typical echopattern changes, with reflective and sonolucent nodules. There is frank angle sign and quite obvious hump sign.

reflecting nodules (hailstorm pattern), but this pattern is far from being specific. Simultaneous discovery of the hepatic metastatic deposits and the primary tumor is an easier way to histological correlation—as a matter of fact, rather often the same liver scan displays both the metastases and a renal or colonic carcinoma (Fig. 8-16, *A*).

I have already pointed out that the ultrasonic investigation is never purely hepatic, but rather of the whole upper abdomen, including the spleen and retroperi-

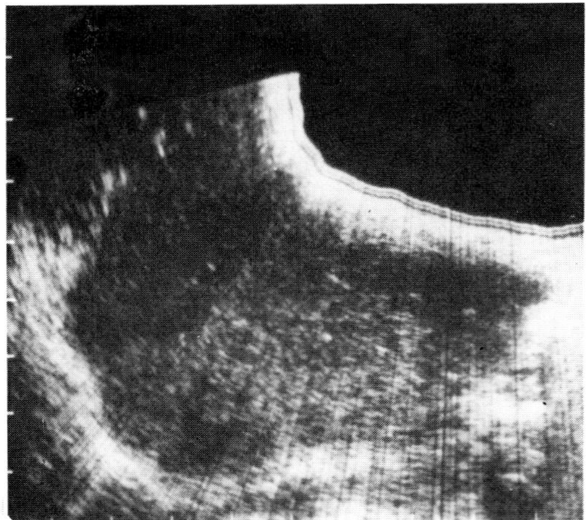

Fig. 8-26. Infiltrative pattern. There is field of increased reflectivity with moderate echopattern changes except for few small sonolucent nodules. Note posterior and diaphragmatic humps.

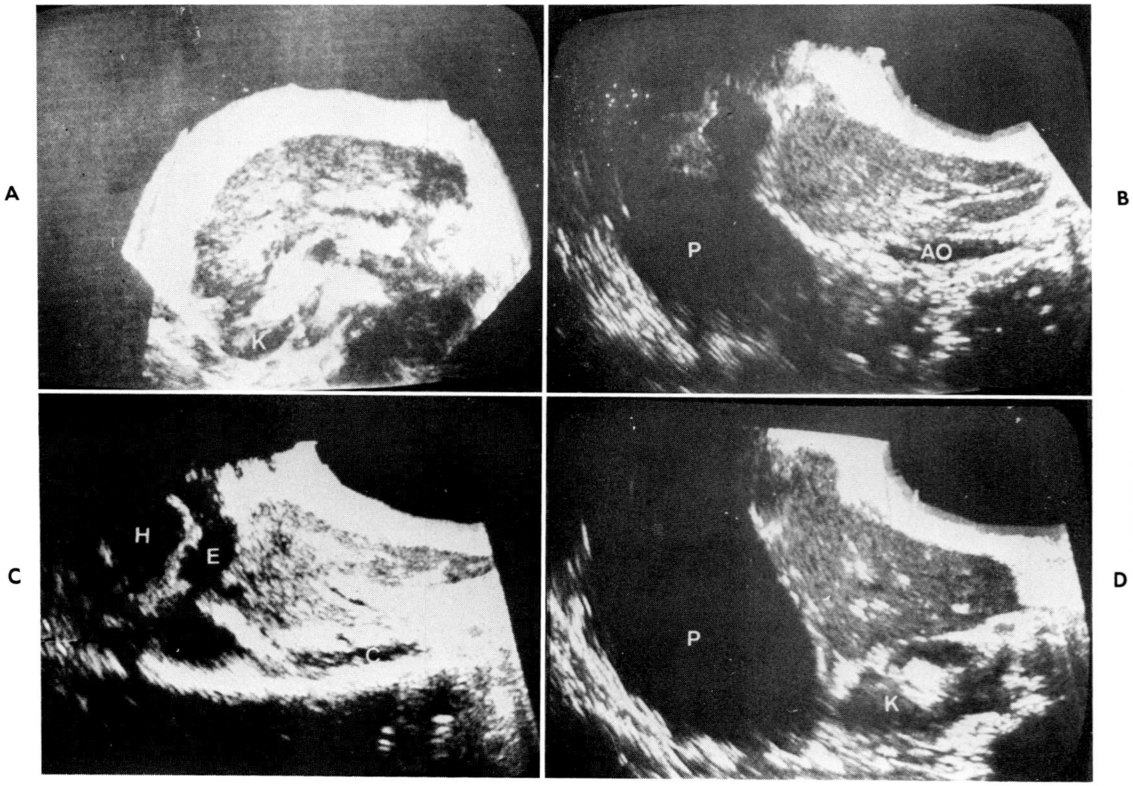

Fig. 8-27. Hepatomegaly due to lymphoma: associated signs. **A,** Transverse scan showing enlarged left hepatic lobe, tangent sign, and edge sign. **B,** Sagittal scan passing through aorta *(AO)* displays quite obvious hepatomegaly, with inferior edge sign. Above diaphragm is pleural effusion *(P)*. **C,** Sagittal scan passing through vena cava *(C)* displays heart *(H)*. There is double cardiac wall image, due to pericardial effusion *(E)*. **D,** Another sagittal scan displaying right kidney *(K)* again shows pleural effusion.

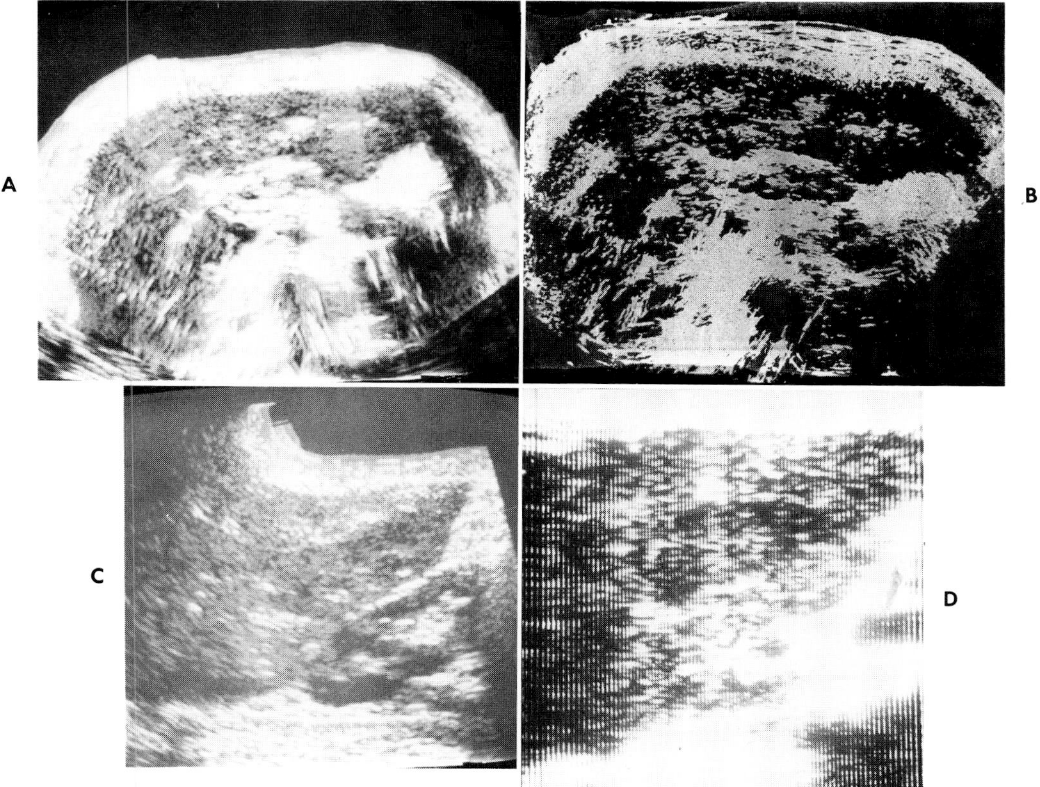

Fig. 8-28. Hepatomegaly in a case of acute myeloblastic leukemia. **A** and **B,** Transverse scans showing enlarged left hepatic lobe, with angle sign, edge sign, and multiple areas of abnormal reflection. **C,** Sagittal scan passing through right kidney displays mottled pattern. **D,** Real-time display better showing mottled pattern with oval bull's-eye nodule.

toneum. This allows one to record associated signs that are particularly important in lymphomas.

Lymphomas

Hepatic signs. In some cases, nonspecific hepatomegaly is the only hepatic sign with lymphomas. In such cases the hepatic margins remain sharp, but with a frankly infiltrative process an edge sign may be recorded (Fig. 8-27), as with metastases. There may also be definite changes in the echopattern, with the appearance of micronodular areas or composite images (mottled pattern) (Fig. 8-28). In my experience, purely sonolucent lesions are exceptional. Rapid necrosis may occur under chemotherapy (Fig. 8-29).

Associated signs. The most common associated sign is splenomegaly, which may be homogeneous or heterogeneous (Chapter 28). It may be possible to display retroperitoneal lymph nodes (Fig. 8-29 and Chapter 25). Finally, there may be pleural (Fig. 8-27, *B*), pericardial (Fig. 8-27, *C*), or, very rarely, peritoneal effusions.

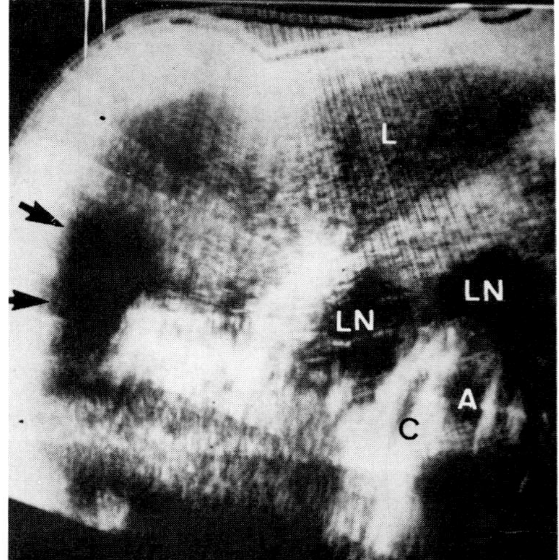

Fig. 8-29. Transverse scan of liver in case of lymphoblastosarcoma. Previous ultrasonogram had shown sonolucent nodule. Twenty-four hours after beginning of chemotherapy, liquid pattern due to necrosis was displayed in abnormal area *(arrows). L,* liver; *LN,* lymph nodes; *C,* cava; *A,* aorta.

A summary of the different ultrasonic signs of *liver metastases* and the ultrasonic signs in *lymphomas* follows.

8 : 1 ULTRASONIC SIGNS OF LIVER METASTASES AND LYMPHOMAS

I. Liver metastases
- A. Fundamental signs
  1. Hump sign
  2. Edge sign
  3. Sonolucent nodule
  4. Reflective nodule and "bull's-eye" nodule
  5. Increased reflectivity in fields
- B. Different types
  1. Solitary nodule
     - a. Sonolucent
     - b. Reflective
  2. Multiple nodules
     - a. Sonolucent: sieve pattern
     - b. Reflective: hailstorm pattern
     - c. Associated: mottled pattern
  3. Infiltrative pattern

II. Lymphomas
- A. Liver signs
  1. Nonspecific hepatomegaly
  2. Hailstorm pattern (sieve pattern exceptional)
  3. Mottled pattern
- B. Associated signs
  1. Enlarged spleen
  2. Retroperitoneal lymph nodes
  3. Pleural effusion
  4. Pericardial effusion

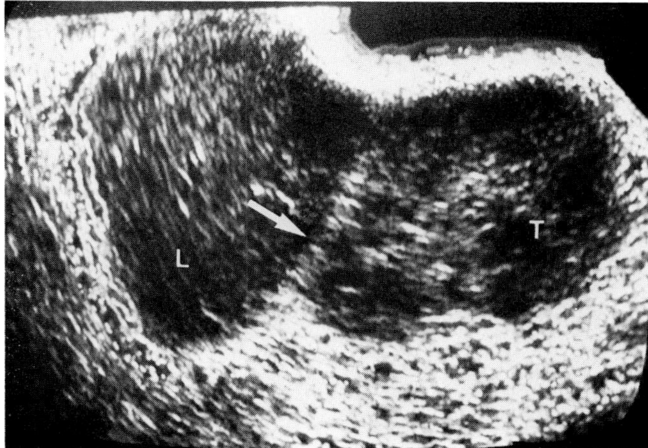

Fig. 8-30. Interpretation pitfall—palpable mass in right upper quadrant. Mass displays mottled echopattern. It was first thought to belong to metastatic peripheral deposit, bulging under liver. However, this sagittal scan displays interface image *(arrow)* between mass *(T)* and liver *(L)*. It proved to be renal carcinoma.

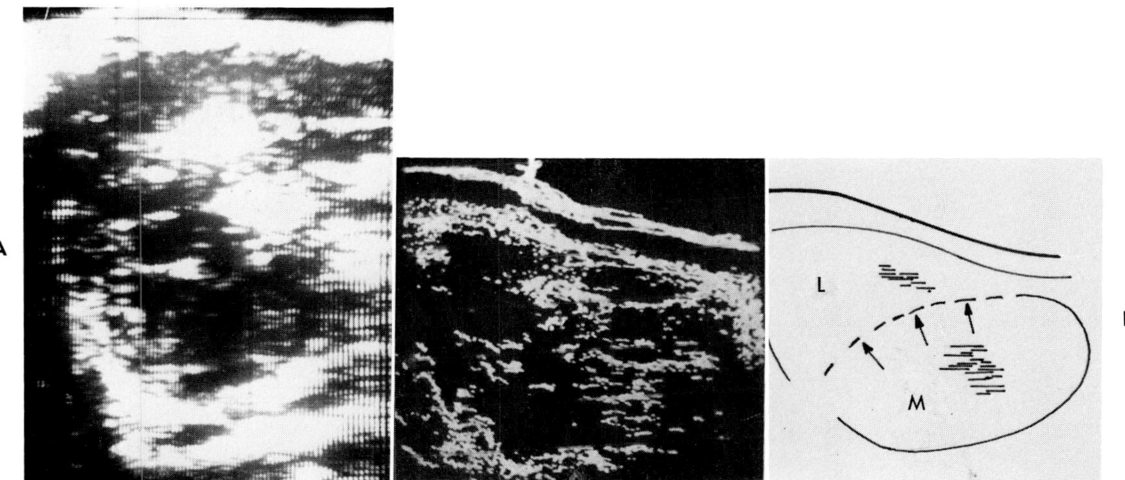

Fig. 8-31. Interpretation pitfall. **A,** Oblique recurrent subcostal scan of enlarged liver in 27-year-old man displays typical tumoral echopattern. Selective celiac angiography showed vascular anomalies indicating presence of hepatoma. As a matter of fact, surgery disclosed, instead of hepatic tumor, adrenal carcinoma with cleavage plane between tumor and liver tissue. **B,** Retrospective analysis of this bistable sagittal scan and schematic drawing discloses interface image *(arrows)* between tumoral mass *(M)* and liver *(L)*.

DIFFERENTIAL DIAGNOSIS

The ultrasonic differential diagnosis of hepatic lesions will be considered systematically in Chapter 12. However, before discussing the differential diagnosis, one must make sure that the abnormalities are really hepatic changes. This is not always easy. Although there is usually an interface image between tumors of the right kidney and the liver (Fig. 8-30), we have mistaken an adjacent adrenal tumor invading the liver for a liver tumor (Fig. 8-31).

RELIABILITY OF ULTRASONIC EXAMINATION

A recent study (Rouhier, 1975) reported 70% correct positive diagnoses of metastases (i.e., the same percentage as with scintigraphy). In fact, with improved gray scale display, combined with the use of real-time scanning, and by using objective criteria of normality and abnormality, one can now achieve better results. The smallest lesion that can be shown reliably is 5 mm in diameter, but most of the time the displayed nodules, or humps, are over 1 cm in diameter.

REFERENCES

Ardle, C. R.: Ultrasonic diagnosis of liver metastases, J. Clin. Ultrasound **4:**265-268, 1976.

Barnett, E., and Morley, P.: Abdominal echography, Borough Green, England, 1974, Butterworth & Co. (Publishers), Ltd.

Floyrac, G., Planiol, T., Mauléon, F., and Feil, C.: Exploration ultrasonore du foie. Les tumeurs hépatiques, J. Radiol. Electrol. Med. Nucl. **57:**604-606, 1976.

Goldberg, B. B., Kotler, M. N., Ziskin, M. C., and Waxham, R. D.: Diagnostic uses of ultrasound, New York, 1975, Grune & Stratton, Inc.

Hassani, N.: Ultrasonography of the abdomen, Heidelberg, Germany, 1976, Springer-Verlag.

Holm, H. H., Kristensen, J. K., Rasmussen, S. N., Pedersen, J. F., and Hancke, S.: Abdominal ultrasound, Copenhagen, 1976, Munksgaard, International Booksellers & Publishers, Ltd.

Holmes, J. H.: Uses of ultrasound for diagnostic study of the abdomen, Ultrasonographia medica, vol. 3, Vienna, 1971, Verlag der Wiener Medizinischer Akademie.

Leopold, G. R., and Asher, W. M.: Fundamentals of abdominal and pelvic ultrasonography, Philadelphia, 1975, W. B. Saunders Co.

Pritchard, J. H., Winston, M. A., Berger, H. G., and Blahd, W. H.: Diagnosis of focal hepatic lesions. Combined radioisotope and ultrasound techniques, J.A.M.A. **229:**1463-1465, 1974.

Rettenmaier, G.: Ultrasound in the differential diagnosis of circumscribed hepatic processes and the occlusive syndrome, Therapiewoche **20:**1827-1832, 1970.

Rouhier, D.: L'échotomographie du foie. Résultats et valeurs diagnostiques à propos de 201 observations, thesis, Lyons, France, 1975, Claude Bernard University.

Taylor, K. J., Carpenter, D. A., and McCready, V. R.: Grey scale echography in the diagnosis of intrahepatic disease, J. Clin. Ultrasound **1:**284-287, 1973.

Taylor, K. J., and McCready, V. R.: A clinical evaluation of grey-scale ultrasonography, Br. J. Radiol. **49:**244-252, 1976.

Weill, F., Becker, J. C., Kraehenbuhl, J. R., Heriot, G., and Walter, J. P.: Clinical atlas of ultrasonic radiography, Paris, 1973, Masson & Cie., Editeurs.

Weill, F., Ricatte, J. P., Prevotat, N., and Bonneville, J. F.: Séméiologie tomo-échographique hépato-biliaire élémentaire, Ann. Radiol. **13:**567-578, 1970.

CHAPTER 9

PRIMARY TUMORS

This chapter is short and disappointing, since images of primary tumors have no specific characteristics that permit differentiation from secondary tumors.

MALIGNANT TUMORS

Some hepatomas are shown as rather well-delineated nodular areas, with a heterogeneous solid pattern (Figs. 9-1 and 9-2) or a bull's-eye pattern (Figs. 9-3 and 9-4). These features are quite typical, but identical images may be seen in solitary nodular metastatic deposits (Fig. 8-12). Other hepatomas are rather poorly defined (Fig. 9-5). Finally, some hepatomas are diffuse, or multinodular, and indistinguishable from multiple metastatic deposits (Figs. 9-5 to 9-7). The problem becomes even more complicated when a hepatoma develops on the underlying heterogeneous pattern of cirrhosis (Figs. 9-8 and 10-12). In Chapter 17 an example of the rare hepatic cystic cholangiocarcinoma will be seen (Fig. 17-10).

Since hepatomas may possess a multinodular pattern, the signs described in the previous chapter (i.e., hump sign and edge sign) may also be associated with the tissue changes in primary tumors (Fig. 9-6, *D*). *Text continued on p. 138.*

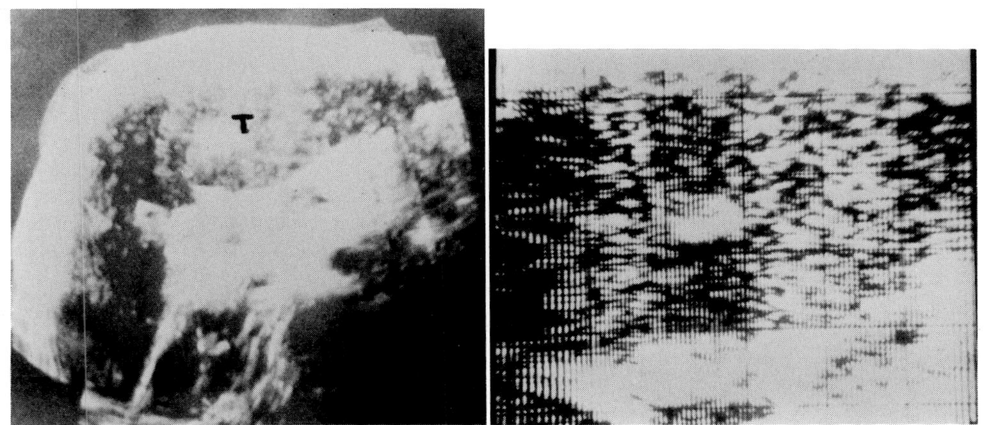

Fig. 9-1. Nodular hepatoma. **A,** Transverse contact scan showing rounded and rather well-marginated reflective area *(T)* in hilar area. **B,** Real-time analysis displaying less specific pattern.

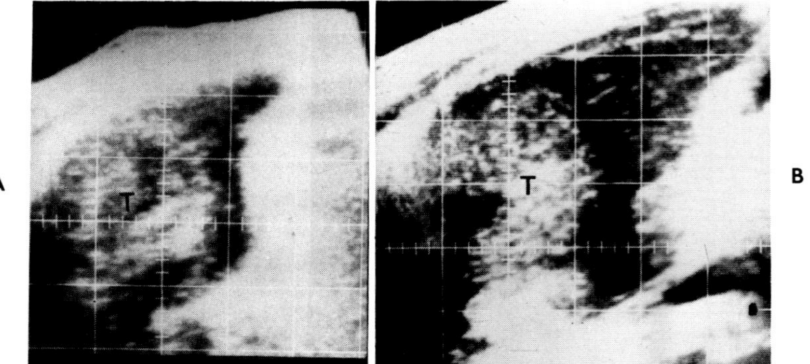

Fig. 9-2. Nodular hepatoma. **A** and **B,** Intercostal scans in two different patients. *T,* tumor. (Courtesy Dr. F. Mauléon, Rouen, France.)

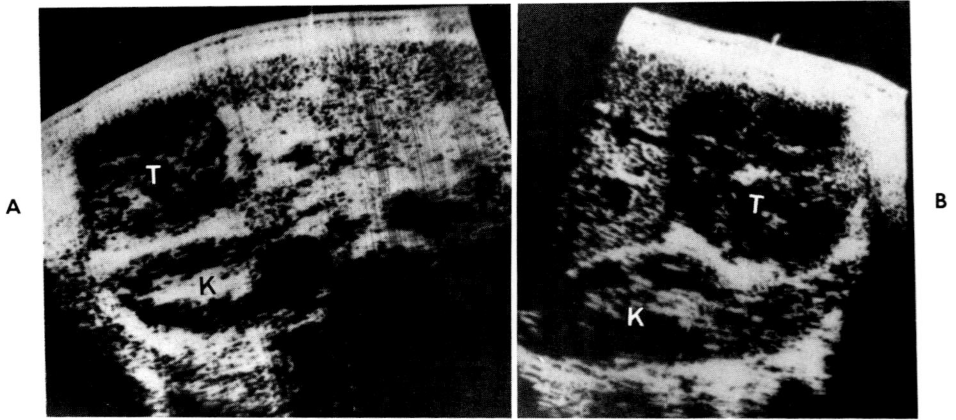

Fig. 9-3. Nodular primary tumor *(T)* (cholangiocarcinoma). **A,** Subcostal scan. **B,** Sagittal scan. *K,* kidney. (Courtesy T. Planiol and C. Feil, Tours, France.)

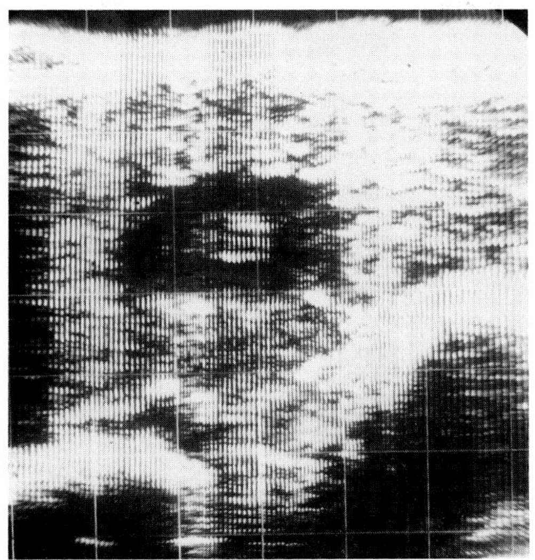

Fig. 9-4. Recurrent subcostal oblique real-time scan displaying intrahepatic well-marginated nodule of bull's-eye pattern, caused by recurrence of surgically treated hepatoma. (From Weill, F., Becker, J. C., Kraehenbuhl, J. R., Heriot, G., and Walter, J. P.: Clinical atlas of ultrasonic radiography, Paris, 1973, Masson & Cie., Editeurs.)

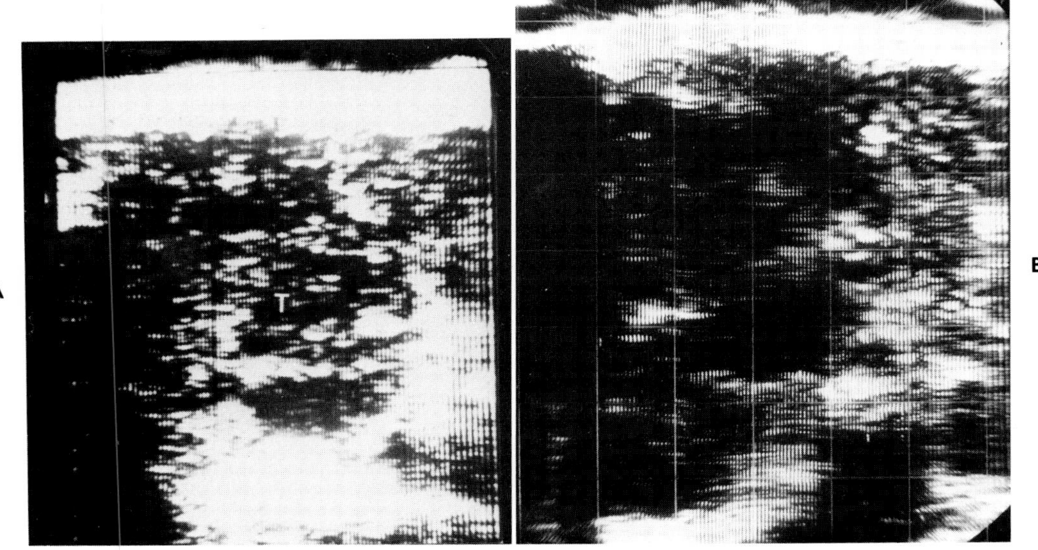

Fig. 9-5. A and **B,** Two examples of multinodular hepatomas, displayed on subcostal oblique recurrent scans. *T,* tumor.

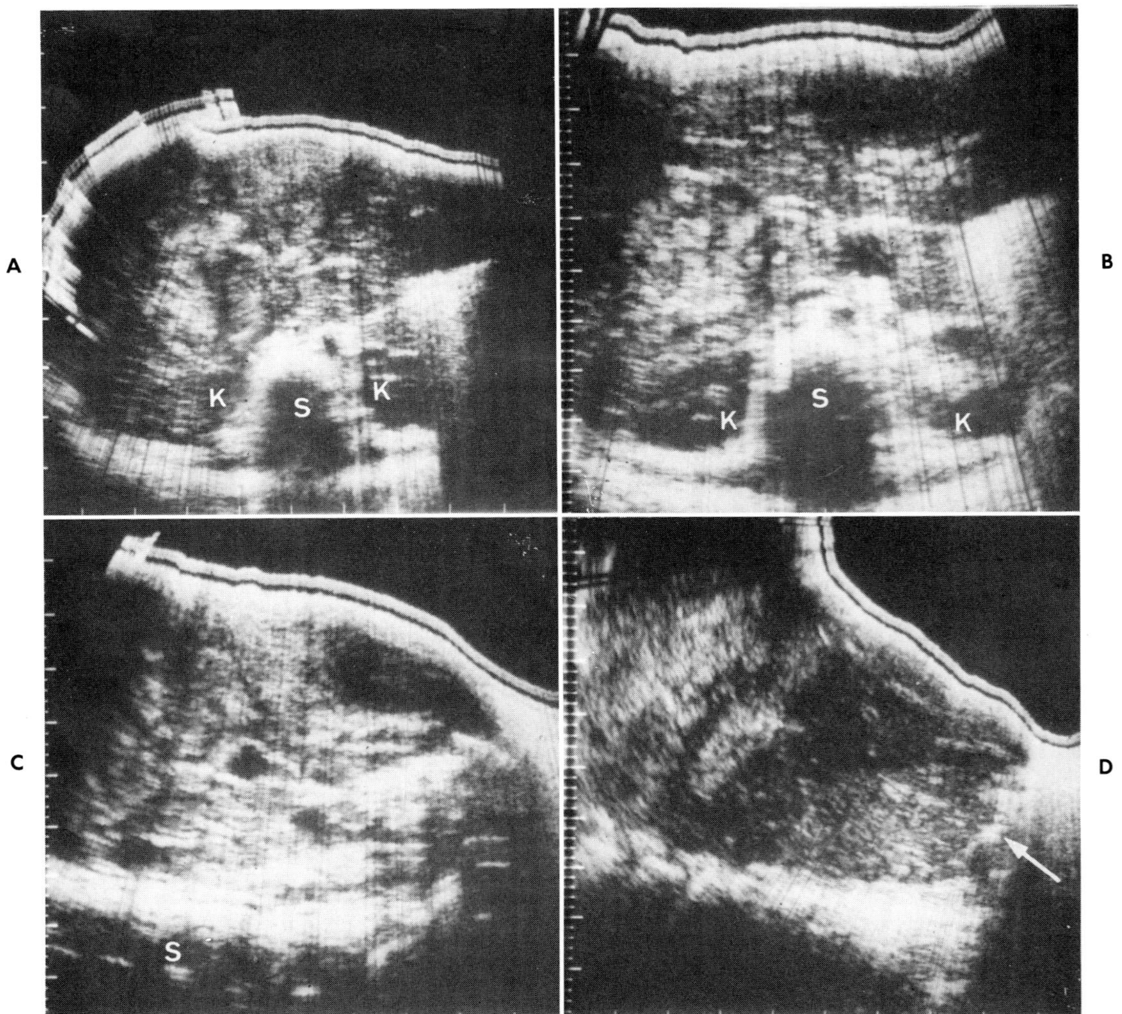

Fig. 9-6. Hepatoblastoma in 5-year-old child. **A** and **B,** Transverse scans. *K,* kidneys; *S,* spine. **C** and **D,** Sagittal scans displaying multiple irregular fields of increased reflectivity, edge sign *(arrow),* and humps.

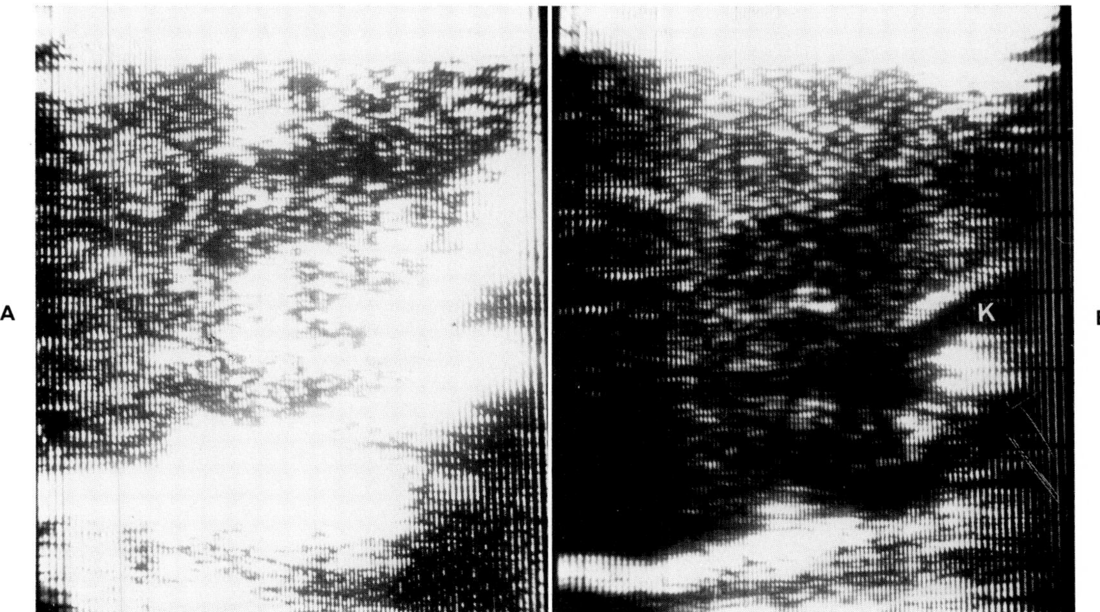

Fig. 9-7. Multinodular hepatoma. **A,** Oblique recurrent subcostal scan displaying heterogeneous echopattern of mottled type, similar to metastatic pattern. **B,** Sagittal scan passing through kidney *(K)* displays same type of echopattern.

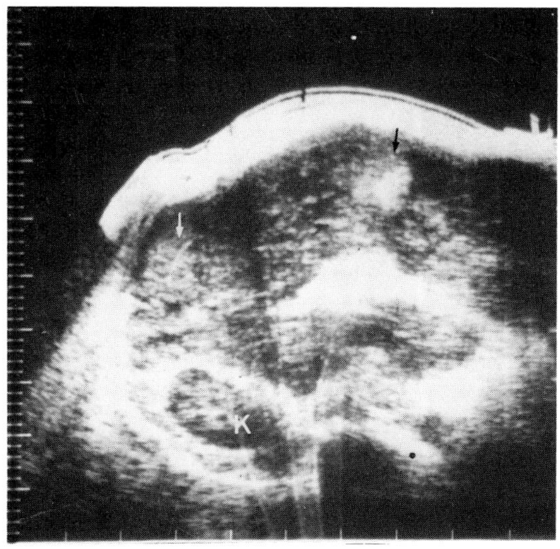

Fig. 9-8. Hepatoma in cirrhotic liver displayed on transverse scan. Left hepatic lobe is enlarged and presents abnormal reflective pattern *(arrows)*. There are several reflective nodules scattered in liver tissue. *K,* kidney.

BENIGN TUMORS

As in angiography, in ultrasonography neither adenomas nor hamartomas give rise to specific benign images. They are displayed as sonolucent or reflective nodular areas (Figs. 9-9 to 9-11).

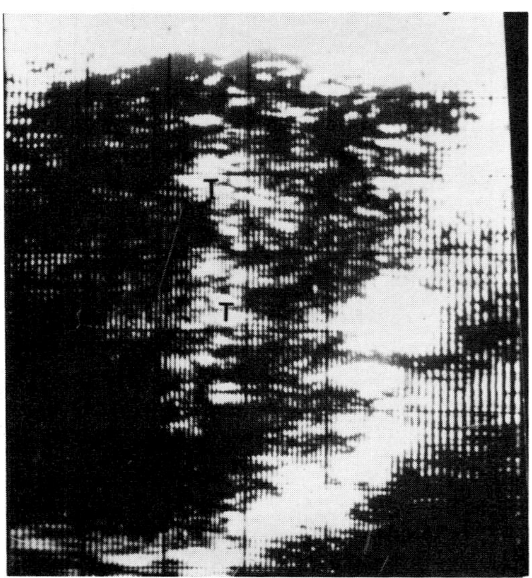

Fig. 9-9. Hamartoma. This oblique recurrent subcostal real-time scan displays different areas *(T)* of abnormal reflectivity in central part of liver.

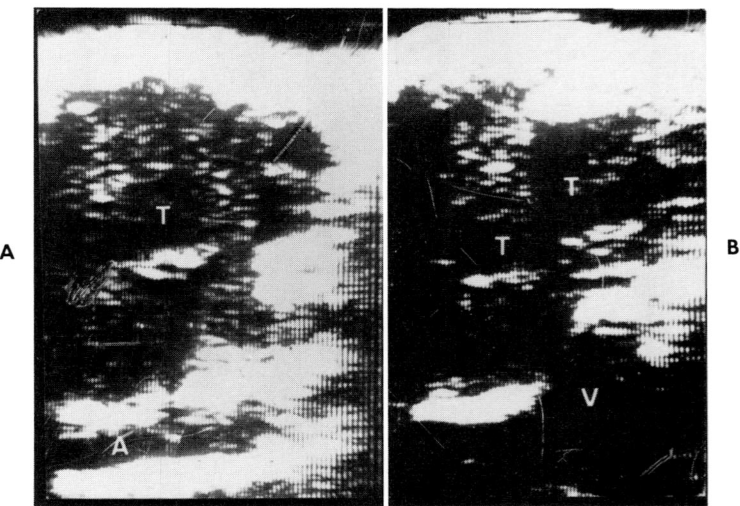

Fig. 9-10. Hamartoma. **A,** Sagittal scan passing through aorta *(A)* displays humps, inferior edge sign, and, above all, sonolucent central nodule *(T)*. **B,** Oblique recurrent subcostal scan showing sonolucent tumoral areas *(T)*. *V,* vertebral body.

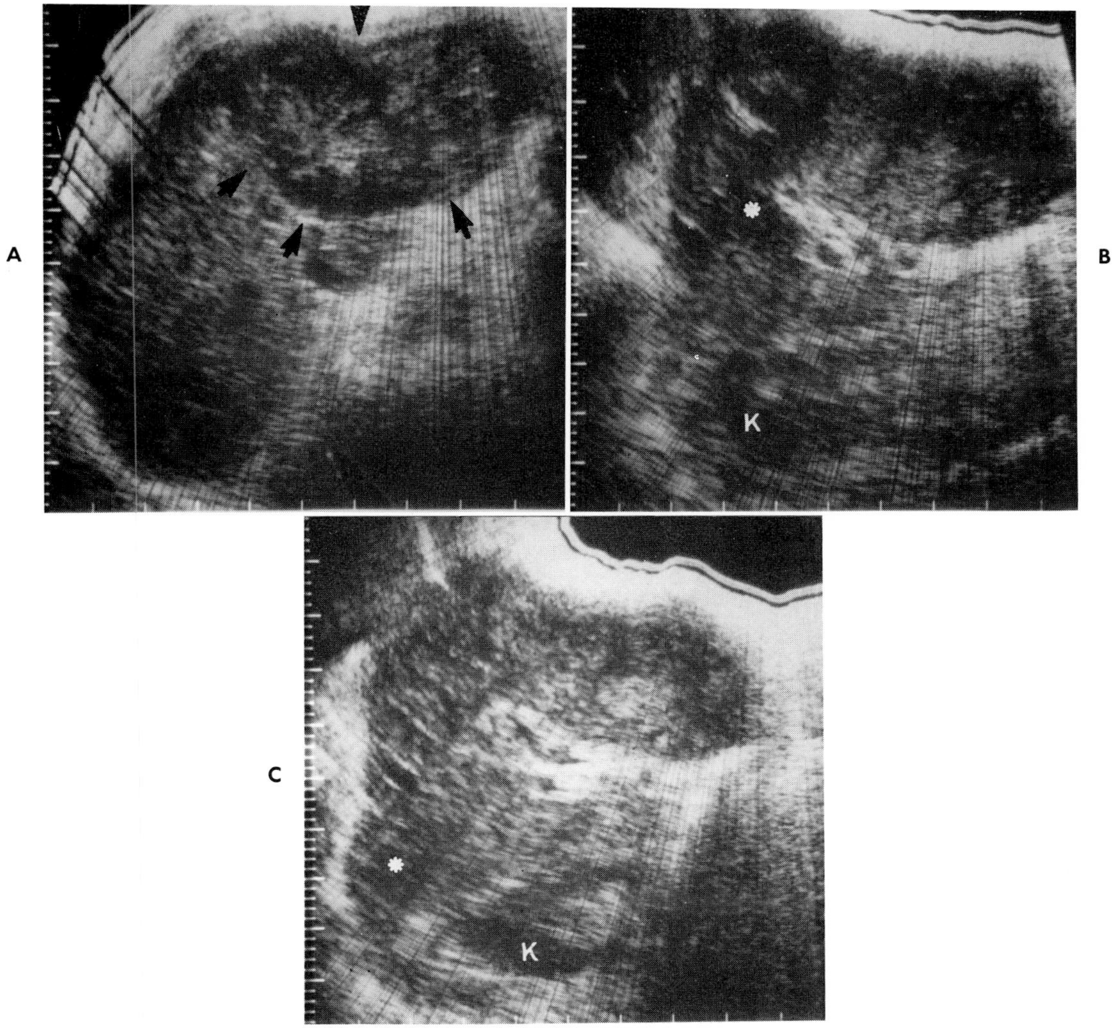

A B C K K

Fig. 9-11. Multiple hamartomas. **A,** Transverse scan showing rounded heterogeneous nodule *(arrows)* occupying left portion of liver. Note left edge sign and tangent sign. **B** and **C,** Two parallel sagittal scans showing multiple smaller nodules, sonolucent or reflective (*). *K,* kidney.

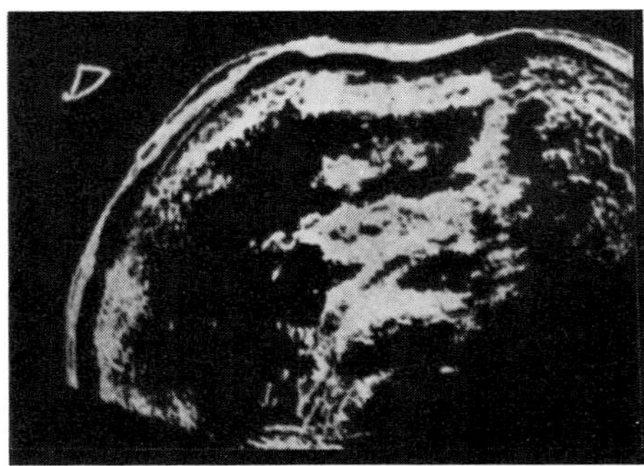

Fig. 9-12. Hemangioma. This old bistable transverse scan displays, in left hepatic lobe, reflective area close to venous branching images of hilus. This image, which lacks specificity, belongs to abnormal arterial network of hemangioma.

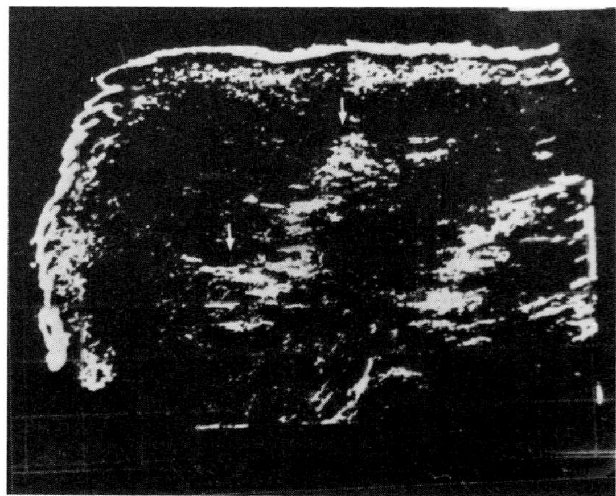

Fig. 9-13. Transverse scan of cirrhotic liver. There are several areas of abnormal reflectivity *(arrows)* without any specificity. They belong to vascular network of arterioportal fistula, due to multiple preoperative blind liver punctures.

Angiomas are displayed as nonspecific reflecting areas, reminiscent of the dense and slightly irregular echopattern of the central pyelovascular area of the kidney (Figs. 9-12 and 9-13). When such an isolated reflective pattern is seen, angiography should be performed before biopsy is attempted.

RELIABILITY

In primary tumors of the liver, ultrasonography does not provide much more information than conventional scintigraphy. However, with particular radionuclides, scintigraphy may give rather specific results. On the other hand, tumoral hyperemia is easily displayed by contrast-enhanced CT scans. Finally, in the diagnosis of primary tumors, scintigraphy and CT scanning may yield more precise results than does ultrasonography. Angiography may display marked hypervascularization in hamartomas but does not always permit a definite diagnosis of malignancy

Table 9-1. Ultrasonic signs of liver tumors

Signs	*Malignant primary tumors*	*Benign primary tumors*	*Metastases*	*Lymphomas*
Solitary nodule				
Reflective	+	+	+	
Sonolucent	+	+	+	±
Multiple nodules				
Hailstorm pattern	+		+	+
Sieve pattern	+		+	
Mottled pattern	+	±	+	+
Infiltrative syndrome	+		+	+
Hump sign	+	±	+	±
Edge sign	+	±	+	+

or benignity. However, angiographic features are much more specific in primary than in secondary tumors; therefore angiography still plays a role in the diagnosis of such tumors. As I have already pointed out, it should be performed before puncture biopsy if an angiomatous lesion is suspected. The biopsy will finally provide the histological diagnosis on which the choice of therapy depends.

I have summarized in Table 9-1 the different ultrasonic signs of liver tumors.

REFERENCES

Barnett, E., and Morley, P.: Abdominal echography, Borough Green, England, 1974, Butterworth & Co. (Publishers), Ltd.

Floyrac, G., Planiol, T., Mauléon, F., and Feil, C.: Exploration ultrasonore du foie. Les tumeurs hépatiques, J. Radiol. Electrol. Med. Nucl. **57:**604-606, 1976.

Goldberg, B. B., Kotler, M. N., Ziskin, M. C., and Waxham, R. D.: Diagnostic uses of ultrasound, New York, 1975, Grune & Stratton, Inc.

Hassani, N.: Ultrasonography of the abdomen, Heidelberg, Germany, 1976, Springer-Verlag.

Holm, H. H., Kristensen, J. K., Rasmussen, S. N., Pedersen, J. F., and Hancke, S.: Abdominal ultrasound, Copenhagen, 1976, Munksgaard, International Booksellers & Publishers, Ltd.

Leopold, G. R., and Asher, W. M.: Fundamentals of abdominal and pelvic ultrasonography, Philadelphia, 1975, W. B. Saunders Co.

Rettenmaier, G.: Ultrasound in the differential diagnosis of circumscribed hepatic processes and the occlusive syndrome, Therapiewoche **20:**1827-1832, 1970.

Rouhier, D.: L'échotomographie du foie. Résultats et valeurs diagnostiques à propos de 201 observations, thesis, Lyons, France, 1975, Claude Bernard University.

Taylor, K. J., Carpenter, D. A., and McCready, V. R.: Grey scale echography in the diagnosis of intrahepatic disease, J. Clin. Ultrasound **1:**284-287, 1973.

Weill, F., Becker, J. C., Kraehenbuhl, J. R., Heriot, G., and Walter, J. P.: Clinical atlas of ultrasonic radiography, Paris, 1973, Masson & Cie., Editeurs.

CHAPTER 10

CIRRHOSIS–PORTAL HYPERTENSION

This is a specifically French chapter. About 20% of patients receiving medical care in a French hospital have, will have, or have had—being then in temporary care in the department of pathology—liver cirrhosis. Despite many years of research, specific ultrasonic patterns peculiar to the abuse of beer, wine, or liquors cannot yet be identified. Hillel's school is sure to have detected differing images in cirrhosis due to Bordeaux and in that due to Burgundy. Schammai's school claims that to be impossible, contending that the present accuracy of the ultrasonic images is insufficient. My opinion is that this unfortunate lack of specificity is related to the fact that patients are so offhand about scientific research as to mix all these causal agents indiscriminately.

HEPATOMEGALIC PHASE OF LIVER CIRRHOSIS

The general criteria of hepatomegaly have already been reviewed in Chapters 6 and 7. In cirrhotic hepatomegaly the transmission of sound, at least at the beginning of the disease, is excellent (Rettenmaier, 1973a; Rettenmaier, 1973b). The demonstration of deep layers of hepatic tissue is therefore easy. The tissue echopattern is homogeneous (Figs. 10-1 and 10-2). I term this type of cirrhotic liver *Type I*. There is often associated splenomegaly, of at least moderate degree.

The progressive development of fibrosis gives rise to increased attenuation of sound (Rettenmaier, 1973a; Rettenmaier, 1973b) (Fig. 10-3). The tissue echopattern remains homogeneous. This is what is called *Type II* of cirrhotic livers. As the disease progresses, the parenchymal texture shows small areas of increased reflectivity, of micronodular type (Fig. 10-4). Such a reflective micronodulation represents Type IIIa of cirrhotic hepatic anomalies.

ADVANCED FIBROTIC PHASE OF LIVER CIRRHOSIS

When fibrosis has progressed, the liver tends to retract, and small contour irregularities appear. These small superficial irregularities correspond to the classic "hobnail" appearance of the cirrhotic liver surface. Retracted areas due to fibrosis may also be encountered (Fig. 10-5), producing a wavy marginal pattern, which is quite different from metastatic humps. At this stage of the disease there are more marked echopattern abnormalities, with definite nodules of intense reflectivity. The diameter of a cirrhotic nodule is usually less than 1 cm. When the various changes in the liver contours and echopattern have occurred, this is referred to as a *Type IIIb cirrhotic pattern*. Finally, when the liver has become very small and retracted above the costal margin, it becomes difficult to display. We term this stage *Type IV* (Figs. 10-6 and 10-7). The anterior approach may have become impossible, since the gas-filled colon has moved up to fill the void and is interposed.

Text continued on p. 147.

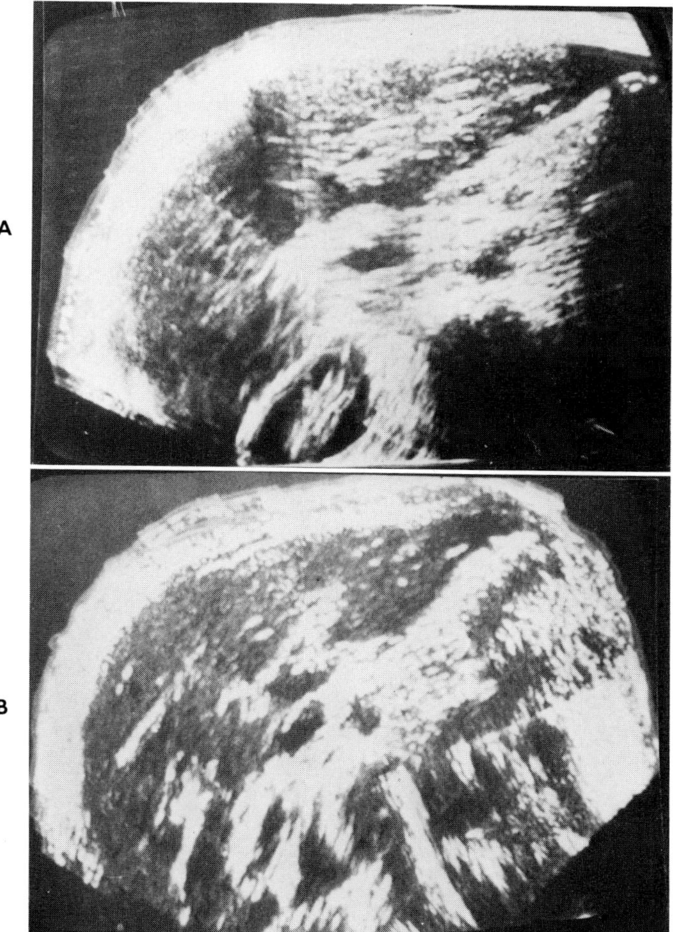

Fig. 10-1. Cirrhotic liver of Type I—nonspecific hepatomegaly. **A** and **B,** Transverse scans.

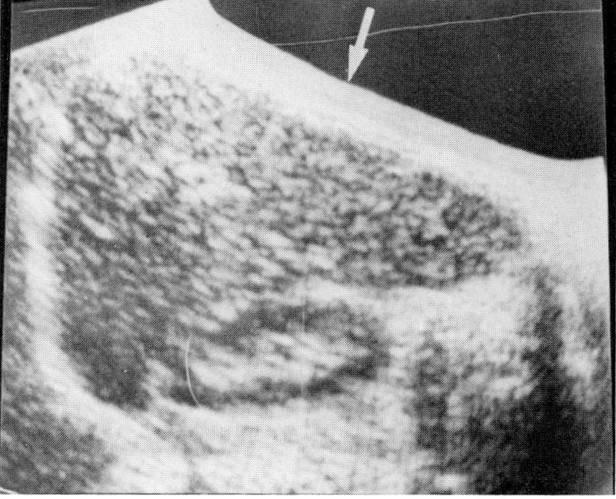

Fig. 10-2. Liver cirrhosis—nonspecific hepatomegaly. This sagittal scan shows liver enlargement. Inferior marginal edge is biconvex, but not frankly rounded. *Arrow,* costal margin.

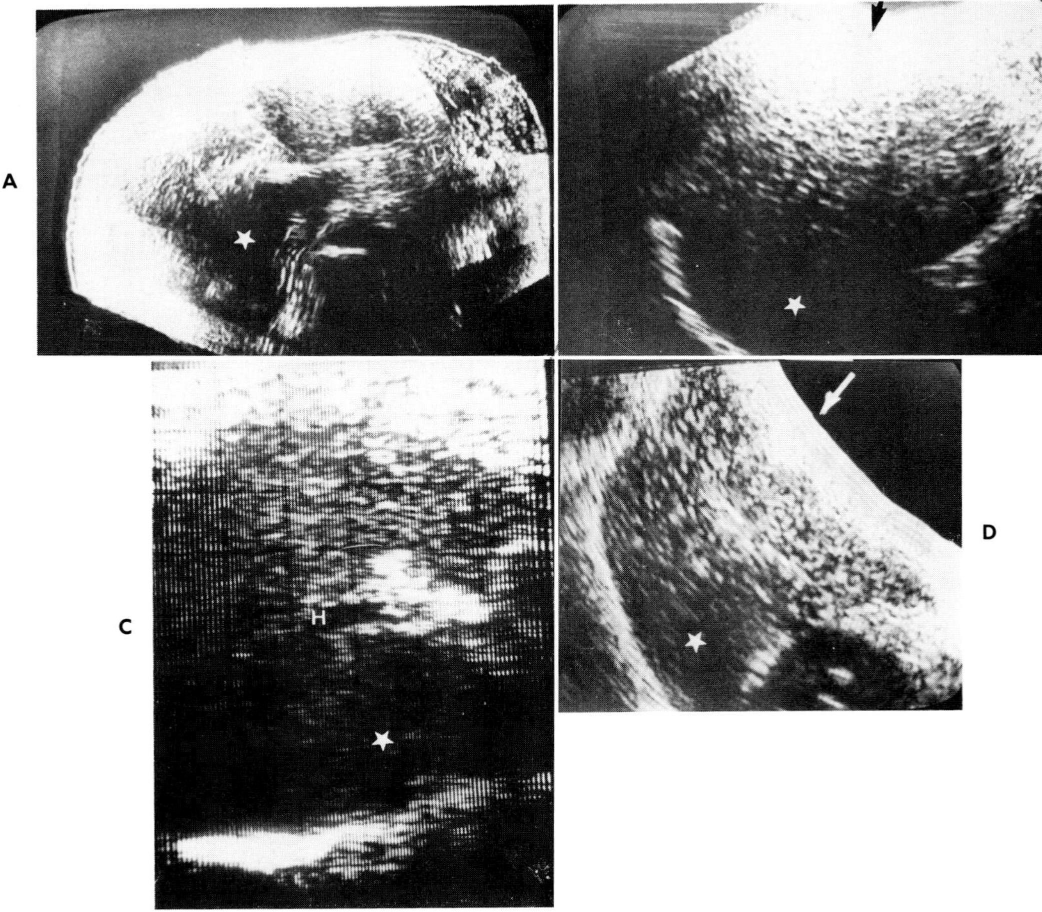

Fig. 10-3. Liver cirrhosis at later stage. Attenuation is increased. Deep layers of tissue *(stars)* are poor in echoes. This echopattern belongs to Type II. **A** to **C,** Transverse, sagittal, and oblique recurrent scans. *H,* hilus. **D,** Sagittal scan of another patient. *Arrow,* costal edge.

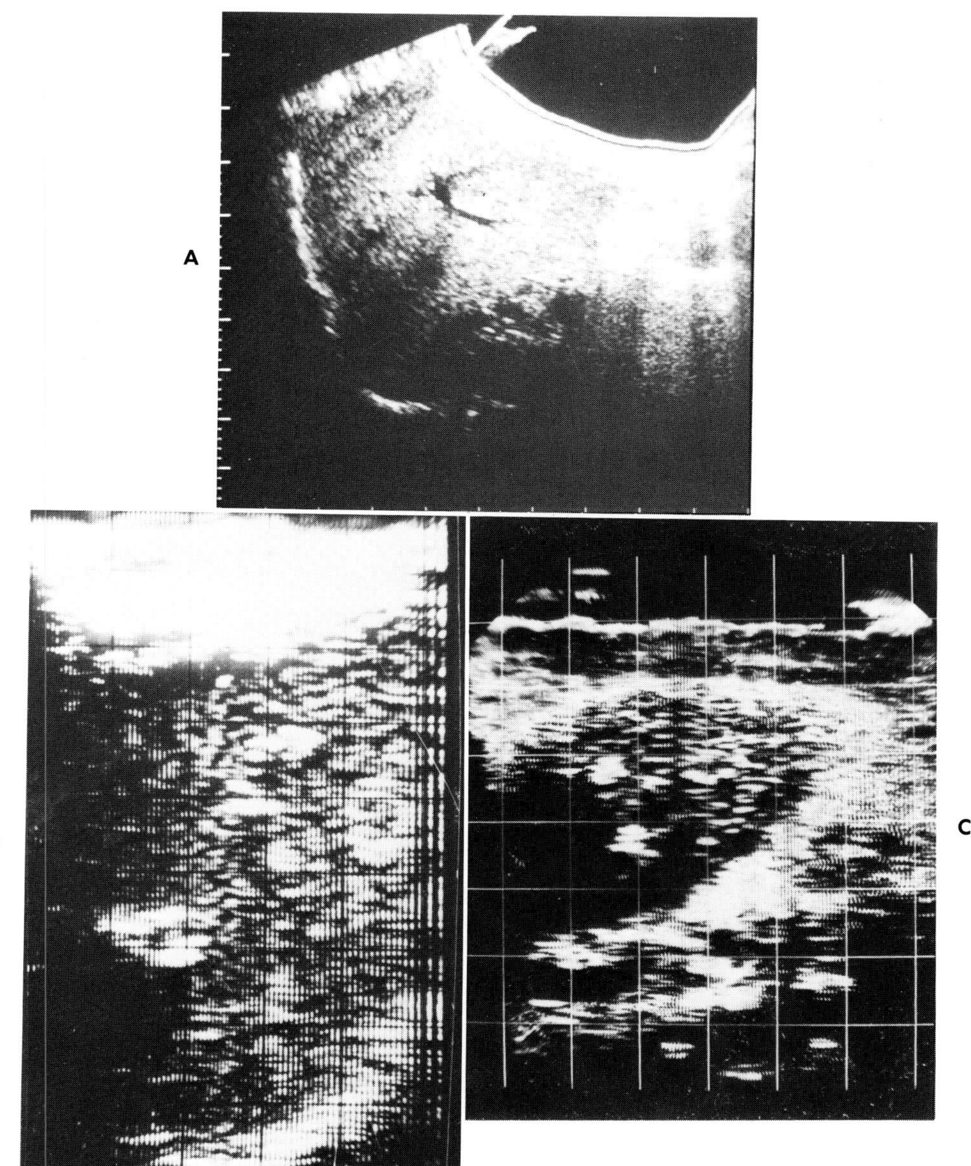

Fig. 10-4. A, Sagittal scan shows increased attenuation, resulting in reduced echoes in deep layers of hepatic tissue. In this case, since tissular echopattern has been displayed in depth, superficial areas are saturated. Rare reflective micronodules are visible (Type IIIa). **B,** Oblique recurrent subcostal real-time scan of another patient showing micronodular echopattern of Type IIIa. **C,** Sagittal scan through left hepatic lobe and aorta, in another case, displays larger nodules and associated increase of attenuation (Type IIIb).

A

B

Fig. 10-5. Retractions: hobnail surface. **A,** Sagittal scan of left hepatic lobe shows deep retraction *(arrow).* On either side of retraction, surface of liver has a curve of large radius, very different from metastatic hump. Anterior aspect has hobnail appearance. **B,** In another case, sagittal scan shows small retraction *(arrow)* on posterior aspect of right hepatic lobe above kidney. Rounded shape of inferior edge of liver belongs to an artifact.

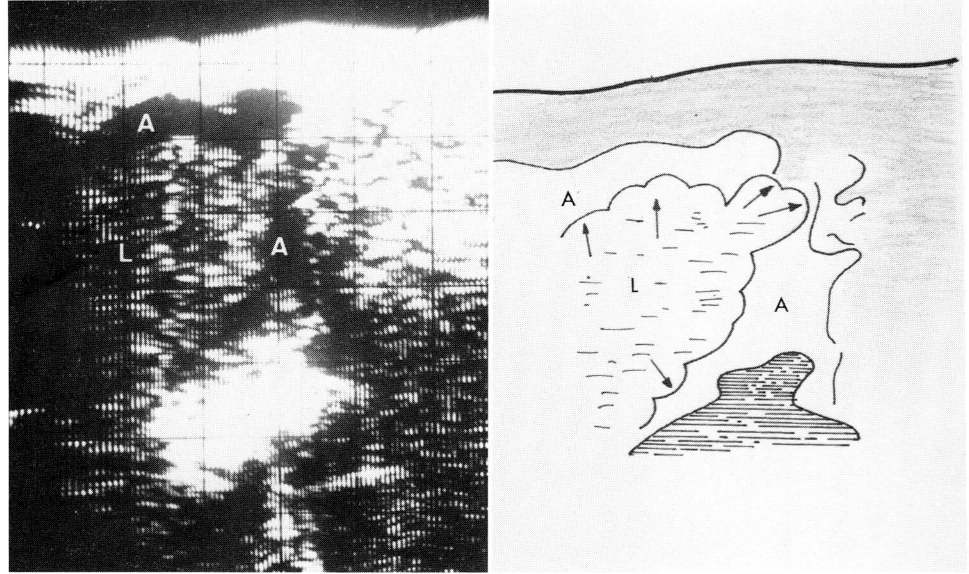

Fig. 10-6. Cirrhosis: contour changes and associated signs. This oblique recurrent subcostal real-time scan, made in terminal phase of liver cirrhosis, and its schematic representation show small retracted liver *(L),* which is bathed in ascitic fluid *(A).* Liver contours are irregular, with small elevations *(arrows),* impressions of which are visible on abdominal wall. Small bulges also deform liver edge and posterior aspect of liver. Such images belong to Type IV.

The only possible approach then is intercostal scanning. By this time the patients have usually lost considerable weight, and it is difficult to obtain satisfactory images in emaciated patients with dehydrated skin. Last, but not least, the attenuation, at this stage, is usually significantly increased. Unfortunately for the patient, but fortunately for the ultrasonographer, associated features facilitate the ultrasonic diagnosis.

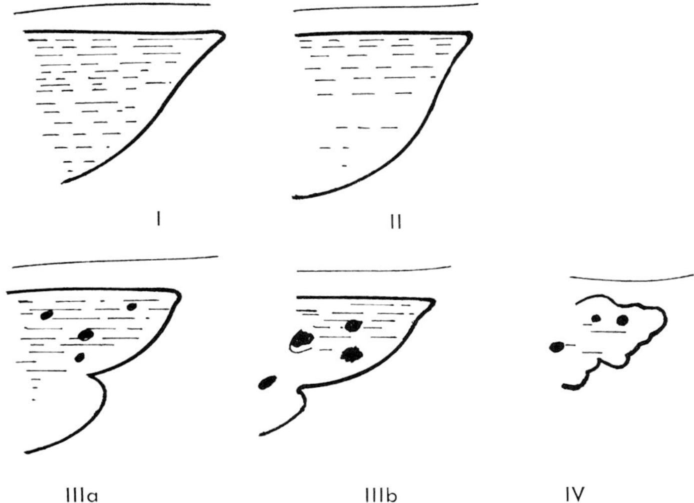

Fig. 10-7. Successive cirrhotic changes. Type *I:* nonspecific hepatomegaly; Type *II:* onset of abnormal increased attenuation; Type *IIIa:* micronodulation with beginning retraction; Type *IIIb:* larger micronodulation; Type *IV:* marked retraction, micronodulation, and possibly ascites.

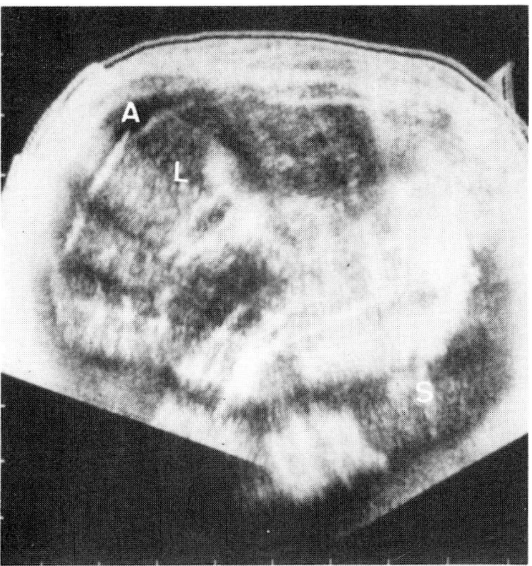

Fig. 10-8. Associated signs. Association of hepatomegaly with ascites *(A)*. Size of spleen *(S)* is slightly increased. *L,* liver.

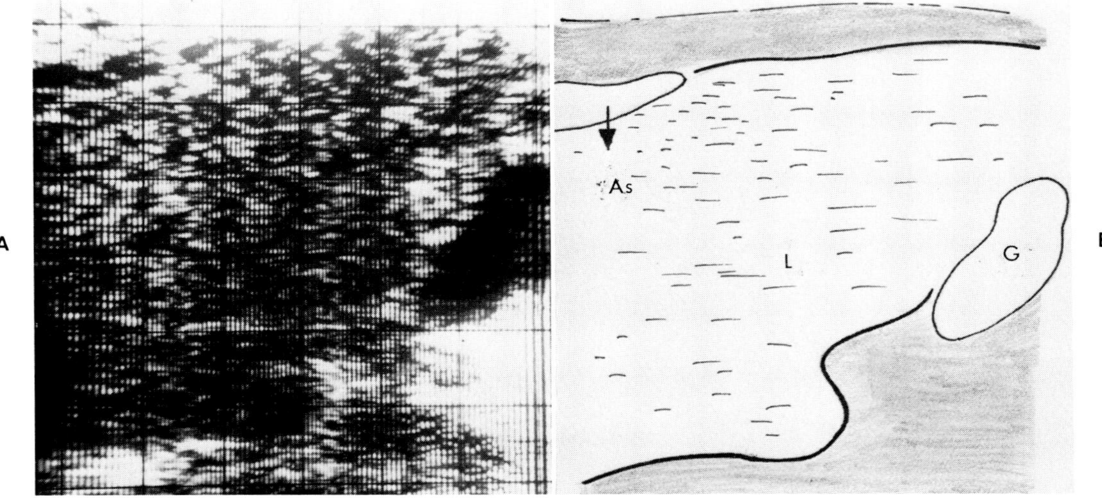

Fig. 10-9. Cirrhosis—early ascites. On sagittal real-time scan, hepatomegaly is displayed. Attenuation has increased. Tissue echopattern is heterogeneous, with micronodules. Narrow sonolucent strip, due to ascites *(As),* appears between anterior aspect of liver *(L)* and anterior abdominal wall. **A,** Scan. **B,** Schematic drawing of **A.** *G,* gallbladder.

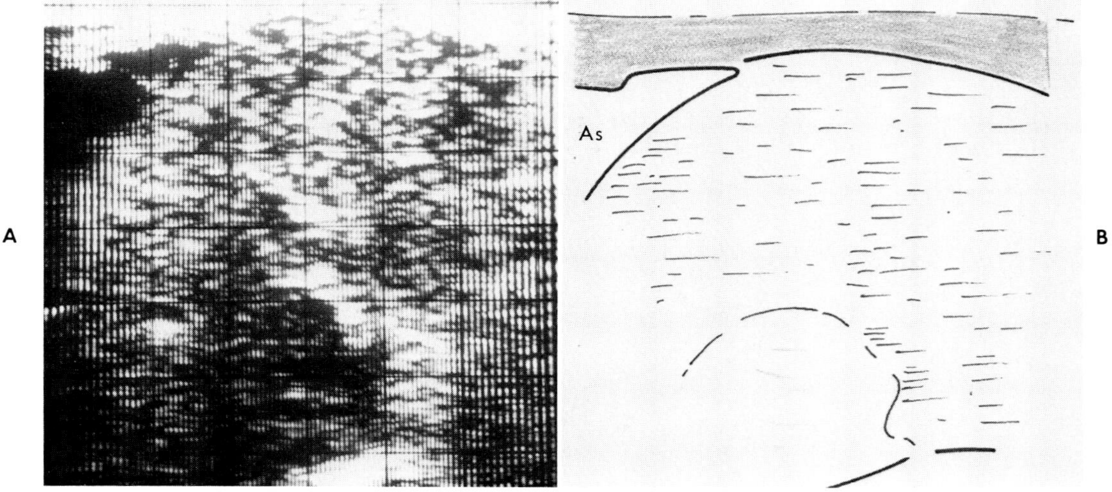

Fig. 10-10. Between cirrhotic liver of Type IIIa and anterior abdominal wall, ascites *(As)* is now evident. **A,** Scan. **B,** Schematic representation.

ASSOCIATED ABNORMALITIES

Splenomegaly

Even if it is usually less pronounced than in lymphoma, splenomegaly can be quite marked in cirrhosis. The splenic tissue echopattern remains sonolucent and homogeneous (Fig. 10-8).

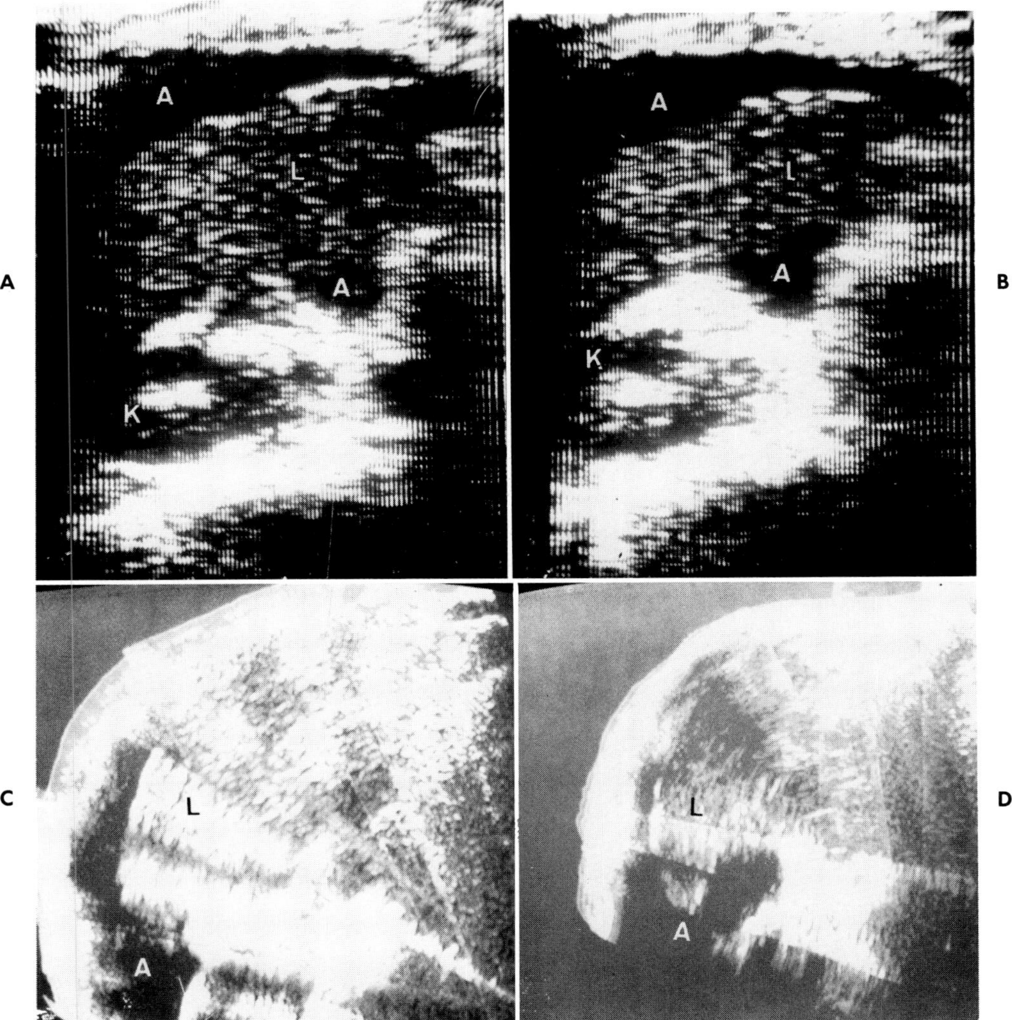

Fig. 10-11. Cirrhosis—abundant ascites. **A** and **B,** Two parallel oblique recurrent subcostal scans. Liver *(L)* is small and retracted, with moderate contour irregularities. It is surrounded by ascitic fluid *(A)*. *K,* right kidney. **C** and **D,** Two parallel transverse gray scale scans again showing ascites between liver and abdominal wall.

Ascites

Ascites rapidly becomes evident, interposed between the liver and the anterior or lateral abdominal wall, as a thin sonotransparent band (Figs. 10-8 to 10-10). When it becomes more abundant, it surrounds the liver, which can then be seen, very well, despite retraction and attenuation (Fig. 10-11). Rettenmaier (1975) emphasizes palpation of the liver under echoscopic real-time control. In such cases of abundant ascites, it is possible to display the mobility of the liver within the ascitic fluid (flow sign). On the other hand, if doubt arises as to the presence of ascites, positional changes should be used. These will be discussed in detail in Chapter 14.

Jaundice

Jaundice of cirrhotic origin has only negative ultrasonic signs, since there is no dilatation of the intrahepatic or extrahepatic bile ducts. This problem will be dealt with in Chapter 26.

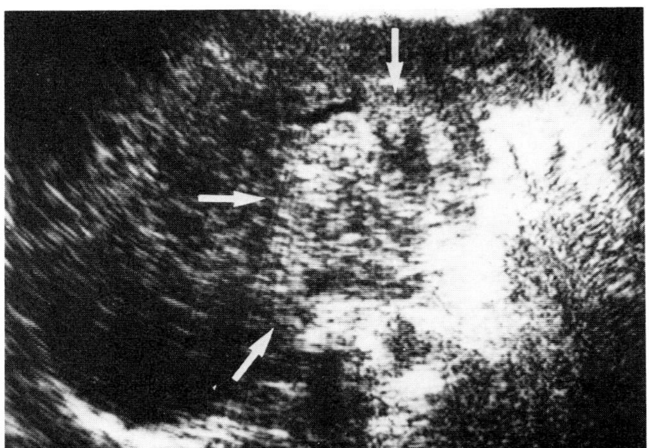

Fig. 10-12. Hepatoma developed in cirrhotic liver. This transverse scan of liver displays very reflective rounded area *(arrows),* giving rise to bulge on posterior aspect of liver. Area of abnormal reflectivity is heterogeneous, with reflective nodules, but also small sonolucent areas. This well-marginated reflective area in cirrhotic liver is rather typical of hepatoma. (Courtesy Dr. G. Triller, Bern, Switzerland.)

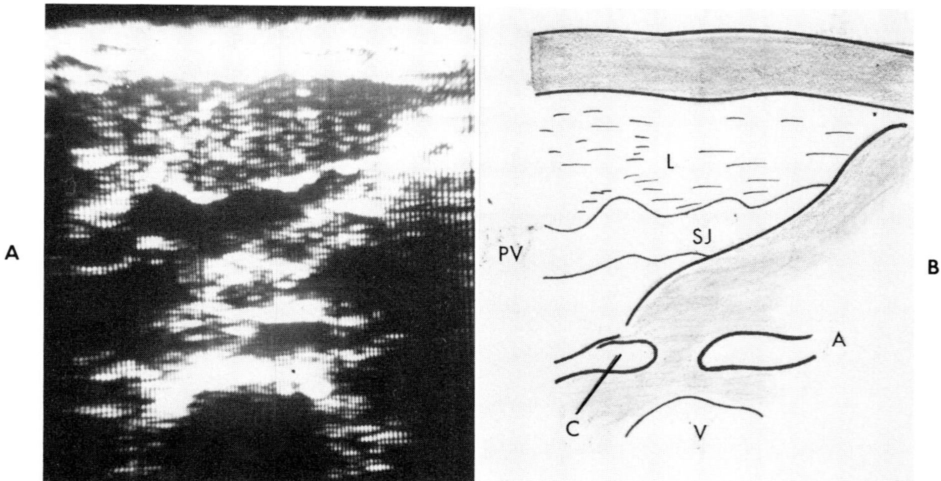

Fig. 10-13. Portal hypertension. **A,** This horizontal scan shows sinuous vessel, belonging to enlarged junction *(SJ)* between splenic vein and portal vein *(PV).* **B,** Schematic drawing of **A.** *C,* vena cava; *A,* aorta; *L,* liver; *V,* vertebral column.

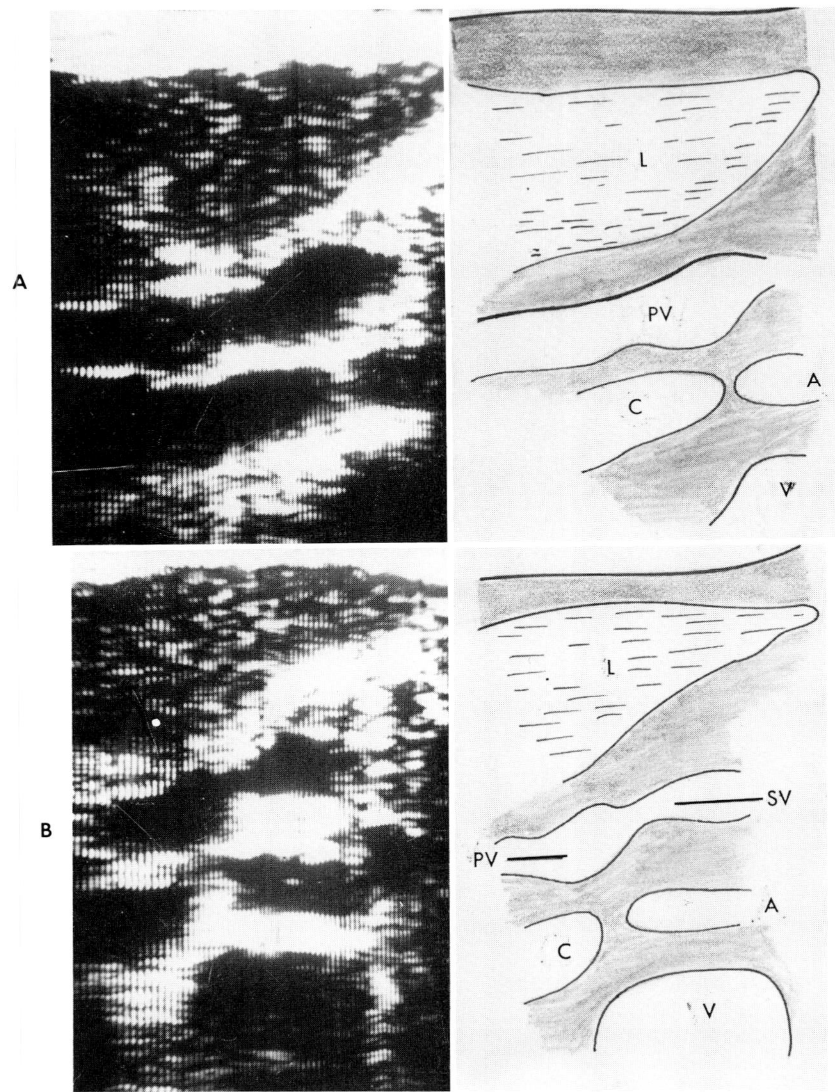

Fig. 10-14. Portal hypertension: real-time scans and schematic drawings of splenoportal axis. **A,** Oblique scan and schematic drawing of right upper quadrant showing portal vein longitudinally. Mesenteric-portal junction and portal vein *(PV)* are dilated. Section of vena cava *(C)* is oblique and therefore oval in shape. *L,* liver; *A,* aorta; *V,* vertebra. **B,** Horizontal scan and schematic drawing of same area showing splenoportal axis *(SV, PV)*. Venous axis is enlarged and tortuous. Vena cava and aorta appear on this transverse scan in more rounded sections. *Continued.*

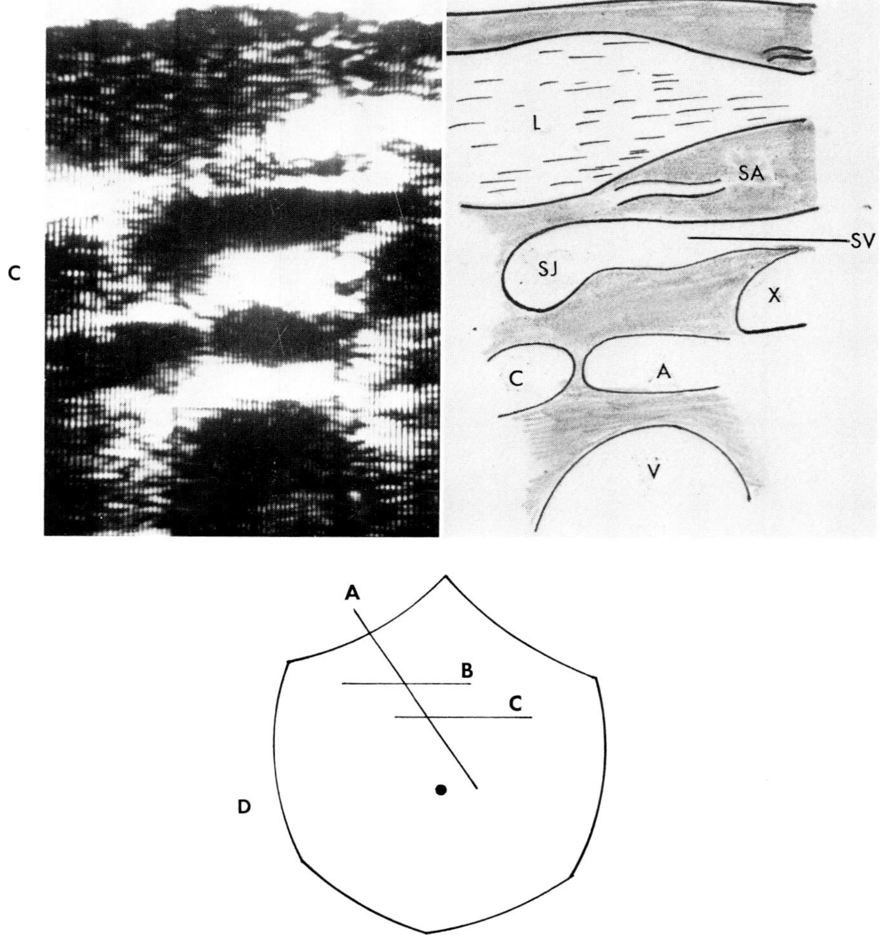

Fig. 10-14, cont'd. C, Another transverse scan and its schematic representation displaying splenic vein *(SV)* and splenoportal junction *(SJ)*. Diameter of splenic vein is 1.5 cm. Just in front of splenic vein is displayed narrow tubular element, likely belonging to splenic artery *(SA)*. Sonolucent area *(X)* represents a varix in splenic hilus. **D,** Scanning planes of **A** to **C.**

Hepatomas

The nodular elements encountered in the cirrhotic echopattern are regularly scattered in the liver tissue. The presence of large areas of abnormal reflectivity is consistent with the development of a hepatoma (Fig. 10-12). Such a diagnosis is, of course, difficult if the liver is retracted, and it may be necessary to resort to other modes of examination, such as scintigraphy, computed axial tomography, or angiography.

Portal hypertension (*with the collaboration of* Albert Eisenscher, M.D.)

The normal ultrasonic pattern of the portal system has already been discussed (Chapter 4). Dilatation of the splenic vein, a rather common feature in portal hypertension, is easily shown (Weill and colleagues, 1973a; Weill and colleagues,

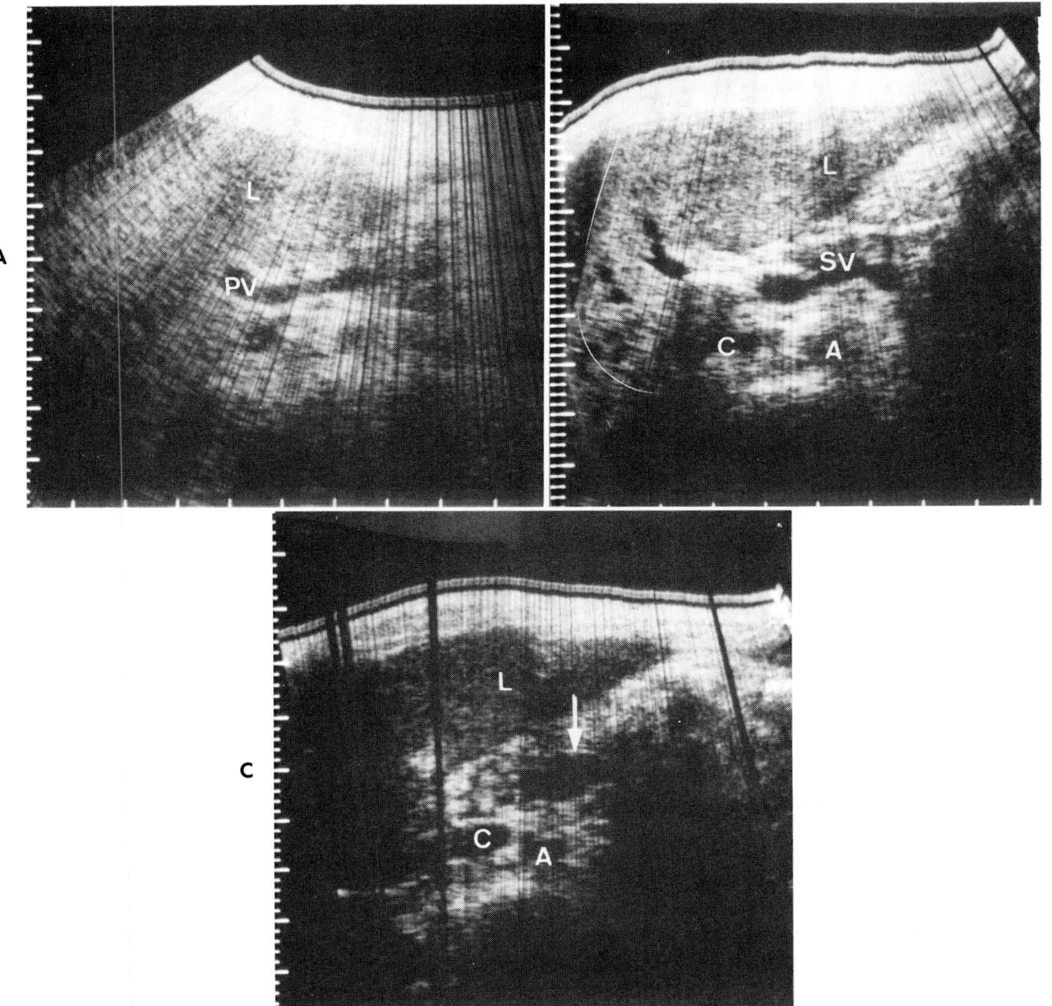

Fig. 10-15. Portal hypertension. **A,** Oblique scan of right upper quadrant showing portal vein *(PV)* in sagittal section. *L,* liver. **B,** Transverse scan displaying sinuous splenic vein *(SV)*. *C,* vena cava; *A,* aorta. **C,** Oblique scan showing frankly dilated splenoportal junction *(arrow)*.

1973b) (Fig. 10-13). Of course, any significant splenomegaly is accompanied by a dilatation of the splenic vein, but, in our opinion, if the diameter of the splenic vein reaches 2 cm, portal hypertension is likely (Figs. 10-14 to 10-16). Since the normal diameter of the portal vein is variable, it is advisable to be careful in the assessment of its enlargement. In some cases, more specific features may be visualized, since collateral circulation may be directly displayed. The umbilical vein (Fig. 10-17) is displayed as a vascular structure, connecting the liver hilus with the abdominal wall and in close contact with the posterior aspect of the right hepatic lobe (Weill, 1976). The venous network of a portal cavernoma gives rise to multiple small vascular-section images of variable sizes and shapes, constituting

Text continued on p. 158.

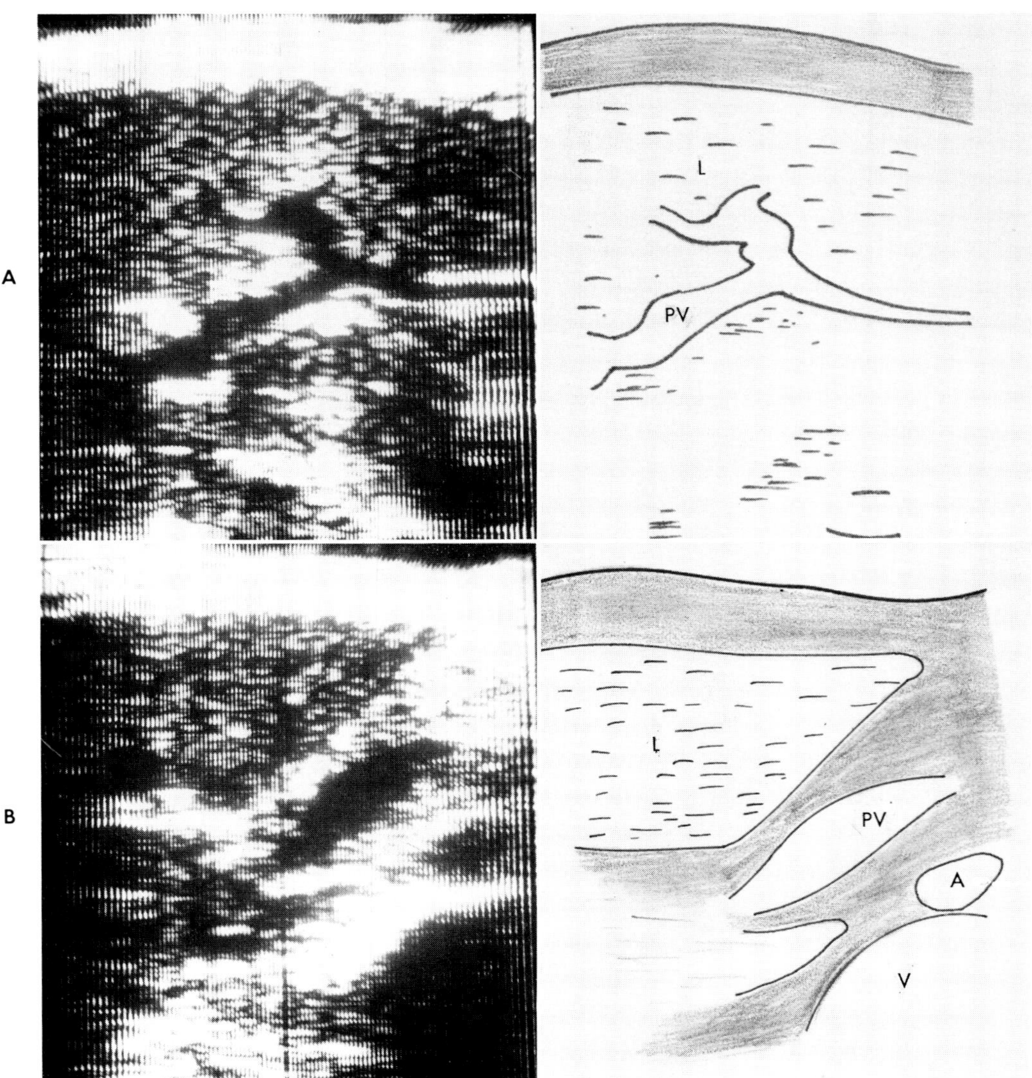

Fig. 10-16. Portal hyptertension. **A,** Oblique recurrent subcostal scan and its schematic representation showing portal division *(PV)* and its branches. *L,* liver. **B,** Oblique scan of right upper quadrant, cutting portal vein *(PV)* longitudinally, and schematic representation. *A,* aorta; *V,* vertebra.

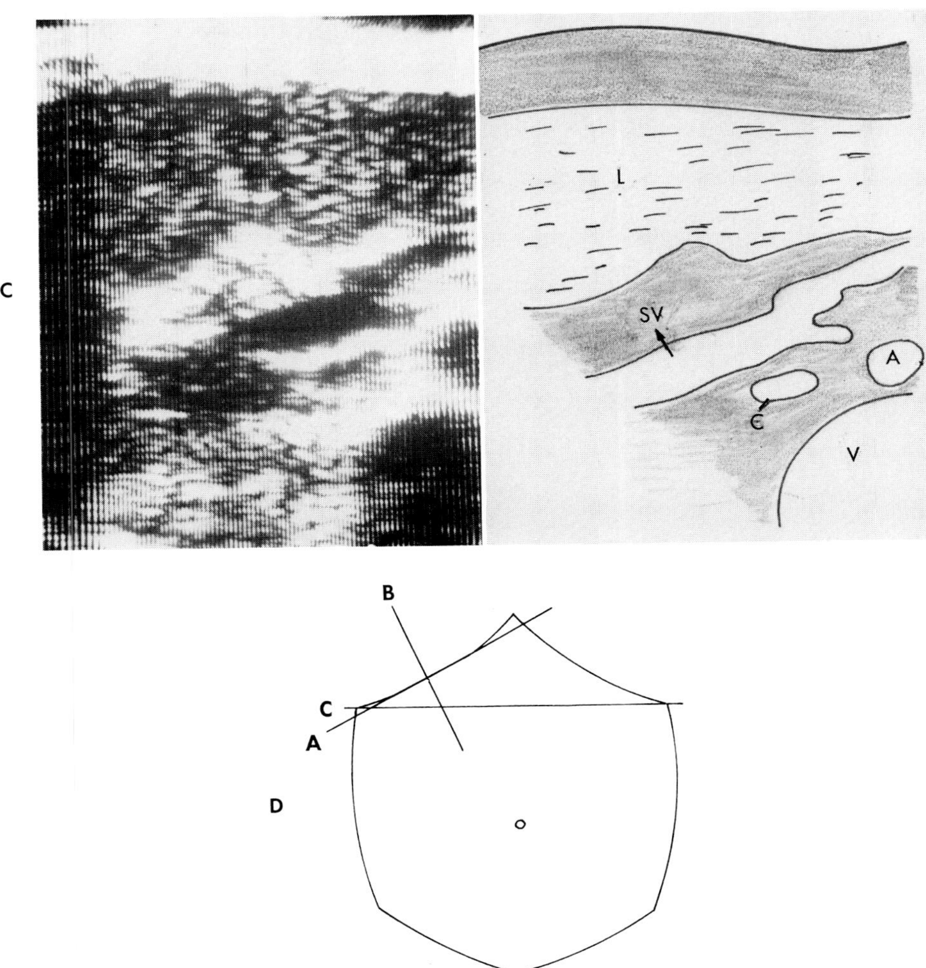

Fig. 10-16, cont'd. C, Horizontal scan and its schematic representation display, between liver *(L)* and vena cava *(C)*, splenic vein *(SV)* and splenoportal junction. Venous axis is dilated and sinuous. *A,* aorta. **D,** Scanning planes.

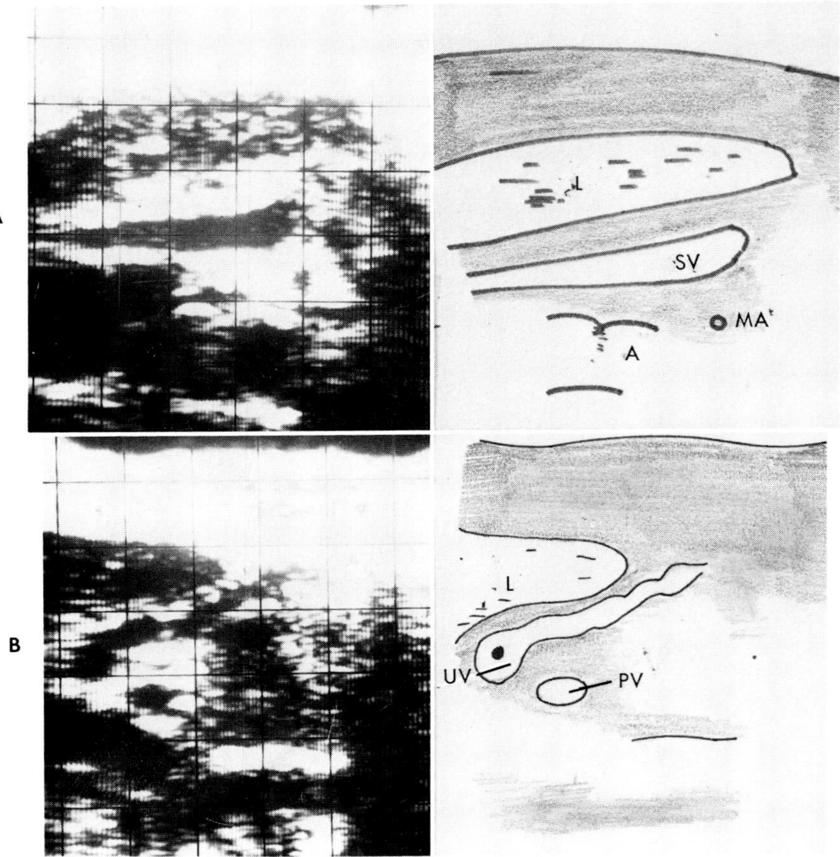

Fig. 10-17. Portal hypertension: patent umbilical vein. **A,** Transverse scan and schematic representation of upper abdomen, displaying, behind liver *(L),* dilated splenic vein *(SV),* as well as splenoportal junction. *A,* aorta; *MA,* mesenteric artery. **B,** Sagittal scan and its schematic representation, showing tortuous vessel in close contact with posterior aspect of liver. This vessel runs from hilus up to abdominal wall and represents umbilical vein *(UV).* This scan also shows portal vein *(PV),* which is now cut obliquely.

C

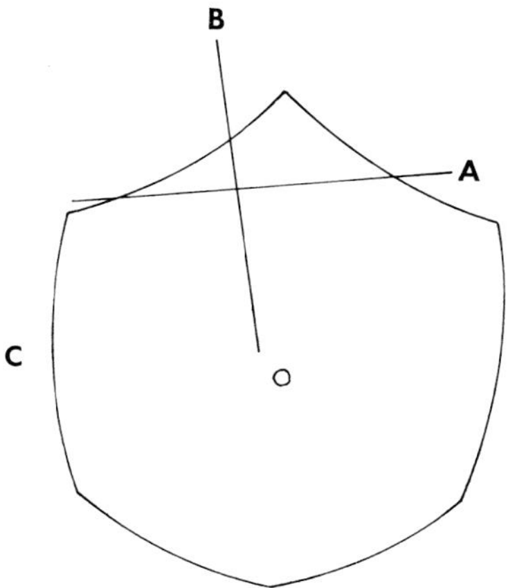

D

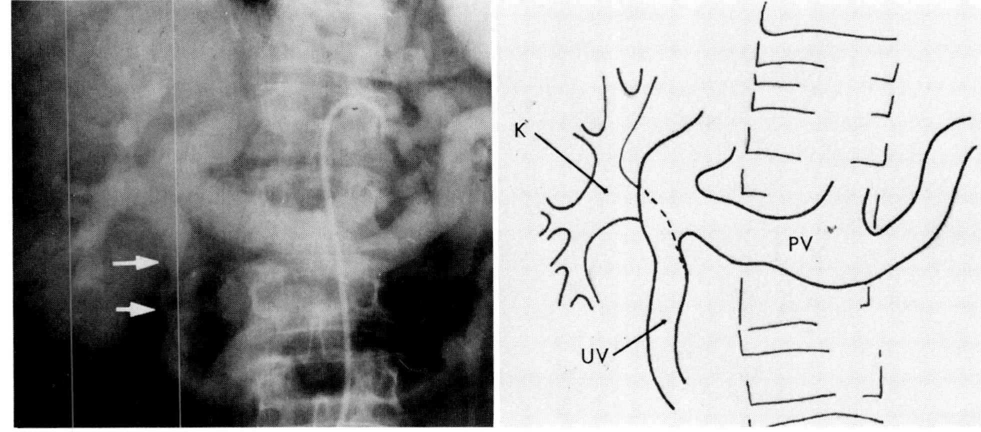

Fig. 10-17, cont'd. C, Scanning planes. **D,** Portal phase of celiacography. Umbilical vein (*arrows* and *UV*) is opacified and partly superimposed on origin of ureter. *K,* kidney; *PV,* portal vein.

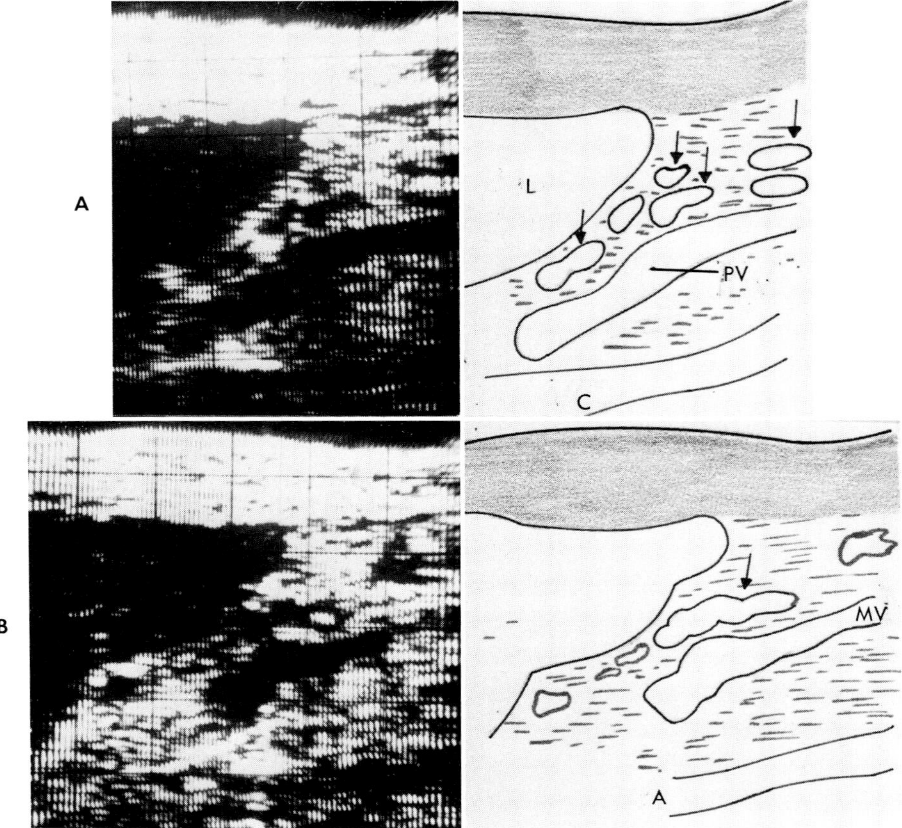

Fig. 10-18. Portal cavernoma. **A,** Oblique, almost sagittal, scan and schematic representation of right upper quadrant, displaying mesenteric-portal axis *(PV)* in sagittal section. Between venous axis and liver *(L)* appear several transparent, well-marginated areas *(arrows),* belonging to collateral venous network. Thrombosis of portal vein is not visible. *C,* vena cava. **B,** Sagittal medial scan and schematic drawing of abdomen displaying mesenteric-portal junction *(MV).* Sections of other abnormal veins are displayed between venous axis and liver *(arrow). A,* aorta.

a honeycomb pattern (Fig. 10-18). Splenic hilar varices may be displayed (Fig. 10-19). An enlarged caudate lobe would be consistent with Budd-Chiari syndrome.

With respect to portal hypertension we should like to quote a recent contribution of Goldberg (1976), who showed that in real time it is possible to check the permeability of a portacaval anastomosis. If the anastomosis is permeable, a Valsalva maneuver will give rise to a portal dilatation secondary to the caval one. Conversely, if the anastomosis is thrombosed, no portal dilatation will appear.

DIFFERENTIAL DIAGNOSIS

During the stage of homogeneous nonspecific hepatomegaly (Type I), only certain associated signs may lead to a specific diagnosis. The presence of increased attenuation (Type II) makes the diagnosis more reliable. When a nodular echopat-

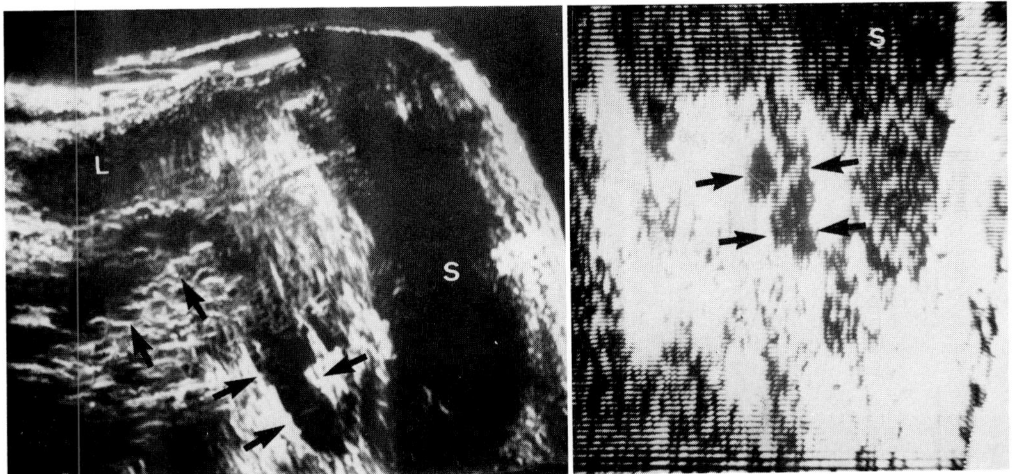

Fig. 10-19. Portal hypertension. **A,** Transverse scan of upper abdomen showing, medial to spleen *(S)*, dilated origin of splenic vein (⇉). Splenic vein itself, also dilated, is visible behind liver *(L)* (↑↑). **B,** Real-time intercostal scan of spleen close to its medial aspect. Enlarged origin of splenic vein *(arrows)* is displayed.

Table 10-1. Differential diagnosis of cirrhotic liver

Signs	*Multinodular metastases*	*Cirrhosis*
Hepatomegaly	+	+
Small liver	0	+
Hailstorm pattern	+	+
Sieve pattern	+	0
Edge sign	+	0
Angle sign	+	+
Humps	+	±
Retracted areas	0	+
Increased attenuation	0	+
Associated signs		
Ascites	+	+
Dilated splenic vein	0	+
Splenomegaly	0 (except for lymphomas)	+

tern has appeared (Types III and IV), metastatic deposits must be considered. Three kinds of morphological features should lead to a differentiation:

- Increased attenuation, which does not exist with metastases.
- The pattern of liver contours: the marginal edge remains angular. It may become biconvex, but without the frankly rounded shape seen in metastases.
- The lack of real marginal humps, with only small surface irregularities. If retraction has occurred, the contour may be wavy, but with curves of greater radius than in metastatic humps.

Finally, the nodular elements are not more than 1 cm in diameter. However, one must keep in mind that, in liver cirrhosis, angiography may display rather large regenerating nodules. Although one would expect large nodules to be displayed by ultrasonography, we have never recorded such large reflective nodules due to regenerative tissue.

Grouped in Table 10-1 are the different elements of the differential diagnosis.

REFERENCES

Barnett, E., and Morley, P.: Abdominal echography, Borough Green, England, 1974, Butterworth & Co. (Publishers), Ltd.

Goldberg, B. B.: Ultrasonic evaluation of portal-caval shunts, World Federation of Ultrasound in Medicine and Biology, San Francisco, 1976, Abstract No. 558.

Goldberg, B. B., Kotler, M. N., Ziskin, M. C., and Waxham, R. D.: Diagnostic uses of ultrasound, New York, 1975, Grune & Stratton, Inc.

Hassani, N.: Ultrasonography of the abdomen, Heidelberg, Germany, 1976, Springer-Verlag.

Holm, H. H., Kristensen, J. K., Rasmussen, S. N., Pedersen, J. F., and Hancke, S.: Abdominal ultrasound, Copenhagen, 1976, Munksgaard, International Booksellers & Publishers, Ltd.

Leopold, G. R., and Asher, W. M.: Fundamentals of abdominal and pelvic ultrasonography, Philadelphia, 1975, W. B. Saunders Co.

Rettenmaier, G.: Echographic diagnosis and differential diagnosis of diffuse liver diseases. Start of quantitative evaluation and results, Verh. Dtsch. Ges. Inn. Med. **79:**962-964, 1973a.

Rettenmaier, G.: Personal communication, 1975.

Rettenmaier, G.: Quantitative criteria of intrahepatic echo patterns correlated with structural alteration. Ultrasonics in medicine, Second World Congress, Amsterdam, 1973b, Excerpta Medica Foundation, pp. 199-206.

Weill, F.: Ultrasonic visualization of an umbilical vein, Radiology **120:**159-160, 1976.

Weill, F., Aucant, D., Bourgoin, A., Eisenscher, A., and Gallinet, D.: Ultrasonic visualization of abdominal veins: vena mesenterica, vena splenica, vena portae, hepatic veins, vena cava, Second European Congress, Munich, Germany, 1975, Abstract No. 103.

Weill, F., Becker, J. C., Kraehenbuhl, J. R., Heriot, G., and Walter, J. P.: Clinical atlas of ultrasonic radiography, Paris, 1973, Masson & Cie., Editeurs.

Weill, F., and Eisenscher, A.: Echo-angiostructure hépatique: étude écho-anatomique des structures canalaires intraparenchymateuses, J. Radiol. Electrol. Med. Nucl. **57:**311-319, 1976.

Weill, F., Eisenscher, A., Aucant, D., Bourgoin, A., and Gallinet, D.: Ultrasonic study of venous patterns in the right hypochondrium, J. Clin. Ultrasound **3:**23-28, 1975.

Weill, F., Kraehenbuhl, J. R., Aucant, D., and Maurat, J. P.: Etude échotomographique des gros troncs veineux abdominaux, Coeur Méd. Interne **12:**431-439, 1973a.

CHAPTER 11

ABSCESSES, CYSTS, AND PARASITOSES

LIVER ABSCESS

Painful hepatomegaly, with pain elicited by the application of the transducer, is suggestive of abscess. Before it collects, an abscess possesses a heterogeneous echopattern, with prevalent sonolucent areas (Fig. 11-1). This pattern is not specific. Later, as the abscess collects, the area of purulent necrosis takes on a true liquid pattern (Figs. 11-2 to 11-5), with floating necrotic debris. The walls of an abscess may be irregular and craggy during the necrotizing phase but tend to become more regularly outlined (Figs. 11-2, 11-4, and 11-5). The posterior wall does not always show strong reinforcement, probably since there is greater attenuation of sound by pus than by fluid. Transparent pseudocystic masses with posterior reinforcement may be encountered, however.

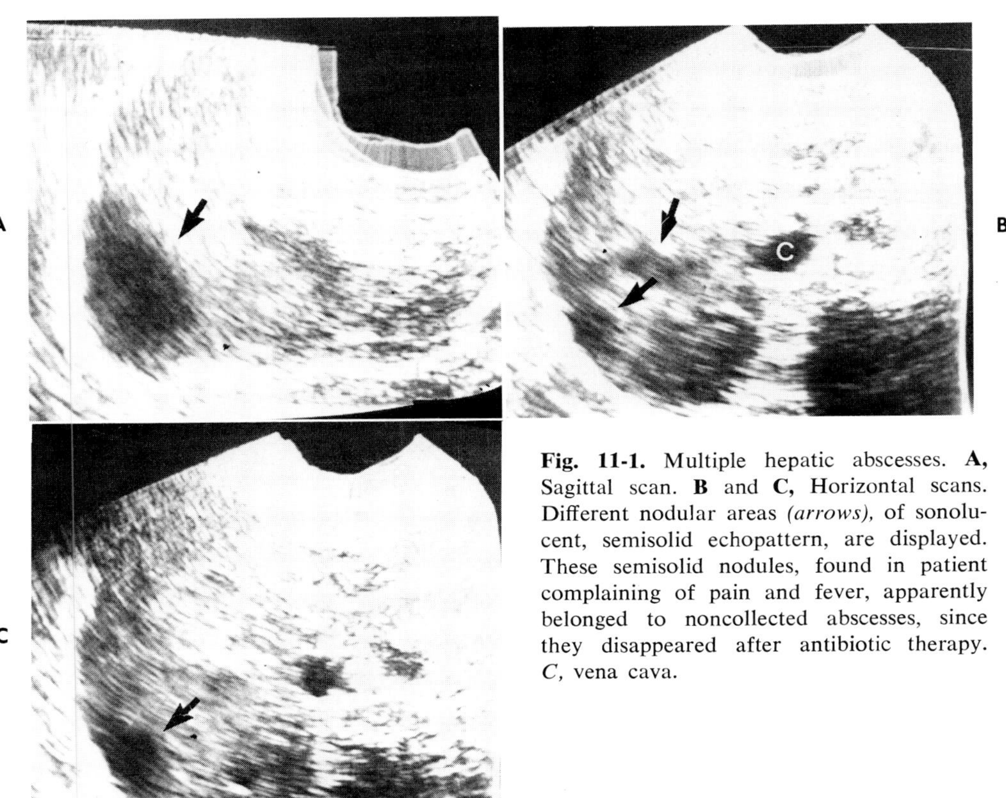

Fig. 11-1. Multiple hepatic abscesses. **A,** Sagittal scan. **B** and **C,** Horizontal scans. Different nodular areas *(arrows),* of sonolucent, semisolid echopattern, are displayed. These semisolid nodules, found in patient complaining of pain and fever, apparently belonged to noncollected abscesses, since they disappeared after antibiotic therapy. *C,* vena cava.

Liver abscesses may be multiple and small; so (Fig. 11-6) even if an obvious lesion has been discovered initially, every part of the liver must be carefully examined for other abscesses. In some cases, specific therapy may cause small abscesses to regress and disappear. This is particularly true in patients with amebiasis treated with antiamebic agents. If surgery is performed, tissue that is strongly reflective may appear (Fig. 11-6, *C*). Some amebic abscesses that are not treated undergo calcification with consequent acoustic shadowing (Fig. 11-7).

I should like to add to this study of liver abscess an observation of liver involvement in Hansen's disease: there was hepatomegaly, and the echopattern was micronodular, with sonolucent micronodules and, at different levels, surrounding reflective areas (Fig. 11-8).

Extrahepatic abscesses will be covered in Chapter 14, but now other sonolucent and transparent liver lesions will be considered.

CONGENITAL CYSTS

Most of these cysts are a part of the syndrome of hepatorenal polycystic disease. Hepatic cysts may be the first manifestation of the disease, but more often the diagnosis of liver cysts is incidental to the diagnosis of polycystic disease of the kidney. In at least 20% of the cases of polycystic disease the liver is involved, as well as the kidney. The cyst of polycystic disease is a typical liquid sonotransparent image, well delineated by wall and separation images, with strong reinforcement of posterior interfaces (Figs. 11-9 to 11-11). The neighboring hepatic tissue presents a normal echopattern. Peripheral cysts produce bulges of the liver contours ("liquid hump"), or they may deform the liver edge. Despite the

Text continued on p. 167.

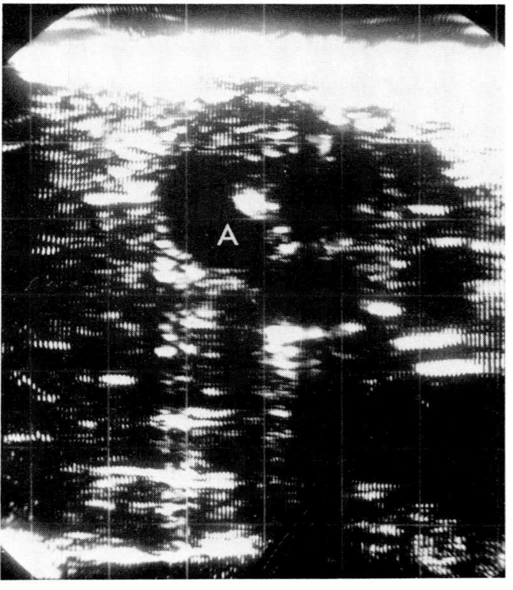

Fig. 11-2. Amebic abscess *(A)*. Oblique recurrent subcostal real-time scan displays rounded, well-marginated cavity with floating debris. Posterior wall image is not really reinforced. (From Weill, F., Becker, J. C., Kraehenbuhl, J. R., Heriot, G., and Walter, J. P.: Clinical atlas of ultrasonic radiography, Paris, 1973, Masson & Cie., Editeurs.)

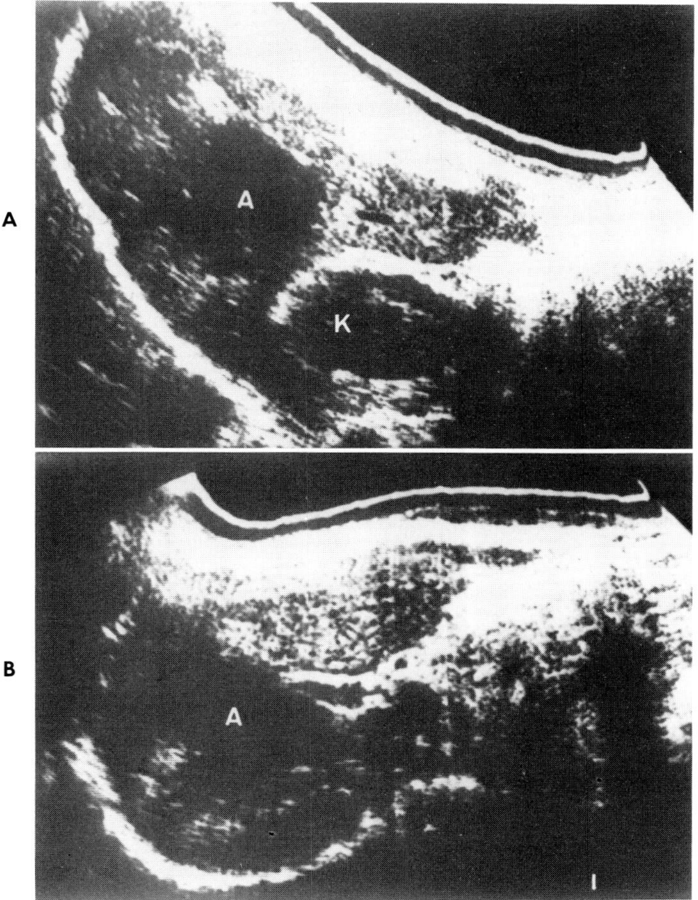

Fig. 11-3. Amebic abscess. **A,** Sagittal scan of right upper quadrant showing rounded sonolucent area *(A)* proximal to upper pole of right kidney *(K)*. There are few echoes inside lesion; posterior wall is not reinforced. This indicates noncollected abscess. **B,** Transverse scan again displaying rounded abscess in right hepatic lobe. Surgery showed amebic abscess. (Courtesy Dr. Triller, Bern, Switzerland.)

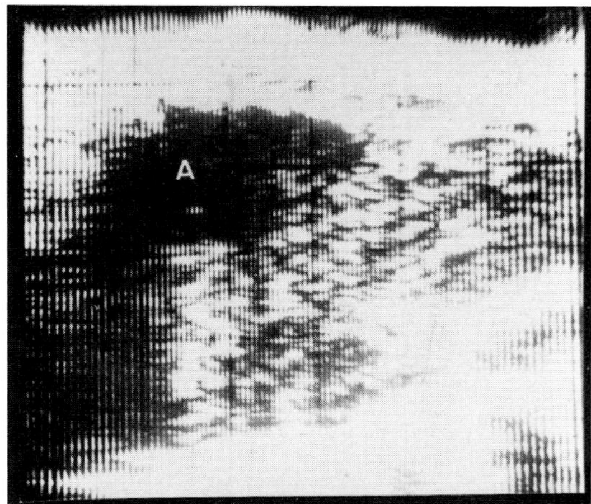

Fig. 11-4. Bacterial liver abscess. Intercostal scan displaying oval sonolucent area *(A)*. Posterior wall image is only slightly reinforced. There are rare scattered echoes amid lesion, indicating noncollected abscess.

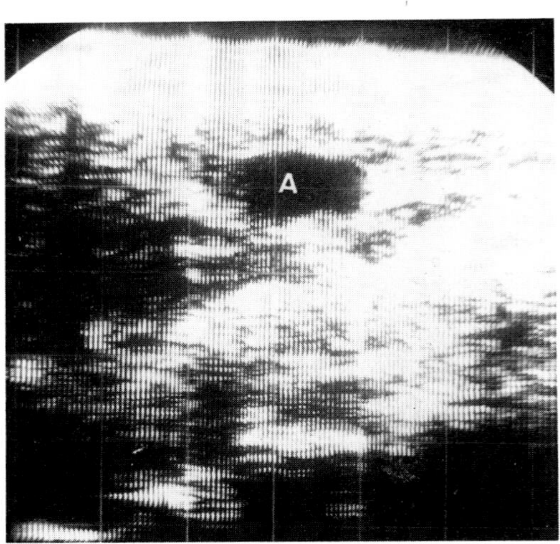

Fig. 11-5. Bacterial abscess. This sagittal scan of left hepatic lobe shows oval nodule of liquid echopattern. This belongs to collected abscess *(A)*.

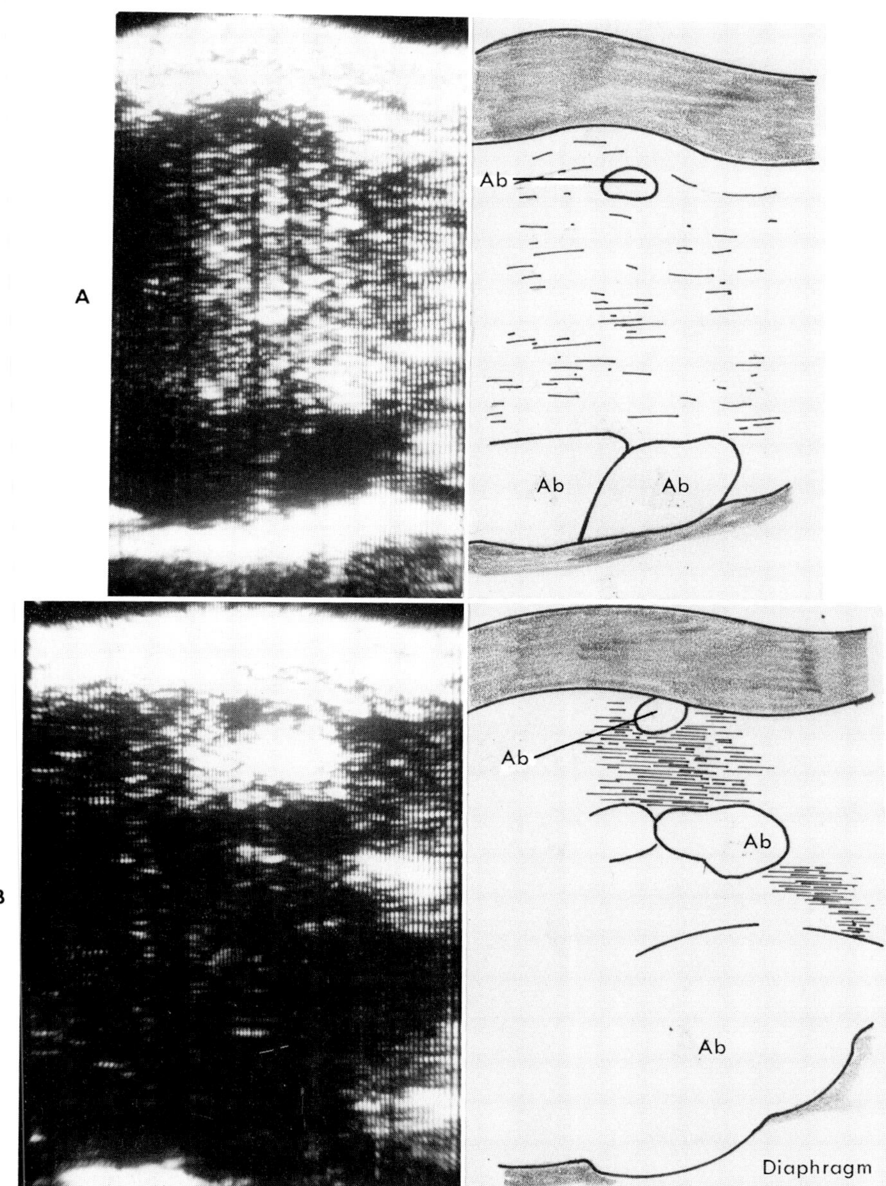

Fig. 11-6. Multiple abscesses. **A,** This oblique recurrent subcostal real-time scan and its schematic representation display several areas of liquid type, indicating collected abscesses *(Ab).* **B,** Second scan and schematic representation displaying other sonolucent areas of same pattern, but different size. In deeper part of liver, just under diaphragm, there is large necrotized area. At surgery, six different abscesses were found.

Continued.

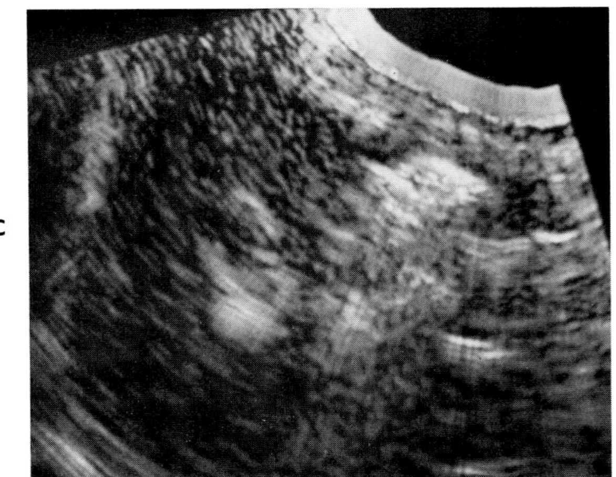

Fig. 11-6, cont'd. C, Follow-up one year later. There are different reflective nodules, which probably represent scar and granulation tissue.

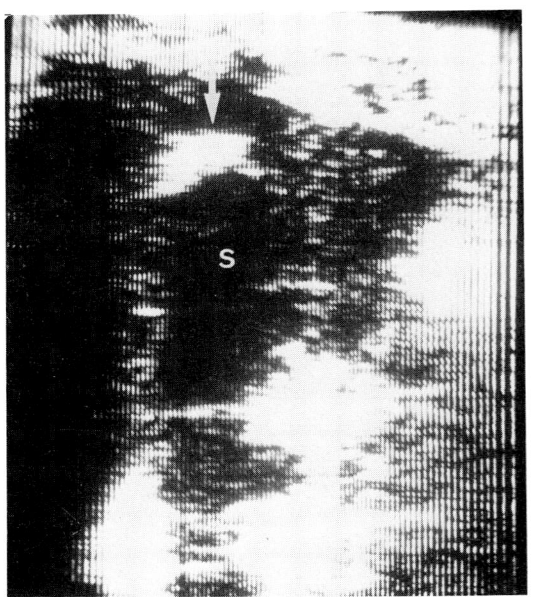

Fig. 11-7. Calcified abscess. This intercostal scan displays reflective strip *(arrow)* behind which is acoustic shadow *(S)*. This is typical of calcified abscess wall (shell sign).

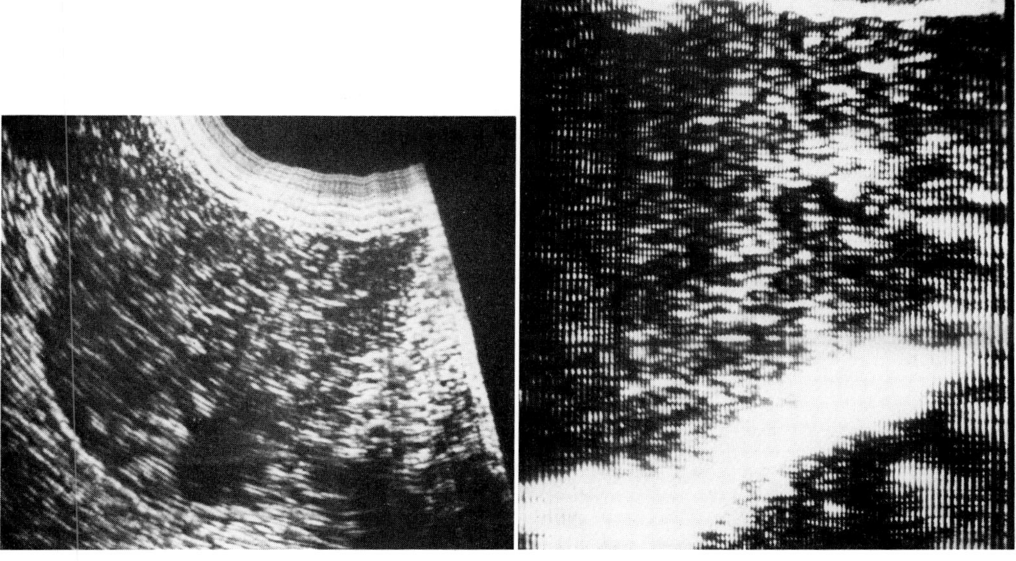

Fig. 11-8. Hansenian lesions (leprosy). **A,** Sagittal scan displaying micronodular tissue echopattern. **B,** Oblique subcostal recurrent scan again showing small sonolucent nodules with marginal echoes.

similarity of the liver contours to those described for metastatic disease, the liquid character of liver cysts is so evident and typical that, even in cases with contour deformity, no diagnostic problem is encountered. A necrotized metastatic deposit could perhaps cause a discussion; but the limits of a necrotic cavity are much less regular than those of a cyst, and the liver tissue proximal to the cavity is abnormal.

In some cases of hepatorenal polycystic disease, it is difficult to differentiate a cyst extending caudally from the liver from a cyst extending cranially from the kidney (Fig. 11-9, *A*). A comparison of the different cuts with an intravenous pyelogram (IVP), if renal insufficiency does not contraindicate that examination, usually permits such a differentiation. However, in polycystic disease the distinction is not of basic importance.

Another problem arises when there is a solitary cyst. If such a cyst has developed within the liver parenchyma, it is easily visualized. (See Fig. 11-12.) However, the only proof of its being congenital is the demonstration of associated renal cysts. Unfortunately, small congenital renal cysts may not be easy to demonstrate. To make solution of the problem even more difficult, liver echinococcal cysts sometimes exist along with renal echinococcal cysts. In countries with endemic echinococcosis or for patients who have a history of exposure, complementary laboratory tests should be carried out. When there is a posterior solitary cyst, it is more important to assess whether the cyst is hepatic or renal (or adrenal) (Fig. 11-13). Again, a thorough study of multiple cuts and comparison of them with IVPs and scintigraphic and even angiographic films may contribute to a correct diagnosis. These different investigations are justified because, although puncture of a renal cyst is legitimate and puncture of a hepatic cyst may, of course, be

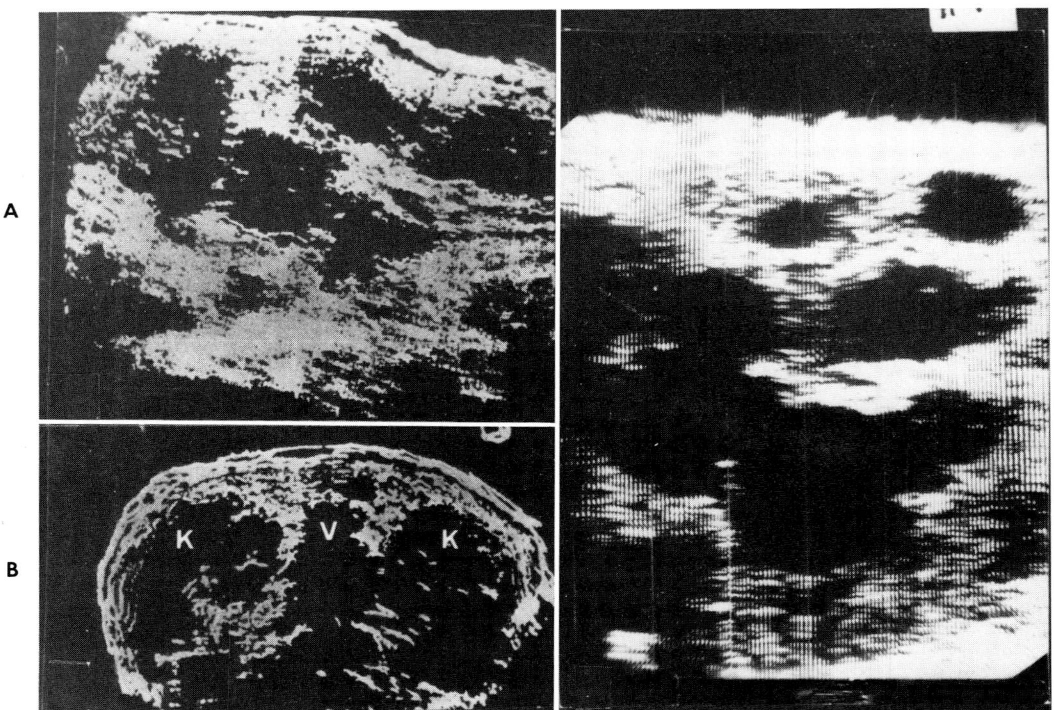

Fig. 11-9. Hepatorenal polycystic disease. **A,** Sagittal scan of enlarged liver displaying multiple liquid collections. **B,** Transverse scan made with patient in prone position shows, on both sides of vertebral body *(V)*, kidney *(K)* diameter to be larger than twice vertebral width. This is typical for polycystic kidneys. **C,** Sagittal scan in real time clearly displays cysts with their septa.

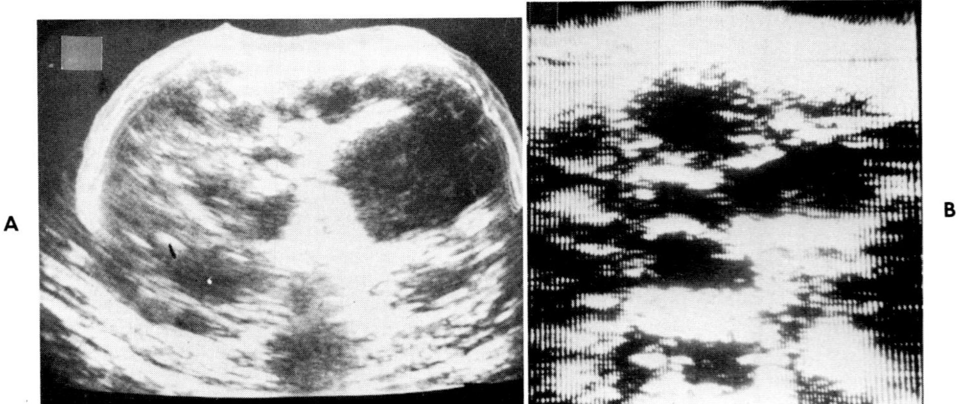

Fig. 11-10. Hepatorenal polycystic disease. **A,** Transverse scan of upper abdomen. Different intrahepatic cysts are displayed. There is large cyst in left lobe of liver. **B,** Oblique recurrent subcostal real-time scan also showing coalescent cysts of variable sizes.

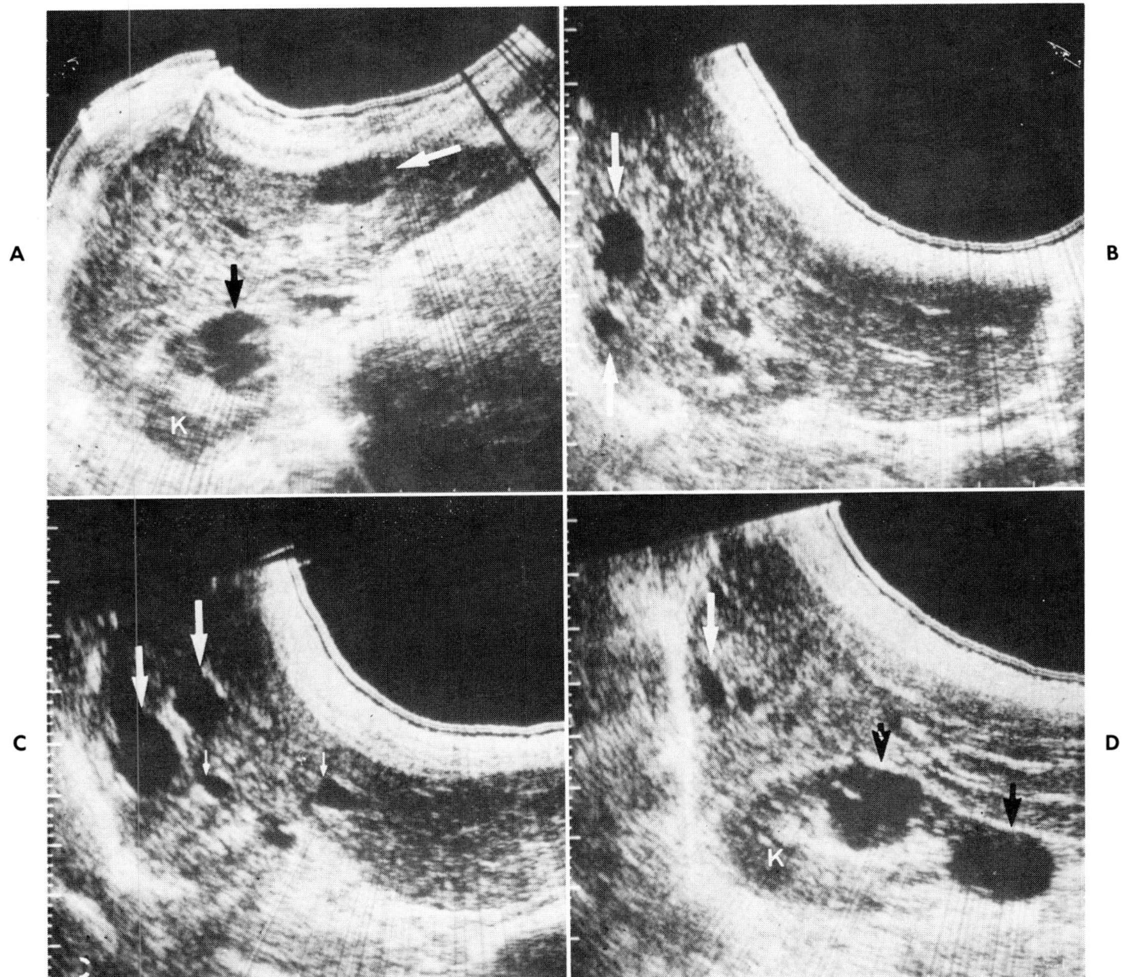

Fig. 11-11. Hepatic and renal congenital cysts. **A,** Transverse scan of right upper quadrant. *K,* kidney. **B** to **D,** Parallel sagittal scans. There are several cysts *(white arrows)* in the liver, which is enlarged. Delineation between renal cysts *(black arrows)* and liver tissue is sharp.

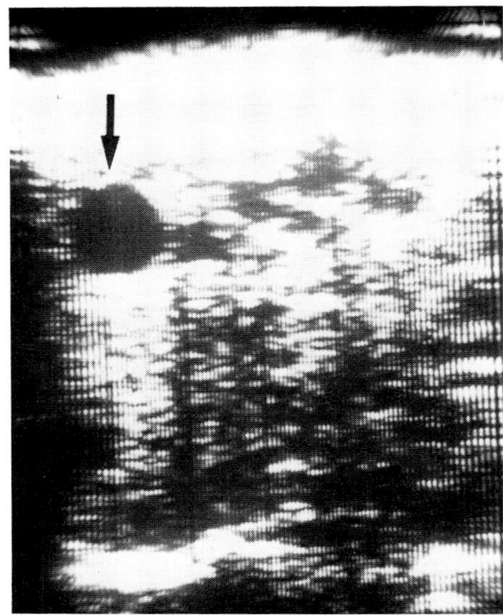

Fig. 11-12. Solitary congenital hepatic anterior cyst *(arrow)*, displayed on oblique recurrent subcostal scan. Such an image may be mistaken for the gallbladder.

performed, puncture of an echinococcal cyst is contraindicated. Follow-up of a cystic lesion may be required. Congenital cysts, even when growing, do not change in echopattern except in case of intracystic hemorrhage, whereas, as will be seen later, echinococcal cysts may increase in size and also change in echopattern.

Another problem arises when there are anteriorly located liquid areas, since a liver cyst may be confused with the gallbladder (Figs. 11-14 and 11-15). The gallbladder may be distinguished by a contraction test and, if necessary, by a comparison with the cholecystogram.

Another confusing problem is the occurrence of a congenital cyst in association with another lesion (Fig. 16-26). Since congenital cysts are usually asymptomatic, if a patient complains of pain in the right upper quadrant, the presence of a congenital cyst is not a satisfactory explanation.

PARASITIC CYSTS AND DISEASES

Most, if not all, parasitic cysts result from classic echinococcal disease; but I shall also mention the cysts that may occur in a related parasitosis, multilocular echinococcosis, which is rather frequent in central Europe, even though rare on the American Continent except in Alaska.

Echinococcal cysts

When young, the echinococcal, like the congenital, cyst is a typical transparent liquid collection with a regular, well-marginated wall (Figs. 11-16 to 11-18). When the cyst is located peripherally, it bulges the hepatic contour. This occurs commonly on the hepatic dome, which is one of the preferred locations of these cysts (Fig. 11-19) and is best seen on sagittal sector scans. Echinococcal cysts may be multiple (Figs. 11-16, *B,* 11-17, and 11-18), resembling polycystic disease, par-

Text continued on p. 175.

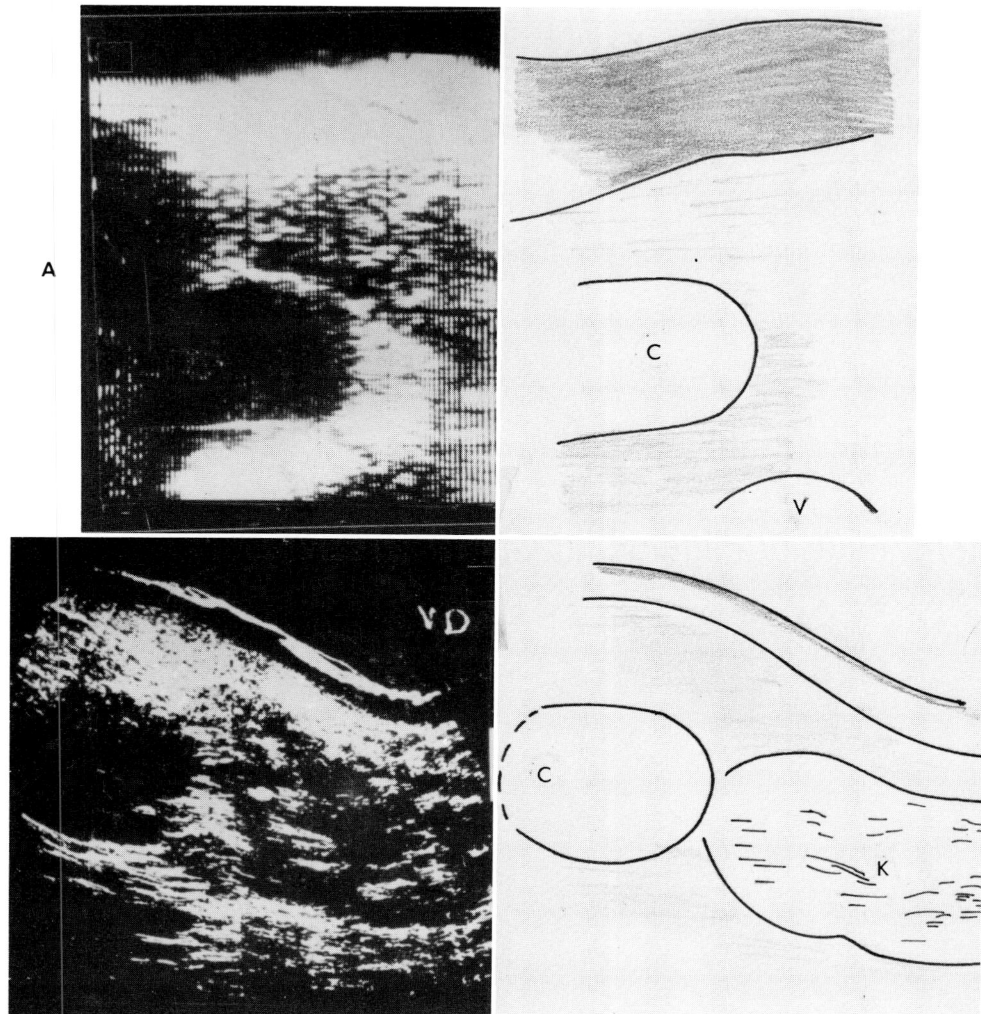

Fig. 11-13. Another example of differentiation betwen renal and hepatic cyst. **A,** Oblique recurrent subcostal scan of right upper quadrant and its schematic representation showing posterior collection *(C)*. *V,* vertebral body. **B,** Sagittal scan, made with patient in prone position, and schematic representation display cyst above upper pole of kidney *(K)*. It possesses proper wall image and is separated from kidney. This, then, is liver cyst.

Continued.

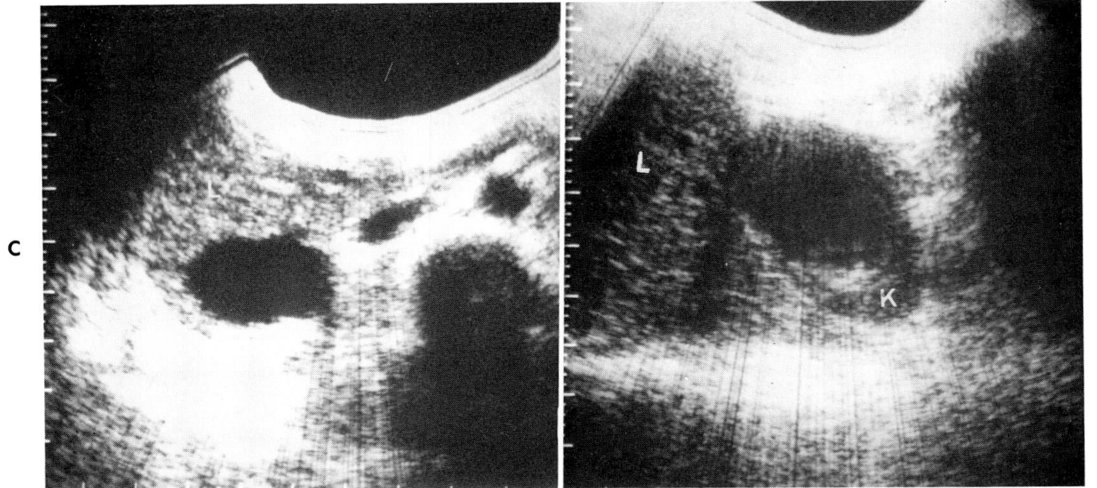

Fig. 11-13, cont'd. C, Transverse scan in another patient, showing, in right upper quadrant, cyst surrounded by liver tissue *(L),* as in **A. D,** Posterior sagittal scan showing relation of cyst to right kidney. Delineation between cyst and liver is sharper than that between cyst and kidney. This cyst is renal.

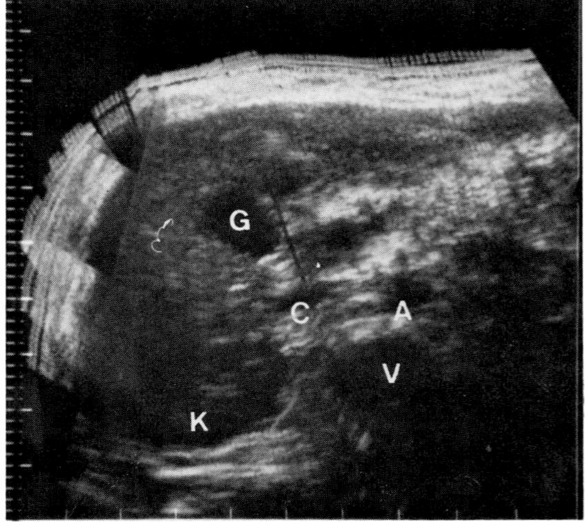

Fig. 11-14. Differentiation between cyst and gallbladder. Transverse scan shows upper abdomen, 3 cm below costal margin. In fasting patients, this kind of scan almost constantly displays, in transverse section, gallbladder *(G),* which may lie deep, in rather close relation with vena cava *(C).* This normal anatomical image is not to be confused with cystic element. In case of doubt, contraction test must be performed. *A,* aorta; *V,* vertebra; *K,* kidney.

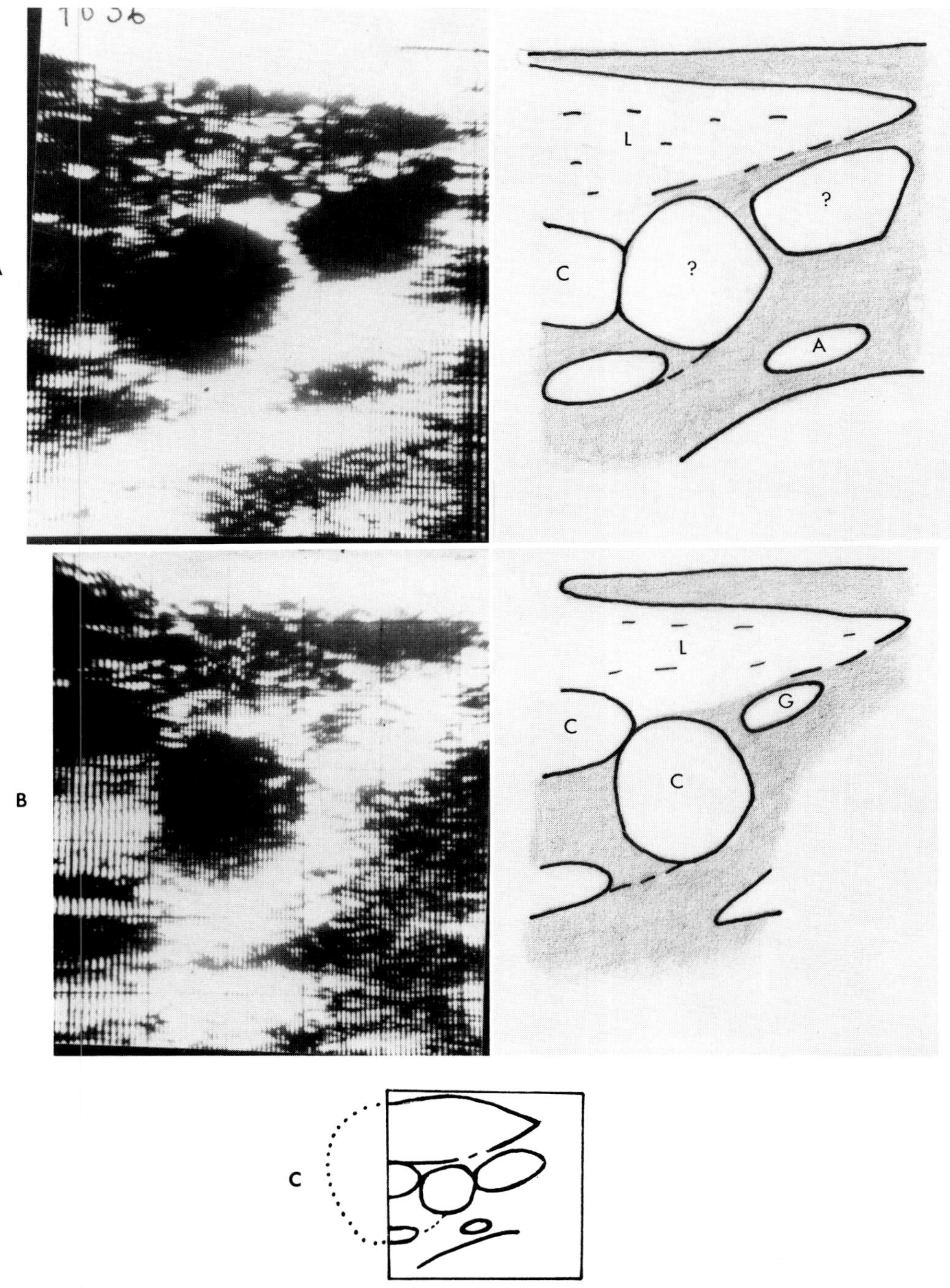

Fig. 11-15. Polycystic disease of liver—differentiation between cyst and gallbladder. **A** to **C**, First example. **A,** Sagittal scan and its schematic representation displaying peripheral cysts *(C)* close to gallbladder. As a matter of fact, it is difficult to tell which collection belongs to cyst and which to gallbladder *(?)*. *L,* liver; *A,* aorta. **B,** Identical scan made after contraction test and schematic representation. Image of gallbladder *(G)* has almost disappeared. **C,** Schematic drawing of liver area displayed.

Continued.

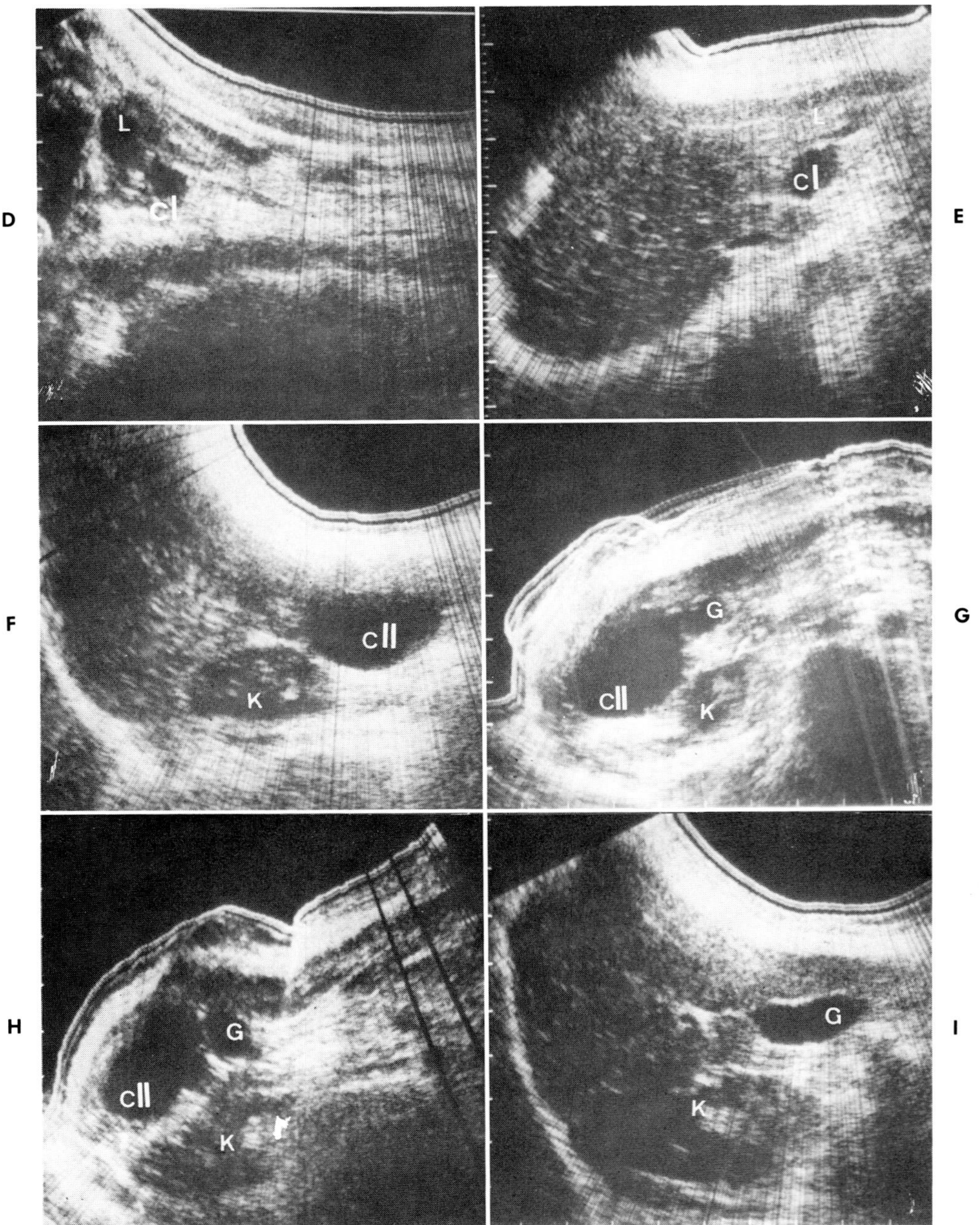

Fig. 11-15, cont'd. D to **I,** Second example. **D** and **E,** Sagittal and transverse scans displaying small cyst *(CI)* in left hepatic lobe. **F,** Right sagittal scan showing large collection *(CII),* which could be gallbladder. *K,* kidney. **G** and **H,** Transverse parallel scans showing gallbladder internal to main collection. **I,** Sagittal scan of gallbladder.

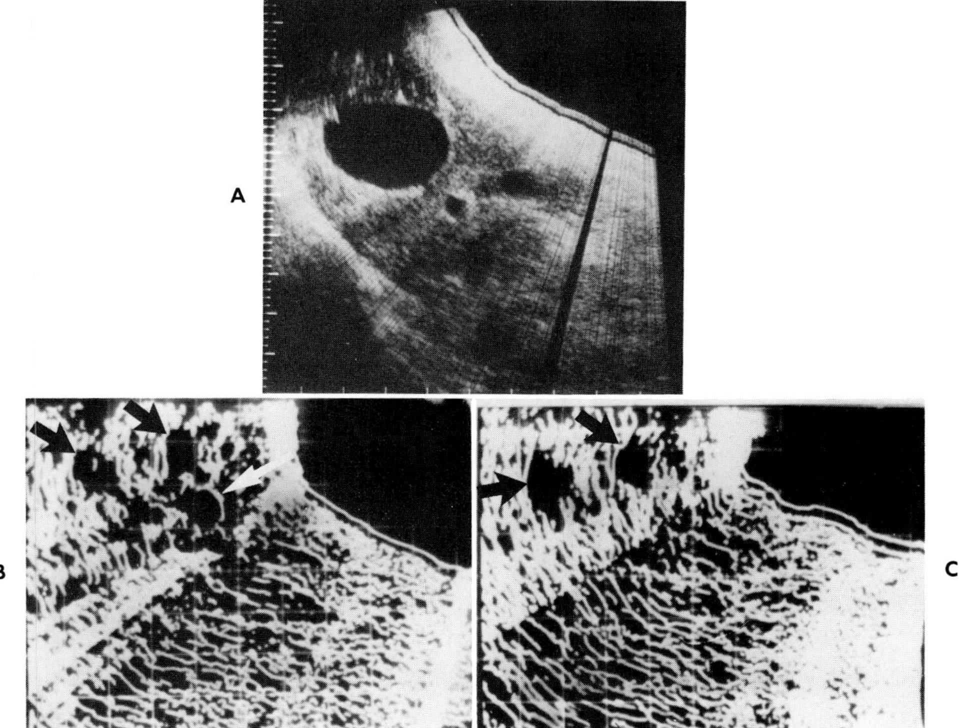

Fig. 11-16. Young echinococcal cysts. **A,** Large solitary cyst. **B** and **C,** Multiple small hydatid cysts shown on sagittal scans. (**B** and **C** courtesy Dr. Roussille and Dr. Duquesnel, Lyons, France.)

ticularly in the rare cases of associated echinococcal cysts of the kidney. If the patient is asymptomatic, the cysts are more likely congenital, since echinococcal cysts are generally painful. If necessary, laboratory tests will, of course, lead to a positive diagnosis. After viewing the typical cystic lesions illustrated in this chapter (Figs. 11-16 to 11-19), one could cherish the illusion that the diagnosis of an echinococcal cyst is always easy. Unfortunately, this is not so. Detachment of the cystic membrane gives rise to deformity of the cyst and to a double wall image (Fig. 11-20). However, the major problem is the change in the echopattern of mature cysts (Weill and co-workers, 1973a; Weill and co-workers, 1973b; King, 1973). As the mother cyst fills with daughter cysts, its liquid echopattern is progressively replaced by an echopattern of solid type. The image of the mature echinococcal cyst is therefore much more difficult to recognize, since such an image is not very different from that of a tumor. (See Figs. 11-21 and 11-22.) The presence of wall calcification on a radiograph of the abdomen is then a precious clue. Scintigraphy is also helpful, since, even at this stage of the disease, a frank defect, rounded and regular, much more consistent with a cyst than a tumor, can be seen. The calcified cyst is thus easier to diagnose by radiography or scintigraphy than by ultrasonography until the calcified cyst wall causes a posterior acoustic shadow. (See Figs. 11-23 and 11-24.) Thus, as the disease progresses, its ultra-

Text continued on p. 182.

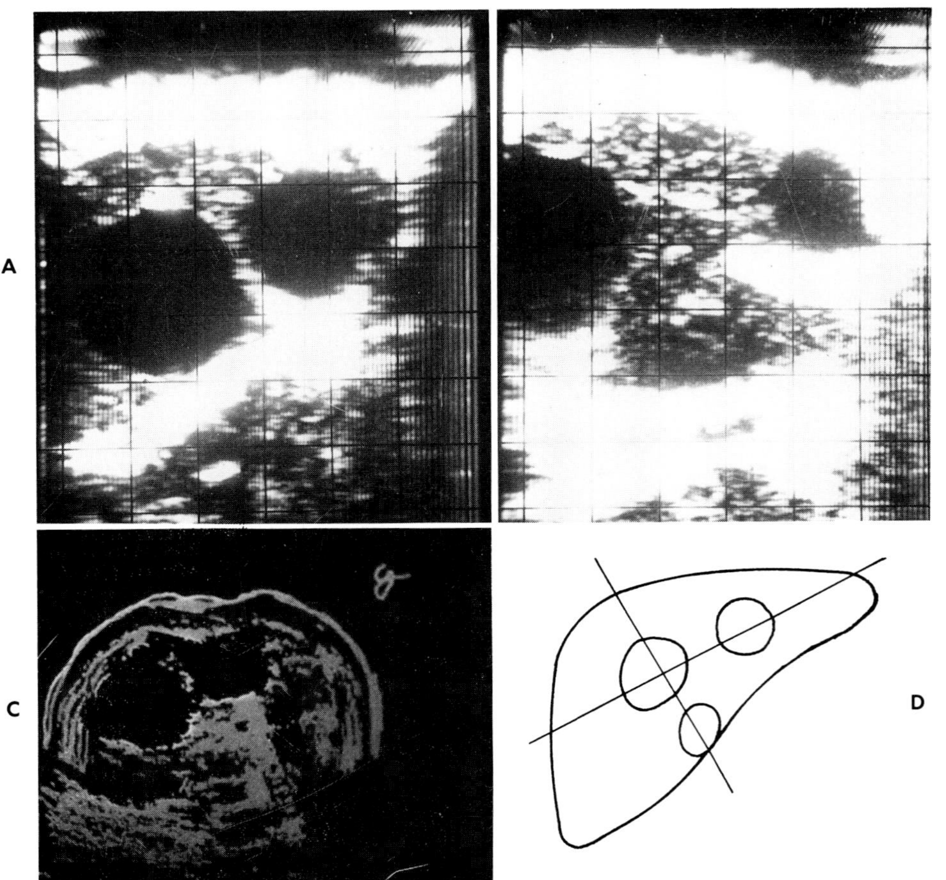

Fig. 11-17. Multiple young hydatid cysts in 7-year-old child of African origin. **A,** Oblique recurrent subcostal real-time scan displaying two typical cysts proximal to one another. **B,** Sagittal scan also displaying two cysts farther apart. **C,** Transverse contact scan again showing two cysts in close relation. **D,** Reconstruction of different scanning planes showing that there are, in fact, three distinct cysts. This was confirmed at surgery.

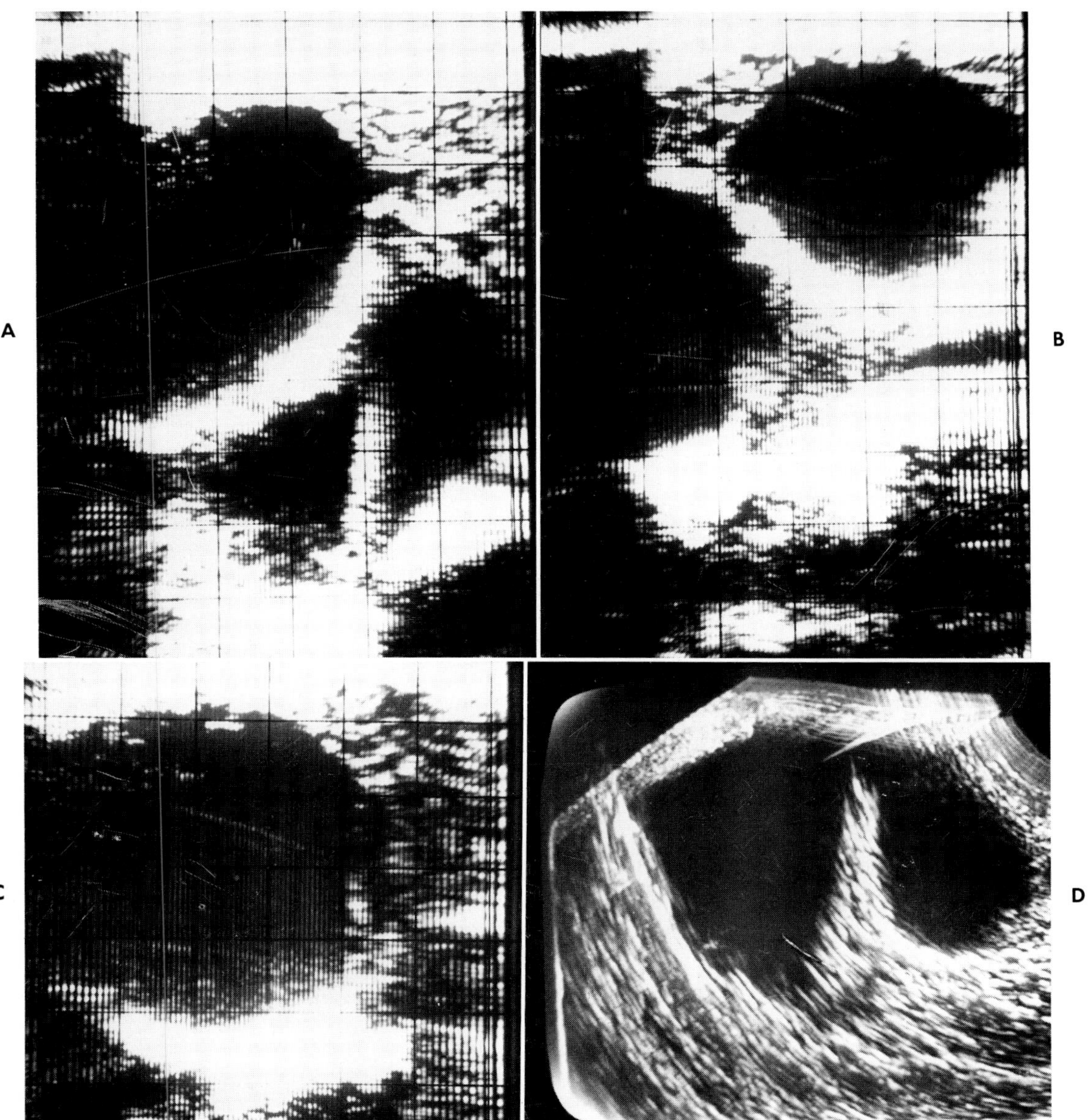

Fig. 11-18. Multiple hydatid cysts in adult. **A,** Subcostal oblique recurrent real-time scan. **B,** Sagittal real-time scan in midline. **C,** Intercostal scan in real time. **D,** Sagittal contact scan. In this case, there are again three distinct echinococcal cysts.

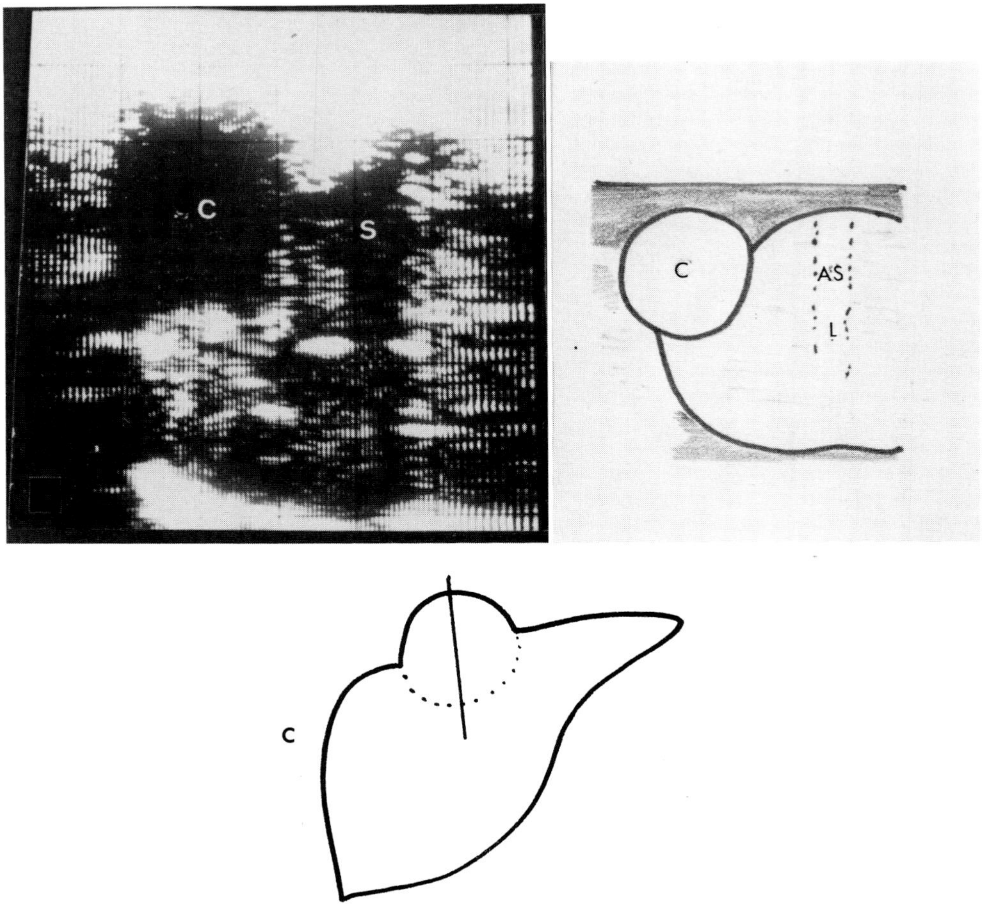

A

B

C

Fig. 11-19. Marginal young echinococcal cyst on liver dome. **A** and **B,** Sagittal real-time scan made with patient in prone position and its schematic representation displaying, despite acoustic shadow *(S, As)* of ribs, transparent image of cyst *(C)*. *L,* liver. **C,** Scanning plane.

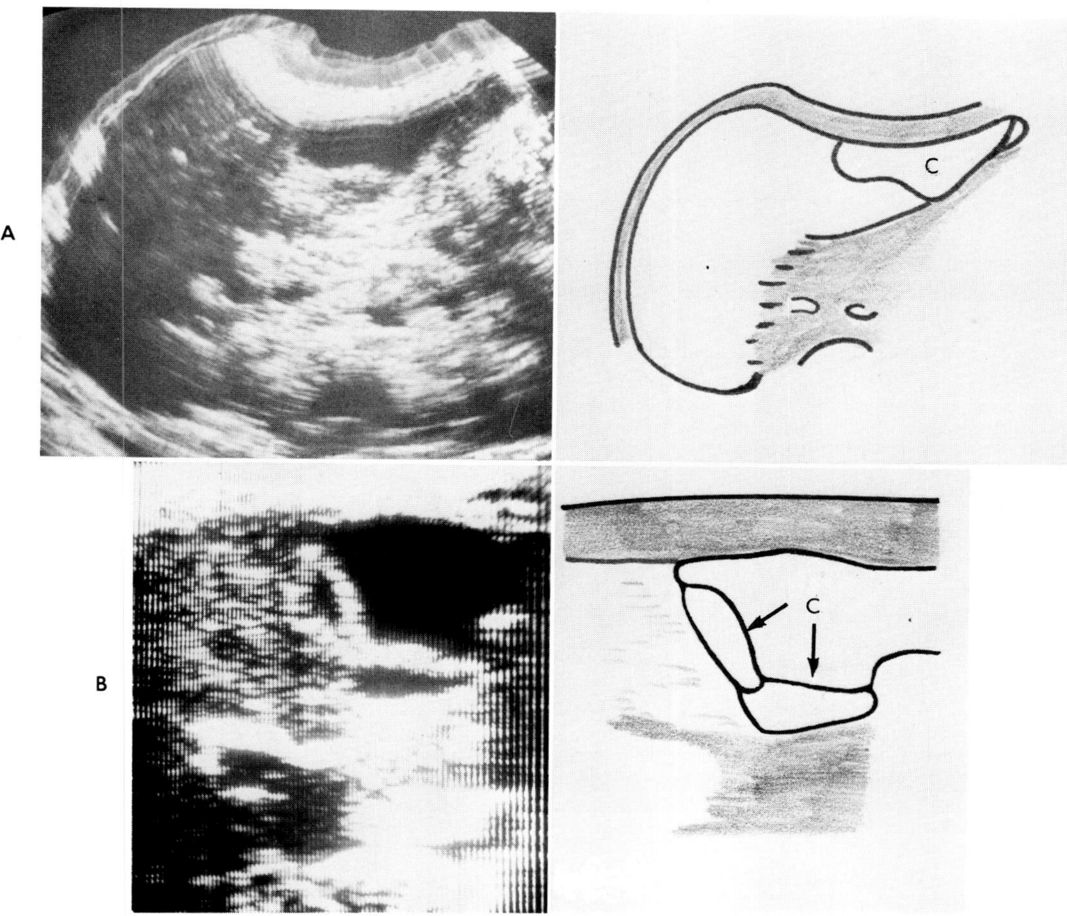

Fig. 11-20. Mature echinococcal cyst. **A,** Transverse scan of upper abdomen and its schematic representation showing flattened cyst *(C)* in left hepatic lobe. **B,** In real time, there is double wall image *(arrows),* which is due to detachment of membrane.

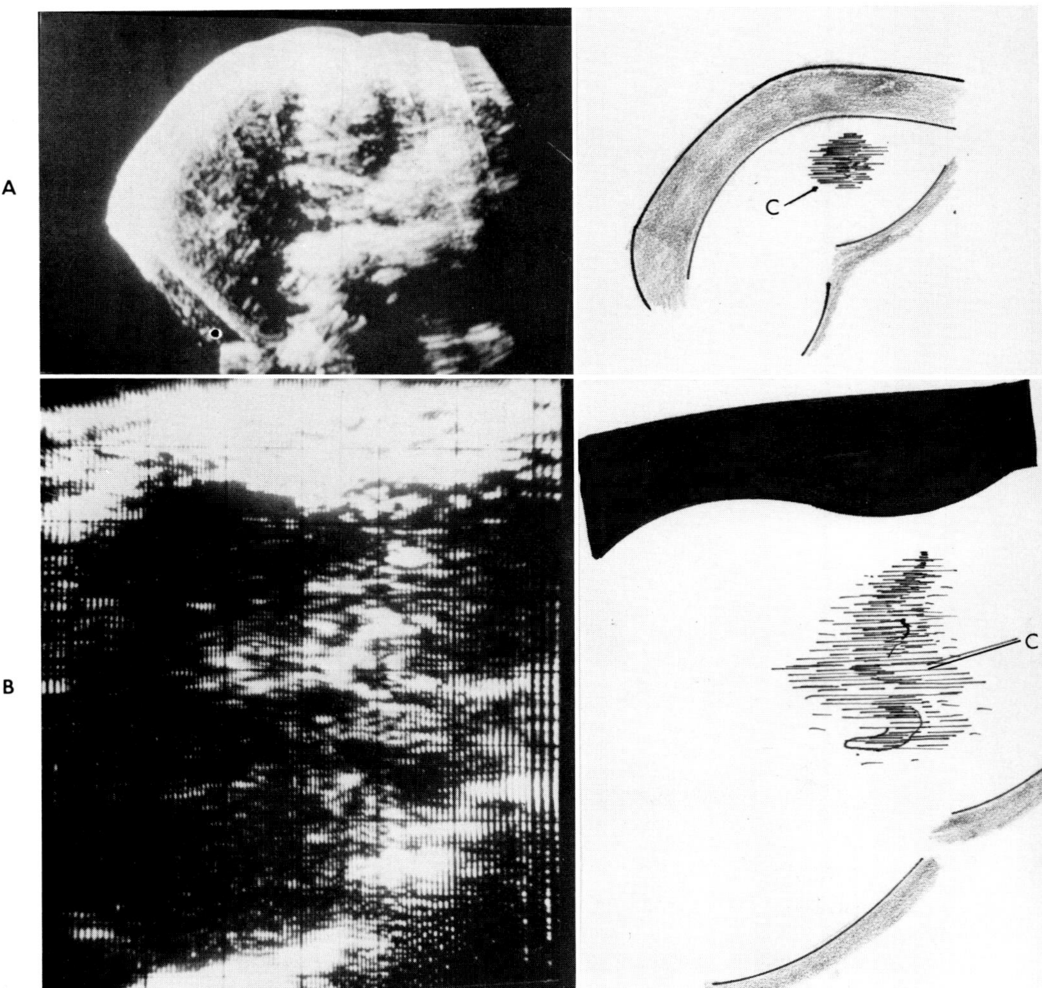

Fig. 11-21. Mature echinococcal cyst. **A,** Transverse scan and schematic representation. Cyst *(C),* filled with daughter vesicles, possesses very reflective pattern, of solid type, quite similar to tumoral echopattern. **B,** Same echopattern on real-time scan and its schematic representation.

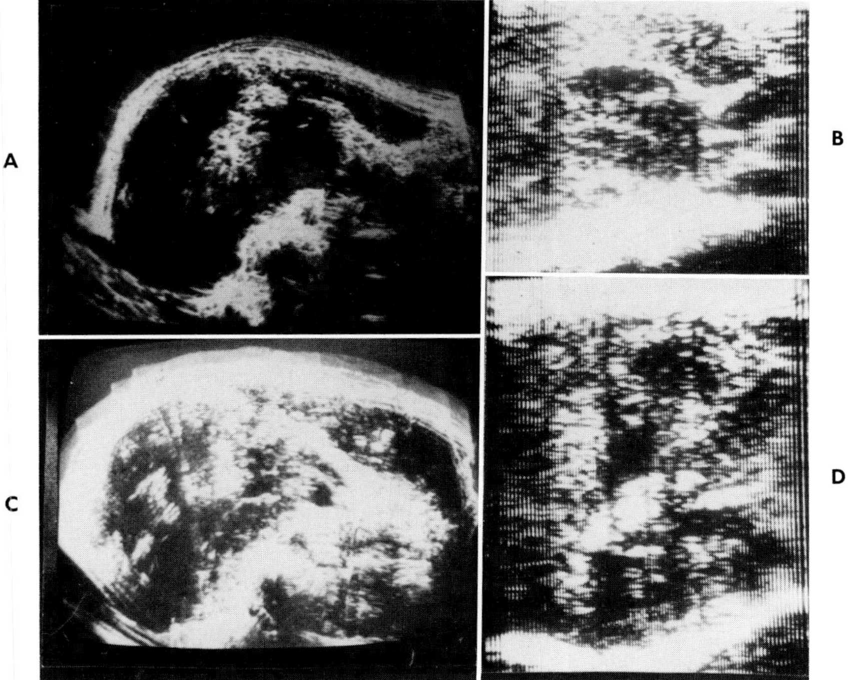

Fig. 11-22. Multiple mature echinococcal cysts. **A,** Transverse scan with low gain, showing abnormal area of reflection in right hepatic lobe. **B,** Same scan with higher sensitivity, displaying multiple abnormal reflective areas. **C** and **D,** Oblique recurrent subcostal real-time scans displaying sonolucent areas proximal to reflecting nodules. At first glance, this liver seems to be invaded by metastases. This patient had lived for several years in central Africa. Immunological tests were positive for hydatid disease.

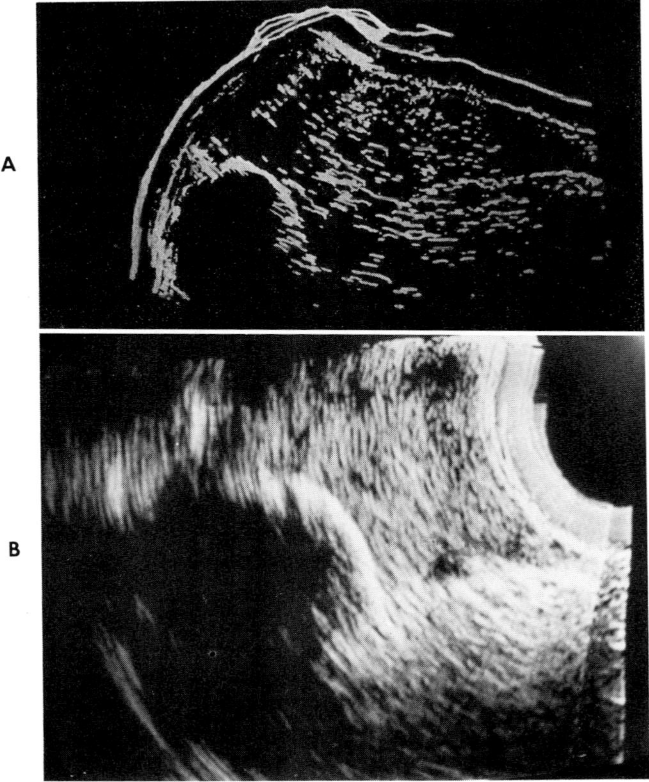

Fig. 11-23. Calcified hydatid cyst. **A,** Transverse scan. **B,** Sagittal scan. Calcified wall is sharply delineated, with posterior acoustic shadow (shell sign).

sonic images lose their specificity, changing from a typical liquid pattern to a tumorlike solid pattern and finally to a line of reflection with an acoustic shadow ("shell sign"). (See also p. 275.)

Multilocular echinococcosis

Common echinococcosis is due to *Echinococcus granulosus,* whereas multilocular echinococcosis is due to the tapeworm *E. multilocularis,* which lives in the intestines of the fox. The eggs of the worm are excreted in the feces of the infested fox. After oral contamination the parasite develops in the human liver (references in Miguet, 1973). In about 30% of the cases a necrotizing process, with cystic elements similar to immature echinococcal cysts, occurs (Figs. 11-25 and 11-26). The cysts are usually located within the liver, but they may also be marginal and cause contour bulging. Since this parasitic process often narrows the hilar or intrahepatic bile ducts, the patient is frequently jaundiced. Thus, in the jaundiced patient, a marginal cyst located on the posterior aspect of the liver may be confused with a dilated gallbladder. (See Fig. 11-25.) In fact, careful study of the liver tissue always discloses tissue abnormalities, such as small areas of heterogeneity (Fig. 11-26). More often, there are more marked changes with areas of intense

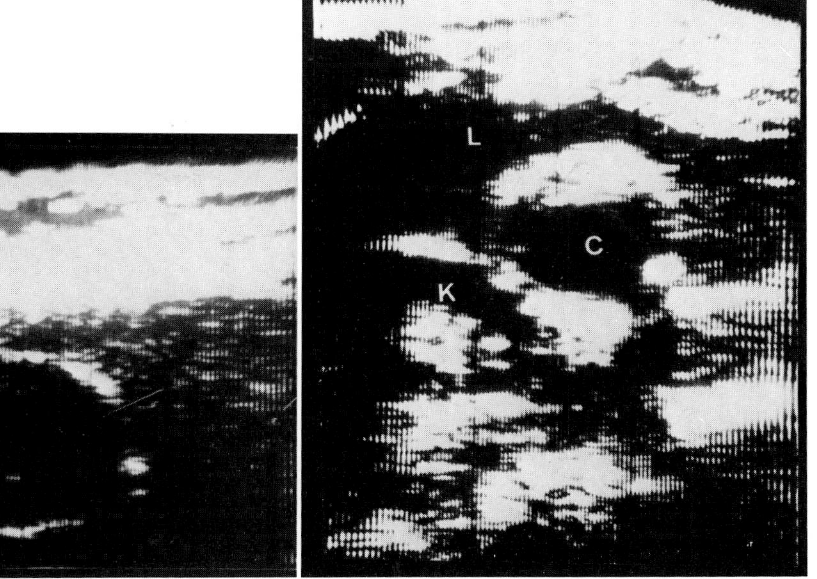

Fig. 11-24. Old calcified cysts. **A,** Oblique recurrent subcostal scan displaying sharply delineated calcified wall of old cyst. Despite acoustic shadow, posterior wall is displayed. Solid echopattern of daughter vesicles is completely erased by acoustic shadow of anterior wall. **B,** Another calcified cyst *(C)* displayed by intercostal scan. *L,* liver; *K,* right kidney.

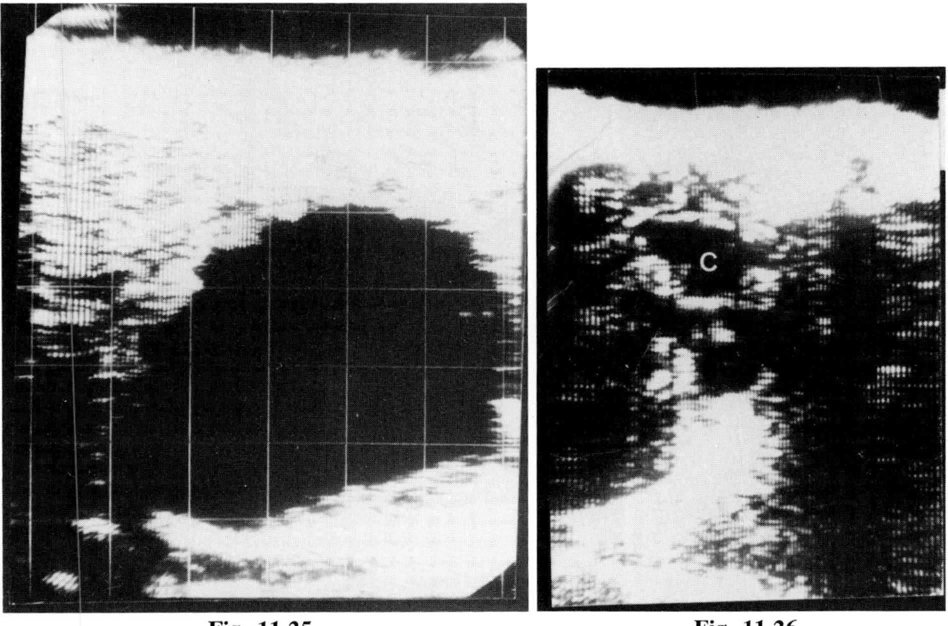

Fig. 11-25 **Fig. 11-26**

Fig. 11-25. Multilocular echinococcosis of cystic type. This cyst originated from posterior aspect of the liver, in jaundiced patient, mimicking enlarged gallbladder. Actually, image belonged to cyst of multilocular echinococcosis.

Fig. 11-26. Another example of necrotizing cyst *(C)* in multilocular echinococcosis, displayed on oblique recurrent subcostal scan. In this case, neighboring tissue is frankly abnormal, displaying multiple reflective areas. This would not be the case if it were common echinococcal cyst.

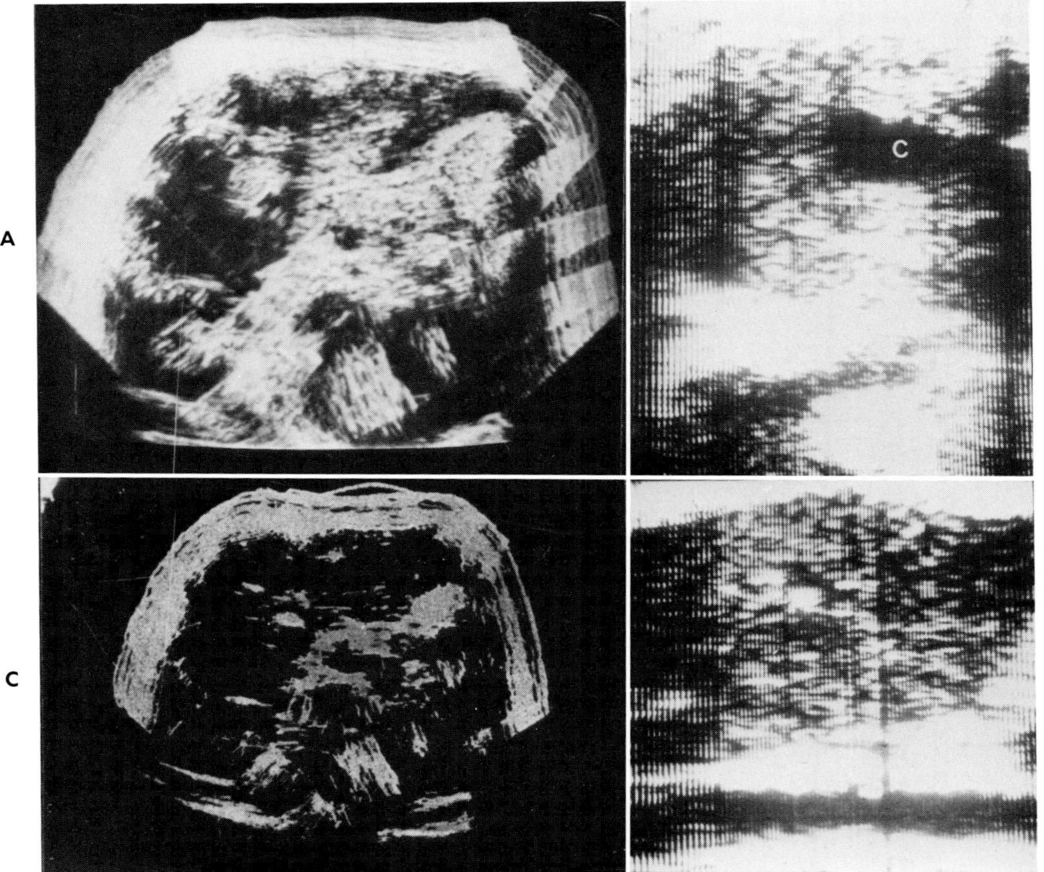

Fig. 11-27. Multilocular echinococcosis. **A,** Transverse scan of upper abdomen displaying several abnormal reflective areas. **B,** Oblique recurrent scan disclosing liquid collection *(C)*, due to necrosis. **C,** Cranial transverse scan showing hepatomegaly. **D,** Sagittal midline scan, passing through aorta, shows extreme enlargement of left lobe. Echopattern is of mottled type. There is large anterior hump.

reflectivity, similar to the hailstorm pattern of metastatic deposits (Figs. 11-27 and 11-28). The presence of a large cyst may be rather characteristic, but, since necrotic metastases may appear cystic and, in these parasitoses, hump signs (Fig. 11-27, *D*) or edge signs (Fig. 11-28, *C*) may be encountered, the ultrasonic differential diagnosis between metastases and multilocular echinococcosis is sometimes impossible. Nevertheless, regarded as common signs in this type of parasitosis, besides hepatomegaly, are tissue changes, with areas of abnormal reflectivity, large or small nodules, and cystic elements. In regions where this disorder is endemic, if there is any existing environmental or occupational hazard of contamination (as for woodcutters or farmers), the discovery of hepatic images consistent with this diagnosis, in the absence of specific ultrasonic signs, should lead to an angiographic examination. Indeed, angiographic images of multilocular echinococcosis are very specific, showing diffuse narrowing and obstructions of arteries and arterioles.

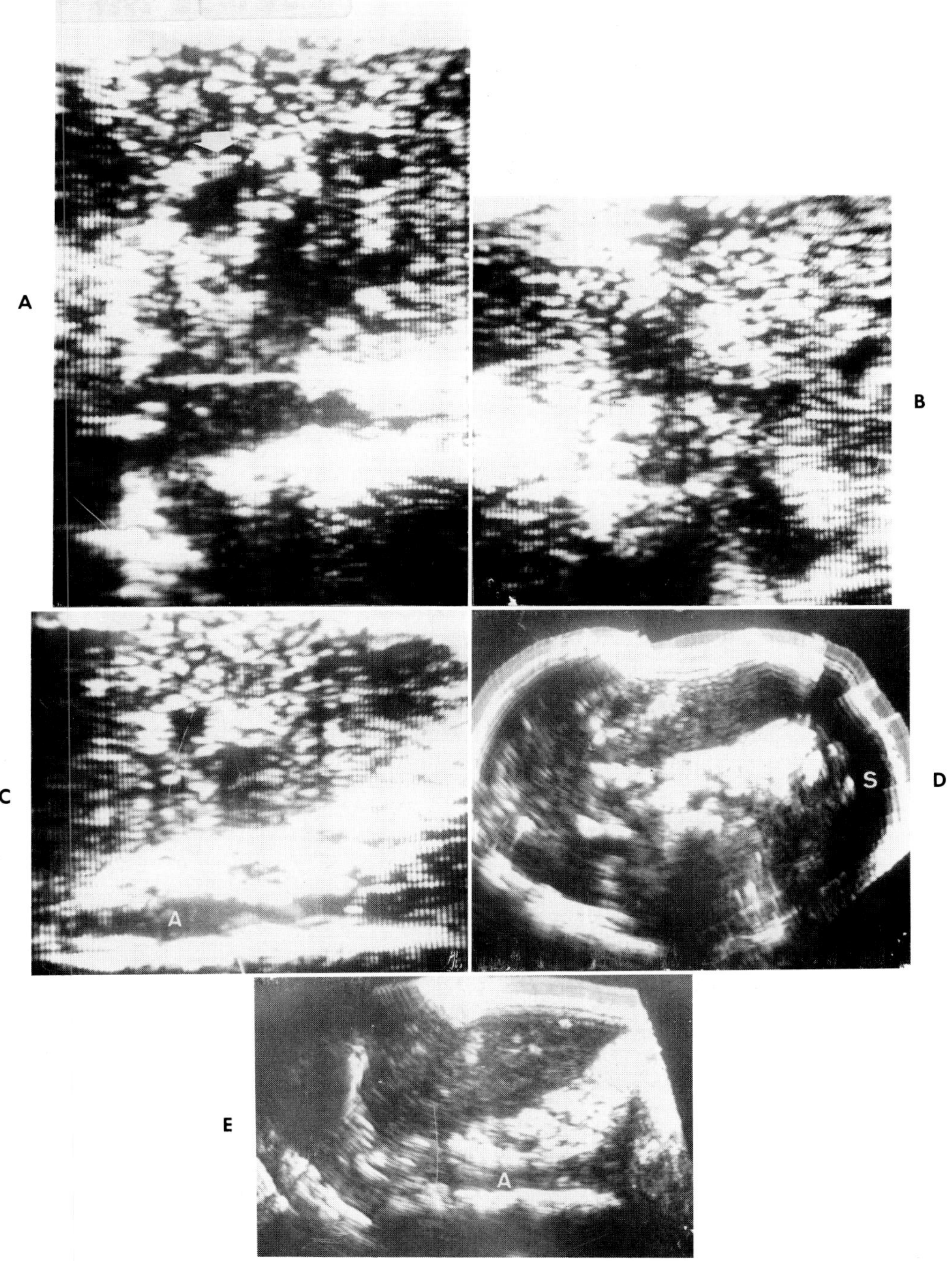

Fig. 11-28. Multilocular echinococcosis. **A** to **C,** Oblique recurrent, intercostal, and sagittal midline scans displaying diffuse mottled tissue echopattern with several small liquid areas due to necrosis. Contour analysis shows small humps in **A** and **B** and edge sign in **C.** *A,* aorta. **D** and **E,** Global transverse and sagittal scans showing hepatomegaly. *S,* spleen.

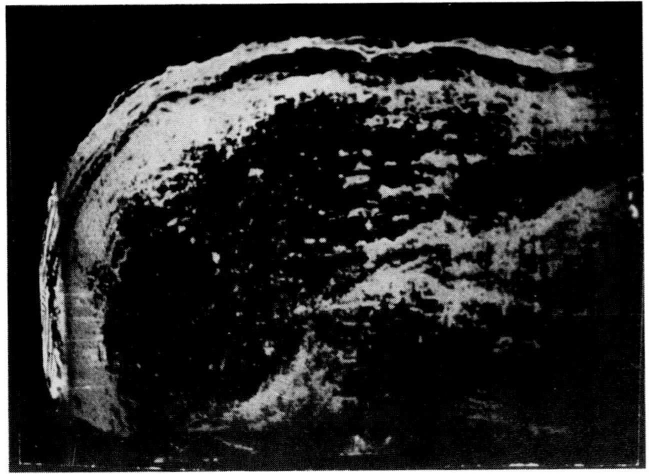

Fig. 11-29. Distomiasis. Old bistable transverse scan displays scattered areas of reflection in enlarged liver.

Distomiasis

I have encountered only one case of distomiasis. The liver was enlarged (Fig. 11-29), and there were small intrahepatic reflective areas without any specificity.

REFERENCES

Barnett, E., and Morley, P.: Abdominal echography, Borough Green, England, 1974, Butterworth & Co. (Publishers), Ltd.

Goldberg, B. B., Kotler, M. N., Ziskin, M. C., and Waxham, R. D.: Diagnostic uses of ultrasound, New York, 1975, Grune & Stratton, Inc.

Hassani, N.: Ultrasonography of the abdomen, Heidelberg, Germany, 1976, Springer-Verlag.

Holm, H. H., Kristensen, J. K., Rasmussen, S. N., Pedersen, J. F., and Hancke, S.: Abdominal ultrasound, Copenhagen, 1976, Munksgaard, International Booksellers & Publishers, Ltd.

Jonas, P.: L'échographie. Sa place dans l'exploration des collections liquidiennes du foie, thesis, Lyons, France, 1975, Claude Bernard University.

King, D. L.: Ultrasonography of echinococcal cysts, J. Clin. Ultrasound **1:**64-67, 1973.

Leopold, G. R., and Asher, W. M.: Fundamentals of abdominal and pelvic ultrasonography, Philadelphia, 1975, W. B. Saunders Co.

Miguet, J. P.: L'èchinococcose alvéolaire en Franche-Comté, thesis, Besançon, France, 1973, Besançon University.

Weill, F., Becker, J. C., Kraehenbuhl, J. R., Heriot, G., and Walter, J. P.: Clinical atlas of ultrasonic radiography, Paris, 1973a, Masson & Cie., Editeurs.

Weill, F., Kraehenbuhl, J. R., Aucant, D., Ricatte, J. P., Miguet, J. P., and Gillet, M.: Le diagnostic échotomographique des kystes hépatiques. Evidences et pièges, J. Radiol. Electrol. Med. Nucl. **54:**345-400, 1973b.

Weill, F., Kraehenbuhl, J. R., Bourgoin, A., Miguet, J. P., and Gillet, M.: Aspects échotomographiques de l'échinococcose alvéolaire, Med. Chir. Dig. **4:**35-37, 1975.

CHAPTER 12

DIFFERENTIAL DIAGNOSIS

The ultrasonic differential diagnosis of hepatic disease proceeds in three stages. The first consists of eliminating confusing extrahepatic images; the second, of identifying nonpathological intrahepatic images; and the third and last, of determining the existing hepatic lesion.

PITFALLS OF JUXTAHEPATIC IMAGES

Difficulties caused by lucent and transparent images. The first of the lucent and transparent images to cause problems in diagnosing hepatic disease is the gallbladder. The details of gallbladder morphology will be studied in Chapter 15, but many films of the gallbladder have already been shown (e.g., Figs. 5-4 to 5-6) demonstrating its close relation to the liver. Some of the diagnostic problems arising from the kidney, such as marginal cysts, have already been examined (Chapter 11). Another pathological liquid image located in the vicinity of the liver—the subphrenic abscess—will be discussed in Chapter 14.

Problems arising from reflective images. I pointed out in Chapter 8 that tumors of the kidney or adrenal could at first glance be confused with tumors of the liver. More careful examination shows a separating interface. A posterior reflective area may appear on a transverse or oblique subcostal recurrent liver cut made just above the upper pole of the right kidney. Such a reflective area may correspond to a transverse section of the upper extension of the perirenal fat, which is often highly reflective. A sagittal cut will then show the continuity of reflective tissue around and above the kidney (Fig. 12-1). In Chapter 17 the appearance of gallbladder tumors will be studied. Gastric tumors and tumors of the ascending part of the colon (Chapter 25) are usually well separated from the liver and do not present diagnostic problems.

INTRAHEPATIC ANATOMICAL IMAGES

Lucent and transparent anatomical images

When cut in transverse sections, the veins and intrahepatic biliary ducts in an individual scan may resemble sonolucent nodules, but the comprehensive information available with the use of real-time technique always enables one to integrate the sectional images of vascular and tubular networks. Strongly reflective venous walls may give rise to acoustic shadows in the hilar area (Figs. 6-9 and 15-6, upper and lower left.) I mentioned (Fig. 8-11) an unusual type of transparent image seen in front of the vena cava just under the diaphragm and probably of a venous nature. Another example of such an image is again depicted in Fig. 12-2.

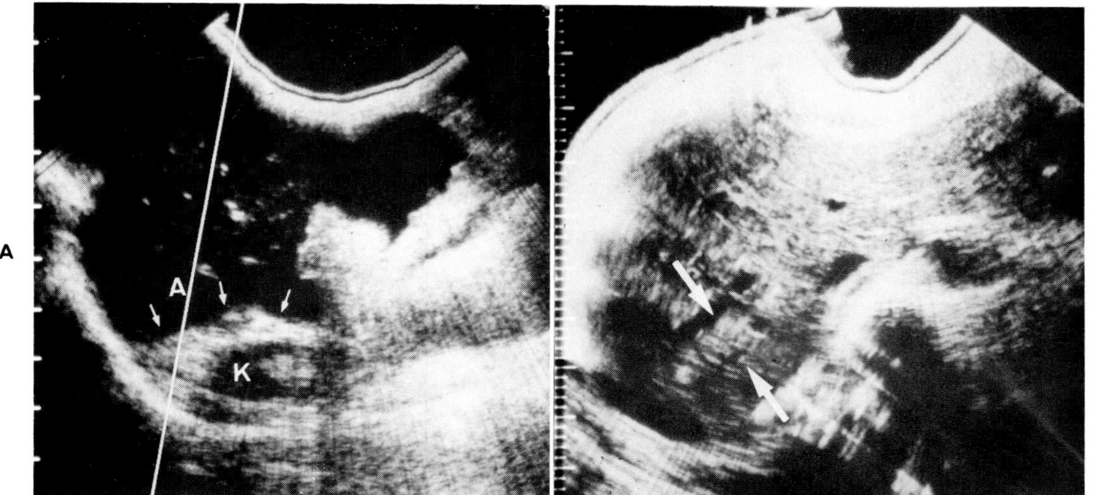

Fig. 12-1. Perirenal fat. **A,** Sagittal scan displaying perirenal fat *(arrows),* underlined by ascites *(A),* around right kidney *(K).* **B,** Scan made along *white line* in **A** showing fat as reflective area *(arrows).*

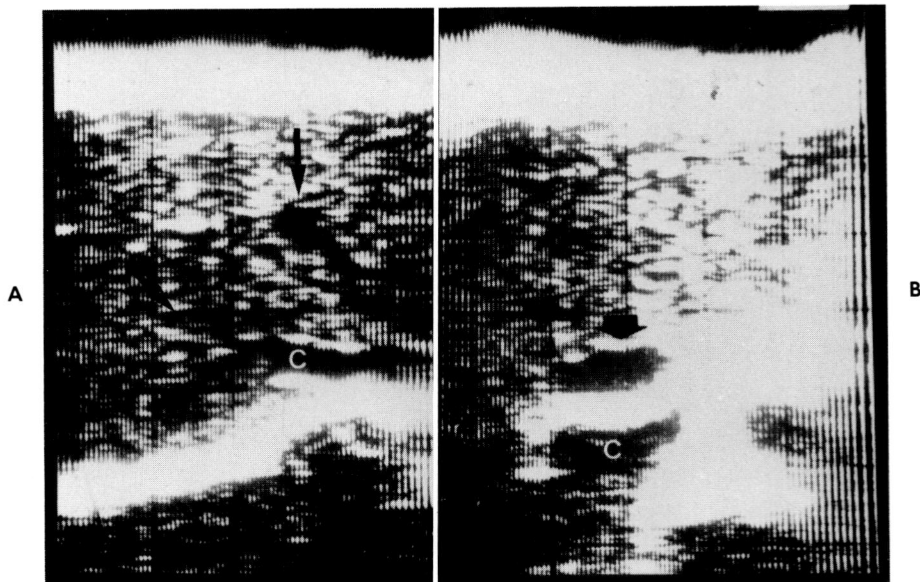

Fig. 12-2. Rare mysterious sonolucent image. (See also Fig. 8-11.) **A,** Oblique subcostal recurrent scan passing through vena cava *(C)* and hepatic veins *(arrows).* **B,** Parallel, more cranial scan. In front of vena cava is sonolucent, well-marginated area *(arrow),* probably of venous nature (and, of course, in this case, different from portal vein).

Table 12-1. Lucent and transparent nodules

	Solitary nodule	*Multiple nodule*	*Hump*	*Edge sign*	*Semi-solid echo-pattern*	*Liquid echo-pattern*	*Neighboring tissue*	
							Normal	*Ab-normal*
Primary tumors	+	+	+	±	+	Excep-tional*	+	–
Metastases	+	+	+	+	+	If necro-tized	±	±
Abscesses before collection	+	+ (rare)	–	–	+	–	+	–
Abscesses after collection	+	+ (rare)	–	–	–	+	+	–
Congenital cyst	+	+	+	–	–	+	+	–
Young echinococcal cyst	+	+ (rare)	+	–	–	+	+	–
Multilocular echinococcosis	+	+	+	+	+	+	–	+

*Cystic cholangiocarcinoma (Fig. 17-10).

Table 12-2. Multiple cystic images

	Directly related cysts	*Neighboring tissue normal*	*Neighboring tissue abnormal*	*Renal involvement*
Polycystic disease	+	+	–	+
Multiple echinococcal cyst	0 (exceptional)	+	–	Exceptional
Multilocular echinococcosis	0	–	+	0

Table 12-3. Reflective areas

	Solitary nodule	*Multiple nodule*	*Hump*	*Edge sign*	*Infiltra-tive pattern*	*Neigh-boring tissue normal*	*Neigh-boring tissue abnormal*	*Attenu-ation*
Primary tumors	+	+	Rare	Rare	–	+	–	N*
Metastases	+	+	+	+	+	+	+ (Infiltra-tive pat-tern)	N
Lymphomas	+	+	–	–	+	±	±	N
Cirrhosis	–	+	–	–	+	–	+	++
Mature echinococcal cyst	+	Rare	Rare	–	–	+	–	N
Multilocular echinococcosis	–	+	+	+	+	–	+	N

*Normal.

Reflective anatomical images

Reflective anatomical images are mainly due to the reflections of the vascular branches, particularly the portal veins. Such reflections may appear as pseudonodules when technique is not optimal. (See Fig. 6-11.) Another type of linear reflection proximal to the hilus has been described in Chapter 6 (Fig. 6-12).

Contours

Contact scanning often builds false edge signs, since the transducer presses down the liver edge while building its image. Thus analysis of the inferior edge of the liver is reliable only in real-time scanning.

DIFFERENTIAL DIAGNOSIS OF HEPATIC LESIONS

Differential diagnosis of different hepatic lesions is summarized in Tables 12-1 to 12-3.

REFERENCES

Barnett, E., and Morley, P.: Abdominal echography, Borough Green, England, 1974, Butterworth & Co. (Publishers), Ltd.

Goldberg, B. B., Kotler, M. N., Ziskin, M. C., and Waxham, R. D.: Diagnostic uses of ultrasound, New York, 1975, Grune & Stratton, Inc.

Hassani, N.: Ultrasonography of the abdomen, Heidelberg, Germany, 1976, Springer-Verlag.

Holm, H. H., Kristensen, J. K., Rasmussen, S. N., Pedersen, J. F., and Hancke, S.: Abdominal ultrasound, Copenhagen, 1976, Munksgaard, International Booksellers & Publishers, Ltd.

Leopold, G. R., and Asher, W. M.: Fundamentals of abdominal and pelvic ultrasonography, Philadelphia, 1975, W. B. Saunders Co.

Weill, F., Becker, J. C., Kraehenbuhl, J. R., Heriot, G., and Walter, J. P.: Clinical atlas of ultrasonic radiography, Paris, 1973, Masson & Cie., Editeurs.

CHAPTER 13

SURGERY

Performance of a partial hepatectomy results in the disappearance of part of the hepatic volume (Figs. 13-1 and 13-2) with a variable degree of compensatory hypertrophy of the remainder (Fig. 13-1). For several months after resection of a tumor or cyst, the hepatic tissue may remain void. A recurrence may then be feared (Figs. 13-3 to 13-6), but successive examinations will show progressive filling of the defect (Figs. 13-3 and 13-4).

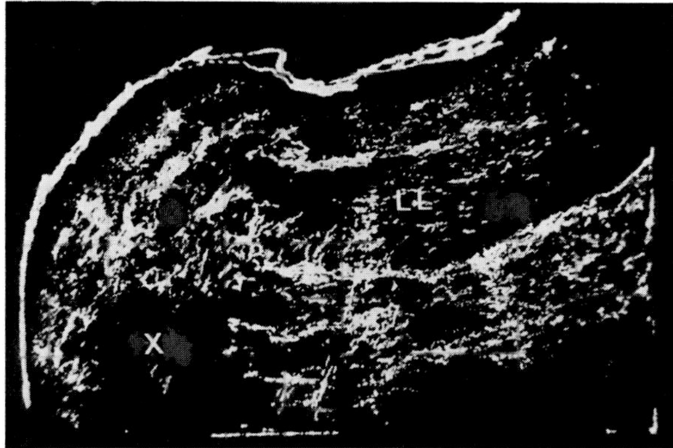

Fig. 13-1. Right hepatectomy in a case of multilocular echinococcosis. *LL,* remaining left lobe; *X,* resected volume. (From Weill, F., Becker, J. C., Kraehenbuhl, J. R., Heriot, G., and Walter, J. P.: Clinical atlas of ultrasonic radiography, Paris, 1973, Masson & Cie., Editeurs.)

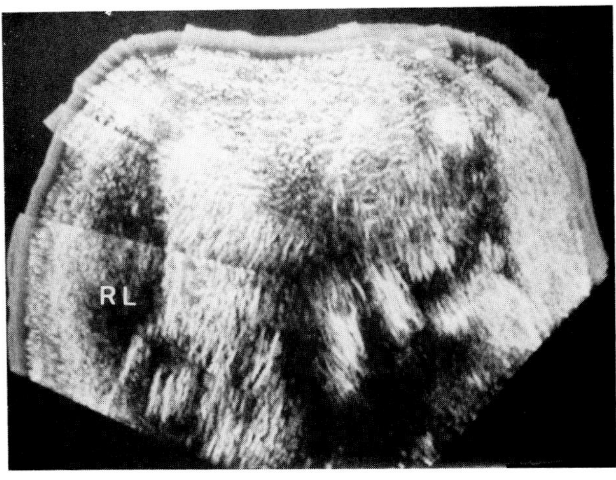

Fig. 13-2. Left hepatectomy for hepatoma. *RL,* remaining right lobe.

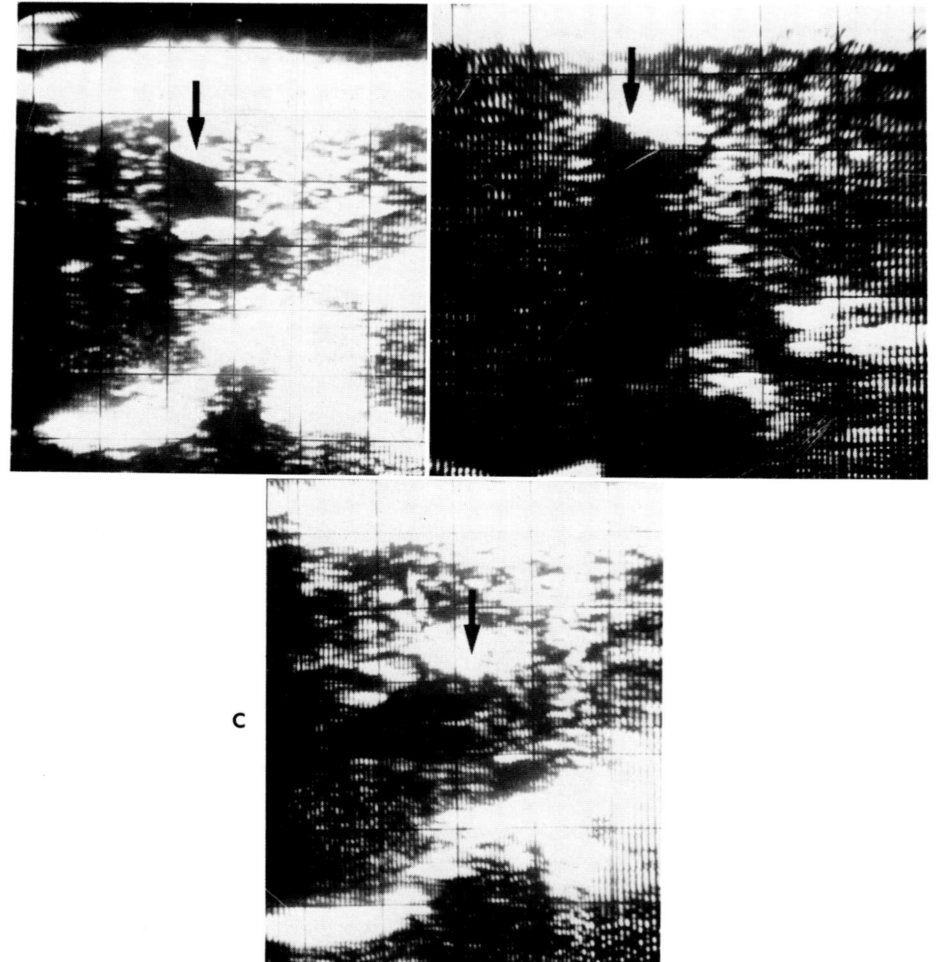

Fig. 13-3. Real-time follow-up scanning after resection of hamartoma (case already reported in Fig. 9-10). **A,** Three months after operation, nodular sonolucent area *(arrow)* can still be seen in central part of liver. **B,** Six months later, this image is still seen. **C,** Almost no change after another delay of 3 months.

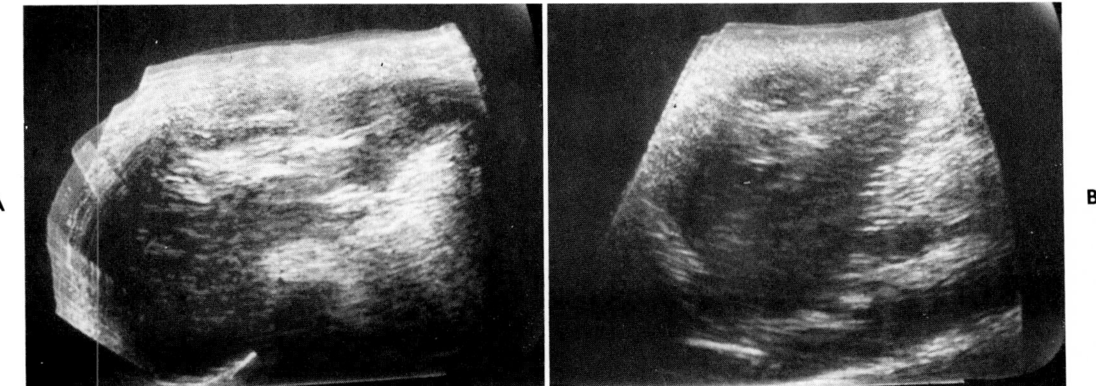

Fig. 13-4. After new delay of 6 months, nodular area has disappeared. Only area of abnormal cicatricial reflection remains. **A,** Transverse scan. **B,** Sagittal scan.

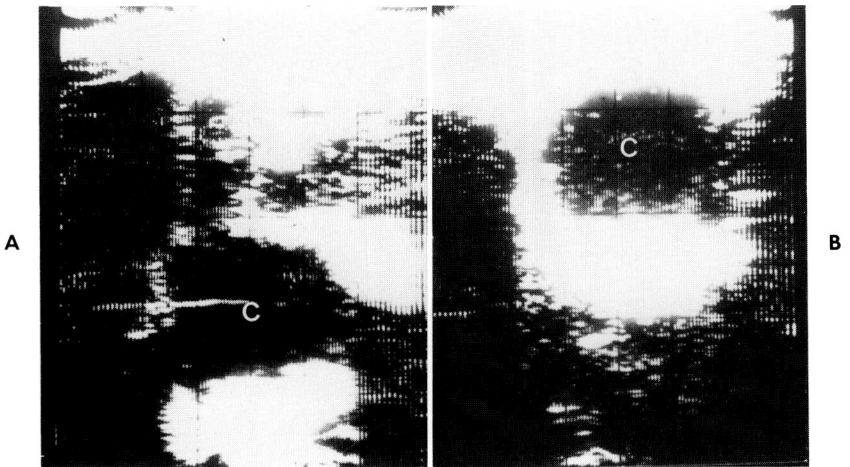

Fig. 13-5. Echinococcal cyst of hepatic dome in 15-year-old girl. This is same case as that in Fig. 11-19. Cyst *(C)* is displayed by subcostal recurrent scan, **A,** and intercostal scan, **B.**

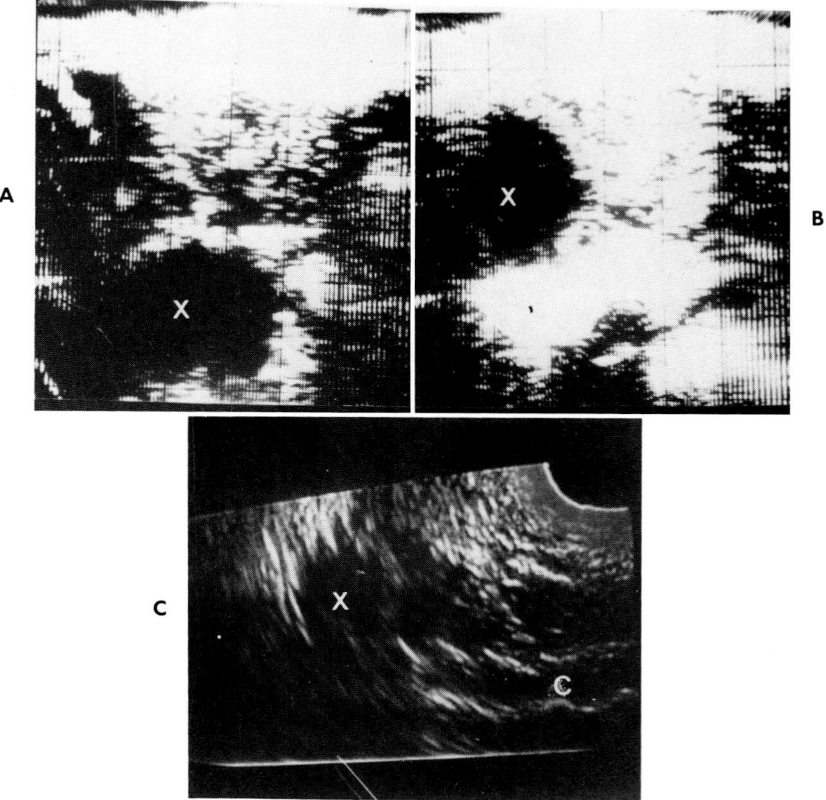

Fig. 13-6. Images similar to those in Fig. 13-5 displayed a month after operation. Sonolucent areas *(X)* are not due to recurrence, but to remaining impression of resected cyst. **A,** Recurrent subcostal scan. **B,** Intercostal scan. **C,** Sagittal scan. *C,* vena cava.

CHAPTER 14

JUXTAHEPATIC FLUID COLLECTIONS: hematomas, abscesses, pleural effusions, and ascites

Different types of liquid collections may be encountered adjacent to the liver. These include lesions close to the liver, such as hematoma of the liver and subphrenic abscess, as well as more peripherally located collections, such as ascites and pleural effusion. To study such perihepatic collections, all the cuts previously described in the liver examination are useful. Two types of scans are, however, particularly important. These are, first, intercostal scanning, which shows the external aspect of the liver, and, second, sagittal subcostal scans to display the diaphragm.

LIVER HEMATOMAS

Ultrasonography is rarely available in emergency wards, but with the development of compact real-time scanners it has become possible to perform portable examinations. Trauma is, of course, the most common cause of liver hematomas. Liver-puncture biopsies usually produce only scant intraperitoneal bleeding, which may, on rare occasions, be followed by a small capsular hematoma. Least commonly, spontaneous hematomas may be encountered in patients receiving anticoagulant therapy or suffering from disorders of blood coagulation.

A hematoma gives rise to a fluid band along one of the surfaces of the liver (Figs. 14-1 to 14-3). The subcapsular location of this fluid band may be recognized by the presence of a well-demarcated peripheral margin. Moreover, this sonolucent band maintains the same relation to the liver during the following different dynamic changes observed in real-time ultrasonography:

- Respiratory liver movements
- Manual displacement of the liver by palpation
- Positional changes, such as the lateral or oblique decubitus

In contrast to the hematoma, collections of ascites change their relation to the liver or disappear from view with positional changes.

Fig. 14-4 shows a large perihepatic fluid collection that seems in close connection with the liver. It is as typical an image of a subcapsular hematoma as one could expect. To our chagrin, surgery showed it to be a pancreatic pseudocyst, which had insinuated itself between the liver parenchyma and the liver capsule.

Intrahepatic hematomas produce heterogeneous tissue abnormalities with semisolid areas (Fig. 14-5). Frank fluid collections seem to be uncommon.

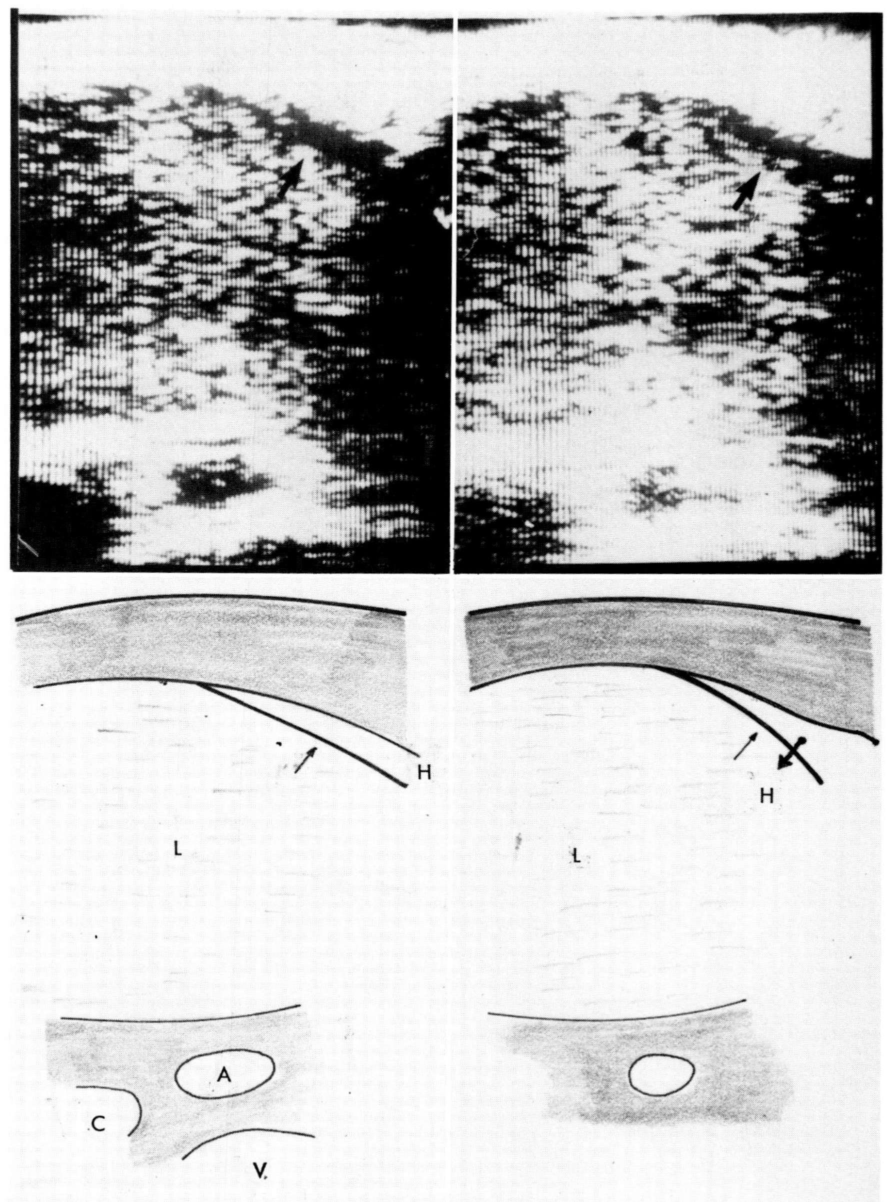

Fig. 14-1. Hematoma after liver puncture. Echo-free band *(arrows)* of hematoma *(H)* is displayed along anterior aspect of liver *(L)* and examined through intercostal scans at two levels. This image is similar to that of early ascites but does not change with position. *A*, aorta; *C*, vena cava; *V*, vertebral body.

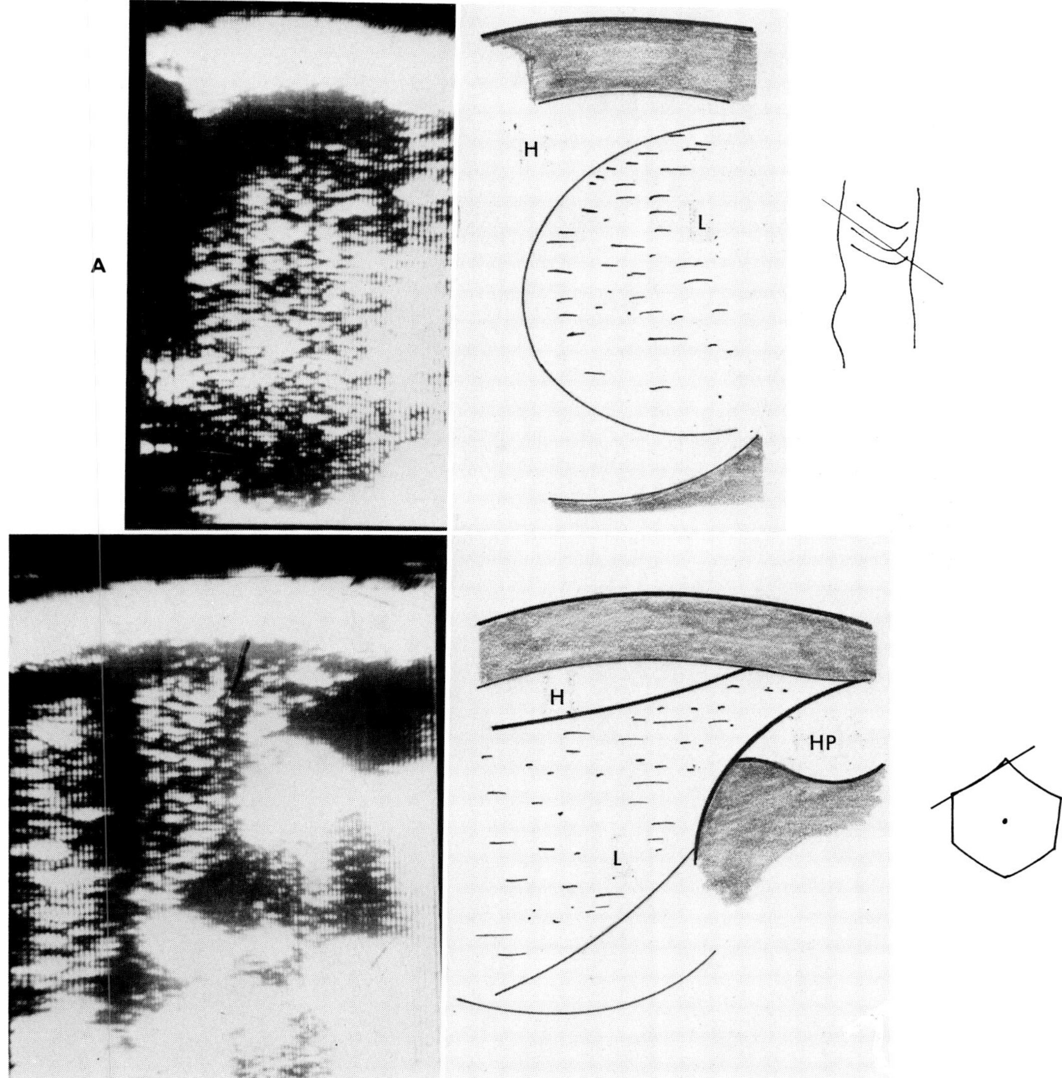

Fig. 14-2. Subcapsular hematoma due to trauma. **A,** Intercostal scan, schematic representation, and scanning plane. Note perihepatic fluid strip *(H). L,* liver. **B,** Recurrent very oblique scan, schematic representation, and scanning plane. Same echo-free strip is found along anterior aspect of liver. This scan also traverses the heart. Note hemopericardium *(HP).*

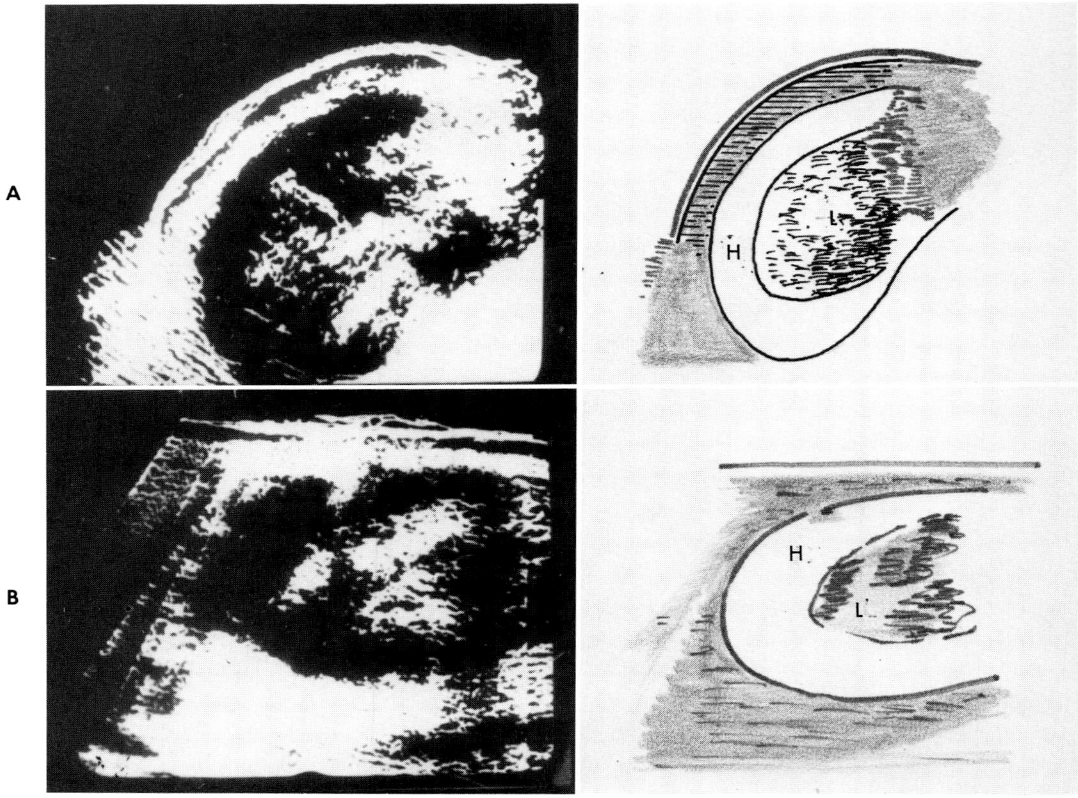

A

B

Fig. 14-3. Subcapsular hematoma of liver *(L)* due to blunt trauma. Note transparent lateral hepatic strip *(H)*. **A,** Transverse scan and its schematic representation. **B,** Intercostal scan and schematic representation.

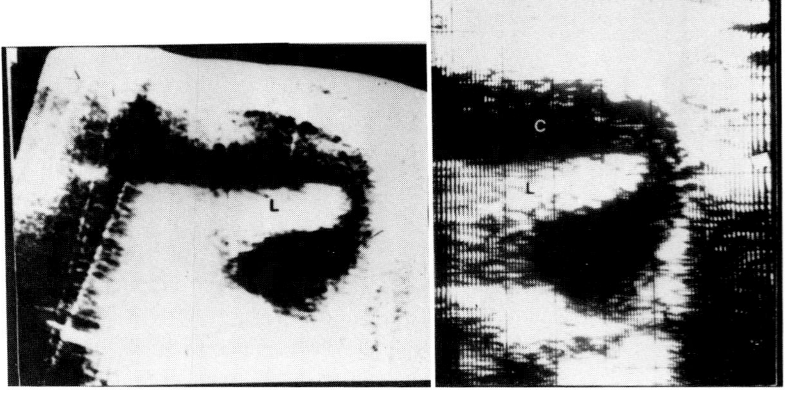

Fig. 14-4. Typical pattern of perihepatic collection *(C)*, which led to diagnosis of hematoma. At surgery, subcapsular infiltration by pancreatic pseudocyst was found. *L,* liver.

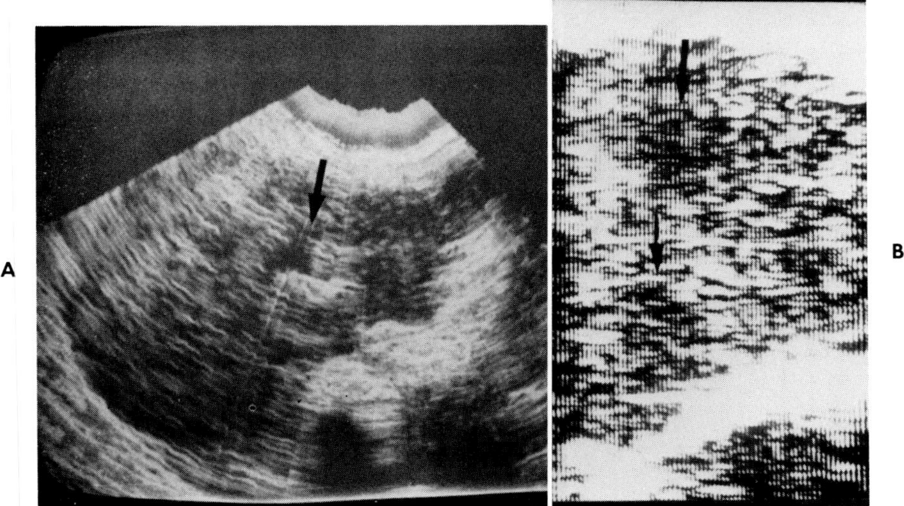

Fig. 14-5. Hepatic contusion. **A,** Horizontal scan. **B,** Oblique recurrent scan. Sonolucent areas *(arrows)* consistent with internal hematomas are displayed within liver tissue. (This patient was not operated on.)

ABSCESSES, WITH SPECIAL REGARD TO SUBPHRENIC AND POSTOPERATIVE TYPES

Since the usual pattern of abscesses is a fluid one, subphrenic abscesses should be easy to diagnose. This is true in the upper right quadrant, where it is easy to image the diaphragm so that even a small fluid collection will be evident between the liver and the abdominal wall (Fig. 14-6) or between the liver and the diaphragm (Fig. 14-7). The pitfall of colonic interposition must be remembered. Such collections are also readily seen in the right hepatic area (Morison's pouch) (Fig. 14-8), but on the left side the colon often interferes with the examination. Positional changes are then necessary, and only positive results have clinical value. A negative result is not reliable. Immobility of the diaphragm, if the patient is breathing normally, is an indirect clue.

It is now appropriate, before proceeding to other perihepatic collections, to consider briefly *other abscesses and collections.* Such entities may appear as frank fluid images (Fig. 14-9, *A* and *B*). Kressel and Fillis (1978) recently described an echogenic pattern of solid type without acoustical shadowing in abdominal abscesses containing gas bubbles. Even a small amount of fluid is suggestive, but not always of infection (Fig. 14-9, *C*). A dilated, occluded *intestinal loop* may mimic a postoperative abscess (Fig. 14-9, *D*). (See Table 25-1, p. 407.) *Chronic or encapsulated abscesses* have a semisolid pattern and are more or less marginated. An example of such an abscess is shown in Fig. 14-10, an appendiceal abscess. Similar images are seen in colon carcinomas, which will be dealt with in Chapter 25. Abscesses in the abdominal wall possess exactly the same pattern as do *wall hematomas* (Figs. 14-11 and 14-12). They constitute superficial collections, appearing ovoid on sagittal scans and variable on transverse scans.

Text continued on p. 204.

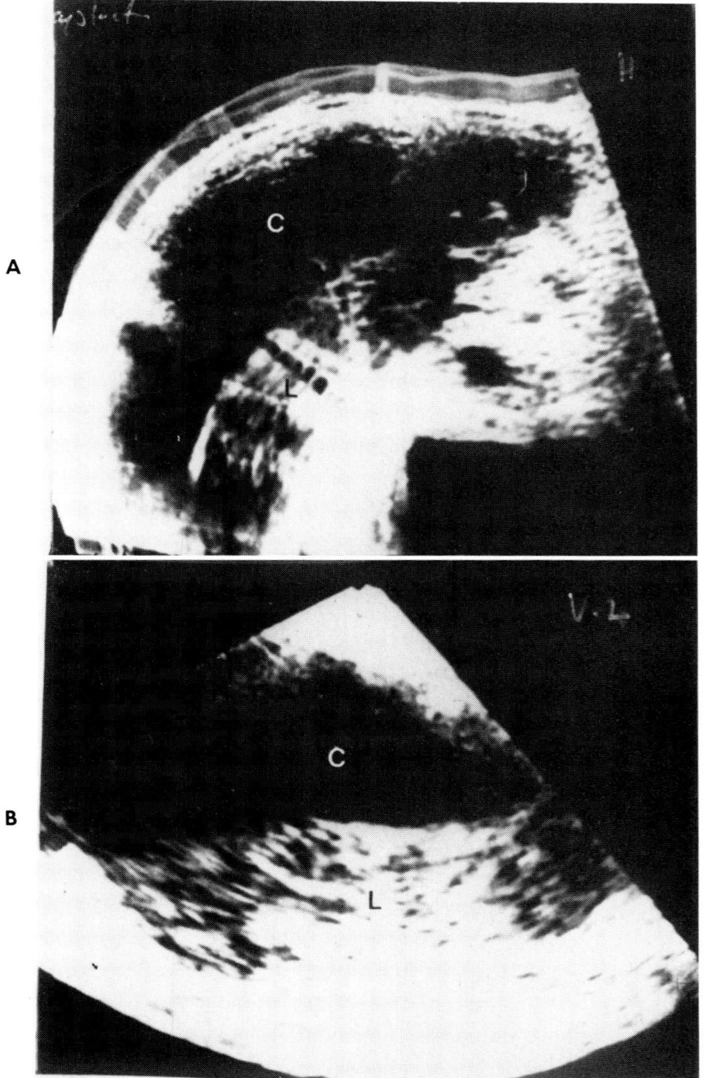

Fig. 14-6. Postoperative subphrenic abscess. Between liver *(L)* and abdominal wall, fluid collection *(C)* is displayed. **A,** Transverse scan. **B,** Intercostal scan.

Fig. 14-7. Clinically suspect right subphrenic abscess. Patient had fever, pain, and basal opacity on chest x-ray film 6 days after gastrectomy. **A,** Subphrenic collection *(A)* located between liver *(L)* and diaphragm *(D)*. Pleural effusion *(PE)* is displayed above diaphragm, which is thus limited by two liquid collections. **B,** Sagittal scan of right upper quadrant showing abscess *(arrows)* located above, rather than below, diaphragm. *K,* right kidney. (**A** courtesy Dr. M. Graham, Montreal.)

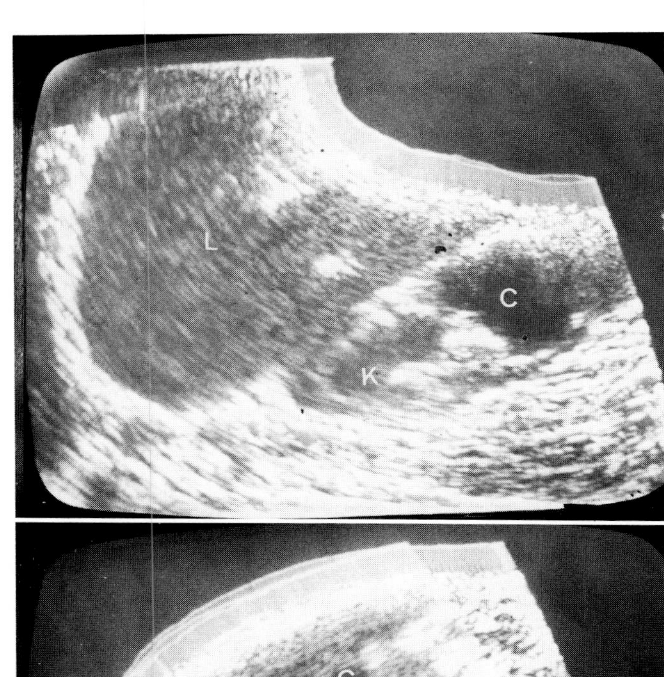

Fig. 14-8. Postoperative subphrenic collection *(C),* which appeared after removal of stone from right renal pelvis. Collection developed between kidney *(K),* liver *(L),* and gallbladder *(G).* **A,** Sagittal scan. **B,** Transverse scan.

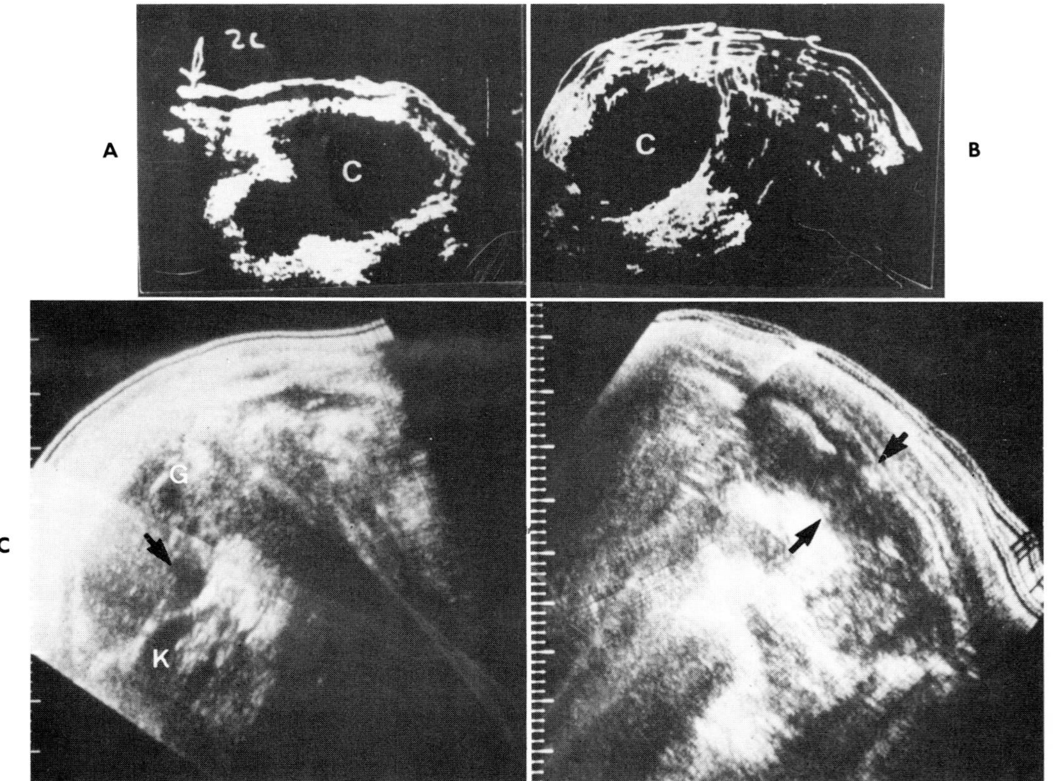

Fig. 14-9. **A** and **B,** Postoperative collection in right abdominal fossa. This is bile collection *(C),* resulting from leakage through drainage orifice of main bile duct. **A,** Sagittal scan. (*Arrow* marks costal edge.) **B,** Transverse scan. **C,** Intraperitoneal fluid. Patient was referred for acute cholecystitis, but gallbladder *(G)* appears normal. There is fluid *(arrow)* between liver and right kidney *(K).* Operation showed, not pus, but blood, from ruptured extrauterine pregnancy. **D,** Semisolid strip found *(arrows)* in contact with abdominal wall of surgical patient at two successive examinations. Following operation disclosed, not abscess, but dilated, volvulated intestinal loop. (**D** courtesy Dr. F. Zeltner, Besançon, France.)

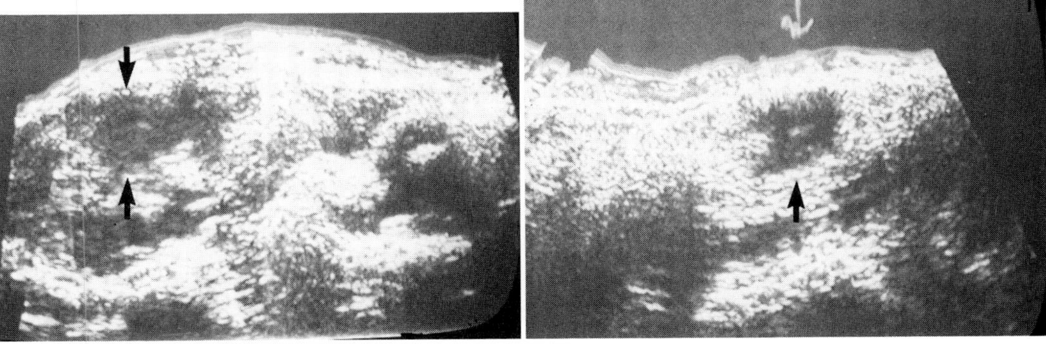

Fig. 14-10. Inflammatory mass, which appeared in right iliac fossa several months after appendectomy and persisted for over a year. **A,** Transverse scan displaying semisolid mass *(arrows)* just under abdominal wall. **B,** Sagittal scan with *arrow* indicating palpable mass. Surgery disclosed chronic encapsulated abscess.

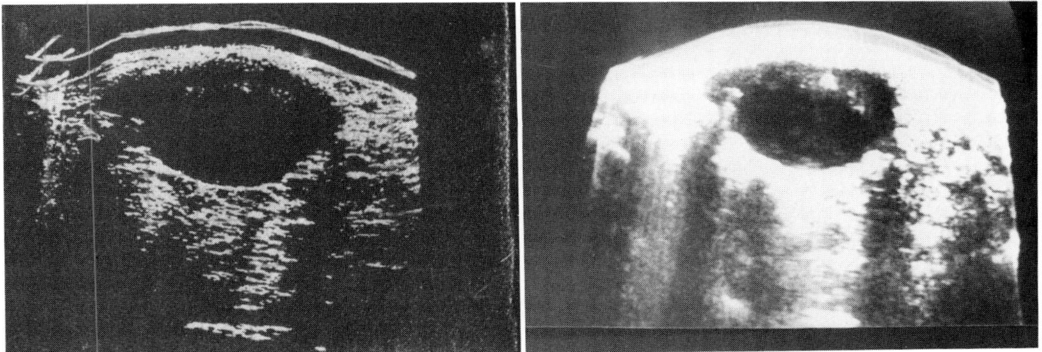

Fig. 14-11. Postoperative wall abscess. Note crescent-shaped superficial collection.

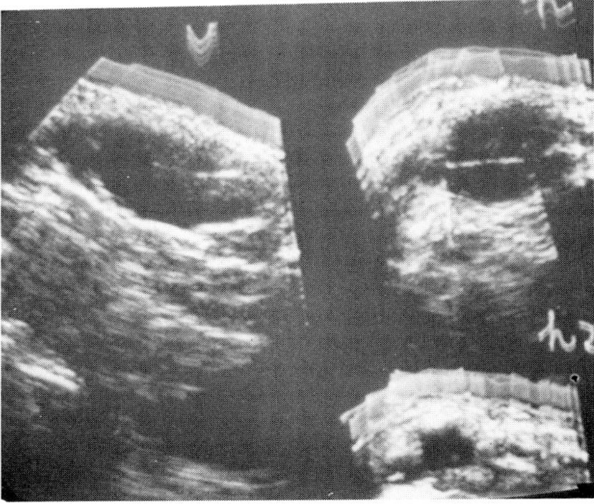

Fig. 14-12. Similar image representing hematoma, which appeared under anticoagulant therapy.

PLEURAL EFFUSIONS

As indicated in Chapter 10, ascites is evident at the beginning of the real-time examination, on an oblique recurrent scan, as a small fluid band close to the liver either laterally or anteriorly (Fig. 14-13, *A*). If the ascites is not abundant, usually no fluid is found between the posterior aspect of the liver and the posterior abdominal wall, since in the recumbent position the weight of the liver tissue displaces fluid from that posterior area. When a wide crescent of fluid is seen behind the liver (Fig. 14-13, *B* to *D*), this crescent is due, not to ascites, but to a pleural effusion that in the recumbent position has gathered in the posterior pleural gutter. This typical posterior crescent is confirmed in sagittal sector scans, in which the appearance resembles a lateral chest radiograph turned 90 degrees, so that the spine is below (Figs. 14-14 to 14-16).

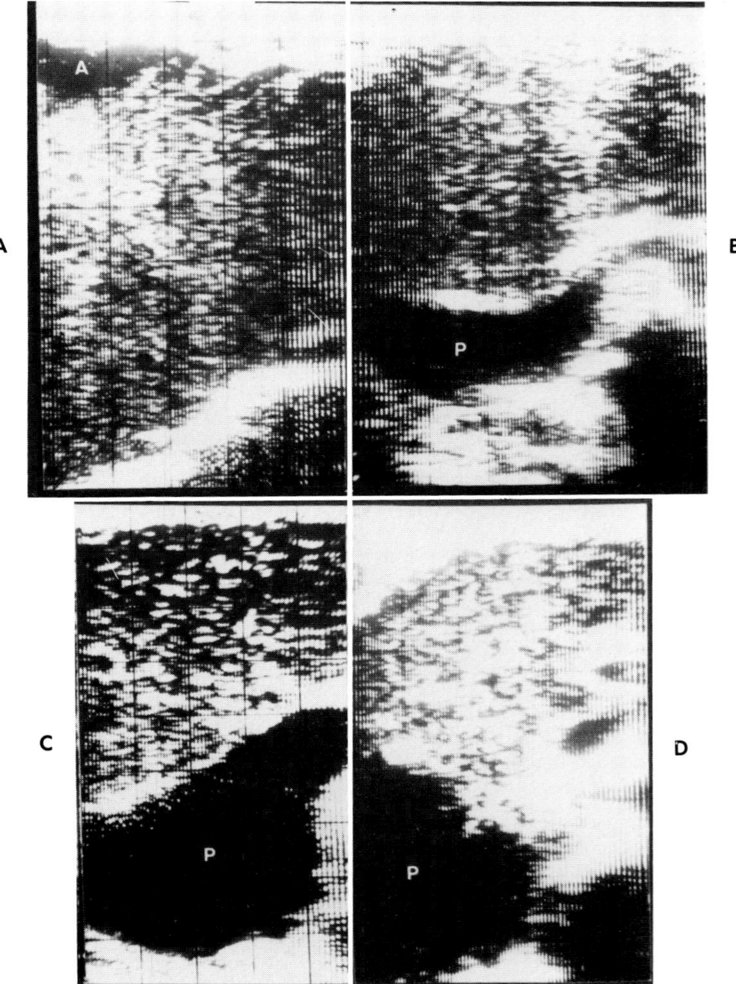

Fig. 14-13. Comparative patterns of ascites and pleural effusions on real-time oblique recurrent scans of liver. **A,** Anterior fluid band of ascites *(A)*. **B** to **D,** Posterior fluid-type band caused by pleural effusions *(P)*.

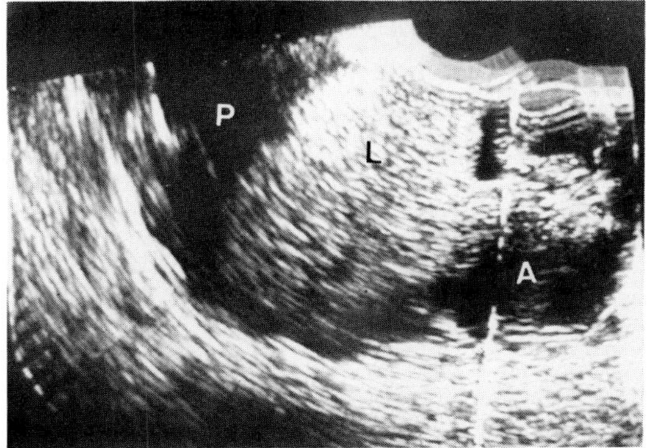

Fig. 14-14. Multiple effusions, displayed on sagittal scan of right upper quadrant in cirrhotic patient. Above liver *(L)* and diaphragm, pleural effusion *(P)* appears; below liver is ascites *(A)*.

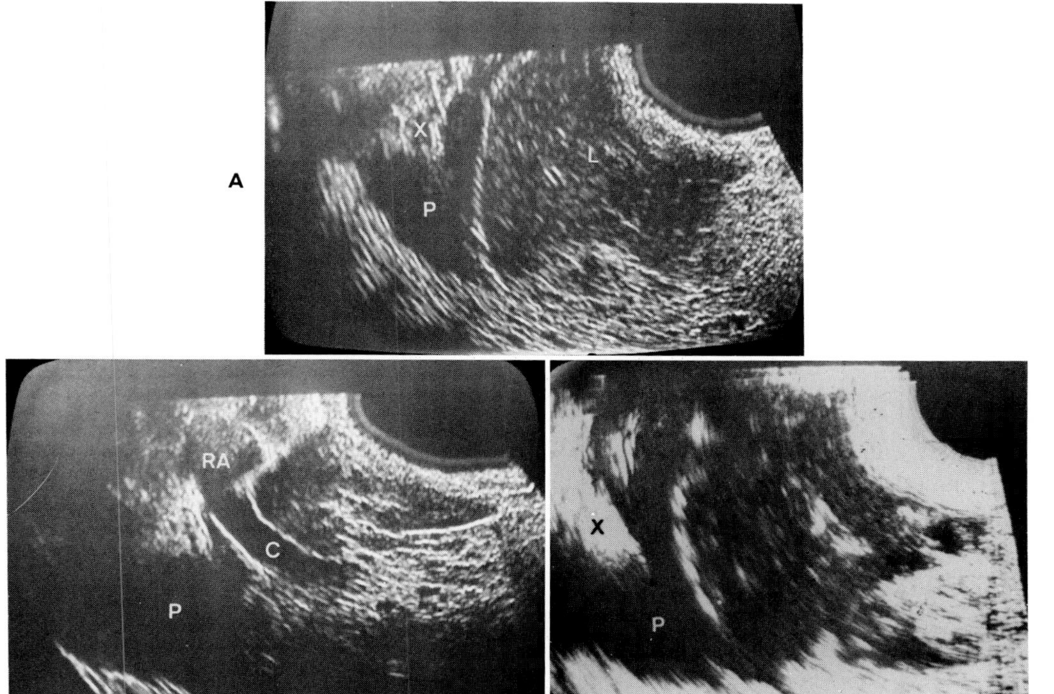

Fig. 14-15. Pleural effusions. **A,** Sagittal scan of right upper quadrant. Pleural effusion *(P)* is displayed above liver *(L)* and diaphragm; above pleural effusion is reflective area *(X)* corresponding to metastatic lung deposit. Both pleural effusion and lung deposit are due to ovarian carcinoma. **B** and **C,** Pleural effusion of cardiac origin. **B,** Sagittal scan of right upper quadrant shows vena cava *(C)* and right atrium *(RA)*. Effusion is also displayed. **C,** Scan is more lateral and better displays pleural effusion. Reflection belongs to normal lung.

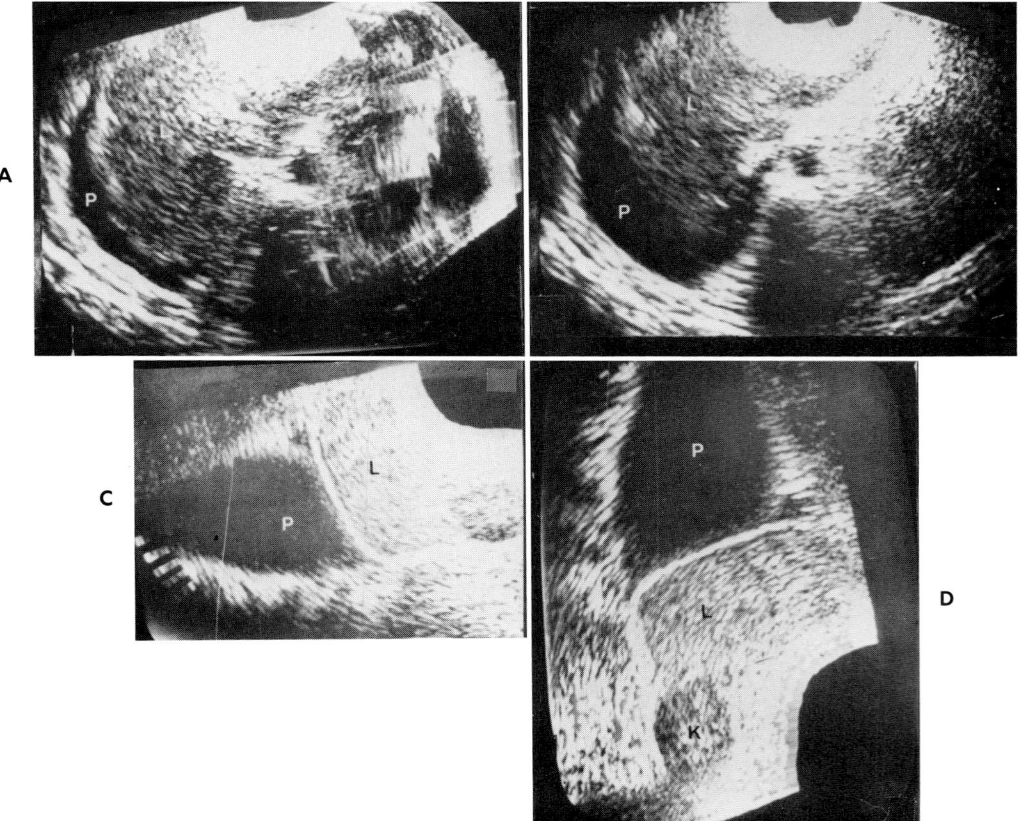

Fig. 14-16. Pleural effusion due to lymphosarcoma. **A** and **B,** Two transverse scans displaying posterior accumulation of pleural effusion *(P)*. Fluid images appear between liver *(L)* and thoracic wall. **C** and **D,** Sagittal scans better showing location of liquid collection above diaphragm. These images are similar to lateral films of thorax. *K,* kidney.

ASCITES

Ascites has already been discussed (Chapter 10) in relation to cirrhosis of the liver, at which time small effusions were emphasized primarily.

In such cases, a narrow sonolucent band is seen between the liver and the abdominal wall. A small peritoneal effusion may also be demonstrated in a recumbent patient in the flank, where it outlines a sonolucent crescent along the abdominal wall. In doubtful cases, positional changes produce significant differences in the location, shape, and size of the liquid image (Fig. 14-17, *A* to *C*). In exceptionally heavy patients, extraperitoneal fat may mimic a thin strip of ascitic fluid until the patient is examined in another position. A small amount of ascites may also

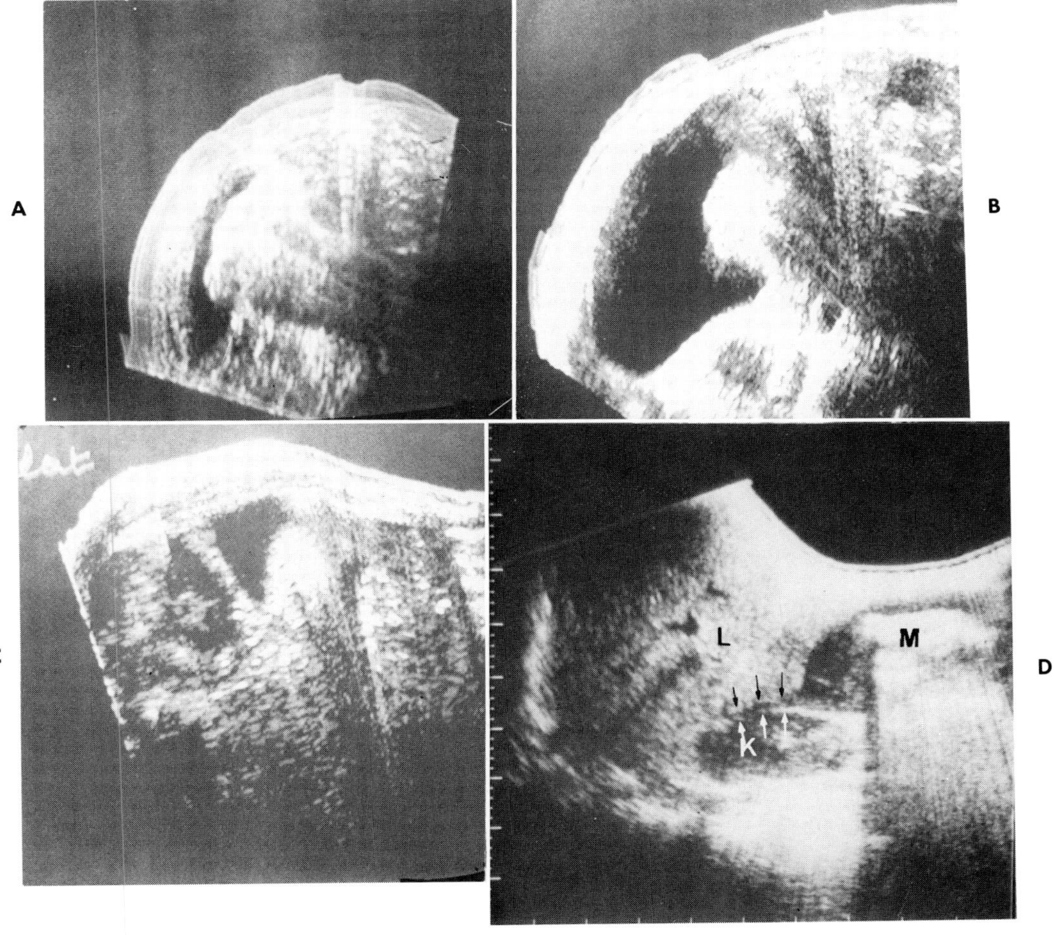

Fig. 14-17. Ascites. **A,** Small fluid collection displayed in right flank, with patient recumbent. **B,** More abundant ascitic collection displayed in right flank. **C,** Same region. Patient was examined this time on left side. Fluid collection seems less abundant, since fluid has moved—sign of free ascites. **D,** Sagittal scan showing ascites as thin sonolucent strip *(arrows)* between liver *(L)* and kidney *(K)*. Mass *(M)* corresponds to gelatinous ascites around carcinoma of ascending part of colon. Note acoustic shadow of intestinal gas.

be displayed in Morison's pouch on sagittal liver scans (Fig. 14-17, *D*). In abundant ascites the liver can be seen floating in a large amount of perihepatic fluid (Fig. 14-18). The liver can be displaced by palpation under echoscopic real-time control (Rettenmaier, 1969). Transverse scans performed below the liver show a fluid crescent between the anterior abdominal wall and the intestinal loops, which outlines an anteriorly convex curvature (Figs. 14-19 to 14-21), whereas the restricted collection of a giant ovarian cyst has an anteriorly concave limit. This is called the *curvature sign* (Figs. 14-22 to 14-24, and 14-27). The curvature sign is not the only sign on which to rely for a differential diagnosis between ascites and a giant ovarian cyst. As already seen, in cases of ascites there is always fluid between the liver and the anterior or lateral abdominal wall. With a giant cyst, on the contrary (Fig. 14-23), there is no fluid at all around the liver. The distinction between a giant cyst of the ovary and ascites is not academic. Every year we see several patients, often young, referred to our hospital for endlessly recurrent ascites, who, in reality, have giant ovarian cysts. The curvature

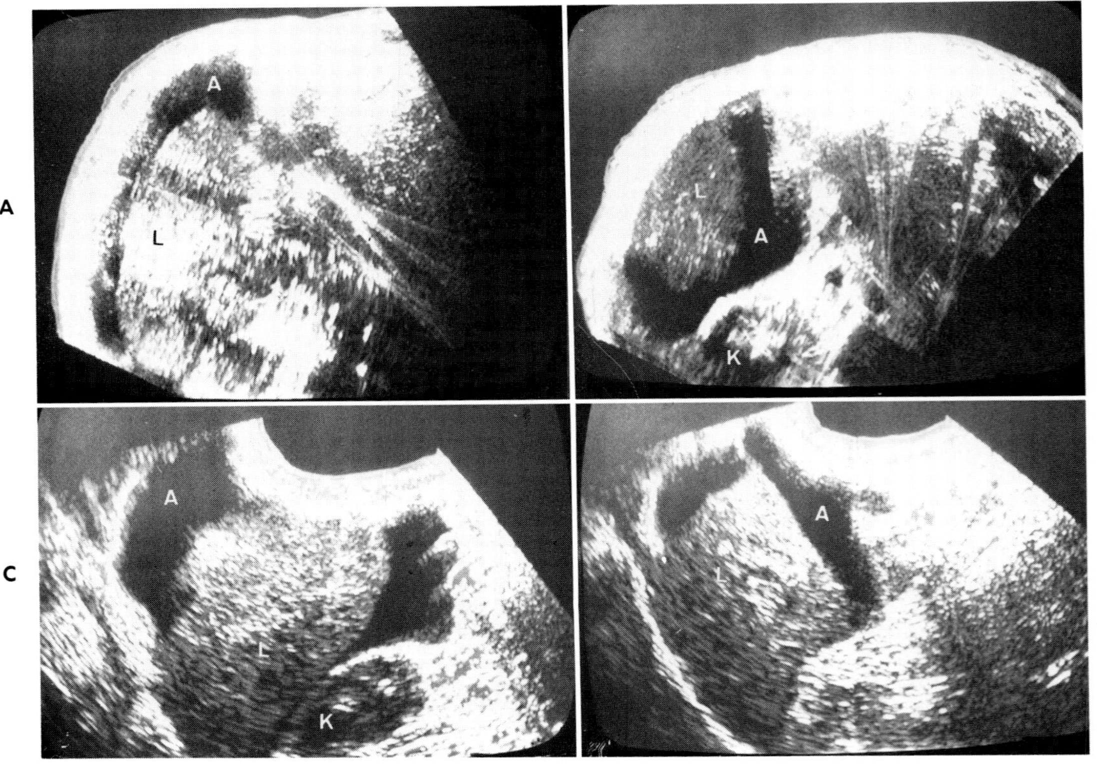

Fig. 14-18. Abundant perihepatic ascites. **A** and **B,** Two horizontal scans at different levels. *L,* liver; *K,* right kidney; *A,* ascites. **C** and **D,** Two sagittal scans. In **C,** hump on superior aspect of liver displays abnormal reflective pattern, which is due to metastatic deposit. Ascites is malignant.

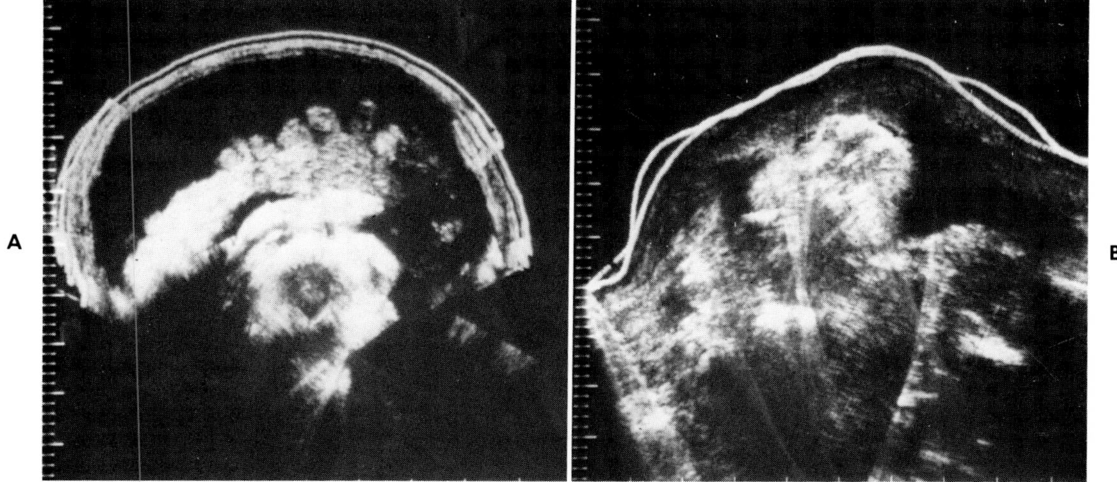

Fig. 14-19. Typical pattern of free ascites. Intestinal loops outline limits convex to anterior (curvature sign). **A** and **B,** Parallel transverse scans.

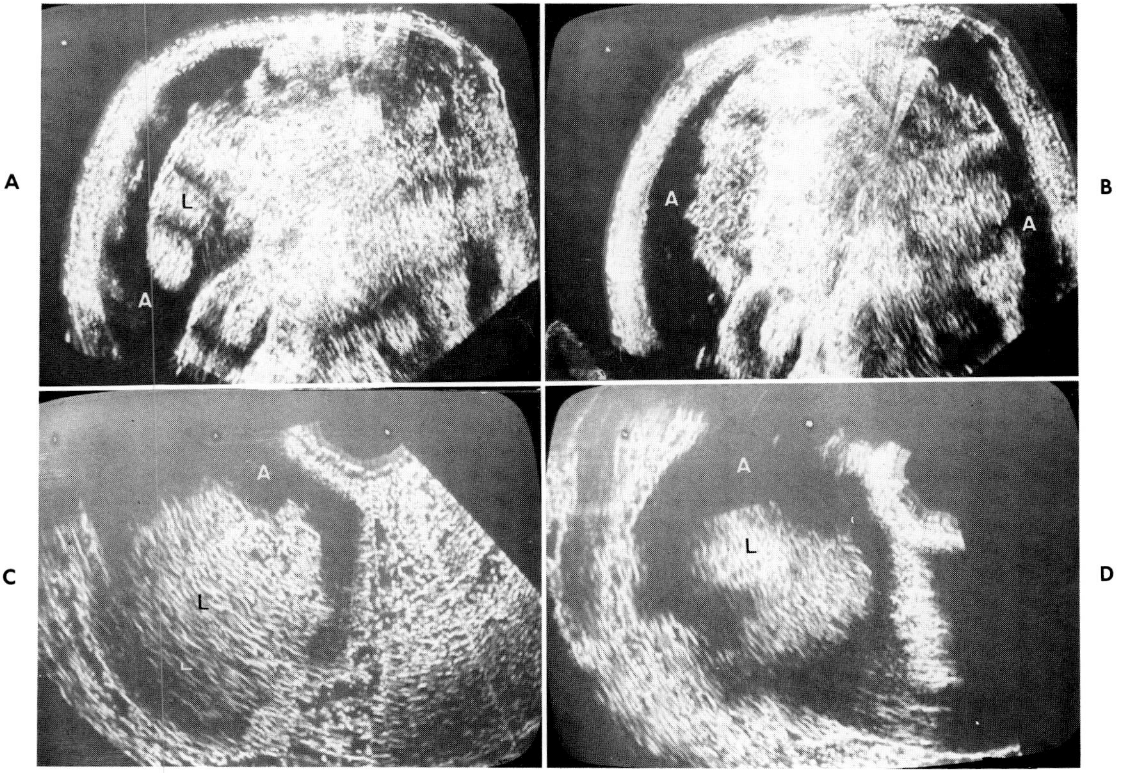

Fig. 14-20. Curvature sign. **A,** Transverse scan at level of umbilicus displaying fluid collection *(A)* in each flank. On right side, collection is perihepatic; on left, it is barely visible between intestinal loops and abdominal wall. **B,** Transverse scan below level of umbilicus. Image of fluid collection is more evident than in **A.** Intestinal anterior curvature remains frankly convex to anterior. **C** and **D,** Two sagittal scans showing liver *(L)* floating in ascites.

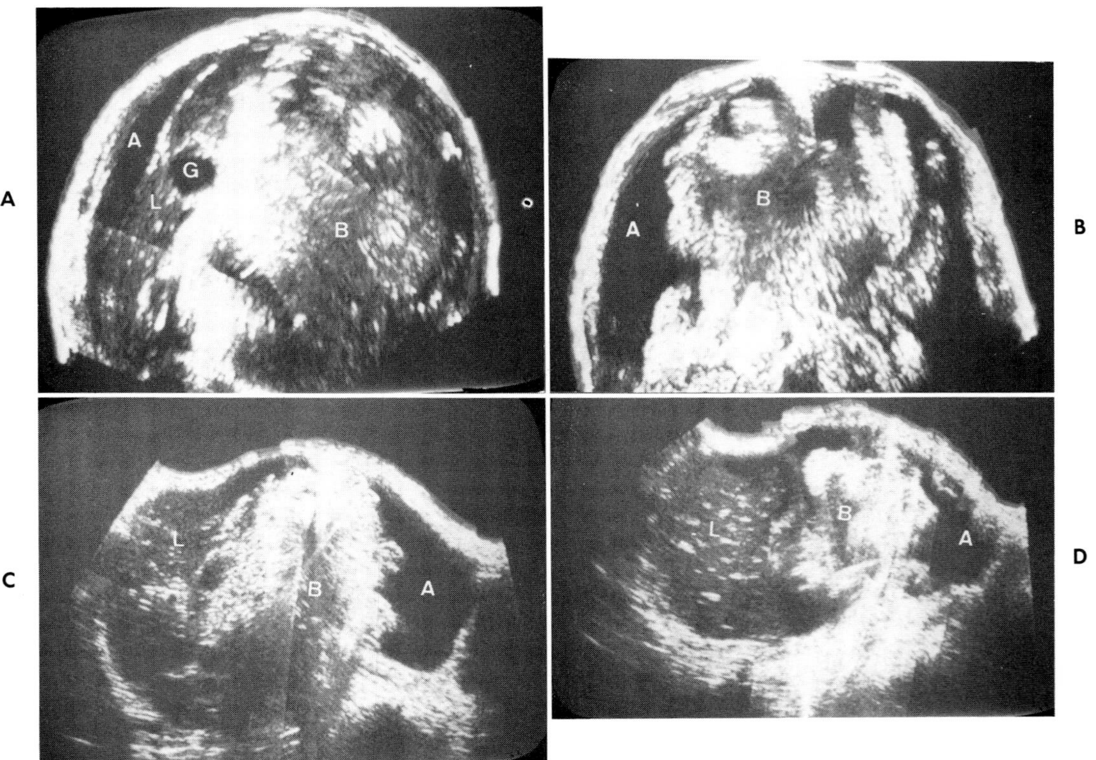

Fig. 14-21. Ascites (curvature sign). **A,** Transverse scan in liver area. Fluid band *(A)* appears between liver *(L)* and right abdominal wall; another is displayed along left abdominal wall. Rounded transparent image close to liver is gallbladder *(G)*. *B,* bowel. **B,** Transverse scan at level of umbilicus. Two fluid bands can be seen, one in each flank. **C** and **D,** Two sagittal sections displaying ascitic fluid around liver and in pelvis.

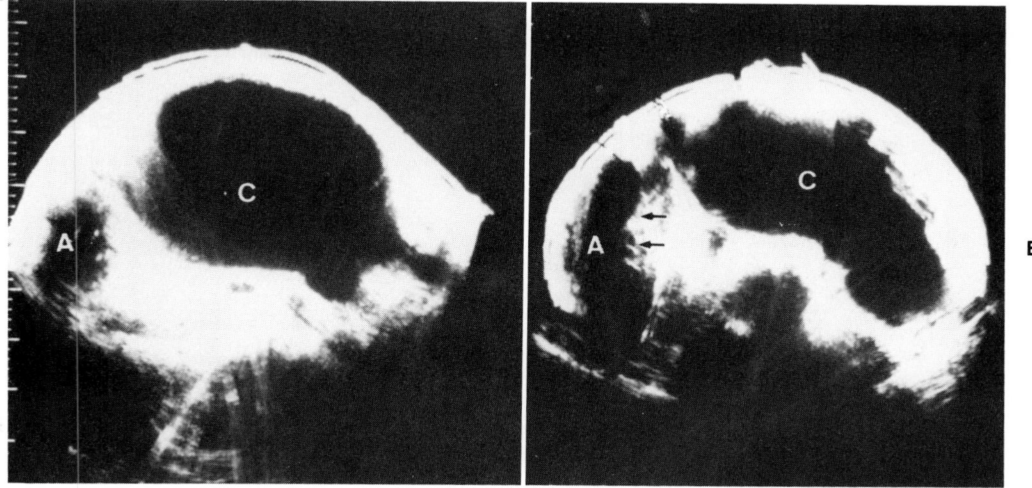

Fig. 14-22. Cyst and ascites (curvature sign). **A,** Transverse scan of abdomen displaying large fluid collection *(C),* with posterior concave limit. Small lateral fluid accumulation *(A)* is also present. **B,** Parallel, more caudal scan again showing cyst and lateral fluid accumulation. Deep limit of latter is convex *(arrows),* as is usual case in ascites. Ascites associated with cyst is consistent with ovarian carcinoma.

sign is usually reliable, except in loculated ascites, when the fluid collection may have a cystic pattern (Figs. 14-24 and 14-25). Most of those loculations are due to peritoneal extension of ovarian carcinoma. In such cases it is difficult to distinguish the cystic tumor from the associated loculated ascites (Fig. 14-22). In the lateral decubitus or the Trendelenburg position, there may be a change in size or shape of the collection, so that differentiation between a cyst and ascites is possible. Another sign consistent with septate ascites is the presence of the acoustic shadow of intestinal gas (Fig. 14-17, *D*); such acoustic shadows, of

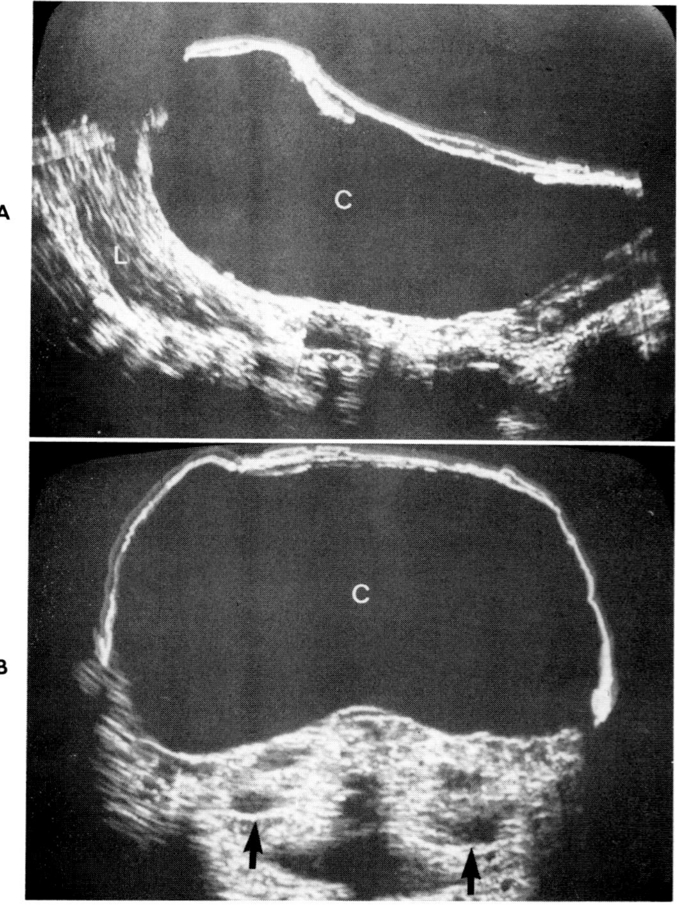

Fig. 14-23. Giant cyst of ovary in young girl referred for celiac angiography. This examination was supposed to demonstrate portal hypertension, suspected because of "abundant recurrent ascites." **A,** Sagittal scan displaying liver *(L)* posteriorly displaced and laminated. No fluid is present between liver and abdominal wall; therefore fluid collection belongs to cyst *(C)* and not to ascites. **B,** Transverse scan. *Arrows,* kidneys.

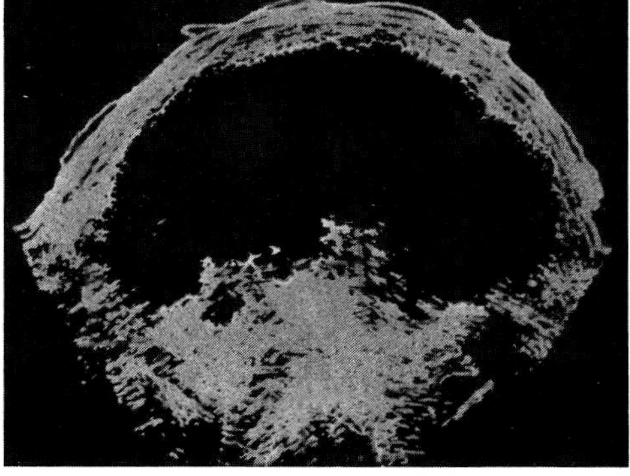

Fig. 14-24. Septate (malignant) ascites. Posterior limit of ascites in pelvis is irregular and convex to anterior. Therefore this fluid collection is due to ascites and not to cysts, despite what appears at first glance to be cystic pattern of collection.

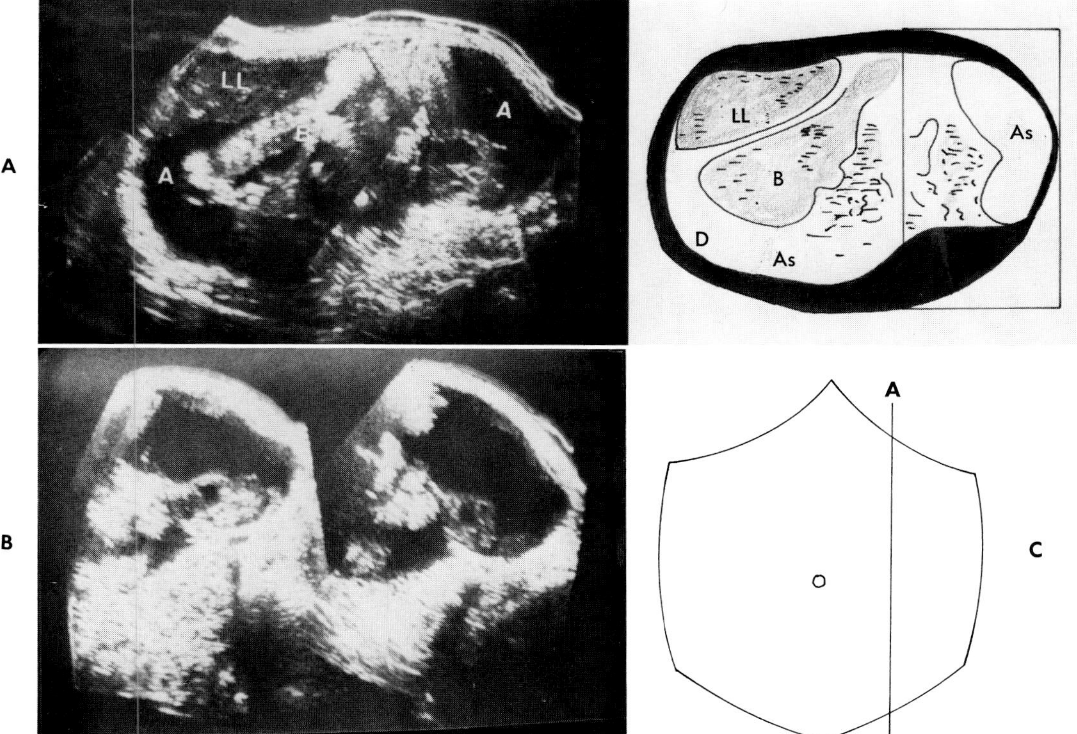

Fig. 14-25. Possible failure of curvature sign in septate ascites. **A,** Sagittal scan of left side of abdomen and its schematic representation displaying ascites *(A, As)* between left hepatic lobe *(LL)* and diaphragm *(D)*. Bowel *(B)* is floating within fluid. There is abundant cystlike fluid collection in pelvis. **B,** Sagittal scan of pelvis made with patient in Trendelenburg position shows that ascites is loculated. In such cases, curvature sign is reversed and becomes similar to that of a cyst. **C,** Scanning angle of **A.**

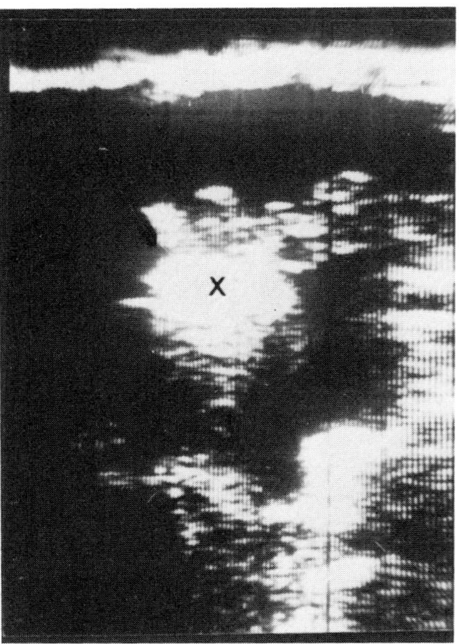

Fig. 14-26. Malignant ascites. Abnormal reflective area *(X)* on intestinal loop is surrounded by ascites. Such reflective area, associated with fixation of intestines, palpated under echoscopic control, is strongly suggestive of peritoneal metastases.

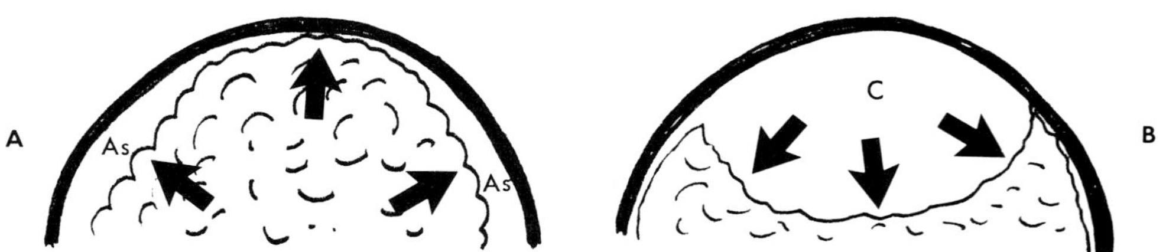

Fig. 14-27. Schematic representation of curvature sign. **A,** Anterior convexity of intestinal images in case of ascites *(As).* **B,** Posterior convexity in case of cyst *(C)* or, exceptionally, septate ascites.

course, can also be present in an ovarian cyst containing calcified areas, but calcifications are then evident on a plain x-ray film of the abdomen. This type of image may be encountered in Krukenberg's tumor—a return to the field of digestive pathology. Other features of malignant ascites with peritoneal metastases include areas of abnormal reflection on some intestinal loops (Fig. 14-26) and fixation of the loops when palpated under echoscopic real-time control.

The only case of gelatinous ascites, due to a carcinoma of the ascending part of the colon in a 19-year-old girl, that I have encountered had the appearance of a plain septate ascites (Figs. 14-17, *D,* and 14-28).

Another cystlike pattern appears when fluid accumulates in lesser omental sac (Chapter 25).

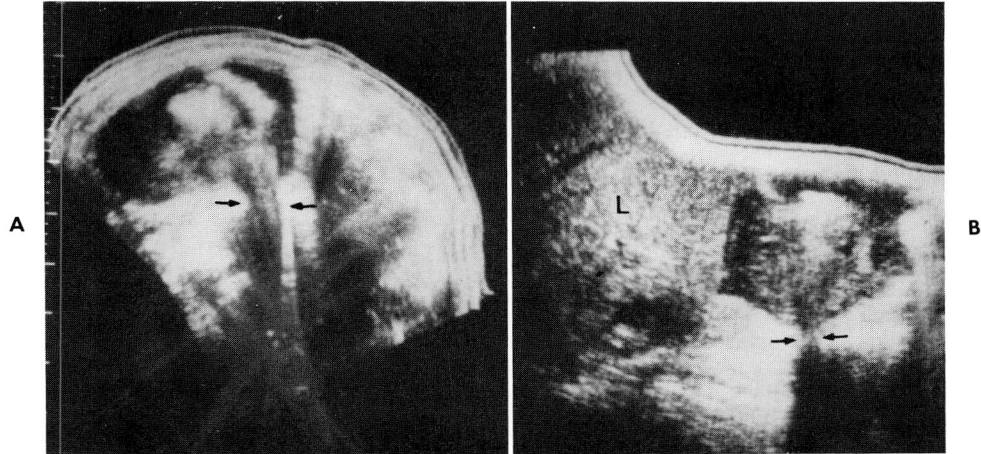

Fig. 14-28. Gelatinous ascites. **A,** Transverse scan. **B,** Sagittal scan. Note acoustic shadows *(arrows)* due to intestinal gas. In this case, gelatinous ascites developed around carcinoma of ascending part of colon. *L,* liver. (See also Fig. 14-17, *D.*)

I have summarized in the following outline the different types of perihepatic and abdominal collections studied in this chapter.

Closely related perihepatic collections
- Subcapsular hematomas
- Subphrenic abscesses
- Pleural effusions
- Ascites (and intraperitoneal blood)

Less closely related collections
- Abdominal postoperative collections and abscesses
- Wall hematomas and abscesses
- Septate ascites
- Giant ovarian cyst

Other types of fluid collections (retroperitoneal hematomas and abscesses, mesenteric hematomas, and mesenteric cysts) will be discussed in Chapter 25.

REFERENCES

Barnett, E., and Morley, P.: Abdominal echography, Borough Green, England, 1974, Butterworth & Co. (Publishers), Ltd.

Goldberg, B. B., Kotler, M. N., Ziskin, M. C., and Waxham, R. D.: Diagnostic uses of ultrasound, New York, 1975, Grune & Stratton, Inc.

Hassani, N.: Ultrasonography of the abdomen, Heidelberg, Germany, 1976, Springer-Verlag.

Holm, H. H., Kristensen, J. K., Rasmussen, S. N., Pedersen, J. F., and Hancke, S.: Abdominal ultrasound, Copenhagen, 1976, Munksgaard, International Booksellers & Publishers, Ltd.

Kressel and Fillis: Am. J. Roentgenol. Radium Ther. Nucl. Med. **130:**71-73, 1978.

Leopold, G. R., and Asher, W. M.: Fundamentals of abdominal and pelvic ultrasonography, Philadelphia, 1975, W. B. Saunders Co.

Rettenmaier, G.: Personal communication, 1969.

Weill, F., Becker, J. C., Kraehenbuhl, J. R., Heriot, G., and Walter, J. P.: Clinical atlas of ultrasonic radiography, Paris, 1973, Masson & Cie., Editeurs.

PART III

BILIARY TRACT

CHAPTER 15

EXAMINATION TECHNIQUES AND ECHOANATOMY

TECHNIQUES OF EXAMINATION

The gallbladder

In most subjects the gallbladder clears the anterior costal margin sufficiently to be demonstrated readily, *provided the patient is fasting*. This is a compulsory condition. The patient lies in the recumbent position; the RTH is moved along the upper right quadrant, with a sagittal orientation, from right to left and left to right (Fig. 15-1, *A*). The orientation of the head is adjusted to the axis of the gallbladder as soon as it is identified (Fig. 15-1, *B*). Close sections parallel to that axis are then scanned, with an alternating sweeping movement. Transverse scans, perpendicular to that axis (Fig. 15-1, *C*), may then be performed. Other gallbladder images will appear on subcostal oblique recurrent scans of the liver.

If the gallbladder is not immediately apparent in the recumbent position, a left oblique posterior positioning of the patient is helpful; but, above all, it is necessary to employ deep inspiration, as in examining the liver, to displace the gallbladder below the costal margin. If after these additional maneuvers the gallbladder is still not visible, this may be due to its high, retrocostal location. The patient must then be placed in left lateral decubitus or at least in a frankly oblique left posterior position for right intercostal scans (Fig. 15-2, *A*). If even intercostal scans fail to show the gallbladder, it is advisable to check whether the patient is indeed fasting. To do this, do not ask the patient, "Did you have breakfast this morning?" but rather, "How much butter did you have with your toast this morning?" If the patient really is fasting and is breathing as deeply as possible and nevertheless real-time scans are unsuccessful in demonstrating the gallbladder, contact scanning with sagittal subcostal sector scans may produce the desired image (Fig. 15-2, *B* and *C*). However, real-time examination of the gallbladder is so reliable, easy, and quick that we use contact scanning only as a complementary method or to obtain better-looking images. A better appearance is the only reason that in this chapter many gallbladder images are gray scale contact scans. In fact, they were performed after real-time images had already disclosed the diagnosis.

In a few cases it is useful to follow the recumbent phase of the examination by scanning the standing patient. As will be discussed later, the reason for this is to observe the gravitational displacement of gallstones. Moreover, it may be helpful to resort to a contraction test, either by the patient's ingesting a fatty meal or by injection of cholecystokinin* if available.

Finally, I would like to emphasize that my colleagues and I greatly prefer the real-time technique for the gallbladder examination. All the views just described

*Or cerulein.

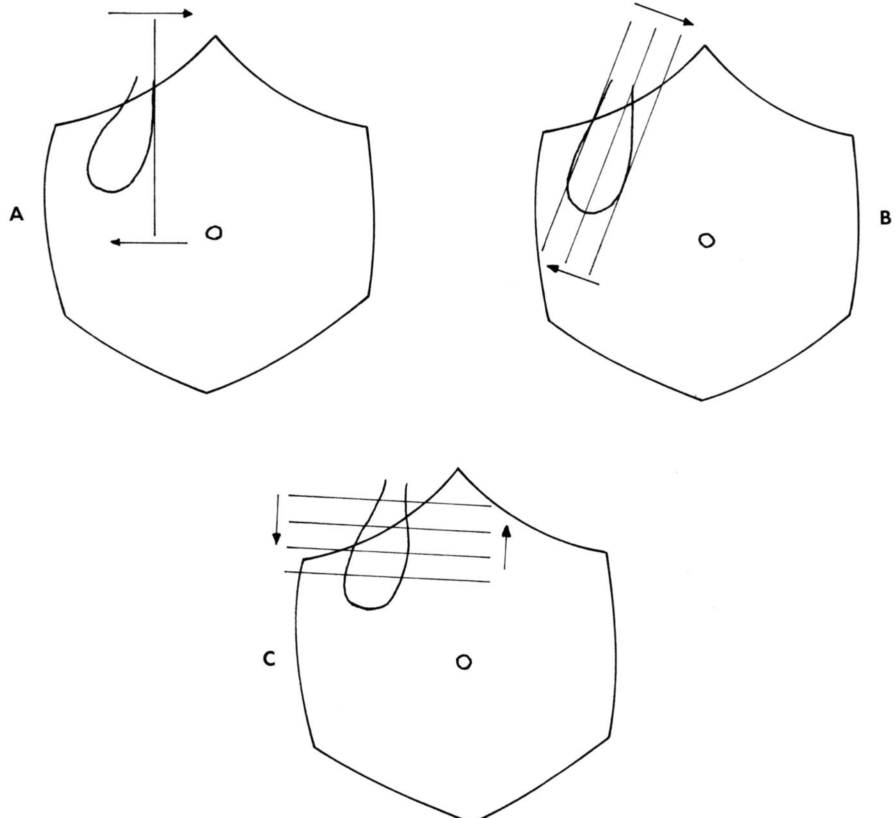

Fig. 15-1. Positions in real-time ultrasonic investigation. **A,** Sagittal scanning. Rocking movement of real-time ultrasonic head is made on surface of right upper quadrant. **B,** Adjustment of scanning direction to sagittal axis of gallbladder, with rocking movements of RTH. **C,** Transverse scanning.

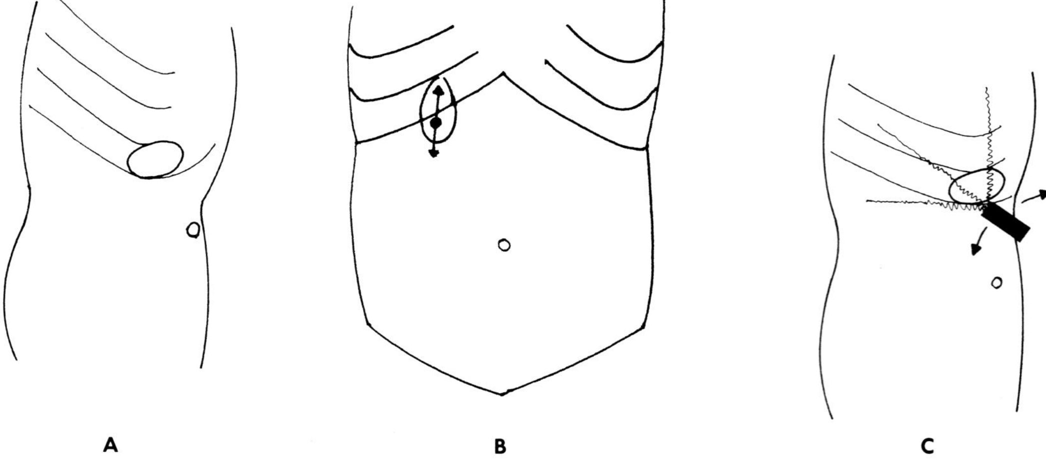

Fig. 15-2. Additional views. **A,** Intercostal real-time scanning. **B** and **C,** Subcostal contact sagittal sector scans.

are taken systematically, a process that in real time requires only a few minutes. If the patient is really fasting, the examination was made during deep inspiration, and no scan visualizes the gallbladder, one may conclude that a pathological condition exists—the rarest being total aplasia. Following are the different steps in ultrasonic examination of the gallbladder:

With a fasting patient
- In the recumbent (or possibly erect) position and during deep suspended inspiration
  - Sagittal scans
  - Transverse scans
- In the left posterior oblique position
  - Intercostal scans
  - Subcostal recurrent scans

Extrahepatic biliary tree

With improved ultrasonic imaging it is now regularly possible to see the normal main bile duct,* whereas until recently it was thought that only the abnormally dilated main bile duct could be seen on ultrasonic scans. Because of the close relation of the common hepatic duct and the proximal common bile duct to the portal vein, the views for the main bile duct are the same as those used for the portal vein, that is, oblique scans of the upper right quadrant (Chapter 4).

Intrahepatic bile ducts

As I pointed out in presenting the different hepatic echoangiographic structures, intrahepatic bile ducts of normal caliber are usually too thin to be displayed on hepatic scans. The only element of the upper part of the biliary tree that is regularly seen in a normal patient is the convergence of the two main hilar biliary ducts. This convergence is outlined in front of the portal division on intercostal, horizontal, or oblique subcostal recurrent scans. It is worthwhile to search for this tubular junction, since it is the best place to detect early dilatation of the biliary tree. (See Chapter 26.)

The ultrasonic examination of the biliary tree is not, of course, an isolated procedure. Examination of the gallbladder and the extrahepatic and intrahepatic bile ducts proceeds in sequence. Moreover, it must be correlated with the ultrasonic examination of the liver and pancreas, as well as the findings of other radiological investigations.

ECHOANATOMY

The gallbladder

The radiological image of the gallbladder is so well known and its ultrasonic image on sagittal scans is so similar that detailed description is not necessary. The

---

*In this context the main bile duct includes the extrahepatic biliary tree, from the biliary junction down to the ampulla of Vater. It includes the common hepatic duct and the common bile duct. Unfortunately, there is no English term for this anatomical segment, which is called in French *voie biliaire principale*.

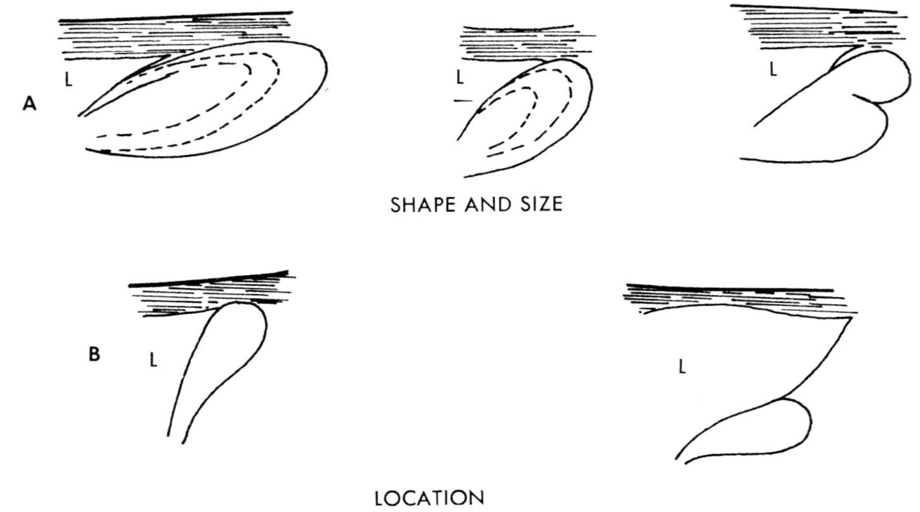

A

SHAPE AND SIZE

B

LOCATION

Fig. 15-3. Schematic drawings of different types of gallbladders. **A,** Different shapes and sizes. **B,** Different locations and relations to liver and abdominal wall.

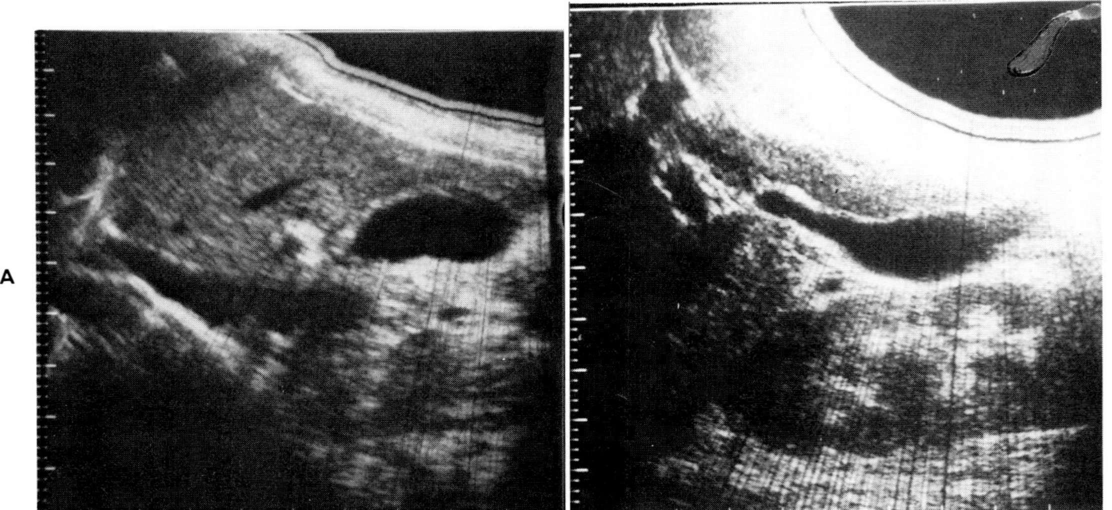

Fig. 15-4. Normal gallbladders displayed on two sagittal scans. **A,** Infundibulum lies proximal to cava. **B,** Gallbladder is in direct relation to right kidney.

gallbladder may be briefly described as usually superficial, clearing the liver edge and in close contact with the abdominal wall. It may also lie more posteriorly, in a retrohepatic position. Its sagittal section is elongated and oval or, on occasion, almost circular. (See Figs. 15-3 to 15-8.) Multiple close parallel scans permit one to outline the infundibulum (Figs. 15-7 and 15-8). The transverse section of the gallbladder is usually circular (Figs. 15-8, *B,* and 15-9) and appears

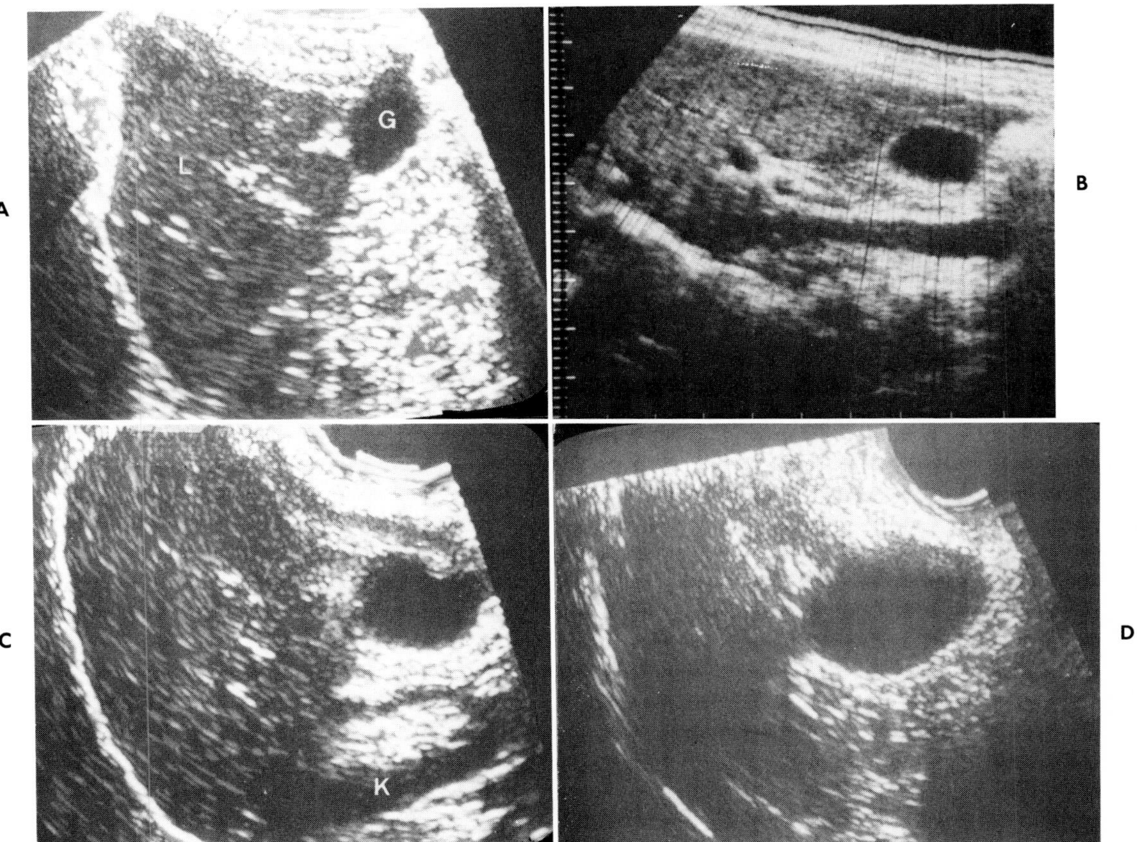

Fig. 15-5. Different types of gallbladders. **A** to **D,** Sagittal scans displaying variable shapes, sizes, and locations with regard to abdominal wall. *G,* gallbladder; *L,* liver; *K,* right kidney.

closely related to the neighboring hepatic parenchyma. This is also the case in gallbladder images on oblique recurrent sections. These pass through the gallbladder along its sagittal axis and display it as an elongated ovoid, lying within the hepatic parenchyma. (See Fig. 15-10.) Some high gallbladders are hidden by the ribs and cannot always be shown on sagittal sector scans (Fig. 15-11). In such cases, intercostal scans are usually helpful (Fig. 15-12). Gallbladders that are visible only on intercostal scans are generally small, but sometimes such scans are needed to show much longer gallbladders (Fig. 15-12, *D*), which use of the anterior approach has failed to display.

The angulated, bilobate, or trilobate shape of some gallbladders, so commonly seen on cholecystograms, is, of course, also found with ultrasonography, especially on oblique recurrent scans (Figs. 15-13 and 15-14). A contraction test can be readily performed (Fig. 15-15).

Size. The size of the gallbladder is extremely variable. Criteria of normality would be helpful, since the diagnosis of gallbladder enlargement is important. An unpretentious gallbladder does not exceed 10 cm in length, but it is possible to see

Text continued on p. 231.

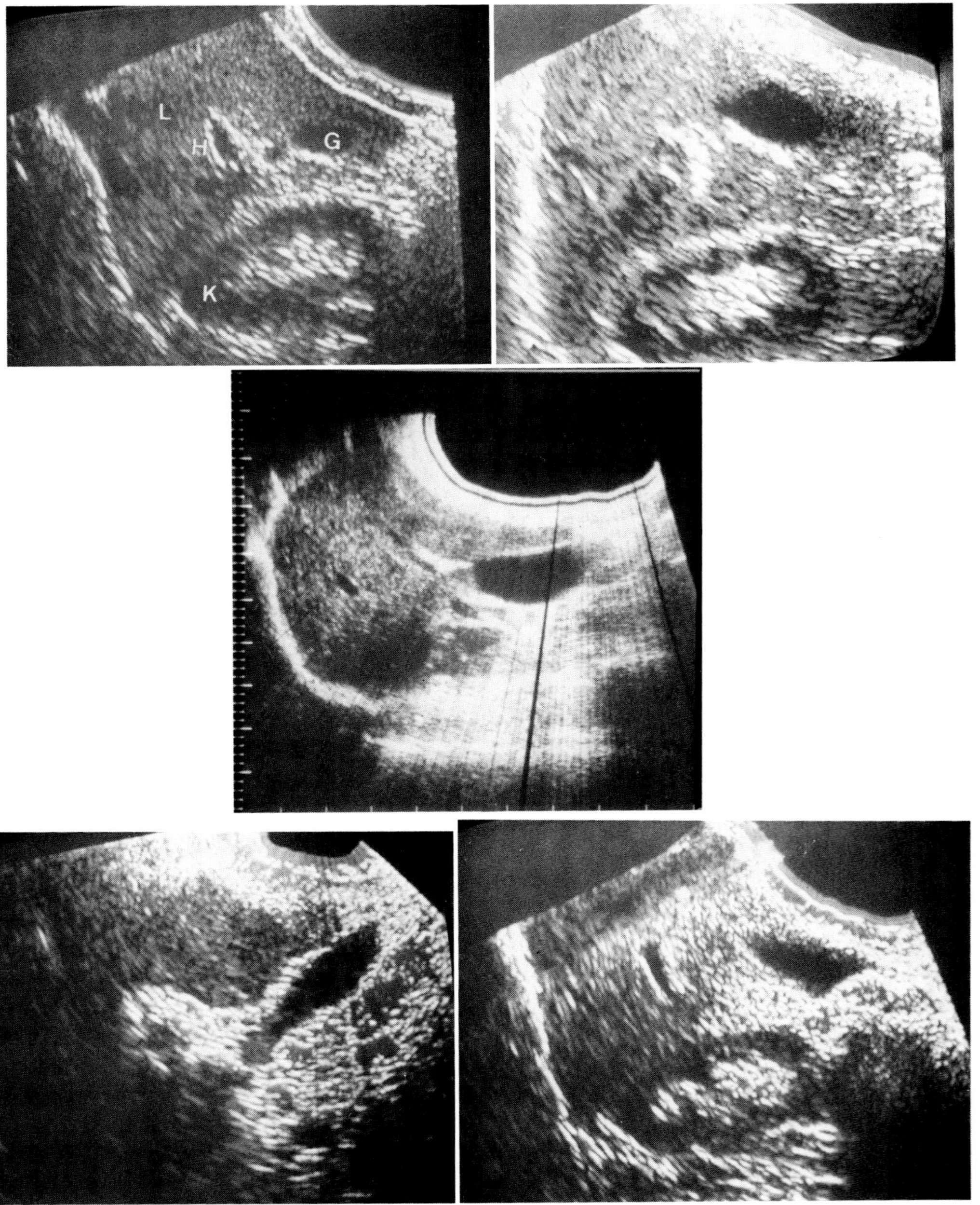

Fig. 15-6. More examples of normal gallbladders. *G,* gallbladder; *L,* liver; *H,* hilus; *K,* right kidney.

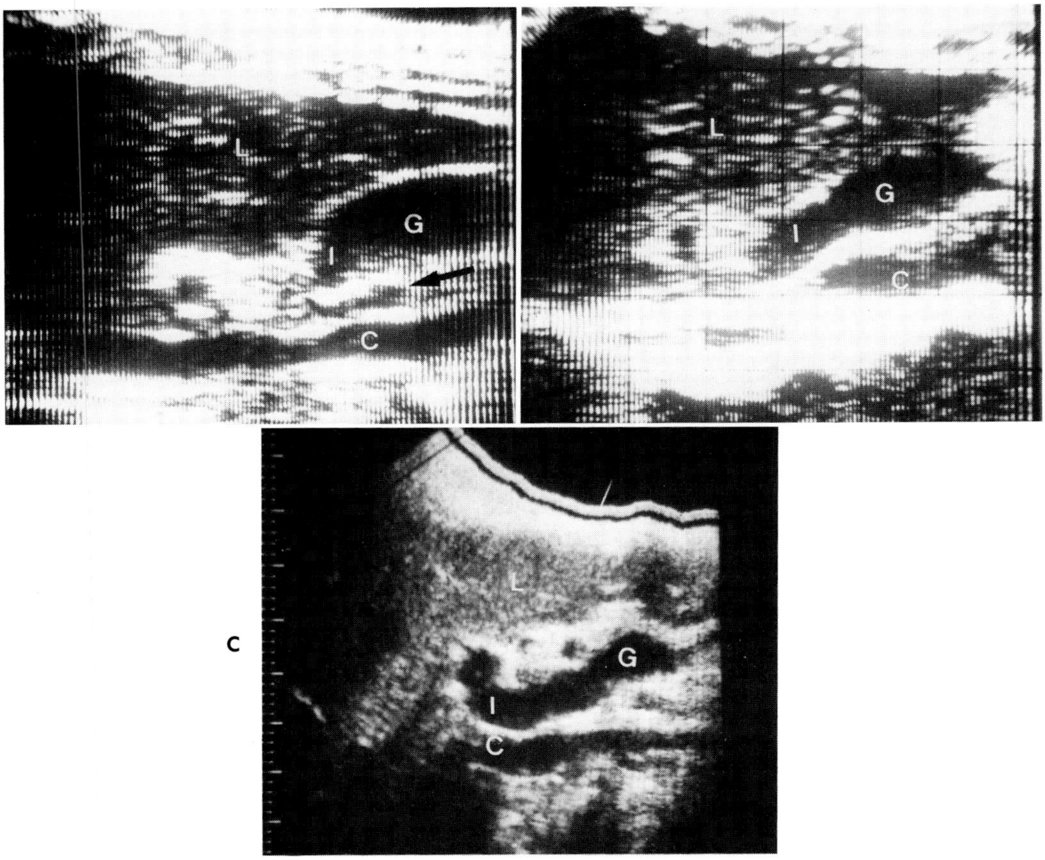

Fig. 15-7. Examples of normal posterior gallbladders. Gallbladder *(G)* is in close contact with liver *(L)*. Note, in **A**, relation of infundibulum *(I)* to portal vein *(arrow)* and, in **B**, vena cava *(C)*. **C**, Another precaval infundibulum.

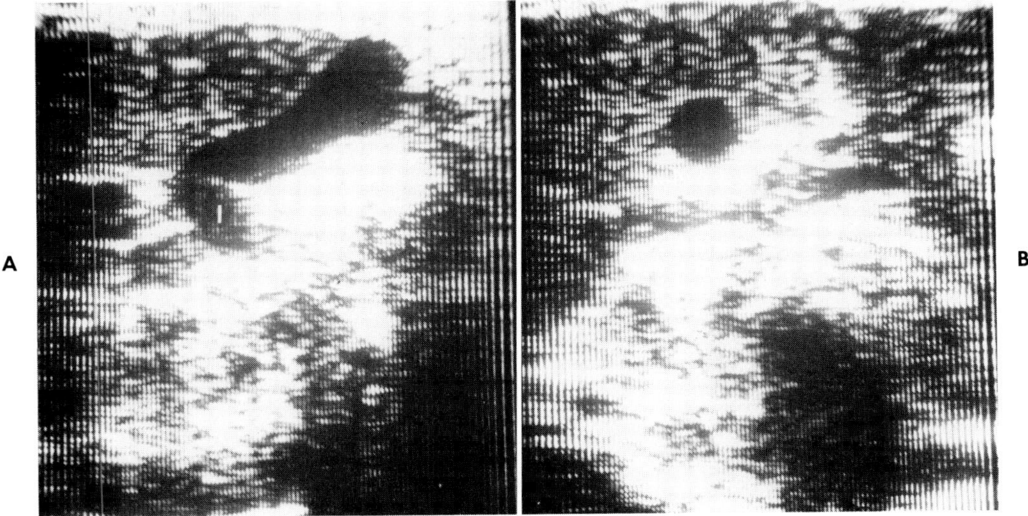

Fig. 15-8. Normal gallbladder. **A**, Sagittal scan displaying angled infundibulum *(I)*. **B**, Transverse scan. Note close relationship of gallbladder section with liver parenchyma.

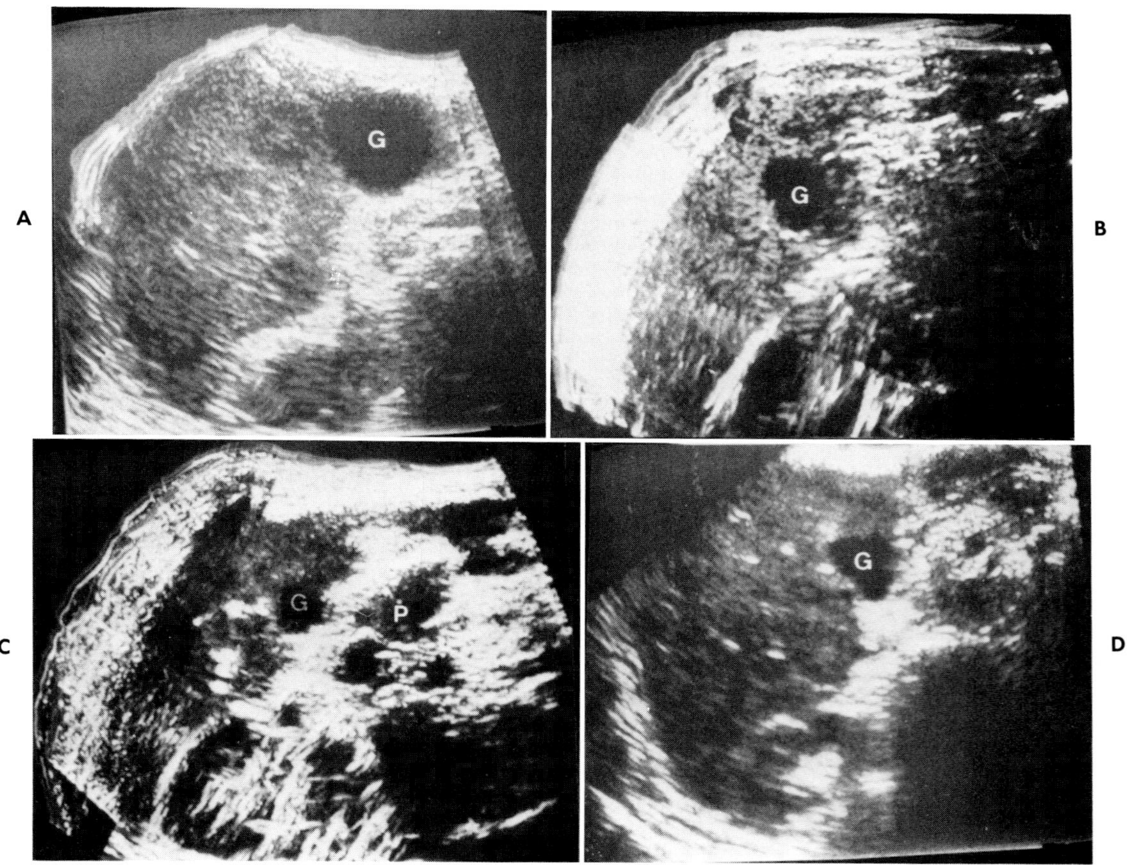

Fig. 15-9. Examples of transverse sections of gallbladder *(G)*. **A,** Superficially located large gallbladder. **B** to **D,** Deeply located gallbladder. *P,* pancreatic head.

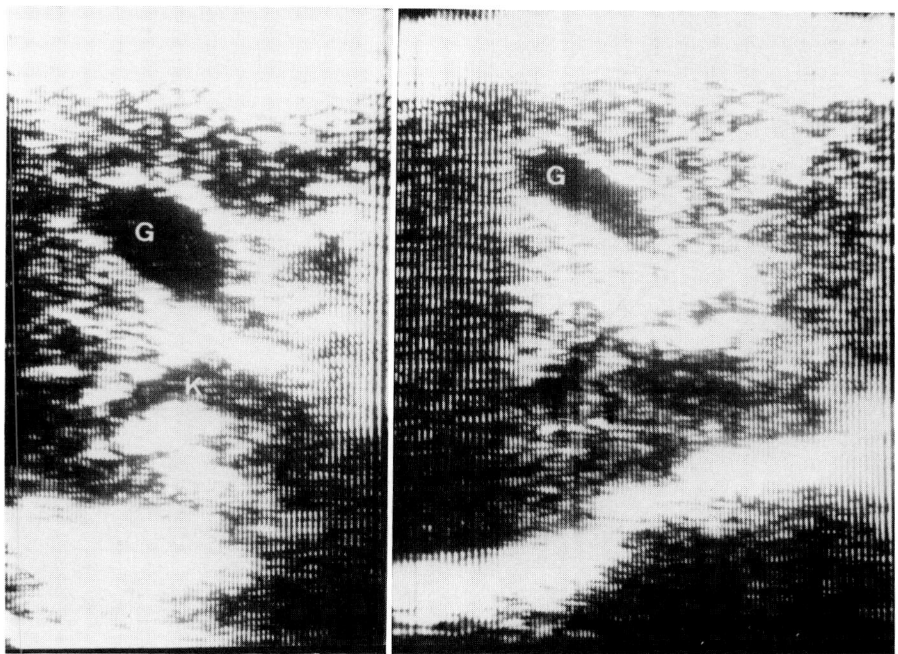

Fig. 15-10. Normal gallbladder *(G)* displayed on oblique recurrent subcostal scans. Note close relationship of gallbladder to surrounding liver tissue. *K*, right kidney.

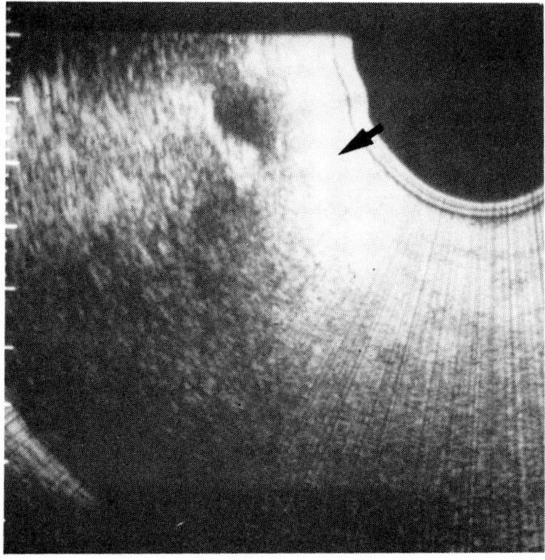

Fig. 15-11. Retrocostal gallbladder. Costal edge is marked by arrow. Ascending sagittal contact sector scan was necessary to display this high gallbladder.

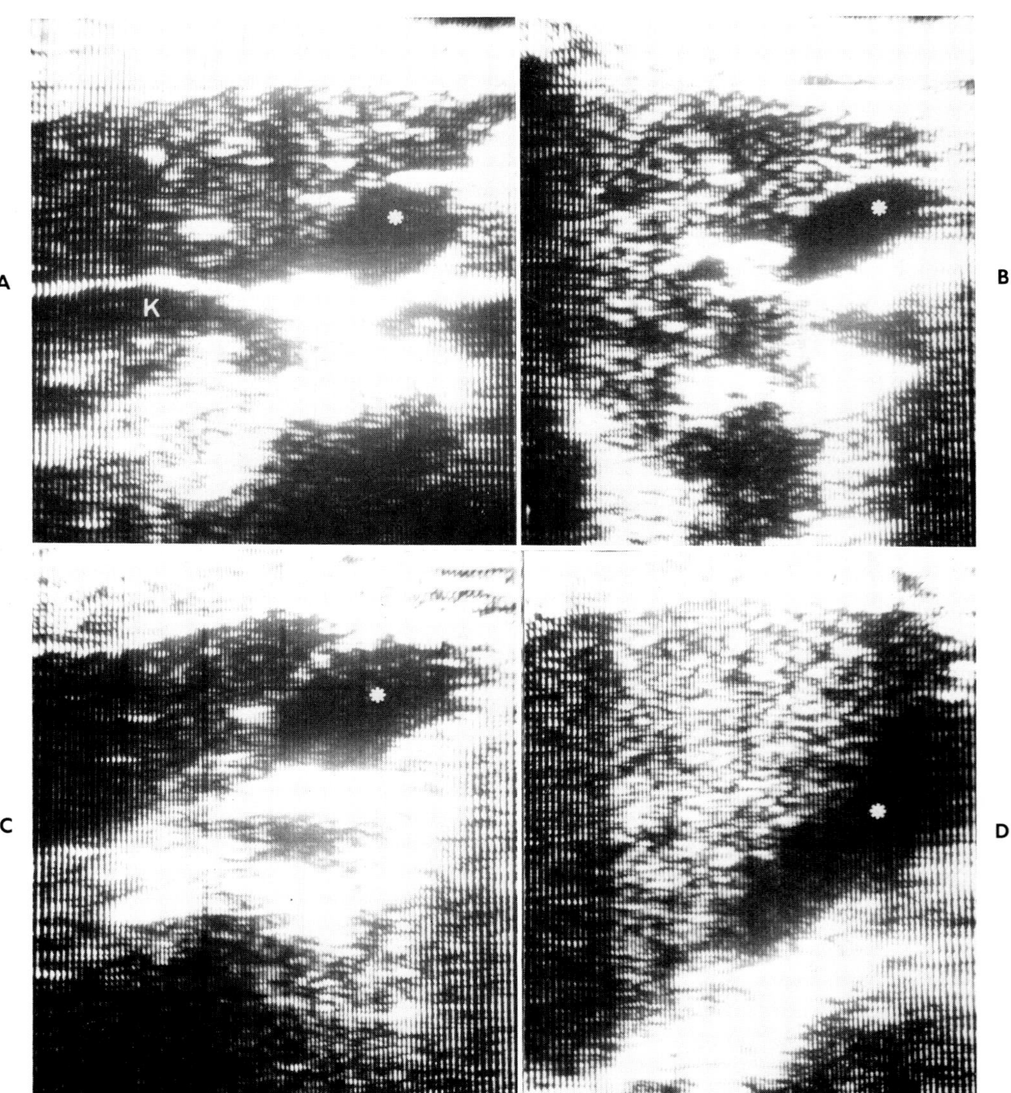

Fig. 15-12. Examples of normal gallbladder (*) displayed on intercostal real-time scans. Even largest of these gallbladders could not be displayed by anterior scanning. *K*, right kidney.

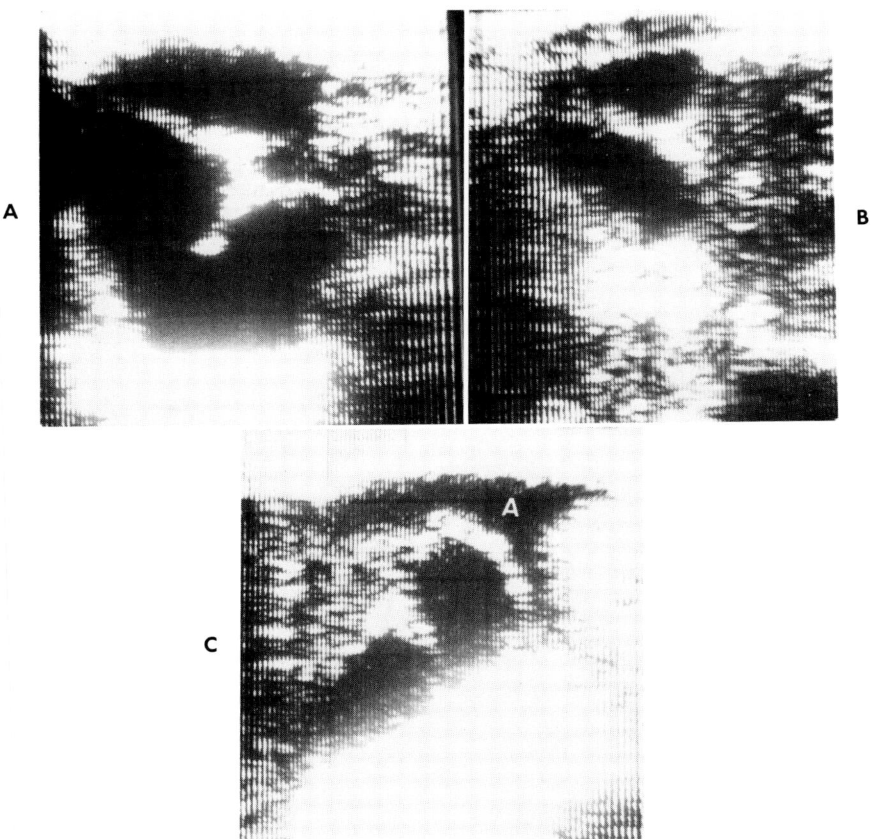

Fig. 15-13. Examples of septate gallbladders. **A,** Oblique recurrent scan of trilobate gallbladder. **B,** Oblique recurrent scan of bilobate gallbladder. **C,** Sagittal scan of bilobate gallbladder. Note ascitic fluid *(A)* between gallbladder and anterior abdominal wall.

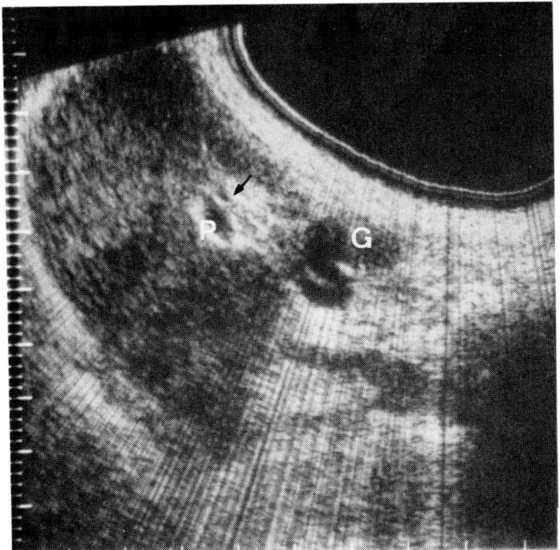

Fig. 15-14. Sagittal scan of septate gallbladder *(G)*. Note biliary junction *(arrow)* in front of portal division *(P)*.

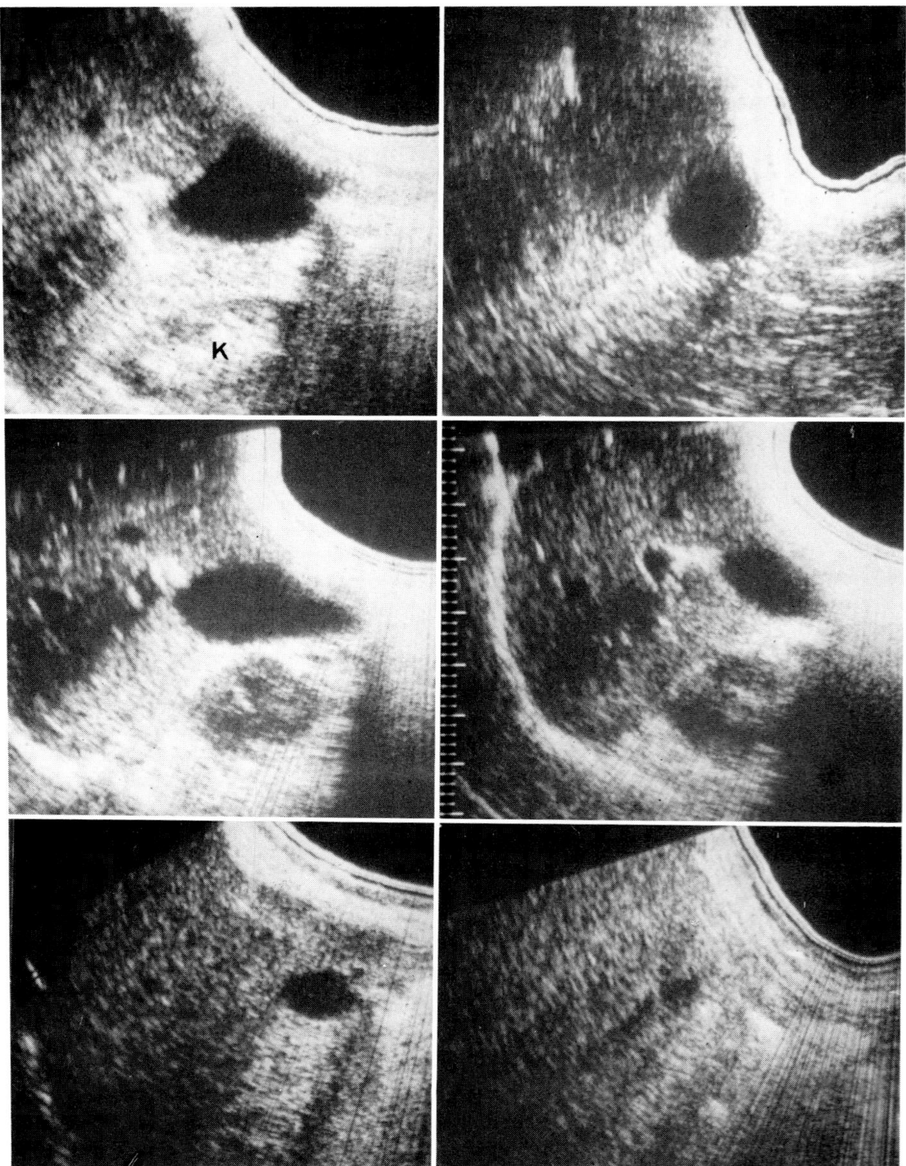

Fig. 15-15. Three examples of contraction test (left, before; right, after). In last example, contraction agent was chocolate pie.

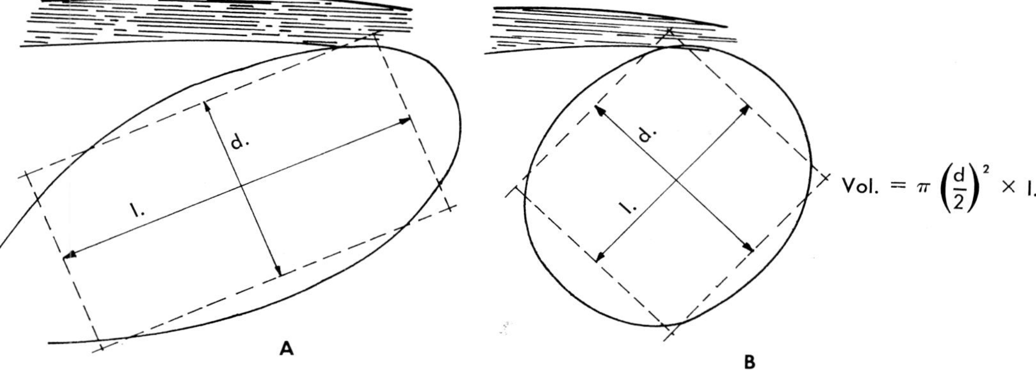

Fig. 15-16. Approximate evaluation of gallbladder volume. **A,** Elongated gallbladder. **B,** Round gallbladder. *l,* length; *d,* diameter.

normal, undilated gallbladders that are much longer. The longest gallbladder that we have encountered in a normal patient with a normal contraction test was 13 cm. The diameter of such long gallbladders does not usually exceed 4 cm, whereas in shorter and broader gallbladders the diameter may reach 5 cm. Such dimensional variations result in significant variations in gallbladder volume, and volume would seem to be the best way to evaluate enlargement. I shall now attempt to estimate the volume of the gallbladder but would discourage anyone who possesses the least knowledge of mathematics from reading the remainder of this paragraph. In most cases, one commits a tolerable error by comparing the gallbladder to a cylinder, disregarding the infundibular and the fundal areas. That means in practice that the height of the cylinder is the maximal length of the gallbladder minus 2 cm. (See Fig. 15-16.) As for the diameter, it is that of the middle of the gallbladder when it is an elongated type (Fig. 15-16, *A*). If the gallbladder has a more rounded shape, as seen on a sagittal scan, an average diameter has to be employed (Fig. 15-16, *B*). If a section through the gallbladder is considered circular, one calculates the volume by multiplying the area of the circle (πr^2) by the height. In the usual honest gallbladder this volume is less than 100 ml. Unfortunately this figure is not useful, since there are dishonest gallbladders that are normal but large, the volume of which may be as great as 160 ml. To avoid false diagnoses of enlargement, it is thus necessary to consider 200 ml the upper limit of normal. Now, many gallbladders that are dilated owing to biliary obstruction do not attain that volume, even after several weeks, so that even a volumetric criterion of normality proves unsatisfactory. One must consider not only the size of the gallbladder but also the diameter of the other elements of the biliary tree. It is also useful to estimate the tension of the gallbladder by palpation under echoscopic real-time control (Rettenmaier, 1975) and resort to a contraction test in doubtful cases.

The wall. The gallbladder wall as displayed on ultrasonic sections is regular and well delineated. Normally, it is difficult to evaluate its thickness except perhaps in the area of contact between the gallbladder and the liver. (See Figs. 15-4 and 15-5, *B*.) Even then one must remember that the pattern of ultrasonic wall images

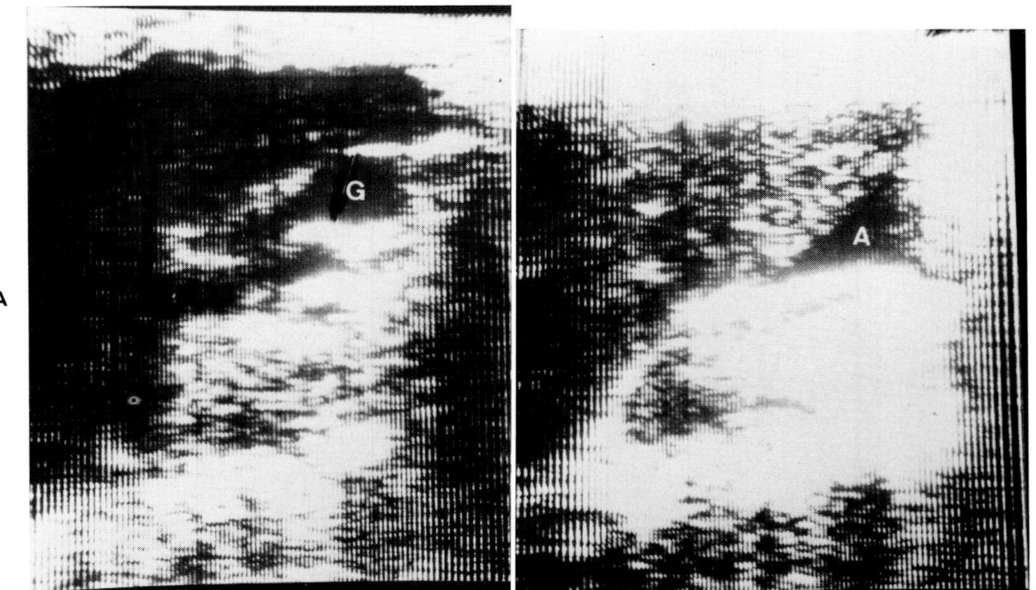

Fig. 15-17. False gallbladder image caused by ascites. **A,** Sagittal scan of right upper quadrant displaying gallbladder *(G)* under liver. **B,** Slightly more medial scan showing retrohepatic fluid collection that could belong to gallbladder but is, in reality, ascitic fluid *(A)*.

depends on the angle at which the ultrasonic beam approaches the wall. The wall image is clearer if the beam is perpendicular (Fig. 15-12, *A* to *C*) than if it is very oblique (Fig. 15-12, *D*). The thickness of a normal wall is less than 4 mm.

Anatomical relations. An ultrasonic sagittal scan of the gallbladder often passes through the right kidney (for example, Figs. 15-5, *C,* 15-6, and 15-12, *A*). The gallbladder may lie rather far from the kidney or, on the contrary, be in close contact with it (Fig. 15-4, *B*). The close relation between the gallbladder and kidney is even more evident if the gallbladder is enlarged. The infundibulum may also be in close contact with the vena cava and the portal vein (Fig. 15-7, *A*). The gallbladder lies just above the colon. When the latter is filled with air, it gives rise to a juxtavesicular shadow, which must not be confused with the shadow produced by a gallstone (Chapter 16). A gas-filled duodenum may also produce an acoustic shadow in the vicinity of the gallbladder.

Visualization. The gallbladder image is a constant feature of the ultrasonic examination of the upper right quadrant in a fasting patient. As I have already suggested, if all the required scans have been performed and the gallbladder is still not visible, it must be considered diseased. It is always uncomfortable not to find the gallbladder, since one then has to rely on a negative sign; but it may also be disconcerting to find several gallbladders, although vesicular duplication is, of course, a well-known dysplastic entity. In fact, an apparent duplication of the gallbladder may be due to the presence of an intrahepatic cyst in the vicinity of the gallbladder (Fig. 11-15). More often, the "second" gallbladder is really a pseudogallbladder

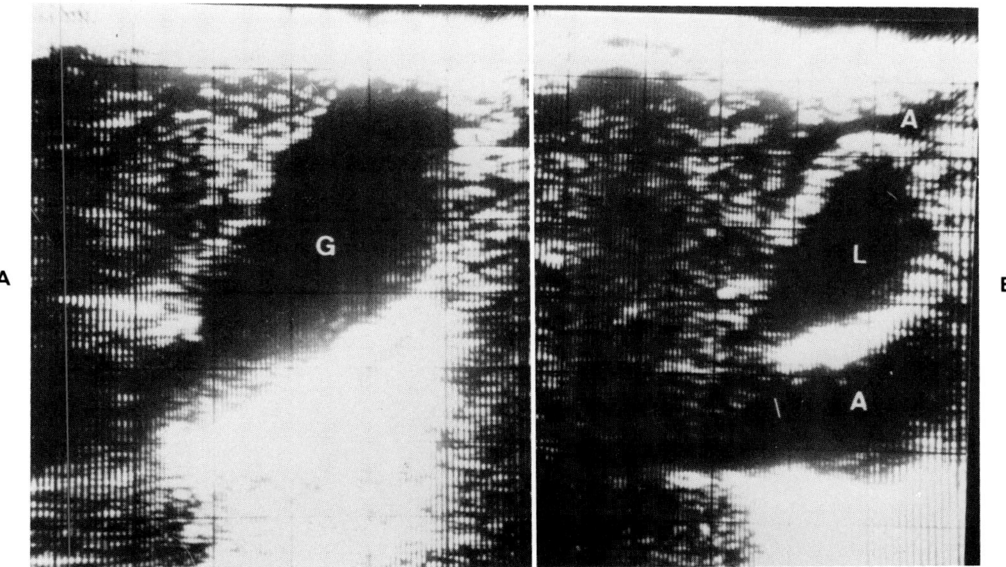

Fig. 15-18. Another false gallbladder image caused by ascites. **A,** Sagittal scan of elongated gallbladder *(G)*. **B,** More lateral scan displaying another oval pattern that looks like a gallbladder. In fact, this image represents intestinal loop *(L)* floating in ascitic fluid *(A)*.

caused by ascites. This is because a small liquid pouch exists between the liver, the gallbladder, and the colon (Fig. 15-17); or an intestinal loop, floating in the ascites just below the liver, may mimic the gallbladder (Fig. 15-18). Rarely a postoperative abscess may masquerade as the gallbladder. If such a finding is a complication of cholecystectomy, it is easily recognized to be consistent with an abscess. (See Fig. 15-19.) Another rare problem is an obstructed or enlarged right colonic loop that may take the shape of an enlarged gallbladder.

Main bile duct

As I have already pointed out, because of the improvements in ultrasonographic imaging, the image of the main bile duct is now regularly obtained. The threshold of visibility is now about 4 mm. The common hepatic duct and proximal common bile duct are displayed as a canal situated immediately in front of the portal vein, in close contact with its anterior wall (Figs. 15-20 to 15-23). As indicated earlier in this chapter this portion of the biliary tree in relation to the portal vein is referred to as the *main bile duct.* Recent imaging improvements now often enable one to display distal parts of the common bile duct on pancreatic transverse scans (Fig. 15-24).

Intrahepatic bile ducts

The intrahepatic bile ducts are, as already mentioned, usually not visible beyond the hilus, but this will probably change with improved equipment. In the

Text continued on p. 238.

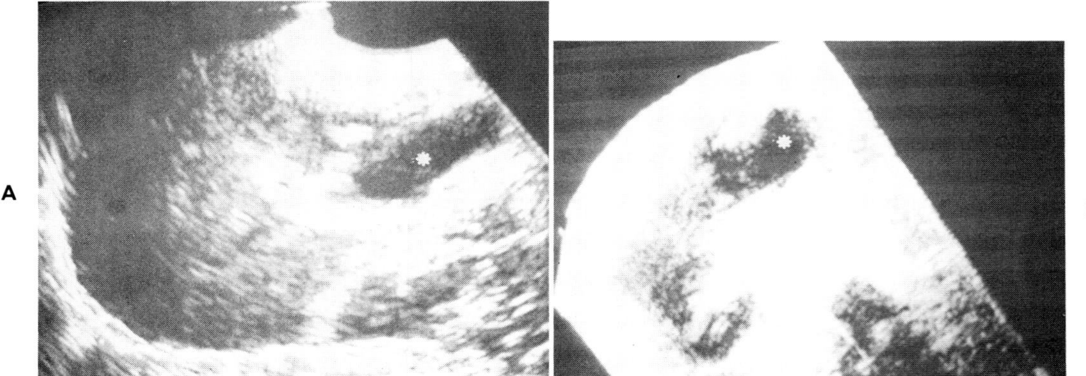

Fig. 15-19. False gallbladder image caused by postoperative abscess. **A,** Sagittal scan of right upper quadrant displaying oval sonolucent area (*) below liver. **B,** Same sonolucent area found on transverse scan. This area resembles gallbladder; however, since patient had undergone cholecystectomy, this is postoperative abscess.

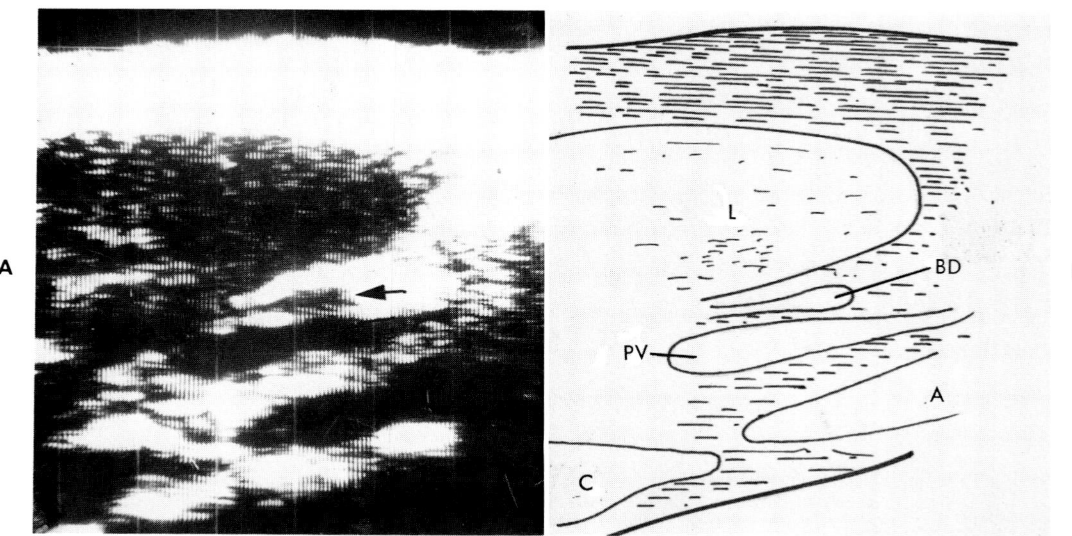

Fig. 15-20. Sagittal cut of main bile duct between liver *(L)* and portal vein *(PV)* displayed on oblique scan of right upper quadrant and schematic drawing. Narrow tubular structure is main bile duct, indicated in **A** by *arrow* and in **B** as *BD*. Vena cava *(C)* and aorta *(A)* are seen in oblique section.

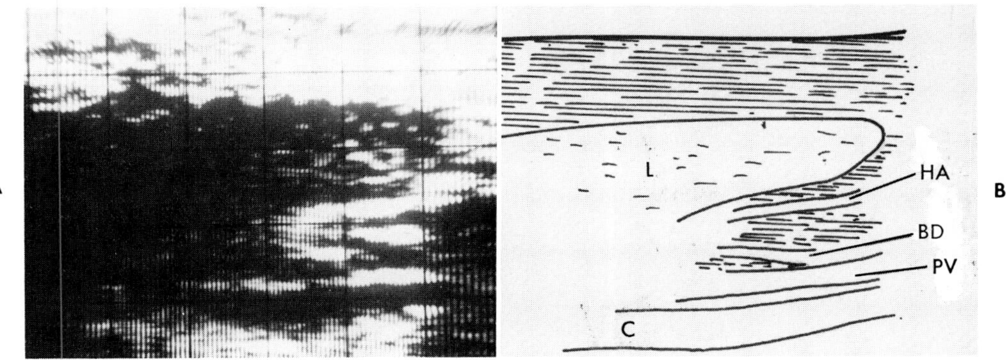

Fig. 15-21. Sagittal cut of normal main bile duct. This oblique scan, **A,** and schematic representation, **B,** of right upper quadrant shows several parallel tubular structures between liver *(L)* and vena cava *(C)*. Deepest is portal vein *(PV)*; two others, which are more anteriorly located, represent hepatic artery *(HA)* and bile duct *(BD)*.

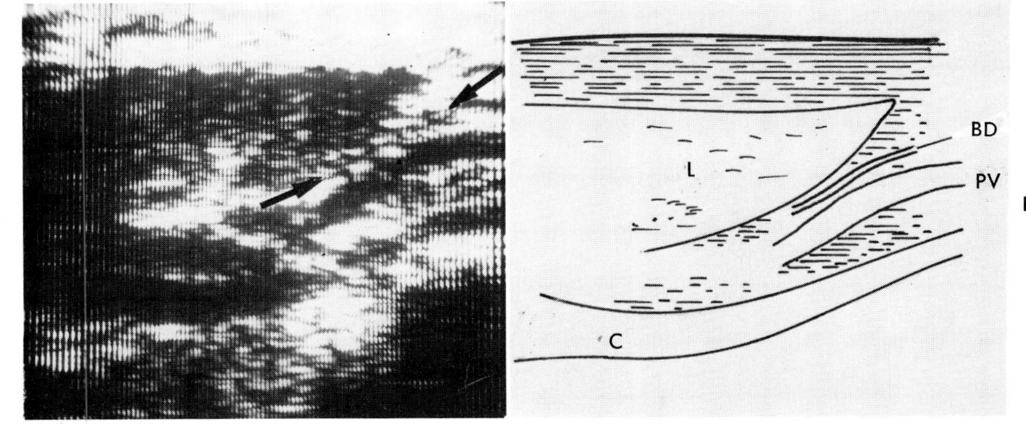

Fig. 15-22. Normal bile duct. This oblique, almost sagittal scan, **A,** and schematic drawing, **B,** of right upper quadrant show, from bottom to top, vena cava *(C)*, portal vein *(PV)*, and a narrow bile duct (*arrows* and *BD*), the image of which lies in close contact with posterior aspect of liver *(L)*.

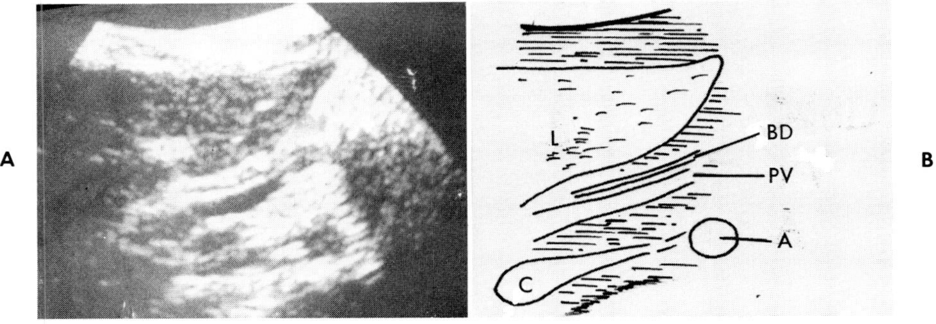

Fig. 15-23. Another normal bile duct. This oblique scan, **A,** and schematic drawing, **B,** of right upper quadrant display narrow tubular element representing main bile duct *(BD)* between liver *(L)* and portal vein *(PV)*. *C,* vena cava; *A,* aorta.

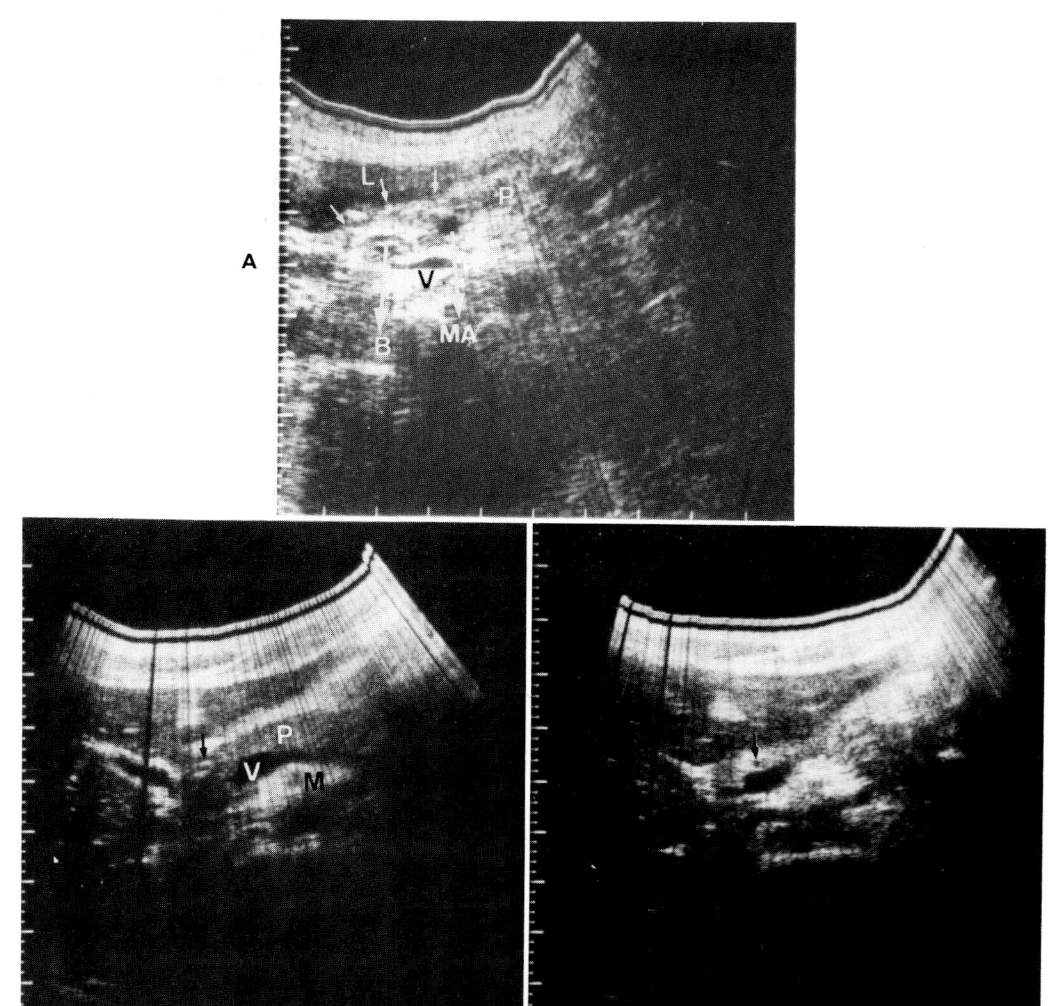

Fig. 15-24. Juxtapancreatic and intrapancreatic common bile duct. **A,** Short segment of intrapancreatic common bile duct *(B)* displayed on transverse section of pancreatic head *(P* and *arrows)*. *MA,* mesenteric artery; *V,* splenoportal junction; *L,* liver. (See also Figs. 19-5 and 19-19, *C.*) **B,** Transverse scan of pancreas *(P)* displaying tubular structure *(arrow)* representing extrapancreatic common bile duct, proximal to external aspect of pancreatic head. **C,** Parallel, more caudal scan showing transverse section of intrapancreatic bile duct *(arrow).*

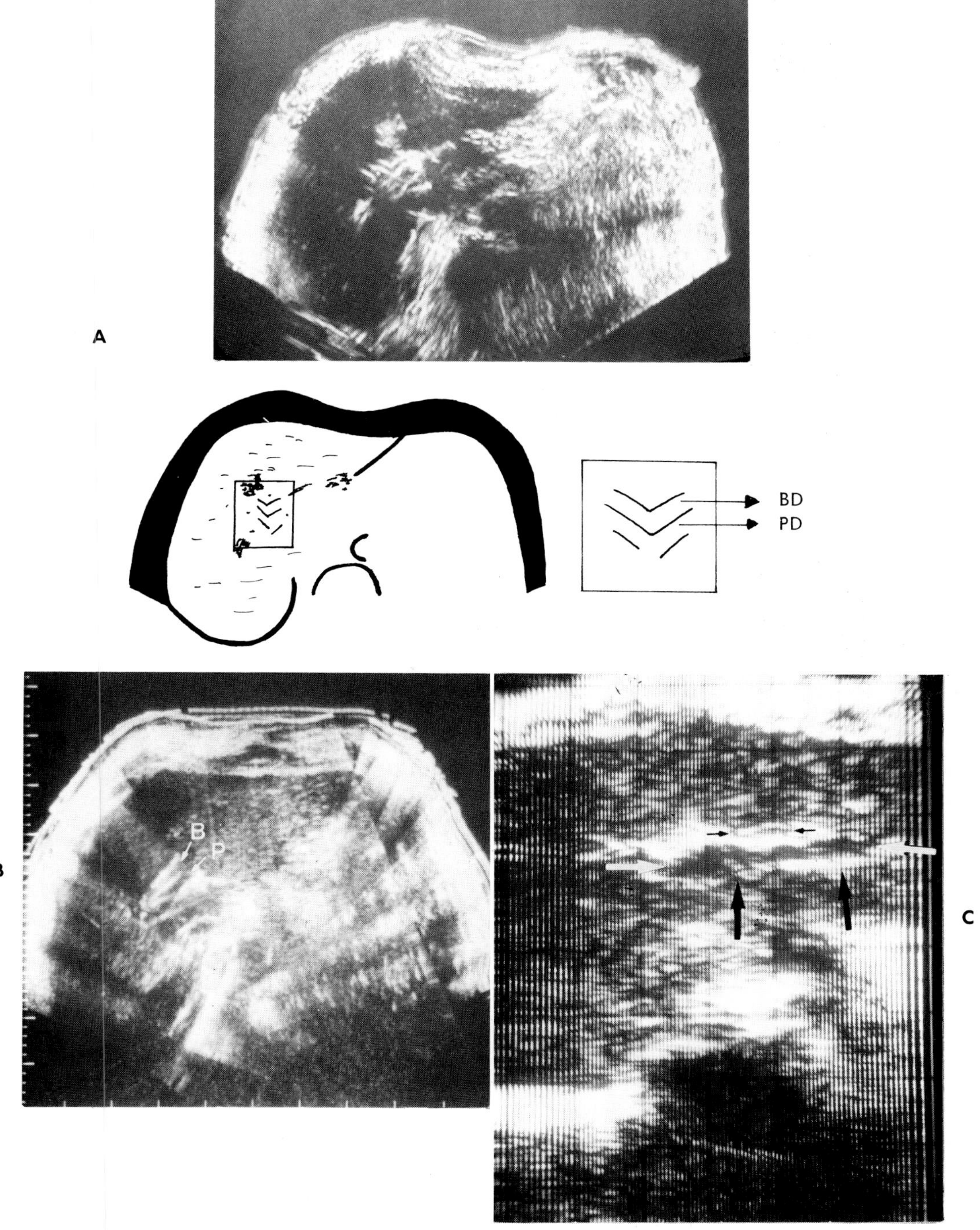

Fig. 15-25. Hilar biliary junction. **A,** Transverse scan and schematic drawing. Biliary duct *(BD),* with portal division *(PD),* outlines chevron-shaped group of parallel lines. **B,** Another example of adjacent normal biliary junction *(B)* and portal division *(P)* on transverse scan of liver hilus. **C,** In fact, display of hilar elements *(arrows)* is usually much easier with real-time technique on oblique recurrent subcostal cuts. *Continued.*

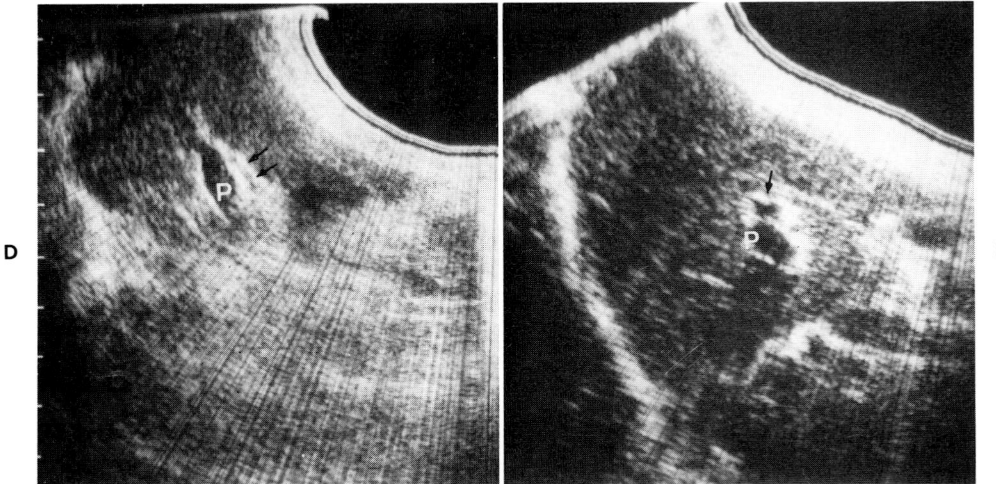

Fig. 15-25, cont'd. D and **E,** Biliary junction *(arrows)* and portal division on sagittal sections (Fig. 15-14). On such sections, juxtaportal infundibulum must not be taken for enlarged biliary junction.

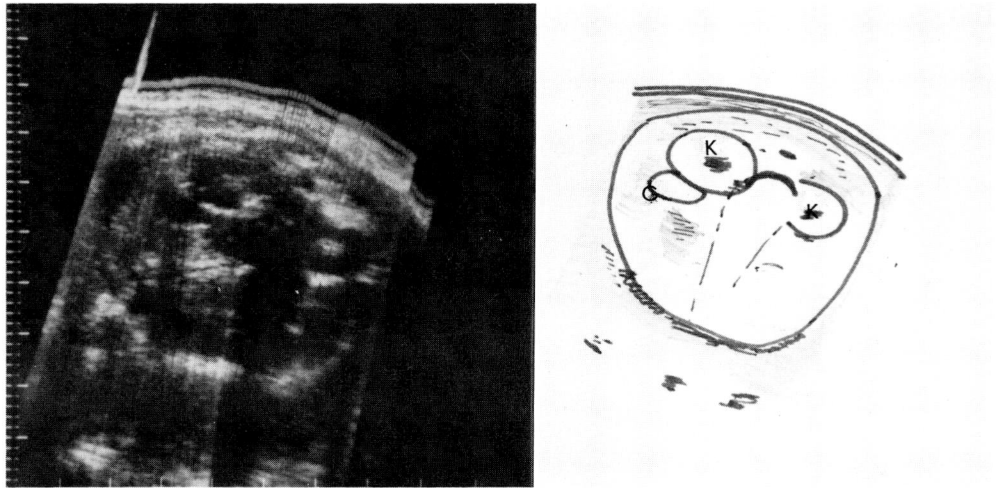

Fig. 15-26. What is this?*

hilus, sagittal, transverse, intercostal, or recurrent scans show the biliary junction anterior to the division of the portal vein (Figs. 15-14 and 15-25). The walls of the biliary ducts and the portal veins produce a group of parallel lines. In this area, early dilatation is most easily discovered. I shall discuss this in more detail in Chapter 26. The unusual visualization of an unenlarged intrahepatic biliary network suggests the possibility of air in the biliary tree (Hassani, 1976), but this is, of course, a simple diagnosis made with ordinary x-ray films.

*Answer: Fetal gallbladder *(G)* outlined in front of right kidney. *K,* kidney.

Resolution of present imaging may lead to other clinical applications (Fig. 15-26).

REFERENCES

Barnett, E., and Morley, P.: Abdominal echography, Borough Green, England, 1974, Butterworth & Co. (Publishers), Ltd.

Goldberg, B. B., Kotler, M. N., Ziskin, M. C., and Waxham, R. D.: Diagnostic uses of ultrasound, New York, 1975, Grune & Stratton, Inc.

Hassani, N.: Ultrasonography of the abdomen, Heidelberg, Germany, 1976, Springer-Verlag.

Holm, H. H., Kristensen, J. K., Rasmussen, S. N., Pedersen, J. F., and Hancke, S.: Abdominal ultrasound, Copenhagen, 1976, Munksgaard, International Booksellers & Publishers, Ltd.

Leopold, G. R., and Asher, W. M.: Fundamentals of abdominal and pelvic ultrasonography, Philadelphia, 1975, W. B. Saunders Co.

Rettenmaier, G.: Personal communication, 1975.

Weill, F., Becker, J. C., Kraehenbuhl, J. R., Heriot, G., and Walter, J. P.: Clinical atlas of ultrasonic radiography, Paris, 1973, Masson & Cie., Editeurs.

CHAPTER 16

CHOLELITHIASIS AND CHOLECYSTITIS

CHOLELITHIASIS

Cholelithiasis may present two quite different ultrasonic patterns. The gallbladder may be completely filled with stones or may contain only one or a few stones, so that a large part of it is filled with fluid. The latter situation, which is the more common, will be discussed first. When the gallbladder is only partially occupied by stones, two kinds of ultrasonic signs may be encountered—direct and indirect.

Direct sign

The direct sign is the image of the stone itself, well displayed as a reflective area surrounded by transparent bile (Figs. 16-1 to 16-3). This appearance occurs with a solitary stone, as well as an accumulation of smaller stones, either calcified or purely cholesteric. The threshold of visibility for a solitary stone is a diameter of about 3 mm. Stones denser than bile sink to the bottom of the gallbladder, and this condition is usually clearly displayed (Figs. 16-4 and 16-5). The intensity of reflection from the posterior wall of the gallbladder may produce a dense and thick reflective strip, which must be distinguished from calculi. Mucosal folds may also give rise to false images of microlithiasis (Fig. 16-6). As in conventional radiology, placing the patient in the upright position confirms or excludes the diagnosis. In the erect position, stones denser than bile will indeed migrate to the bottom of the gallbladder, as shown in sagittal sections. (See Figs. 16-7 and 16-8.) If the patient is unable to stand, the lateral decubitus position is employed (Fig. 16-8). The dependent position of the stones is also shown in horizontal scans performed with the patient in the erect position. Transverse scans passing through the superior part of the gallbladder show only an echo-free section of the gallbladder. (See Fig. 16-9, *A*.) More caudal scans, closer to the bottom of the gallbladder, pass through the accumulated stones and display their echoes from the gallbladder section (Fig. 16-9, *B*).

In some patients the stones are less dense than bile and float. These give rise to a horizontal line at some distance from the dependent portion of the gallbladder (Figs. 16-10 and 16-11). Floating stones are best shown when the ultrasonic beam is perpendicular to them, that is, when the patient lies in the recumbent position. This is quite different from cholecystography, in which floating stones are best shown in the erect position. A pitfall encountered with dilated gallbladders is the layering of bile of different specific gravity, producing an ultrasonic "fluid level" image (Leopold, 1977). Sludge settles at the bottom of the gallbladder with a well-delineated upper level of separation. (See Fig. 16-12.)

Up to a certain point, the more stones, the better they can be seen (Figs. 16-4,

Text continued on p. 248.

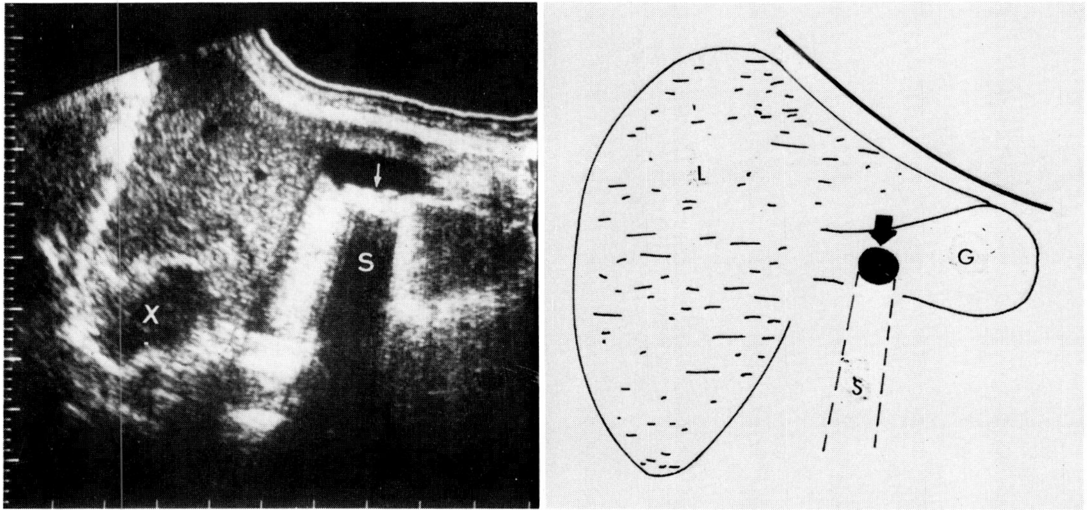

Fig. 16-1. Gallstones: direct image *(arrow)* and indirect image *(S,* acoustic shadow). Patient was referred for fever and pain in right upper quadrant. Are these symptoms now explained?*

*Besides gallstones, there is hepatic abscess *(X)*.

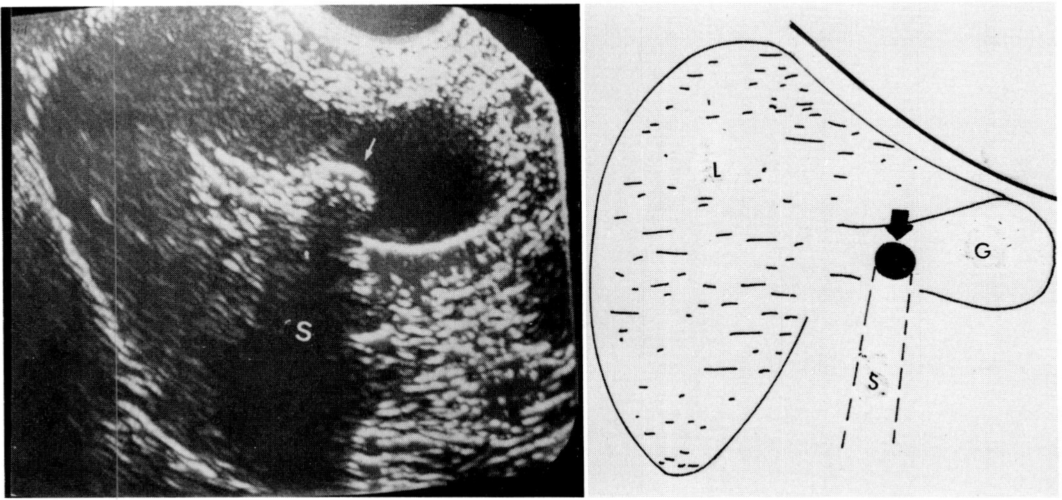

Fig. 16-2. Infundibular gallstone: direct image *(arrows)* and indirect image, acoustic shadow *(S)*. *L,* liver; *G,* gallbladder.

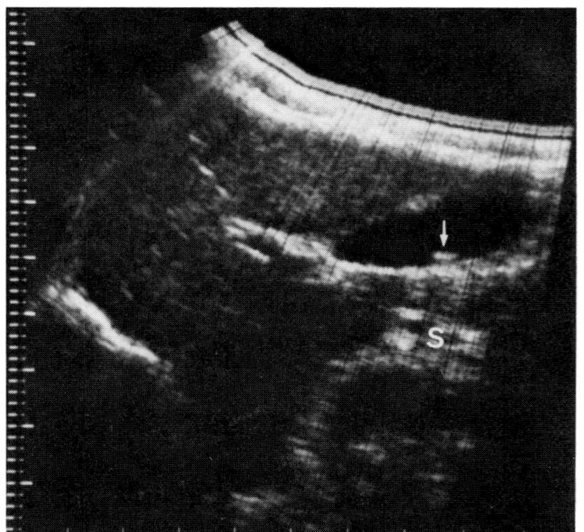

Fig. 16-3. Small gallstone: direct image *(arrow)* and acoustic shadow *(S)*. Stone was not visualized by conventional cholecystography. Note, in hilus, double tubular structure of biliary junction and portal division. (Courtesy Dr. Fred Winsberg, Montreal.)

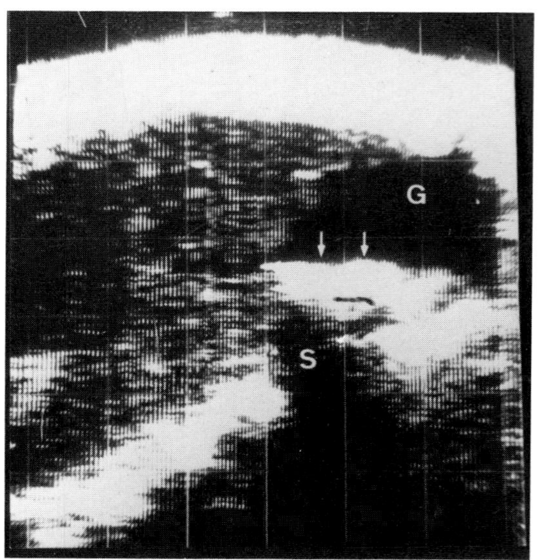

Fig. 16-4. Stones in retrocostal gallbladder *(G)* examined by intercostal scan. Stones are small and gathered in lower part of gallbladder. There is gallstone level *(arrows)*, with acoustic shadow *(S)* behind stones.

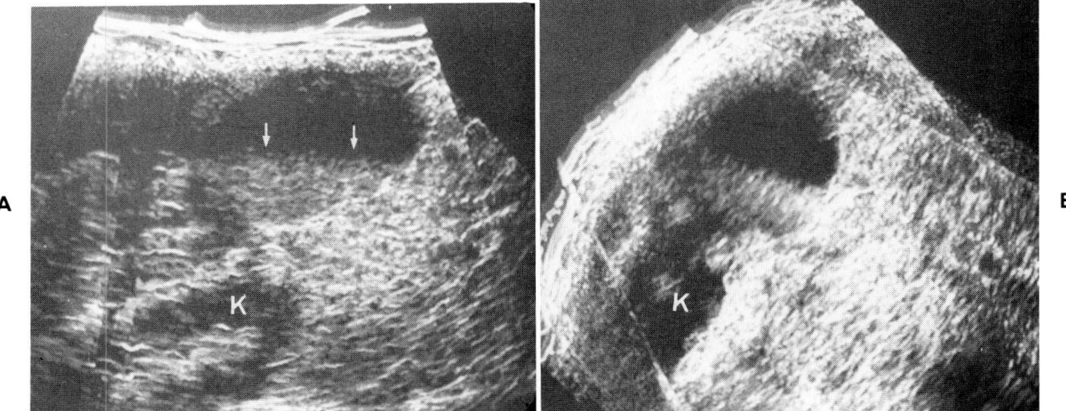

Fig. 16-5. Another example of gallstones settling in dependent part of gallbladder with linear upper limit *(arrows)*. **A,** Sagittal scan. **B,** Transverse scan. *K,* kidney. (Courtesy Dr. Eisenscher, Vesoul, France.)

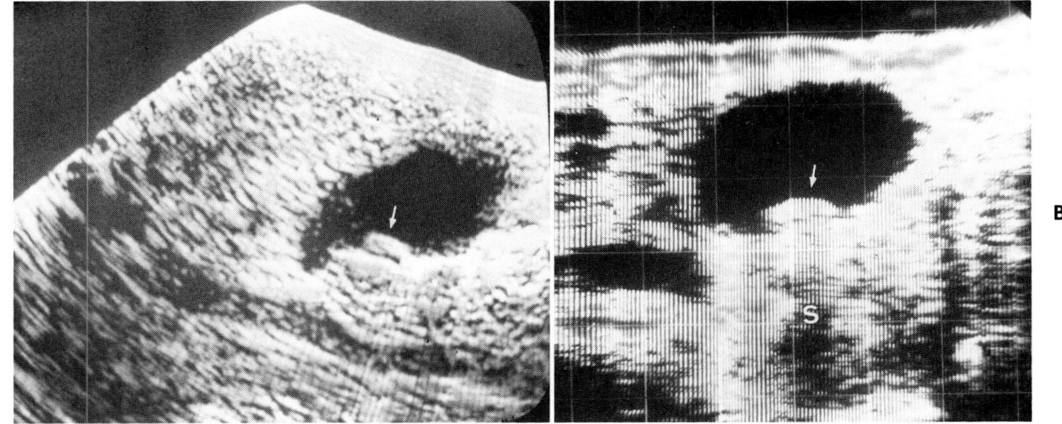

Fig. 16-6. False and true stones. **A,** Sagittal scan of gallbladder displaying small posterior elevation *(arrow)* representing mucosal fold, since it disappeared with patient in erect position. **B,** Quite similar elevation in this gallbladder *(arrow)* with posterior acoustic shadow *(S)*. In addition, when patient was erect, stone migrated to floor of gallbladder.

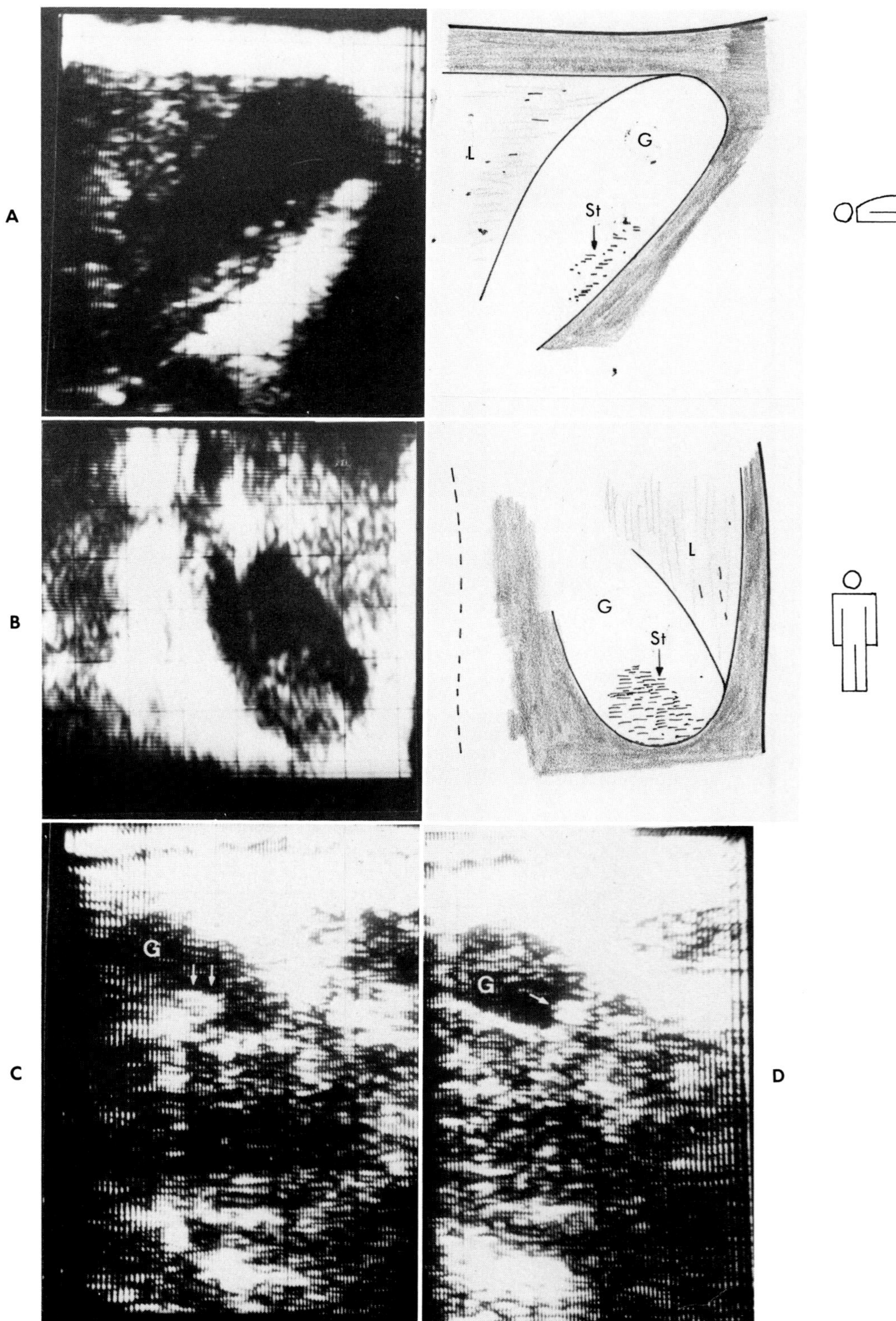

Fig. 16-7. For legend see opposite page.

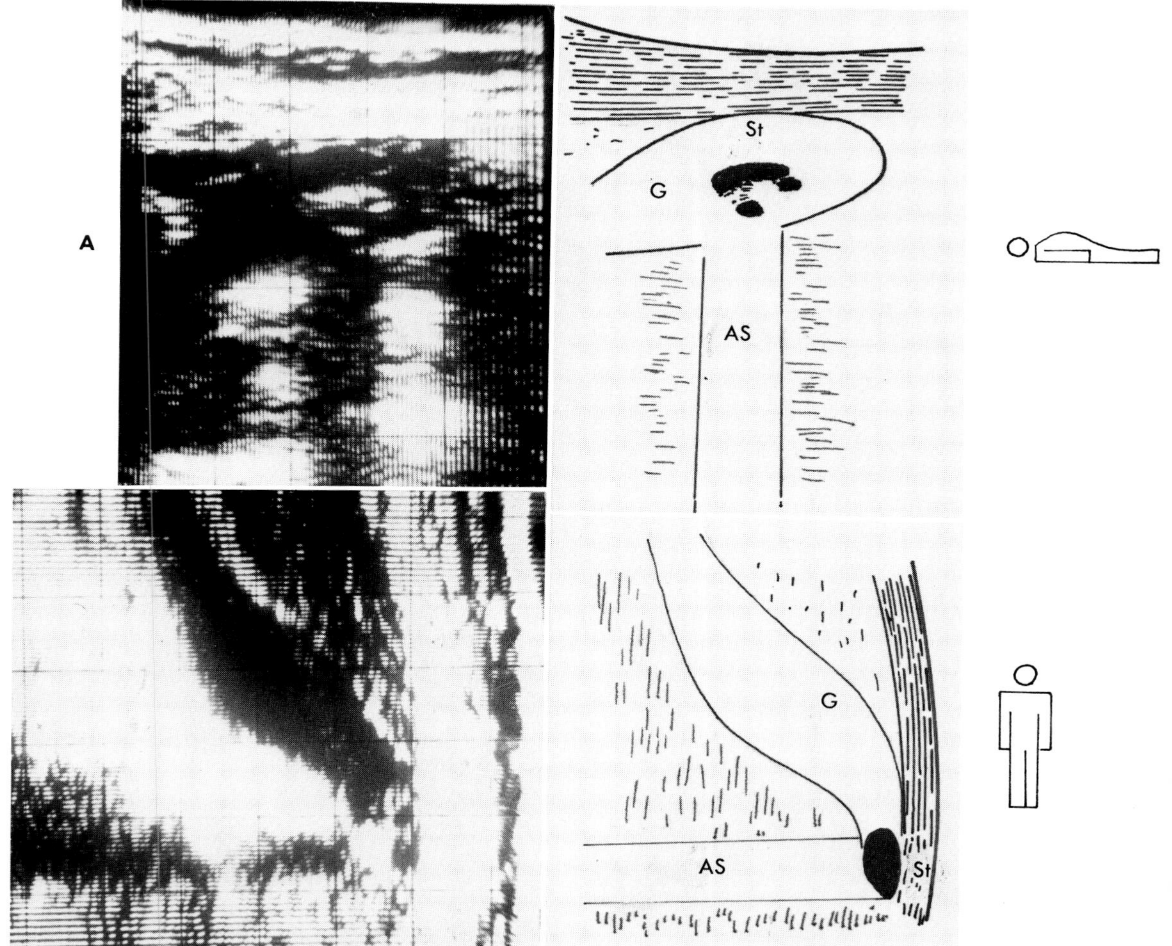

Fig. 16-8. Another example of positional migration of gallstones. **A,** Sagittal scan and schematic drawing of gallbladder *(G)* made with patient in recumbent position, displaying abnormal echoes *(St)* in middle part of gallbladder. Acoustic shadow *(AS)* appears behind stones. **B,** Patient in erect position. Gallbladder seems more elongated, and stone echoes have migrated to bottom of gallbladder. Acoustic shadow appears in direction of ultrasonic beam.

Fig. 16-7. Positional migration of gallstones. **A,** Sagittal scan and schematic drawing of gallbladder *(G),* with patient in recumbent position, displaying small stones *(St)* accumulated in lower part of the gallbladder *(G). L,* liver. **B,** With patient in erect position, stones migrate toward bottom of gallbladder. **C** and **D,** Another example of positional stone migration in 90-year-old patient who could not be positioned upright. Mere rotation to left, from supine to left posterior oblique position, displaced stone *(arrows). G,* gallbladder.

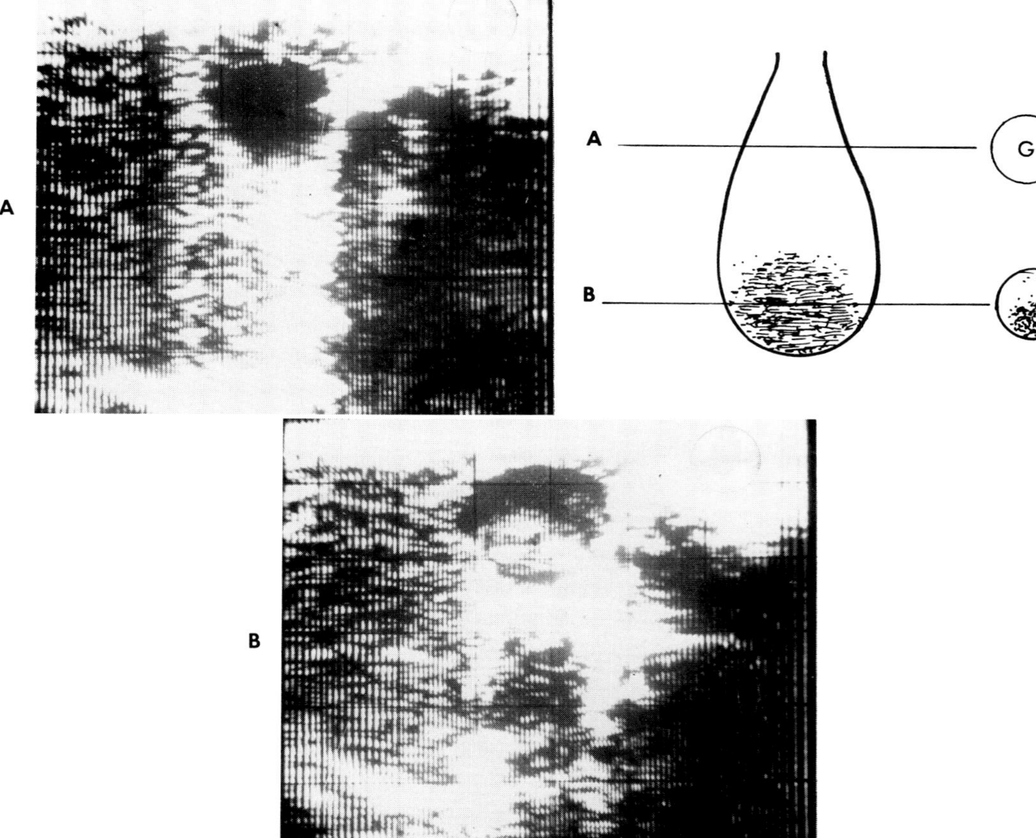

Fig. 16-9. Accumulation of stones in bottom of gallbladder, displayed on transverse scans. **A,** Scan passing above stones, with schematic representation at right. Transverse section of gallbladder shows liquid pattern *(G)*. **B,** Parallel, more caudal scan passing through stones. There are now abnormal echoes within liquid.

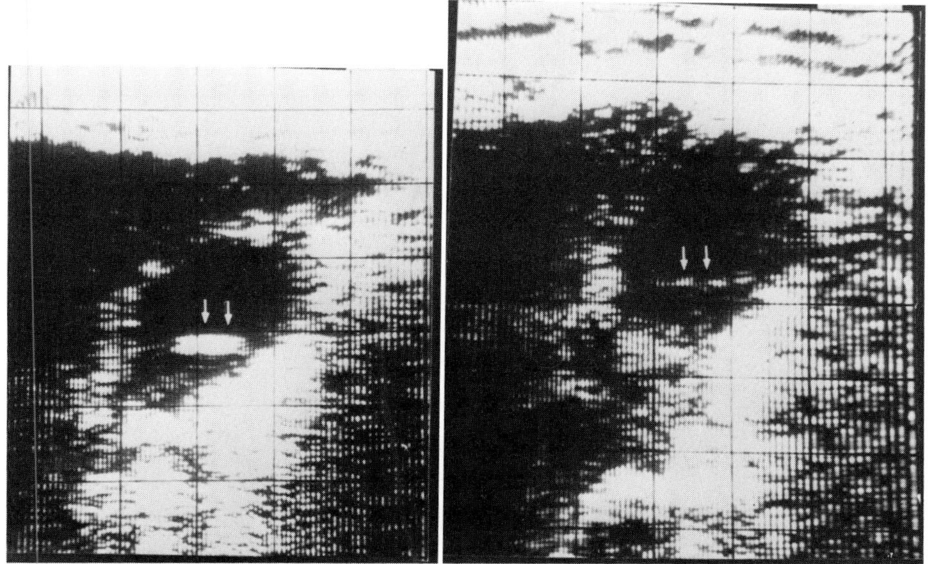

Fig. 16-10. Floating stones in two recumbent patients. Gallbladders are cut sagittally. Stones *(arrows)* outline horizontal levels.

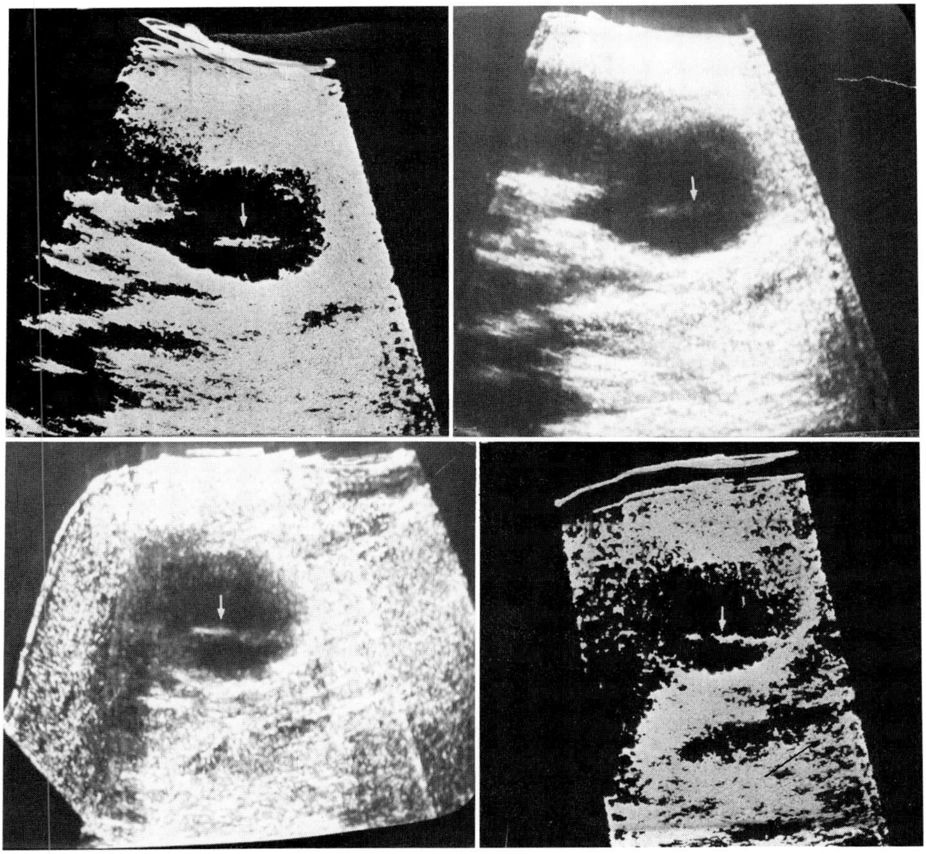

A

B

C

D

Fig. 16-11. Another example of floating stones *(arrows)* seen in examination of patient in recumbent position. **A** and **B,** Sagittal scans. **C** and **D,** Transverse sections.

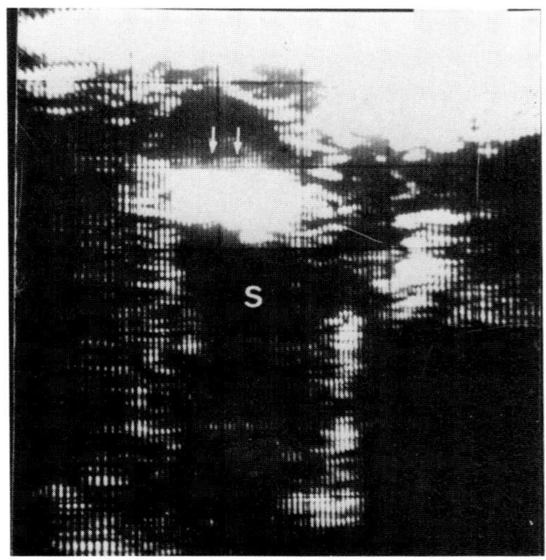

Fig. 16-12. Accumulation of small stones on bottom of gallbladder. Horizontal limit *(arrows)* appears between gravel and bile. Note large acoustic shadow *(S)* behind gravel.

16-5, 16-12, and 16-13, *A* and *B*); but the sharpness of the image depends on the large difference in impedance between the stone-free bile and the stones. As long as a certain portion of the gallbladder remains free of stones, its transparent liquid pattern permits delineation of stones (Fig. 16-13, *A* and *B*). However, when the gallbladder is entirely filled with stones, no surrounding liquid pattern is left. The main source of impedance difference has disappeared. An image of the stones then appears only if a gradient of impedance exists between the stones and the surrounding soft tissues. (See Fig. 16-13, *C*.) This problem will be discussed in more detail later.

Indirect sign

The indirect sign is the acoustic shadow that appears behind the stones in about 80% of the cases (Figs. 16-1 to 16-4, 16-6, 16-8, 16-12, and 16-13, *C*). The observation of an acoustic shadow is not very important when the stone is clearly shown. It is more significant when the stones are small and is especially valuable when it appears in both the recumbent and erect positions (Fig. 16-8). An acoustic shadow in the gallbladder area may also be produced by colonic gas (Fig. 16-14), as will be seen again.

The gallbladder totally filled with stones

As shown in Fig. 16-13, as the number of stones increases, it becomes more difficult to recognize the gallbladder. The stones may possess a proper image, and their grouping may suggest the shape of the gallbladder (Fig. 16-13, *C*). In some cases they give rise to only a nonspecific reflective area, which may also be due to intestinal loops (Fig. 16-14). When no recognizable gallbladder image can be identified, the association of an abnormal reflection with a constant acoustic shadow

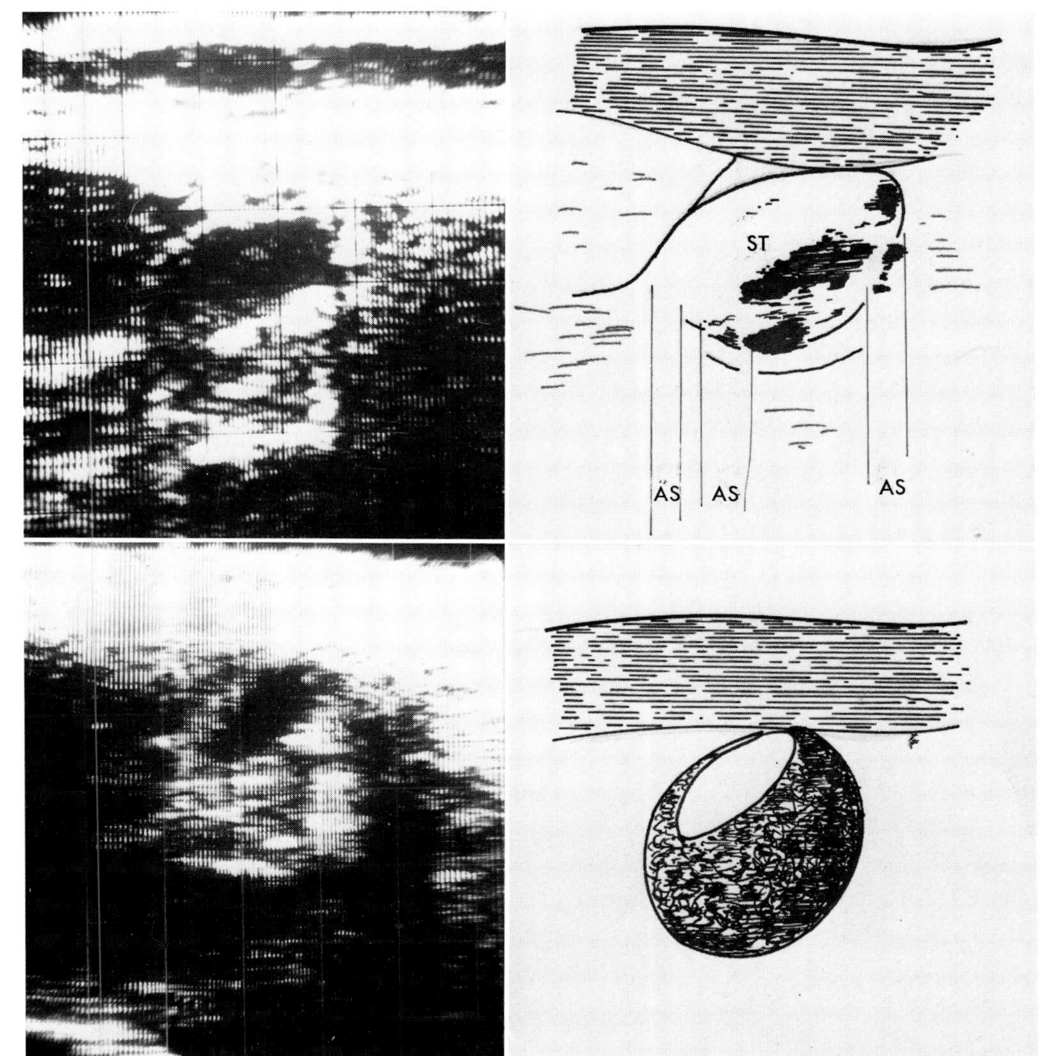

Fig. 16-13. Gallbladder filled with stones. **A,** Sagittal scan and schematic drawing of gallbladder half filled with stones *(St)*. There are several posterior acoustic shadows *(AS)*. **B,** Another gallbladder almost entirely filled with stones. Only its superior part remains free.

Continued.

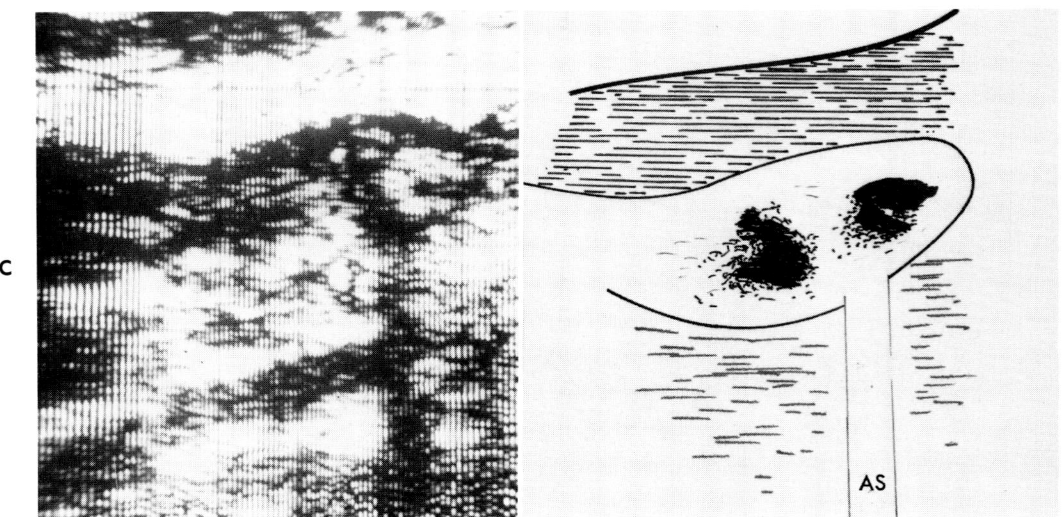

Fig. 16-13, cont'd. C, Gallbladder, displayed on sagittal scan, is completely filled with stones; it is thus more difficult to recognize shape of gallbladder. There is posterior acoustic shadow *(AS).*

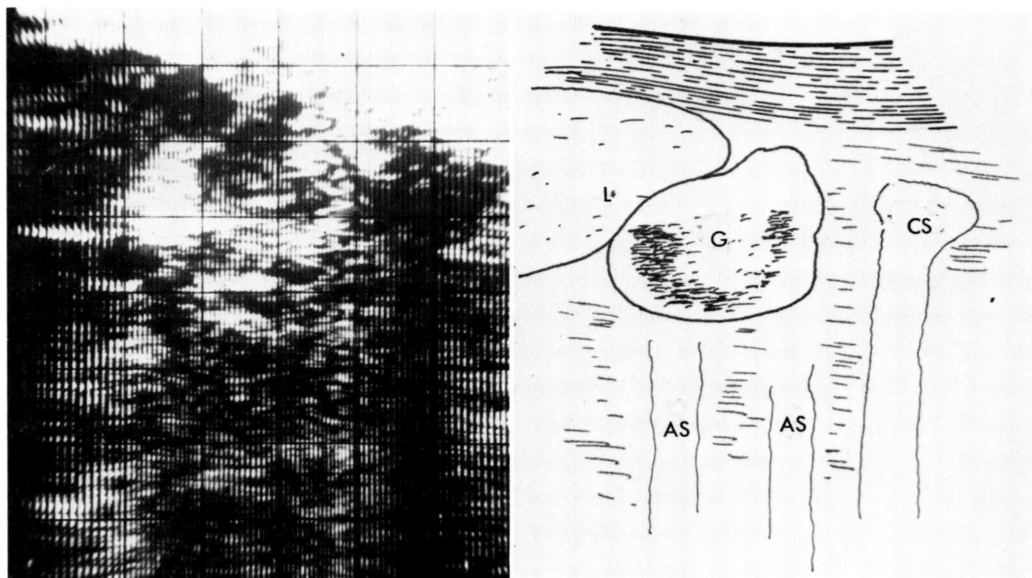

Fig. 16-14. Stone-filled gallbladder. Reflective area *(G)* lies in close contact with liver *(L).* Several posterior acoustic shadows *(AS)* indicate gallstones. Wider strip of acoustic shadow *(CS)* is due to colon.

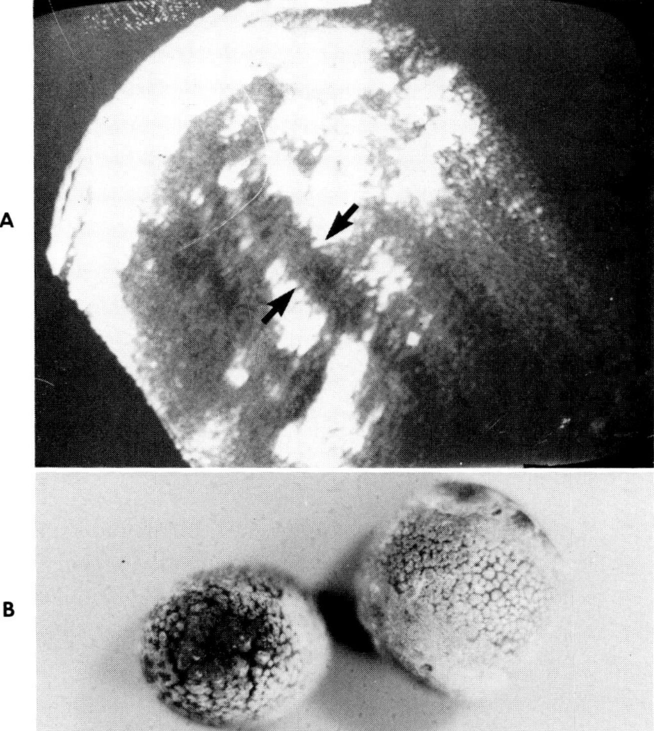

Fig. 16-15. Stone-filled gallbladder (acute cholecystitis). **A,** Transverse scan of right upper quadrant showing typical acoustic shadow *(arrows)* without usual reflective area of gallstones and without recognizable gallbladder image. Such a frank acoustic shadow is consistent with presence of gallstones. **B,** Gallstones after operation.

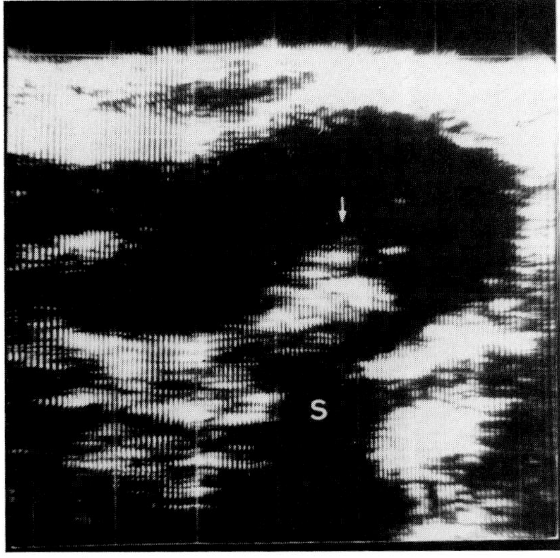

Fig. 16-16. Hydrops with stone. Behind stones *(arrow)* is an acoustic shadow *(S)*. Gallbladder can be considered equivalent to cylinder 10 cm long and 4 cm wide. Estimated volume is only 130 ml, but gallbladder is enlarged.

is a reliable constellation of signs. An acoustic shadow that is clear, well delineated, deep, and permanent in different positions may alone be a reliable sign, even without an abnormal reflective area (Fig. 16-15).

Another indirect sign is hydrops of the gallbladder due to a stone obstructing the cystic duct. The responsible stone may be evident. (See Fig. 16-2.) However, if the stone is small and not very reflective, enlargement of the gallbladder is the only evidence (Figs. 16-16 to 16-18).

Pitfalls in differential diagnosis

Direct images. I have already mentioned the false images of stones caused by an intense reflection in the gallbladder wall. This problem can be resolved by examining the patient in the erect position. If there are multiple small stones, they will migrate downward. *Vesicular papillomas* (Chapter 17) give rise to images that are similar to those of stones, but without acoustic shadow or positional migration. A much more gross error would be to confuse the central echo of a low anterior kidney with a stone lying in an enlarged gallbladder (Fig. 16-19). Such an error can be committed only when the test of positional movement has not been performed, but, as a celebrated predecessor has said, "He who has never sinned, let him cast the first stone"(St. John 8:7).

Indirect signs. An *acoustic shadow* may be of colonic origin, since the hepatic flexure is closely related to the gallbladder (Fig. 16-20). Correct diagnosis is based on the observation, under echoscopic real-time control, of the possible changes of the acoustic shadow and of the neighboring echoes during manual palpation and positional changes. The relations between the acoustic shadow and the abnormal echoes remain unchanged with a stone but change when due to colonic gas. *Diagnosing hydrops of the gallbladder* may be difficult if there is no image of an

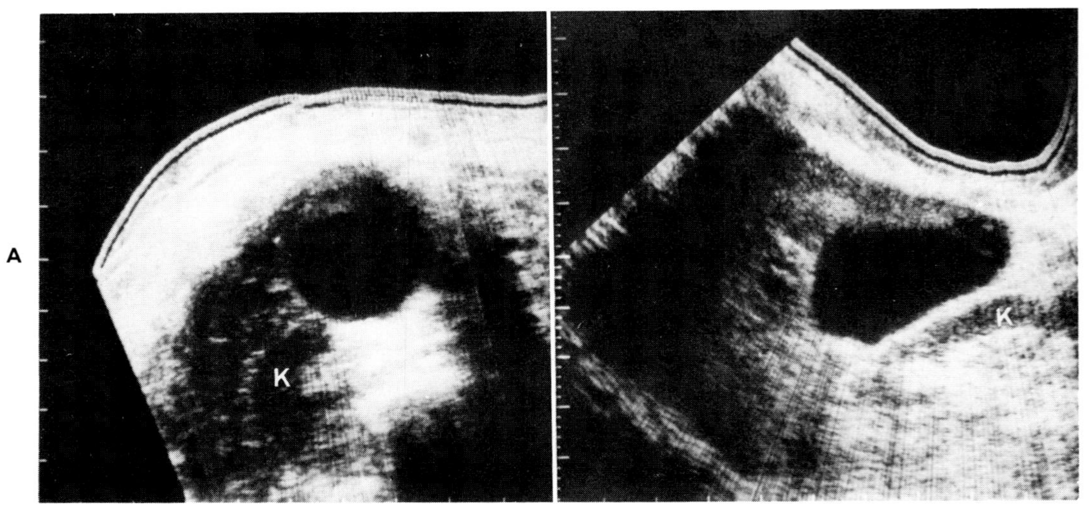

Fig. 16-17. Hydrops due to infundibular stone not visible on these scans. **A,** Transverse scan. **B,** Sagittal scan. *K,* kidney.

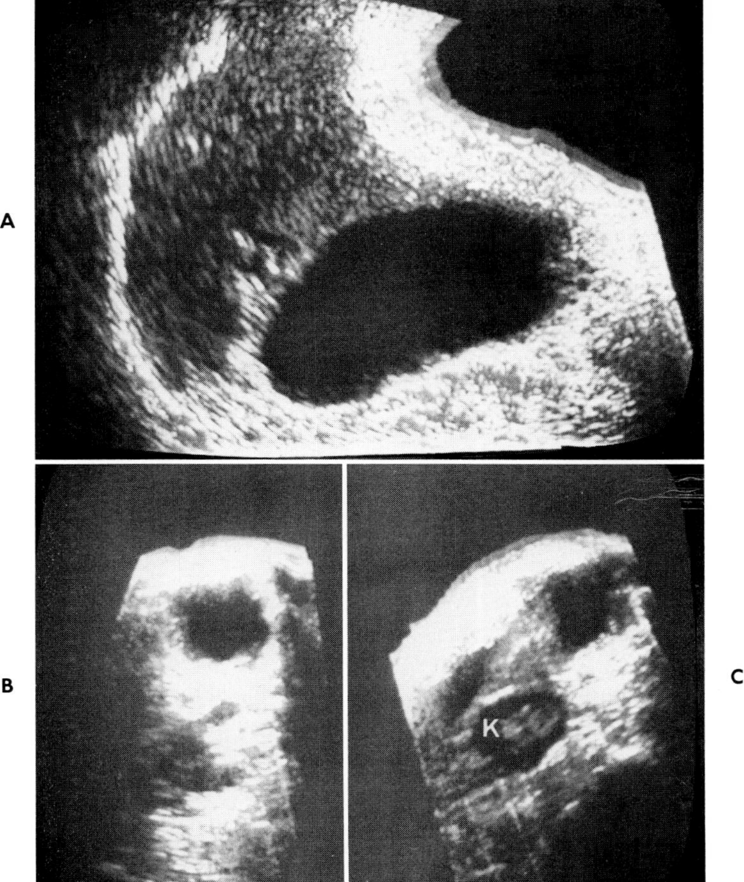

Fig. 16-18. Hydrops due to infundibular stone not visible on these scans. **A,** Sagittal scan. **B** and **C,** Transverse scans at different levels. *K,* right kidney.

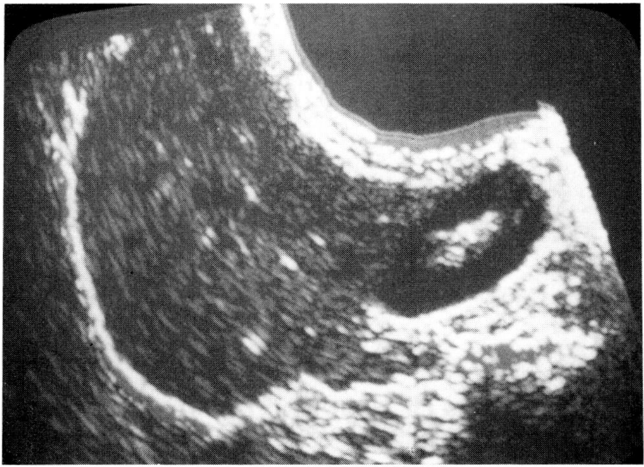

Fig. 16-19. Grossest error in diagnosis of biliary lithiasis. Sagittal scan of right upper quadrant shows sonolucent area with central echoes behind liver. There is no acoustic shadow. This image belongs to normal kidney in low position and not to gallbladder with stones.

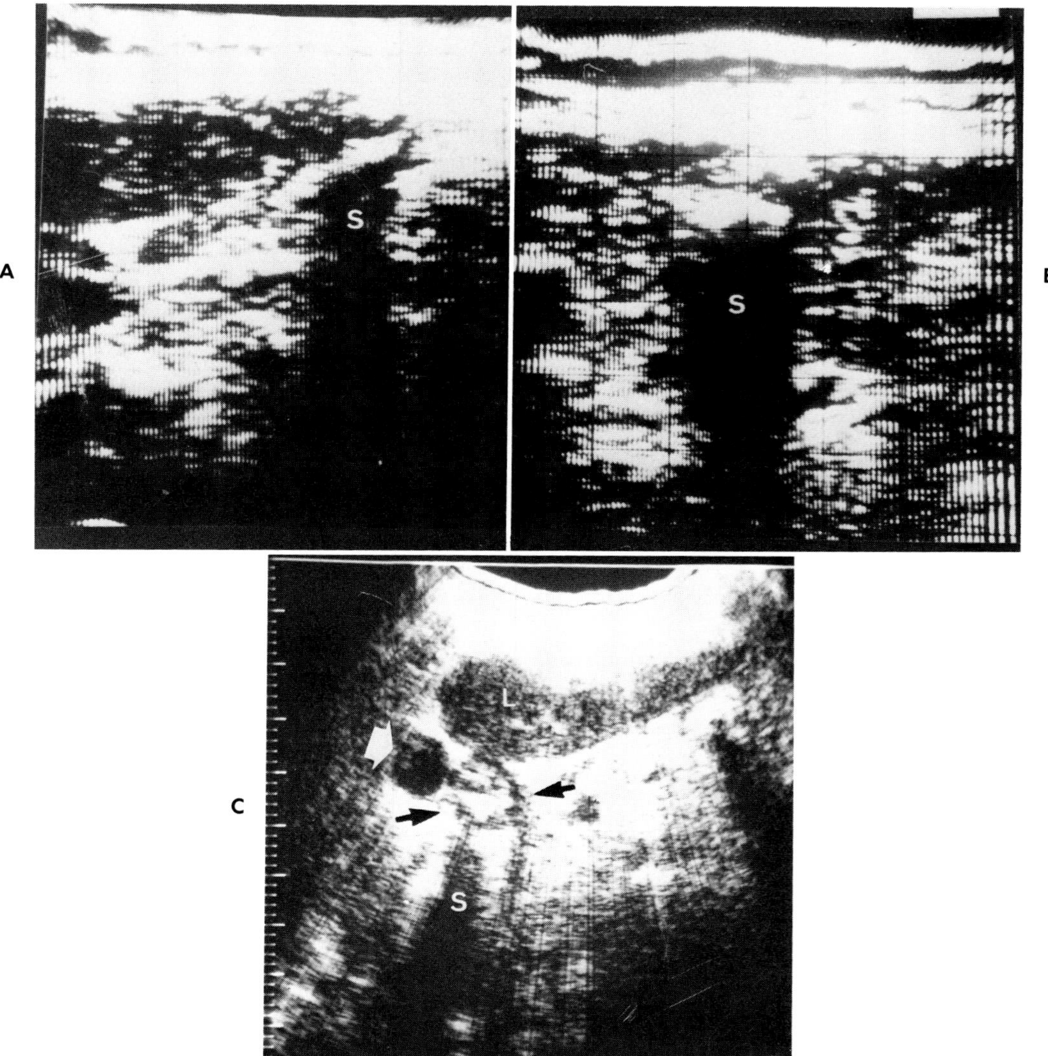

Fig. 16-20. Another pitfall: colonic gas. **A,** Sagittal scan of right upper quadrant showing, behind liver, acoustic shadow *(S)* due to colonic gas. **B,** Horizontal scan, in another case, displaying similar shadow belonging to lithiasis. **C,** Another example of confusing images due to intestine. On this transverse scan, rounded bull's-eye structure *(black arrows)* is displayed with posterior acoustic shadows. Such a pattern could belong to stone-filled gallbladder. In fact, normal gallbladder is also displayed *(white arrow)*. Rounded structure represents duodenum. Gallstones of that size would cast wider acoustic shadows; besides, duodenal pattern changes with patient in standing position. *L,* liver.

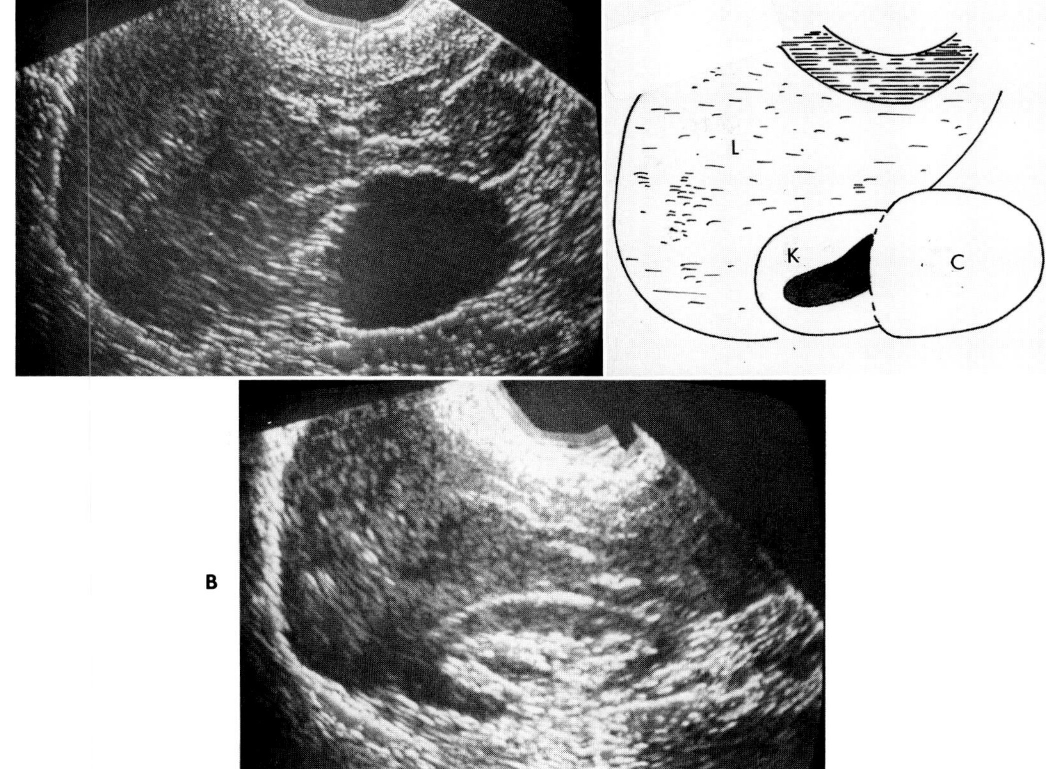

Fig. 16-21. Another important pitfall. Clinical diagnosis was enlarged, palpable gallbladder. **A,** Sagittal scan and schematic drawing of right upper quadrant showing fluid collection *(C)* behind liver *(L)*. As a matter of fact, this collection belongs to inferior pole of right kidney. Upper pole of kidney *(K)* has normal pattern. **B,** After ultrasonically guided puncture, cyst has disappeared, and kidney again presents normal pattern. We were satisfied with that diagnosis. However, as a matter of fact, we overlooked metastatic deposits in enlarged liver.

infundibular stone. As already noted, the volume of the normal gallbladder can be quite large. If the approximation of the volume yields a figure of more than 200 ml, the enlargement is unquestionable. If the estimated volume is less than 200 ml, the cystic duct may still be obstructed, and so a contraction test is necessary. Also, palpation of hydrops of the gallbladder under echoscopic control often produces a feeling of tension (Rettenmaier, 1975). The same consideration applies to the evaluation of jaundice (Chapter 26).

Some more simpleminded problems should be considered, including (Chapter 11) a superficial *hepatic cyst* with an inferior and posterior extension (Fig. 16-26) and a large anterior *renal cyst,* either of which can be confused with the gallbladder (Fig. 16-21). Diagnosis of an enlarged gallbladder, like any other morphological diagnosis, must be based on a gradual and logical analysis of anatomical data from multiple scans. A too rapidly made diagnosis based on a single image often leads to errors. Whatever the differential diagnostic problems, ultrasonic diagnosis of

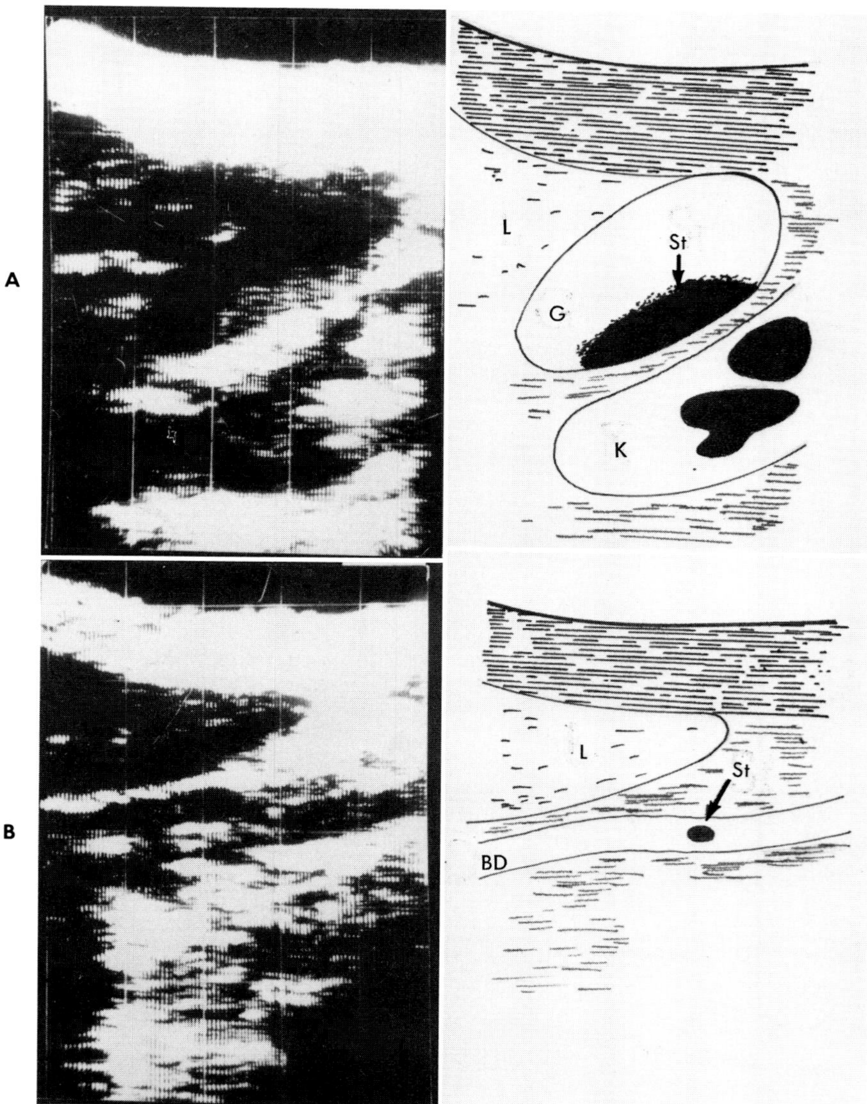

Fig. 16-22. Choledocholithiasis. **A,** Sagittal scan and schematic representation of gallbladder *(G)* showing stones *(St)* that have accumulated in lower part of gallbladder, which lies close to kidney *(K)*. **B,** Slightly more medial and oblique scan and schematic drawing showing, behind liver *(L)*, main bile duct *(BD)*, in inferior part of which small reflective area representing a stone is displayed.

gallstones is usually easy, provided no step of the investigation, particularly the positional changes, has been omitted. With ultrasonography the radiological term *nonvisualized gallbladder* should disappear from medical parlance except, of course, in cases of ultrasonic nonvisualization.

Stones in the common hepatic and common bile ducts. The common hepatic duct is visible when its caliber is 4 mm or greater. Usually, when obstructed, the diameter of the bile ducts increases rapidly, and they become therefore much easier to demonstrate. For a long time it was thought that a main bile duct lithiasis could give rise to a clear image only when there were a few stones lying in a very large duct (Fig. 16-22). Of course, if a bile duct is filled with stones, these are more difficult to display, since the gradient of impedance between the stones and surrounding tissues is less than that between stones and bile. The physical problem is the same as with the gallbladder totally filled with stones. In fact, it is possible to recognize multiple stones in a large bile duct, especially if there is an acoustic shadow. I shall discuss stones in the common hepatic and common bile ducts in Chapter 26.

CHOLECYSTITIS

Acute cholecystitis causes thickening of the gallbladder wall (Figs. 16-23 to 16-26), which is easily visible when diffuse and of sufficient magnitude (Figs. 16-23 to 16-25). Sometimes, the thickened gallbladder wall is ill defined (Figs. 16-25 and 16-26) and difficult to evaluate. The diagnosis is more reliable if thickening is found with real-time, as well as contact, scanning. Stones cannot always be seen in acute cholecystitis. The stones may be small or floating (Fig. 16-26). An indirect sign of great value is exquisite tenderness to palpation of the gallbladder.

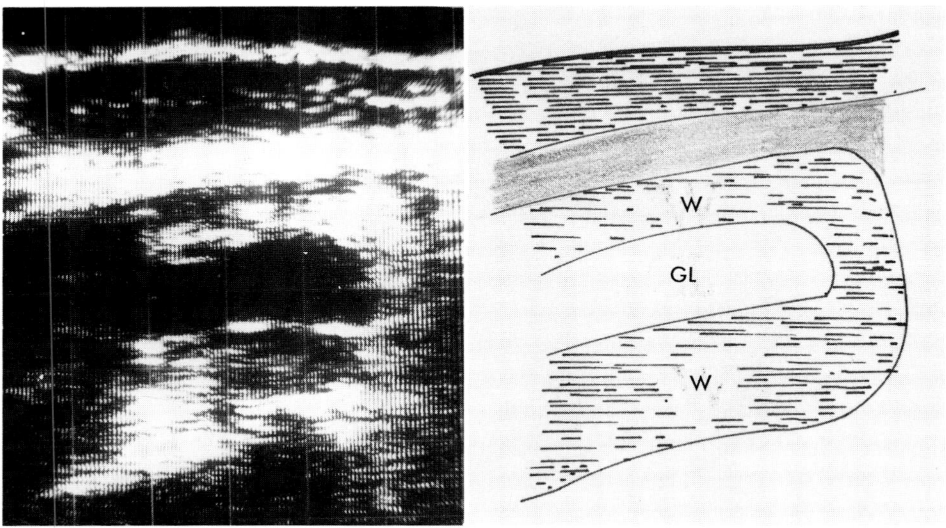

Fig. 16-23. Acute cholecystitis. Patient complained of sharp pain in right upper quadrant. Sagittal scan and its schematic representation show abnormal gallbladder. Gallbladder wall *(W)* is thickened and gallbladder lumen *(GL)* narrowed—a typical pattern for acute cholecystitis.

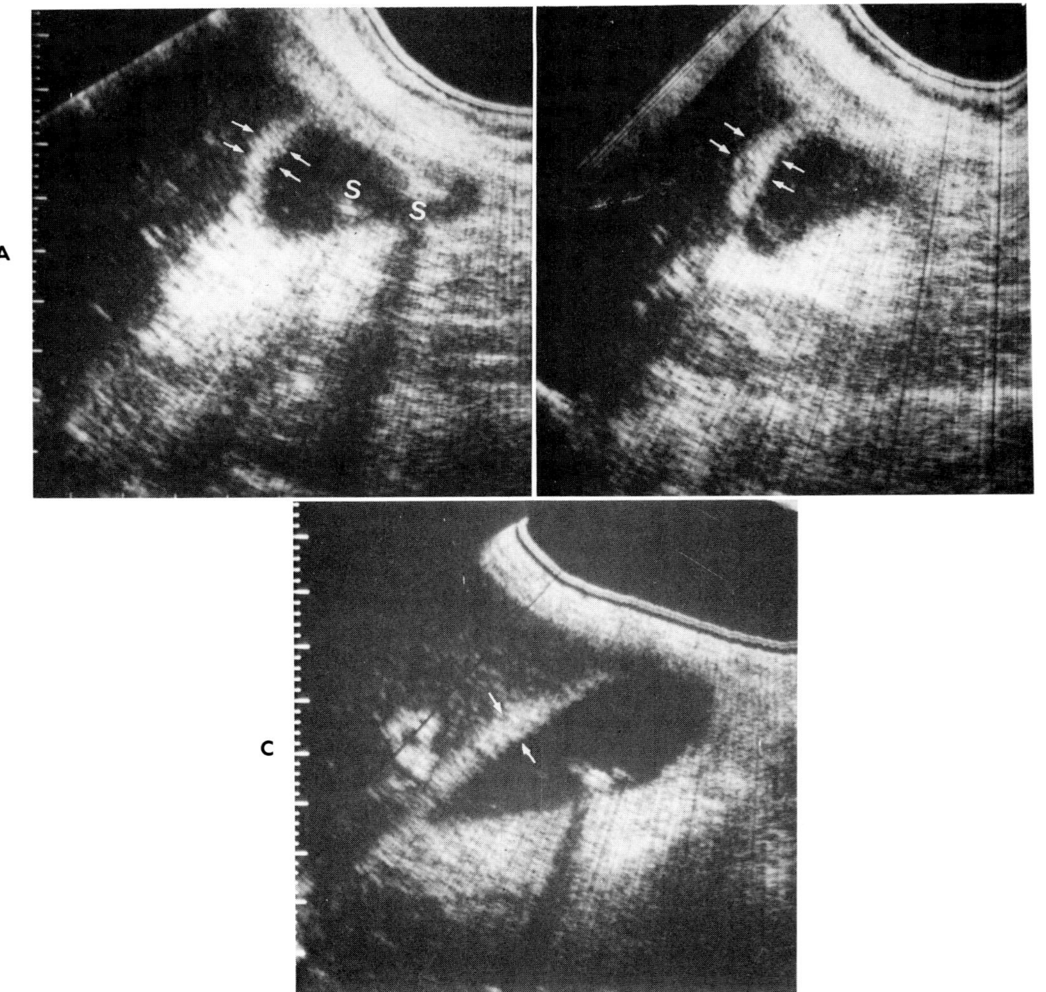

Fig. 16-24. Acute cholecystitis. **A,** Sagittal scan of gallbladder triggered pain and showed two stones *(S)* with acoustic shadow. Gallbladder wall *(arrows)* is 1 cm thick. **B,** Parallel scan again displaying wall enlargement. **C,** Similar case, with gallstones and thickened wall.

Fig. 16-26. Acute cholecystitis. Patient complained of sharp abdominal pain. On palpation, gallbladder was tender. Sagittal scan and schematic drawing show thickening of gallbladder wall *(W)* and floating stone *(St)*. In vicinity of this abnormal gallbladder are several false gallbladder images *(C)* due to polycystic liver disease.

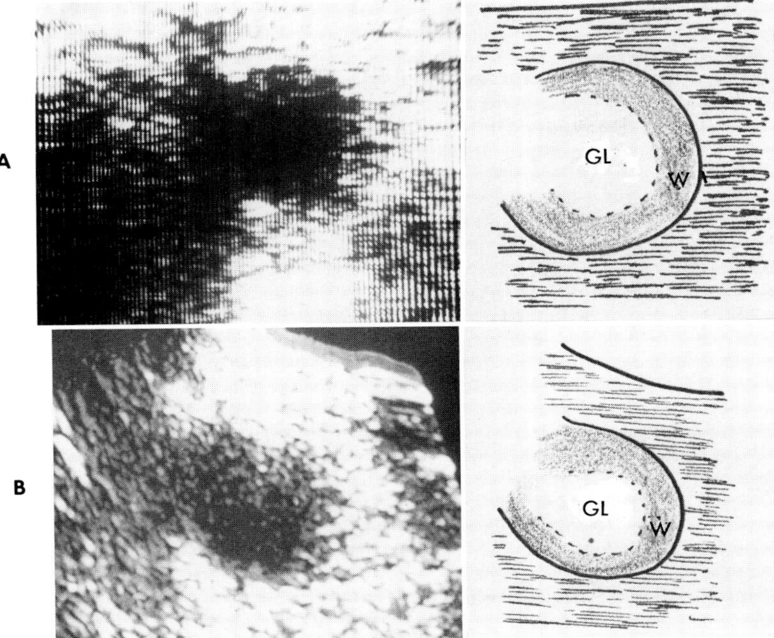

Fig. 16-25. Acute cholecystitis. Small gallbladder is cut sagittally. **A,** Real-time scan and schematic representation showing thickening of gallbladder wall *(W)* and narrowing of gallbladder lumen *(GL)*. **B,** Similar image in contact scanning and its schematic representation.

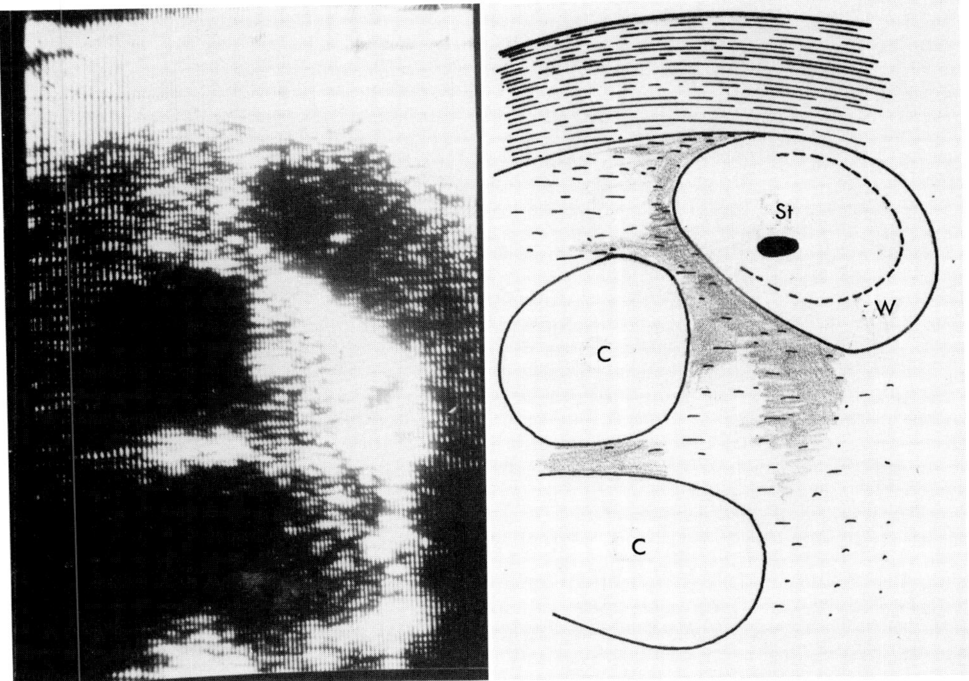

Fig. 16-26. For legend see opposite page.

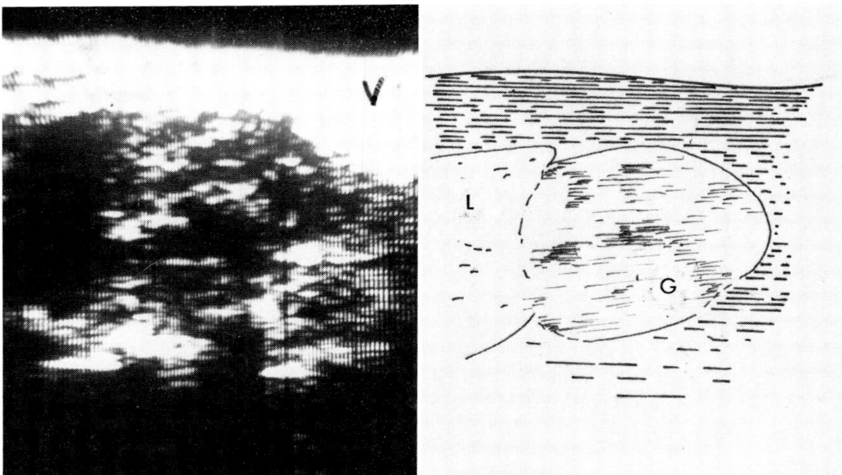

Fig. 16-27. Acute cholecystitis. Sagittal scan and schematic drawing of right upper quadrant show several nonspecific echoes associated with sonolucent areas of semisolid type below liver *(L),* in gallbladder area *(G).* This pattern is rather common in purulent or phlegmonous cholecystitis.

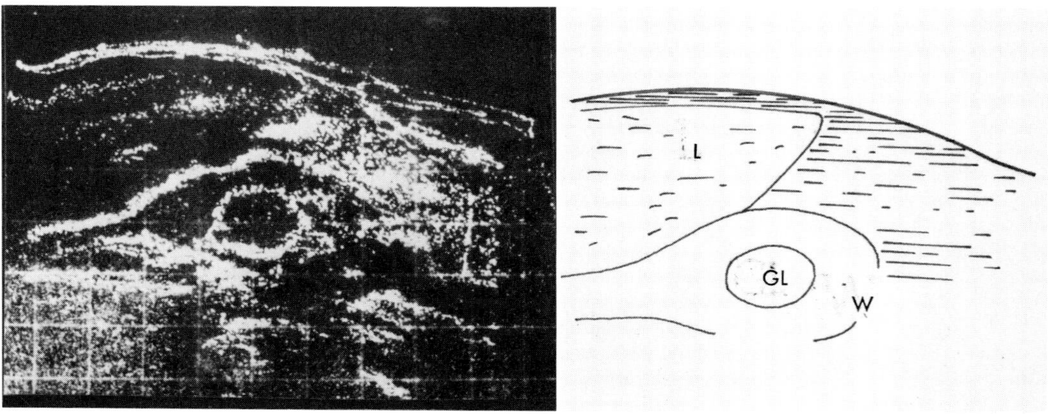

Fig. 16-28. Chronic cholecystitis. Sagittal scan and schematic drawing of right upper quadrant show abnormal gallbladder with thickened walls *(W)* and markedly narrowed lumen *(GL)* behind liver *(L).* Such images of wall thickening are rare in chronic cholecystitis. (Courtesy Dr. Roussille and Dr. Duquesnel, Lyons, France.)

This palpation can be performed manually, under echoscopic real-time control, or directly, with the contact scanning transducer placed on the skin. At the instant when the gallbladder image is displayed on the screen, the patient complains of pain. This contact-induced pain, occurring during an otherwise painless examination, must be taken into account, even if the gallbladder image appears rather normal. The association of gallbladder enlargement with thickening of the wall is a reliable sign of *pyocholecyst.* But the absence of an image of wall thickening in an enlarged gallbladder does not mean that there is no infection. Transducer-

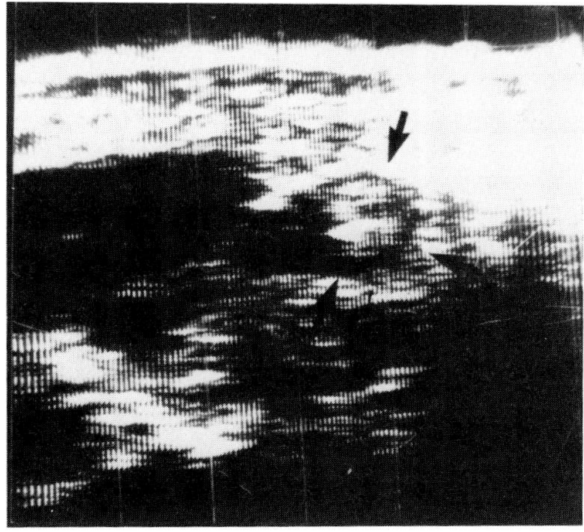

Fig. 16-29. Chronic cholecystitis. Typical pattern produced by small, retracted gallbladder *(arrows)* filled with stones.

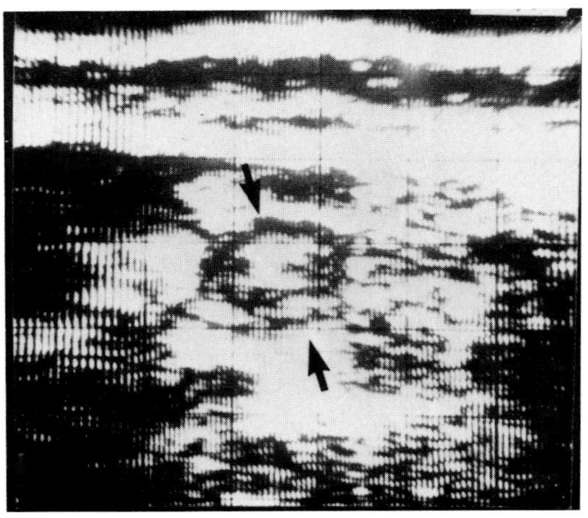

Fig. 16-30. Chronic cholecystitis. Similar image of small, retracted gallbladder filled with stones *(arrows)*.

caused pain is a more frequent sign. In acute cholecystitis, either purulent or phlegmonous, the transparency of the bile may disappear even if the gallbladder is not filled with stones. The gallbladder then appears as a nonspecific heterogeneous mass of semisolid pattern. (See Fig. 16-27.) Acute cholecystitis represents one of the most frequent ultrasonic diagnostic emergencies in digestive pathology, another being acute pancreatitis.

In *chronic cholecystitis,* thickening of the wall is rare (Fig. 16-28). In this condition the gallbladder is usually sclerotic and atrophic. If an accumulation of

Table 16-1. A few ultrasonic signs in cholelithiasis

	Cholelithiasis			*Main bile duct lithiasis*	
	Solitary stone	*Stones totally filling gall-bladder*	*Papilloma*	*Solitary stone*	*Stones totally filling gall-bladder*
Direct sign	+	±	+	+	±
Indirect sign: acoustic shadow	+	+	0	±	±
Positional sign	+	0	0	0	0

stones is associated with such a retraction, the image of the gallbladder is difficult to recognize. In a few cases, however, the image of the small, stone-filled gallbladder is clear (Figs. 16-29 and 16-30). In other cases, only an indirect sign is found, that is, the absence of a gallbladder image no matter what view is used.

A calcified gallbladder gives rise to a shell sign, that is, a strongly reflective strip with a posterior acoustic shadow.

In Table 16-1, some of the ultrasonic signs of cholelithiasis are presented.

RELIABILITY OF ULTRASONOGRAPHY IN THE DIAGNOSIS OF CHOLELITHIASIS

Several studies (Birkenfeld and Otto, 1975; Lutz and associates, 1975; Riegg and Getter, 1975) have shown the reliability of ultrasonic cholecystography. With a trained ultrasonographer the rate of success in the diagnosis of cholelithiasis should be 90%. Of course, false-negative diagnoses of small stones may be made. False-positive results, due to misinterpretation of mural elevations or of acoustic shadows, may also occur. Since conventional cholecystography is easy and essentially noninvasive, this examination, in my opinion, should be used routinely. Ultrasonography should be used when the gallbladder fails to be visualized by cholecystography, in acute cholecystitis, in jaundice, and in case of allergy to iodine or of renal insufficiency. In addition, since the gallbladder is seen in any hepatic or pancreatic investigation provided the patient is fasting, ultrasonography often leads to the discovery of gallstones. As a matter of fact, ultrasonography has become a screening examination for digestive pathology, and therefore ultrasonic cholecystography is also becoming a screening examination. Since ultrasonography cannot show stones less than 2 mm in diameter, this is probably not logical at a time when everyone emphasizes the necessity of achieving the diagnosis of true microlithiasis. The position of biliary ultrasonography with respect to intravenous cholangiography is different. Indeed, cholangiography is not quite harmless. It has a mortality rate of from 1 in 25,000 to 1 in 8,000, according to different statistical studies. Ultrasonography is therefore to be used as the first step, *before* intravenous cholangiography. If cholelithiasis or a pancreatic lesion is disclosed by ultrasonography, it is then possible to avoid using intravenous cholangiography. As for instrumental cholangiography, which will be discussed in Chapter 26, dealing with jaundice, we only rarely use techniques such as this. Ultrasonography is a comprehensive technique of examination, which you may test in Fig. 16-31.

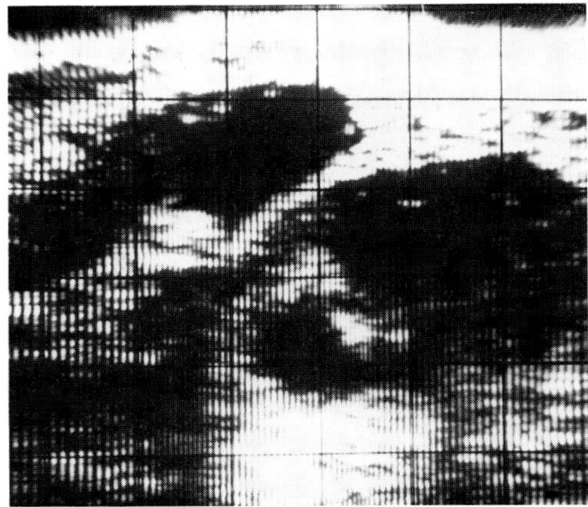

Fig. 16-31. Sagittal scan of gallbladder in real time. What is your diagnosis?*

*There are stones with posterior acoustic shadow, but there is also enlargement of lower pole of right kidney, which is due to renal carcinoma.

REFERENCES

Barnett, E., and Morley, P.: Abdominal echography, Borough Green, England, 1974, Butterworth & Co. (Publishers), Ltd.

Becker, J. C.: Contribution à l'étude tomo-échographique des affections du foie, des voies biliaires et du pancréas, thesis, Besançon, France, 1971, University of Besançon.

Birkenfeld, L., and Otto, P.: The value of ultrasonic tomography in the diagnosis of the gallbladder, Second European Congress, Munich, Germany, 1975, Abstract No. 95.

Crow, H. G., Bartrum, R. J., and Foote, S. R.: Expanded criteria for the ultrasonic diagnosis of gallstones, J. Clin. Ultrasound **4**:289-192, 1976.

Doust, B. D., and Maklad, N. F.: Ultrasonic B-mode examination of the gallbladder. Techniques and criteria for the diagnosis of gallstones, Radiology **110**:643-647, 1974.

Goldberg, B. B., Harris, K., and Broocker, W.: Ultrasonic and radiographic cholecystography. A comparison, Radiology **111**:405-409, 1974.

Goldberg, B. B., Kotler, M. N., Ziskin, M. C., and Waxham, R. D.: Diagnostic uses of ultrasound, New York, 1975, Grune & Stratton, Inc.

Hassani, N.: Ultrasonography of the abdomen, Heidelberg, Germany, 1976, Springer-Verlag.

Holm, H. H., Kristensen, J. K., Rasmussen, S. N., Pedersen, J. F., and Hancke, S.: Abdominal ultrasound, Copenhagen, 1976, Munksgaard, International Booksellers & Publishers, Ltd.

Kitamura, T., Nakagawa, F., Kawai, S., Morii, T., and Kiyoanaga, G.: Ultrasonographic diagnosis of the cholestasis, Med. Ultrasound **9**:24-26, 1971.

Leopold, G. R.: Personal communication, 1977.

Leopold, G. R., and Asher, W. M.: Fundamentals of abdominal and pelvic ultrasonography, Philadelphia, 1975, W. B. Saunders Co.

Leopold, G. R., and Sokoloff, J.: Ultrasonic scanning in the diagnosis of biliary disease, Surg. Clin. North Am. **53**:1043-1052, 1973.

Lutz, H., Seidl, R., Petzold, R., and Fuchs, H. F.: Gallensteindiagnostik mit Ultraschall, Dtsch. Med. Wochenschr. **100**:1325-1331, 1975.

Rettenmaier, G.: Personal communication, 1975.

Riegg, H., and Getter, B.: Sonography or x-ray examination of the gallbladder, Ultrasonics in medicine, Second European Congress, Munich, Germany, 1975, Abstract No. 96.

Weill, F., Becker, J. C., Kraehenbuhl, J. R., Heriot, G., and Walter, J. P.: Clinical atlas of ultrasonic radiography, Paris, 1973, Masson & Cie., Editeurs.

Weill, F., Gisselbrecht, H., Ricatte, J. P., Kraehenbuhl, J. R., Schraub, S., and Becker, J. C.: Diagnostic tomo-échographique des dilatations vésiculaires, Arch. Fr. Mal. App. Dig. **60**: 49-54, 1971.

CHAPTER 17

RARE ANOMALIES: congenital diseases and tumors

BILIARY CYSTS

Biliary cysts give rise to liquid collection images that may mimic the gallbladder (Fig. 17-1). Such images are even more confusing, since gallstones may exist within such cysts and are often found in jaundiced patients. I have also encountered a posterior choledochal cyst mimicking a pseudocyst of the pancreas (Fig. 17-2). Since such cysts are exceedingly rare, they will be diagnosed only if one remembers that a liquid collection in the upper right quadrant does not necessarily belong to the liver, gallbladder, right kidney, or pancreas. Multiple cuts, as well as a combination of real-time and contact scanning, will enable one to display the gallbladder even after a first gallbladder-like liquid area has been displayed in the liver region.

CAROLI'S DISEASE (INTRAHEPATIC BILE DUCT ECTASIS)

Caroli's disease is characterized by images of enlargement of the intrahepatic biliary network. As already stated, this network is not visible at a distance from the hilar region in unjaundiced subjects. The discovery of an enlargement of the biliary network without any other biliary anomaly must, at least, suggest the possibility of Caroli's disease, as stated also by Bass and associates (1977). (See Fig. 17-3, *A*.) A pseudocystic pattern may be typical (Fig. 17-3, *B*), but, of course, other cases of this rare disease should be available for ultrasonic study. Gallstones may be associated (Fig. 17-3, *A*).

GALLBLADDER TUMORS

Benign tumors. Benign tumors appear as small elevations in the gallbladder lumen (Fig. 17-4). These elevations maintain their initial location during positional changes, and there is no acoustic shadow behind a papillomatous elevation.

Malignant tumors. Malignant tumors are encountered in two clinical situations, that is, with a mass in the upper right quadrant and jaundice. In the case of a mass, the first step of the diagnosis is to ascertain that the mass is extrahepatic and does not belong to a metastatic hump. A gallbladder tumor usually gives rise to an area of abnormal reflection, poorly marginated, with at least a partial interface image appearing between the mass and the liver. Amid the mass are found areas of intense reflections, with acoustic shadows, as a result of cholelithiasis, which is always present (Figs. 17-5 to 17-7). If there is no palpable mass, the ultrasonic signs are more discrete. In a few cases the gallbladder preserves its initial shape, and then polypoid elements are present, associated with stones, so

Text continued on p. 271.

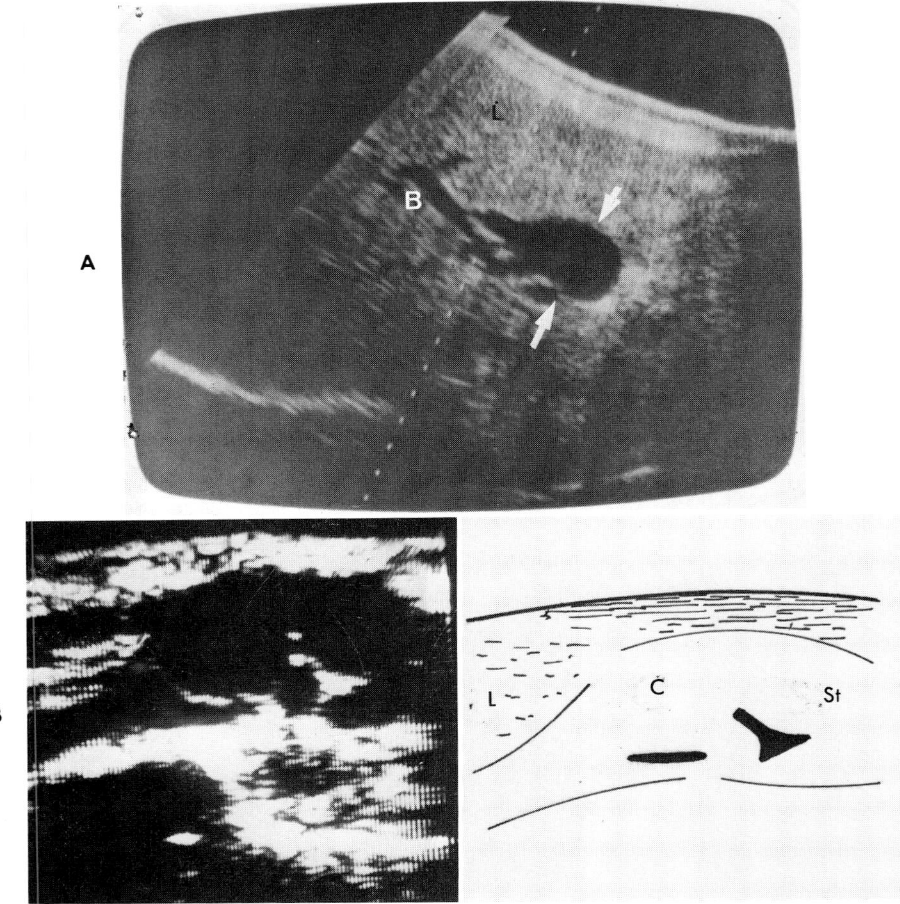

Fig. 17-1. Choledochal cysts. **A,** This pear-shaped, transparent area *(arrows),* which is close to main bile duct *(B),* does not belong to gallbladder, but to choledochal cyst. Gallbladder image was displayed on other scans. **B,** In this jaundiced patient, sagittal scan and schematic drawing of right upper quadrant show oval collection *(C)* below liver *(L).* Echoes *(St)* are scattered amid collection. Diagnosis was enlarged gallbladder with stones. As a matter of fact, more careful study would probably have displayed gallbladder separately, since surgery showed collection to belong to choledochal cyst, with stones. (**A** courtesy Dr. M. Lafortune, Montreal; **B** courtesy Dr. A. Eisenscher, Vesoul, France.)

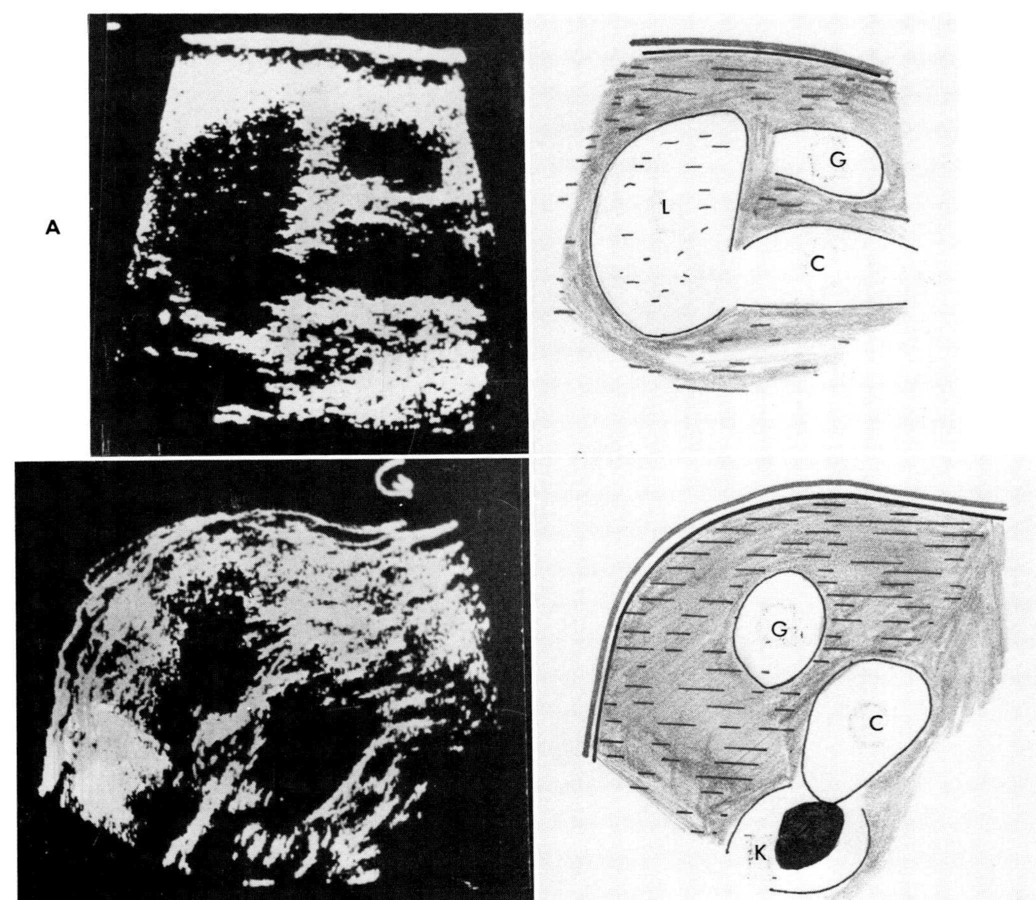

Fig. 17-2. Choledochal cyst. Examination was made to check pancreas in diabetic patient. **A,** Sagittal scan and schematic drawing of right upper quadrant showing enlarged gallbladder *(G)* below liver *(L)*. Behind gallbladder, oval liquid collection *(C)* is displayed. **B,** Transverse scan and its schematic representation also showing this collection behind gallbladder *(G)*, just in front of right kidney *(K)*. Collection was thought to belong to a pancreatic pseudocyst, but surgeon found choledochal cyst.

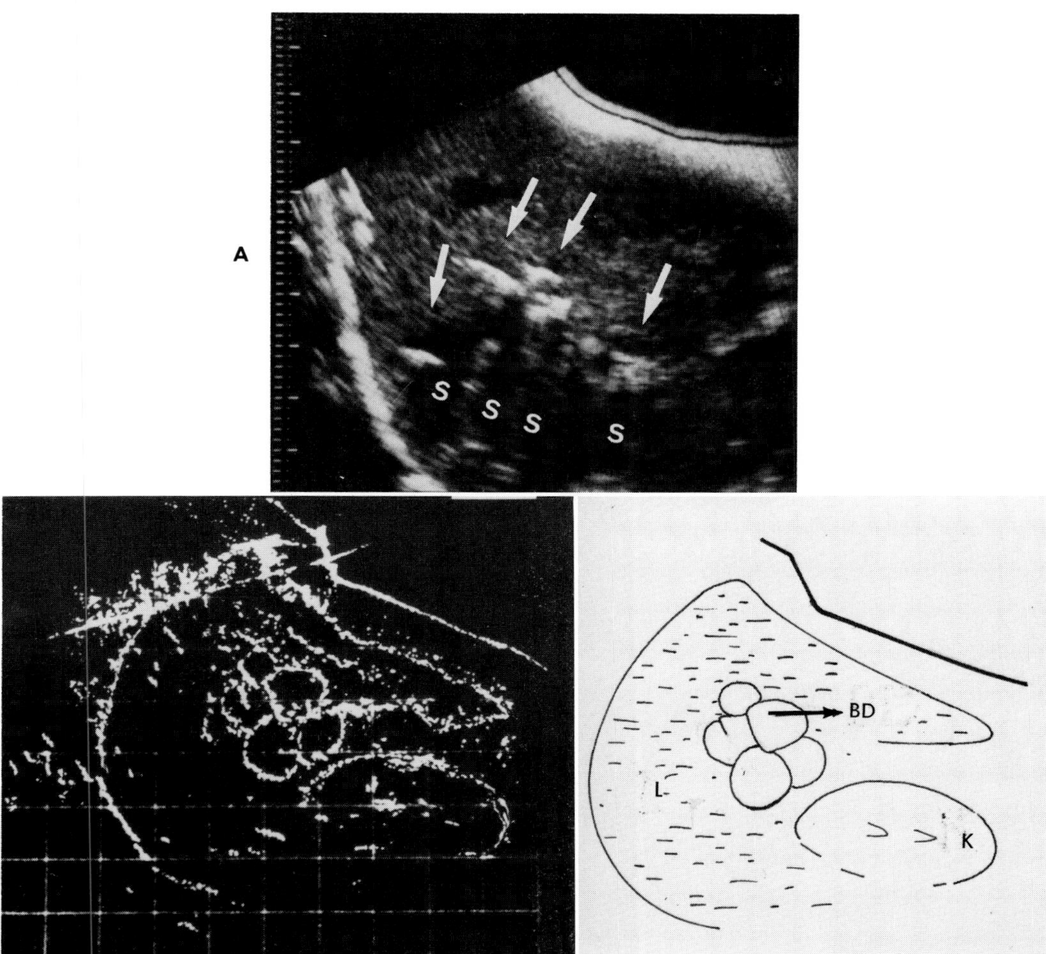

Fig. 17-3. Caroli's disease. **A,** Sagittal scan of liver, displaying sections of enlarged bile ducts. Ducts are partially filled with stones, producing reflective posterior strips *(arrows),* behind which appear several acoustic shadows *(S).* **B,** Sagittal scan and schematic drawing of liver *(L),* showing several cystic elements *(BD)* amid liver tissue *(L).* They belong to enlarged intrahepatic bile duct. *K,* right kidney. (**A** courtesy Dr. F. Winsberg, Montreal; **B** courtesy Dr. Roussille and Dr. Duquesnel, Lyons, France.)

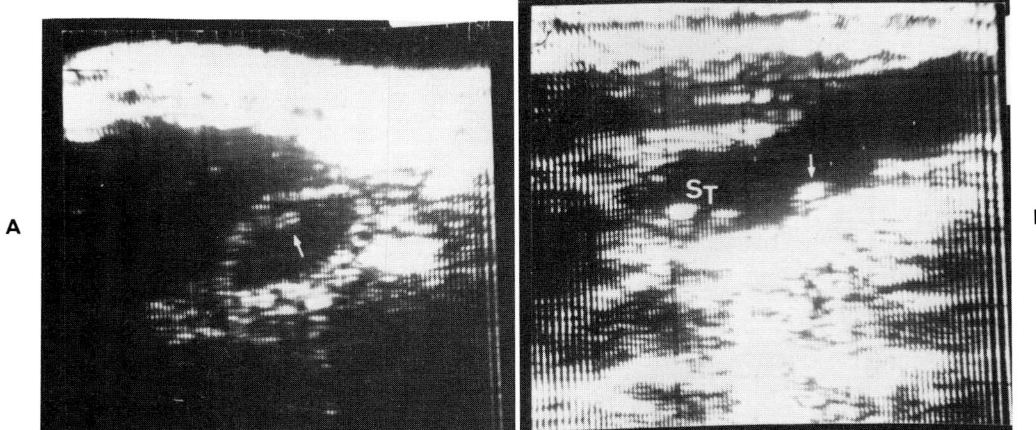

Fig. 17-4. Papilloma. **A,** Small tumor *(arrow)* arising from anterior wall of gallbladder. **B,** In this case, papilloma is posterior *(arrow),* and gallstones *(ST)* are associated.

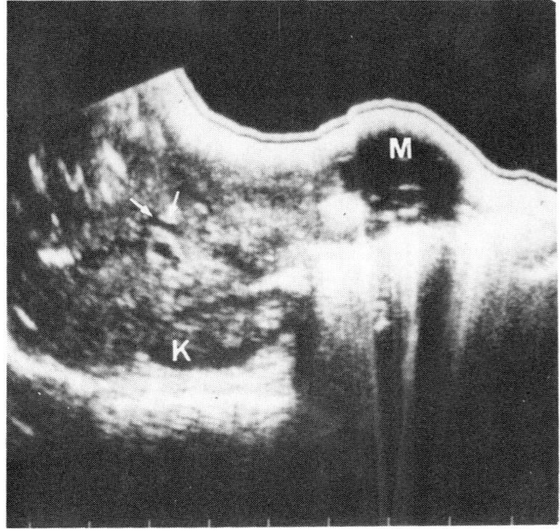

Fig. 17-5. Gallbladder carcinoma: infrahepatic mass *(M),* with reflective areas, due to gallstones casting acoustic shadows. Note enlarged liver with metastatic hailstorm pattern. Enlarged biliary junction *(arrows)* is displayed in front of portal division. *K,* kidney.

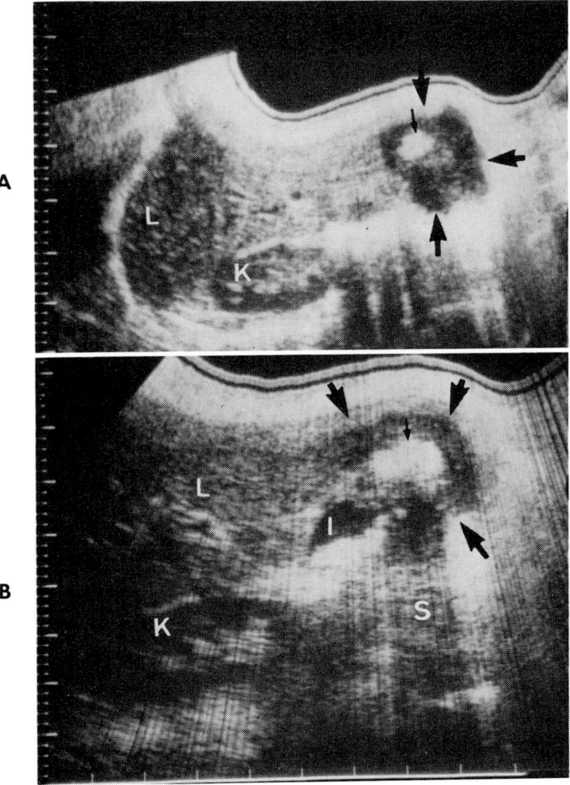

Fig. 17-6. Palpable mass in right upper quadrant of 76-year-old patient. **A,** Sagittal scan showing rounded solid mass *(large arrows)* in close contact with inferior edge of enlarged liver *(L).* In center of mass, dense, reflective area *(small arrow)* is outlined. **B,** Parallel sagittal scan, in larger scale, showing acoustic shadow *(S)* behind that reflective area. It belongs to gallstones located in center of gallbladder carcinoma. *I,* gallbladder infundibulum; *K,* right kidney.

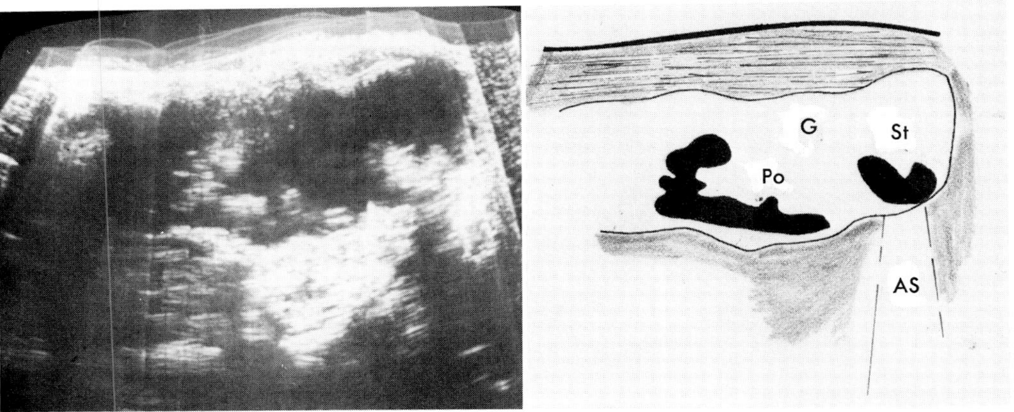

Fig. 17-7. Gallbladder carcinoma. In this jaundiced patient, sagittal scan and schematic drawing of right upper quadrant shows enlarged gallbladder *(G).* Different reflective areas appear in this gallbladder. Some *(St)* bring about acoustic shadow *(AS)*: they belong to stones. Others *(Po)* do not have acoustic shadows: they belong to tumoral polyps. (Courtesy Dr. A. Eisenscher, Vesoul, France.)

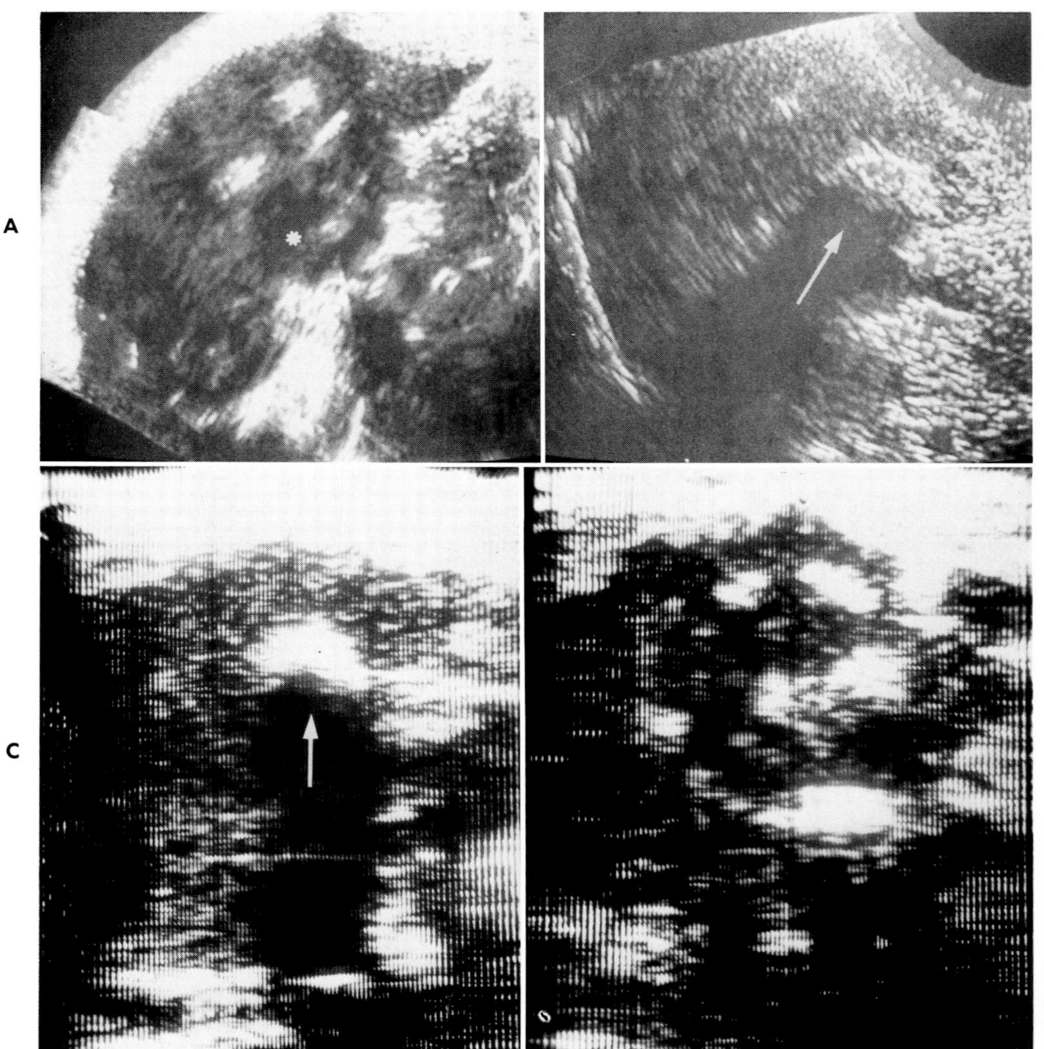

Fig. 17-8. Gallbladder carcinoma in 42-year-old jaundiced woman from Africa. There is no palpable mass. **A,** Transverse scan showing abnormal reflective areas in liver tissue. There is sonolucent area of semisolid type in posterior part of liver (*). **B,** Sagittal scan showing acoustic shadow behind reflective strip *(arrow)*. **C,** This reflective strip, with posterior acoustic shadow, is seen again on oblique recurrent real-time subcostal scan. Presence of reflective strip should lead to diagnosis of cholelithiasis or calcified hydatid cyst. **D,** More cranial real-time scan displaying hepatic hailstorm pattern. Association of hepatic lesions with gallstone images finally led to diagnosis of gallbladder carcinoma, which was verified by surgery.

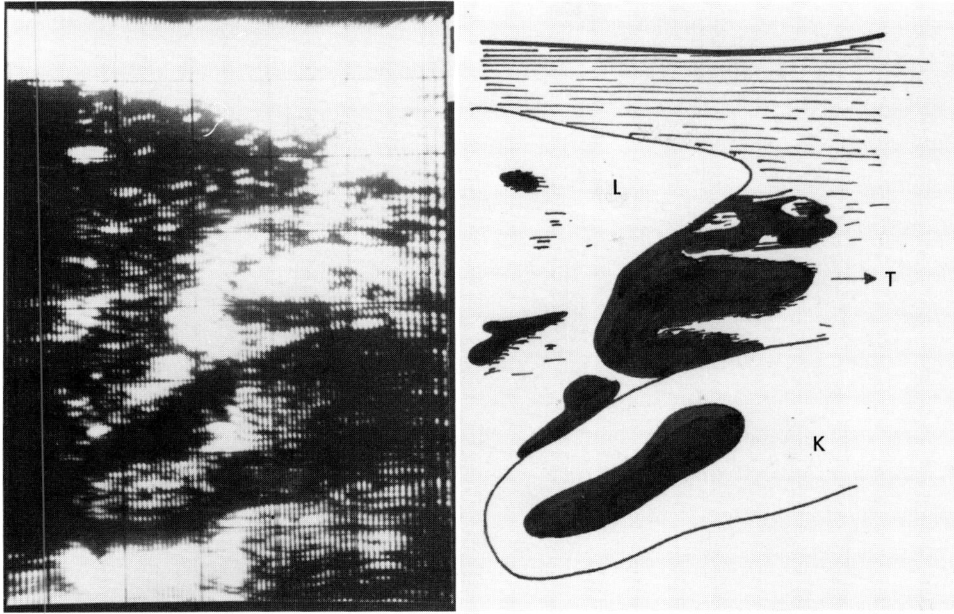

Fig. 17-9. Hilar cholangiocarcinoma. Patient, already operated on for cholangiocarcinoma, had recurrence of jaundice. Sagittal scan and schematic representation of liver *(L)* passing through right kidney *(K)* show strongly reflective tumoral mass *(T)* in hilar region.

that acoustic shadows are displayed behind the stones, but not behind the tumoral elevations (Fig. 17-7). The presence of tumoral extensions toward the hilus and the neighboring liver tissue is also a valuable sign (Fig. 17-8). Tumors originating from the hilus itself give rise to abnormal reflective areas in the hilar region (Fig. 17-9).

With high biliary obstruction due to extension of a gallbladder tumor or to a tumor arising directly from the hilar biliary ducts, an associated sign may of course be encountered. This consists of enlargement of the intrahepatic bile ducts, associated with jaundice. (See Fig. 17-5.) The analysis of such an enlargement of the intrahepatic biliary network is an important diagnostic step, which will be studied in more detail in Chapter 26.

Following are listed the most important ultrasonic signs of gallbladder tumors that I observed in seven cases:

- Specific sign: obvious gallbladder tumoral mass
- Less specific signs: juxtahepatic mass, hilar mass
- Associated signs: acoustic shadow, enlargement of intrahepatic bile ducts

OTHER BILIARY TUMORS

Tumors arising from the common bile duct and ampullary carcinomas have the same ultrasonic features as pancreatic tumors (Chapter 23). Tumors arising from the intrahepatic bile ducts have the same features as primary tumors of the

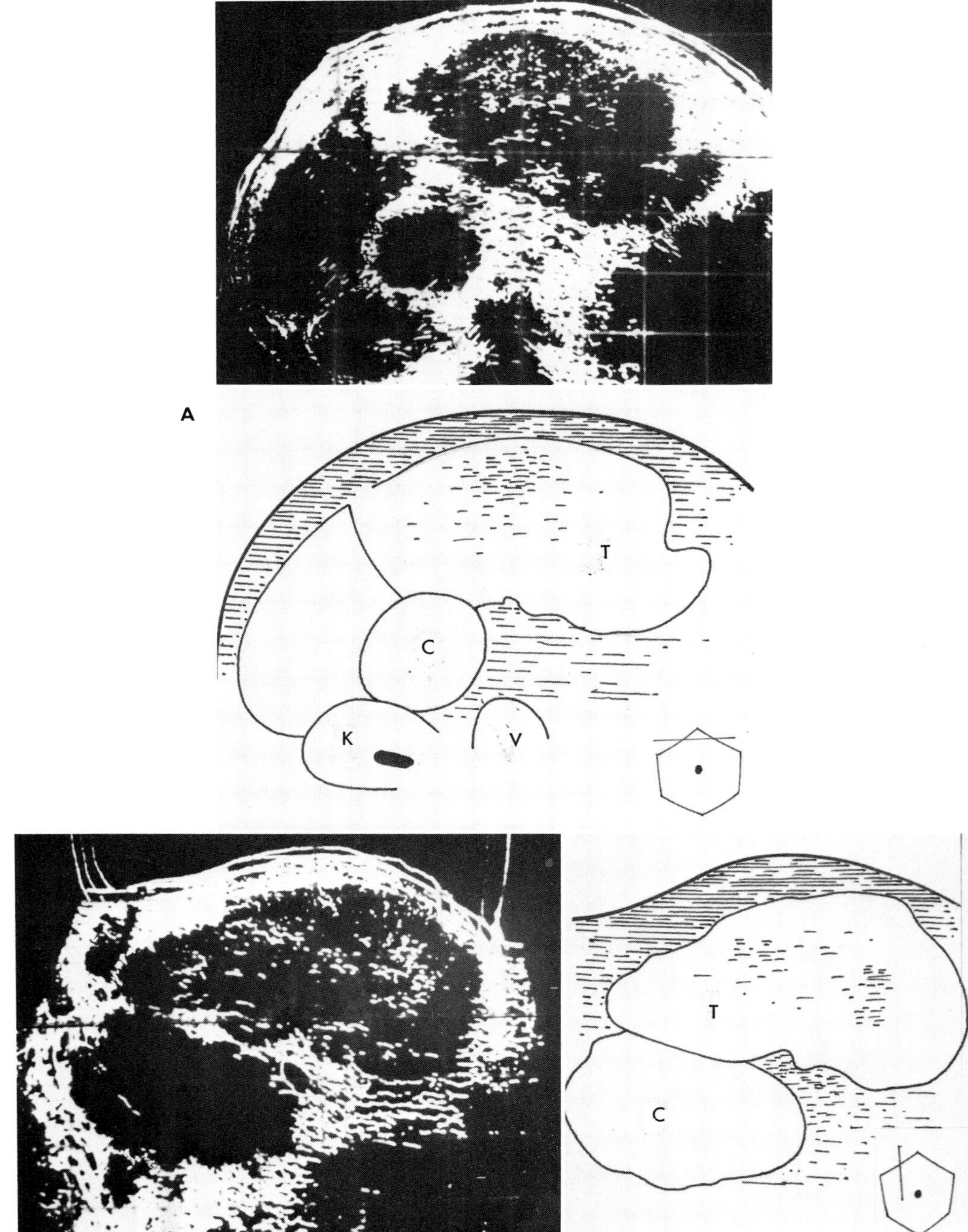

Fig. 17-10. Intrahepatic cystic cholangiocarcinoma. **A,** Horizontal scan and schematic drawing showing enlarged liver. In left lobe, many scattered echoes are displayed in well-marginated circular area. This pattern is rather like that found in mature hydatid cyst. Cystic element *(C)* appears between tumoral area *(T)* and right kidney *(K)*. Small drawing shows scanning angle. *V*, vertebral body. **B,** Sagittal scan and schematic drawing again showing anterior tumoral area and posterior cyst. Small drawing shows scanning angle. (Courtesy Dr. Roussille and Dr. Duquesnel, Lyons, France.)

liver (Chapter 9), that is, an infiltrative or nodular pattern. Only one pattern may be more specific—the pattern of the rare cystic cholangiocarcinoma. In such cases, there are elements of a liquid type, either solitary or multiple. (See Fig. 17-10.) When these cystic elements are of small diameter, their grouping may produce a pattern not very different from a solid pattern and quite similar to that already encountered in old hydatid cysts (Chapter 11).

DIFFERENTIAL DIAGNOSIS

Liquid collections

I have already discussed the problem of the difficult differentiation between a choledochal cyst, an enlarged gallbladder, and a pseudocyst of the pancreas. Caroli's disease is to be considered when there is generalized enlargement of the intrahepatic biliary network. Pseudocystic images, like those shown in Fig. 17-3, *B*, may lead to consideration of a polycystic disease. When one of these rare anomalies is considered, other radiological techniques of investigation (IV cholangiography, contrast-enhanced CT scanning, or percutaneous cholangiography) are used.

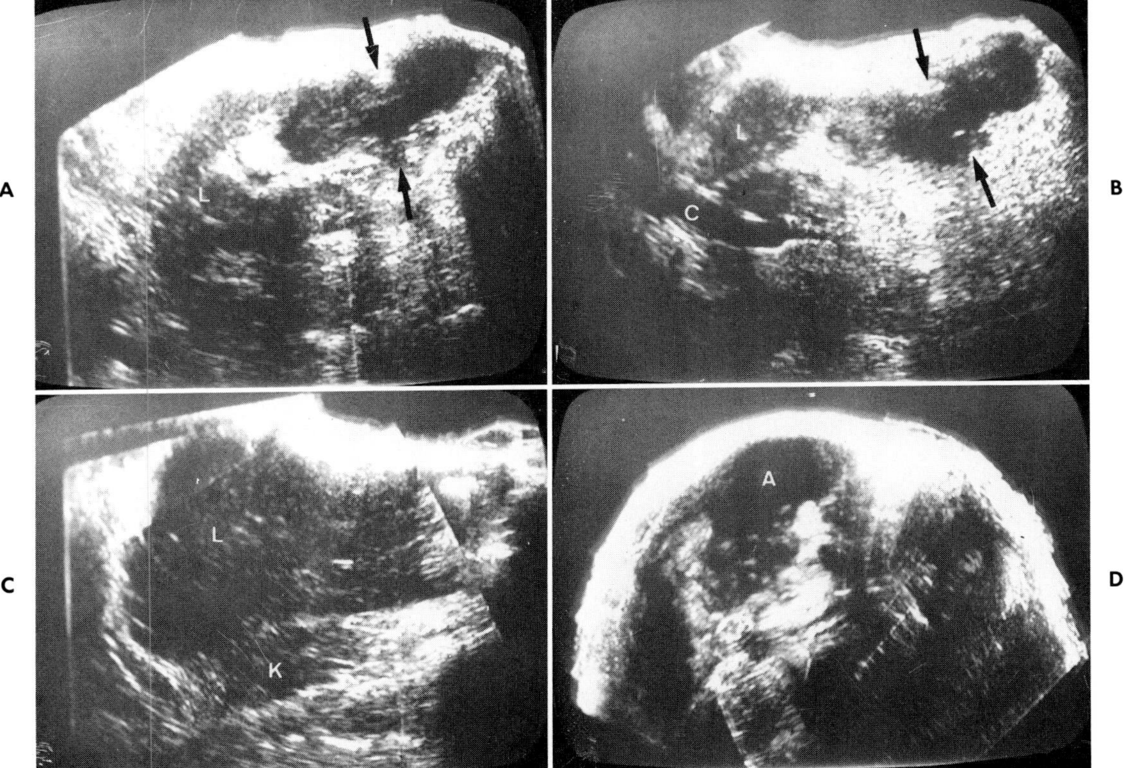

Fig. 17-11. Infrahepatic mass. **A,** Sagittal scan of right upper quadrant displaying heterogeneous mass *(arrows)* inferior to liver *(L)*. **B,** Parallel scan containing vena cava *(C)*. **C,** Another parallel scan also showing this elongated mass. Liver appears enlarged. *K,* kidney. **D,** Transverse scan at level of umbilicus displaying ascites. This mass belongs, not to invasive gallbladder tumor, but to carcinoma of ascending part of colon with dissemination. *A,* ascites.

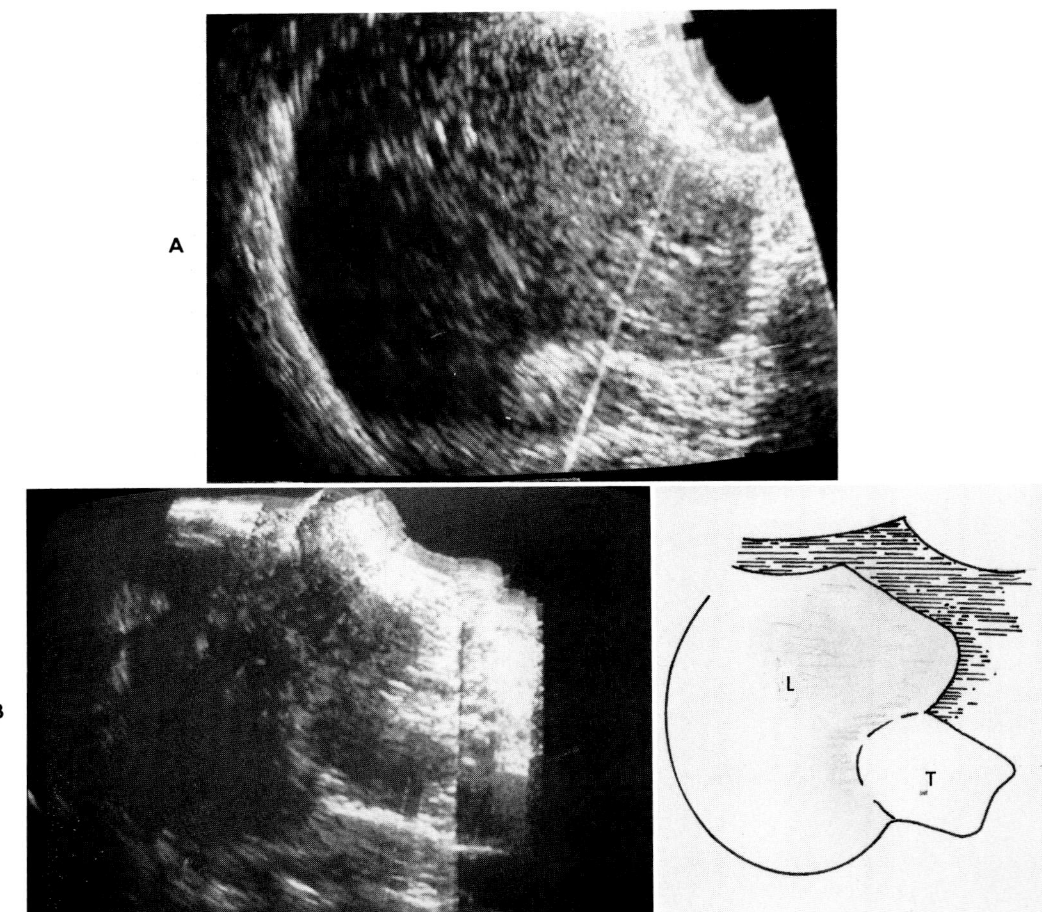

Fig. 17-12. Hilar mass found in jaundiced patient. **A,** Sagittal scan of right hepatic lobe showing hepatomegaly with angle sign. In hilar area, note section of enlarged biliary junction in front of portal division—gun sign (Chapter 26). **B,** Another sagittal scan, passing through hilar region, and schematic drawing show tumoral mass *(T)* below liver *(L).* Mass belonged to metastatic deposits of gastric carcinoma.

Solid elements

Intravesicular tumors. As already mentioned, intravesicular tumors can be differentiated from stones by the absence of positional displacement and of a posterior acoustic shadow.

Juxtahepatic masses. Distinguishing a solid juxtahepatic mass from an enlarged gallbladder image that is liquid is no problem. Purulent lithiasic cholecystitis with a subacute evolution may give rise to a palpable mass of semisolid echopattern. Such a mass could be confused with a tumor. (See Fig. 16-27.) Even the surgeon is sometimes unable to establish a correct diagnosis, even though in direct contact with such a process. In cases of jaundice, especially if the gallbladder is retracted and therefore difficult to visualize, a tumor of the ascending part of the colon

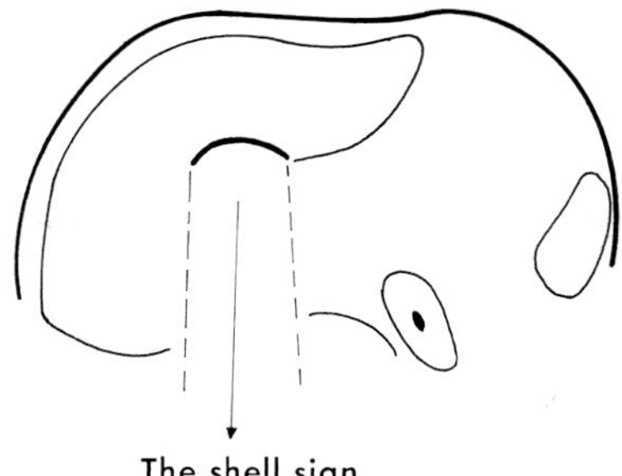

Fig. 17-13. Schematic representation of shell sign.

may be confused with a gallbladder mass (Fig. 17-11), again demonstrating that the ultrasonic information must be correlated with the other radiological data. It would, of course, be a gross error to attempt to diagnose any upper right quadrant mass without using a complementary barium enema.

Hilar masses. Metastatic deposits in hilar lymph nodes, which are rather common in gastrointestinal carcinomas, may produce tumor images quite similar to those of primary hilar tumors (Fig. 17-12). If the primary carcinoma is unknown, diagnosis is impossible before surgery. In a jaundiced patient, a juxtahilar echinococcal cyst may, because of its reflecting wall and acoustic shadow, mimic the association of a cholelithiasis and a gallbladder tumor. This was one of the two diagnoses considered in the patient from Africa whose scans are shown in Fig. 17-8. There was a reflective strip (Fig. 17-8, *B* and *C*) suggestive of an old echinococcal cyst, but the final ultrasonic diagnosis was of gallbladder tumor because of the images of extension of the lesion toward the neighboring liver tissue. Such images would have been absent in the case of a cyst.

Several types of linear reflective images in the hepatic region that are apt to bring about a posterior acoustic shadow have now been discussed. Such a pattern, associating a linear reflection and an acoustic shadow, I term the *shell sign*. (See Fig. 17-13.) Following are possible causes of the shell sign:

- Gas in fixed intestinal loop
- Cholelithiasis and calcified gallbladder
- Old hydatid cyst
- Old calcified amebic abscess
- Cholelithiasis associated with gallbladder tumor
- Forgotten surgical sponge (Fig. 25-39)

REFERENCES

Bass, E. M., Funston, M. R., and Shaff, M. I.: Caroli's disease: an ultrasonic diagnosis, Br. J. Radiol. **50:**366-369, 1977.

Holm, H. H., Kristensen, J. K., Rasmussen, S. N., Pedersen, J. F., and Hancke, S.: Abdominal ultrasound, Copenhagen, 1976, Munksgaard, International Booksellers & Publishers, Ltd.

Marsh, J. L., Dahms, B., and Longmire, W. P.: Cystadenoma and cystadenocarcinoma of the biliary system, Arch. Surg. **109:**41-43, 1974.

PART IV

THE PANCREAS

CHAPTER 18

EXAMINATION TECHNIQUES

This chapter is one of the most important in this ultrasonographic study of digestive pathology. Before the development of computerized axial tomography, ultrasonography was the sole radiological procedure capable of displaying this organ directly. Even now, ultrasonography remains the only simple, inexpensive, and nonionizing procedure for pancreatic examination. Recent technical developments have enhanced the reliability and accuracy of pancreatic ultrasonography. The technical principles of the ultrasonic pancreatic examination are based on anatomical relationships.

ANATOMICAL DATA

Pancreatic orientation is roughly transverse, more often than not slightly ascending to the left, and the pancreas is sometimes crescent shaped (Fig. 18-1). A rather large part of it lies in close contact with the great vessels and is thus located in front of the spine: therefore scanning from behind is impossible. Except for the tail, the only approach is anterior, through sagittal, transverse, and slightly oblique scans. (See Fig. 18-2.)

The tail of the pancreas is in close relationship with the anterior aspect of the left kidney. At this level a posterior approach via the kidney, through sagittal scans, is possible (Pietri and colleagues, 1976). (See Fig. 18-3.) With third-generation

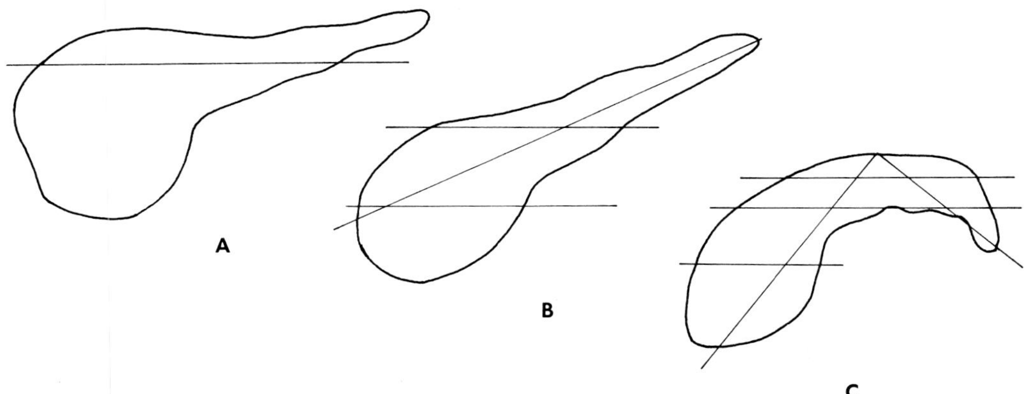

Fig. 18-1. Schematic drawing of frontal view of pancreas. **A,** Horizontal pancreas. In such a pancreas, single horizontal scan contains head, neck, and body. **B,** Oblique pancreas. Slightly oblique scans show pancreas more completely than do horizontal scans. **C,** Crescent-shaped pancreas. In such a pancreas, no scan can display more than part of pancreatic tissue.

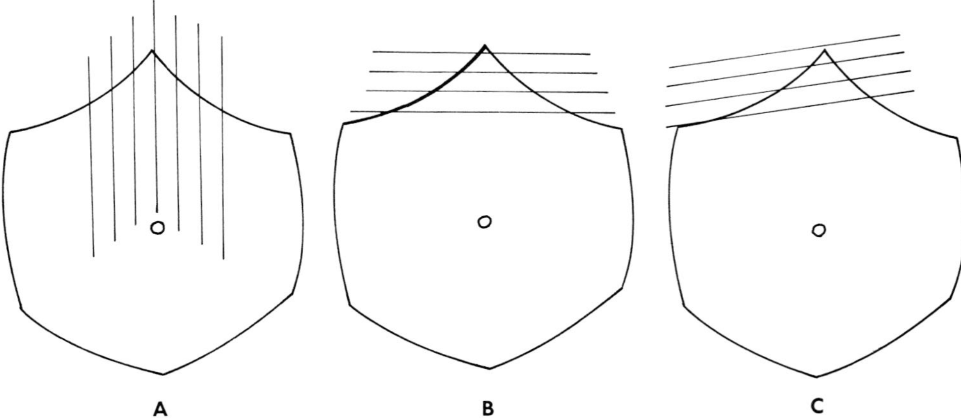

Fig. 18-2. Different section planes used for pancreatic examination by anterior approach. **A,** Sagittal scans. **B,** Transverse scans. **C,** Slightly oblique scans.

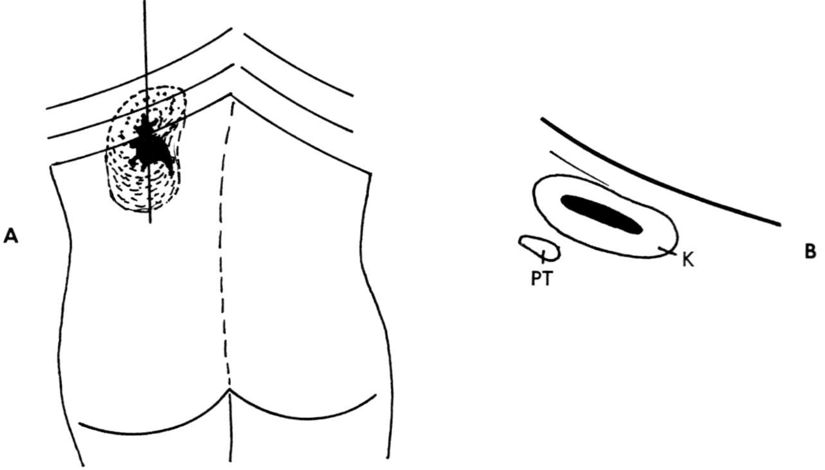

Fig. 18-3. Posterior approach to pancreatic tail across kidney. Transverse posterior approach is also possible. **A,** Scanning plane. **B,** Schematic representation of result. *K,* kidney; *PT,* pancreatic tail.

equipment, it is now possible to visualize the tail of the pancreas by means of a posterior transverse approach.

The pancreas is closely related to various *vessels* (Fig. 18-4, *A*) already discussed in Chapter 4, including the splenic vein, the superior mesenteric vein and artery, the left renal vein, the origin of the portal vein, the vena cava, and the aorta. The scanning planes employed are based on these vascular relations. (See Fig. 18-4, *A* and *B*.)

Splenic vein. As was discussed in Chapter 4, transverse scans of the upper part of the abdomen made with an appropriate technique show the splenic vein. Since

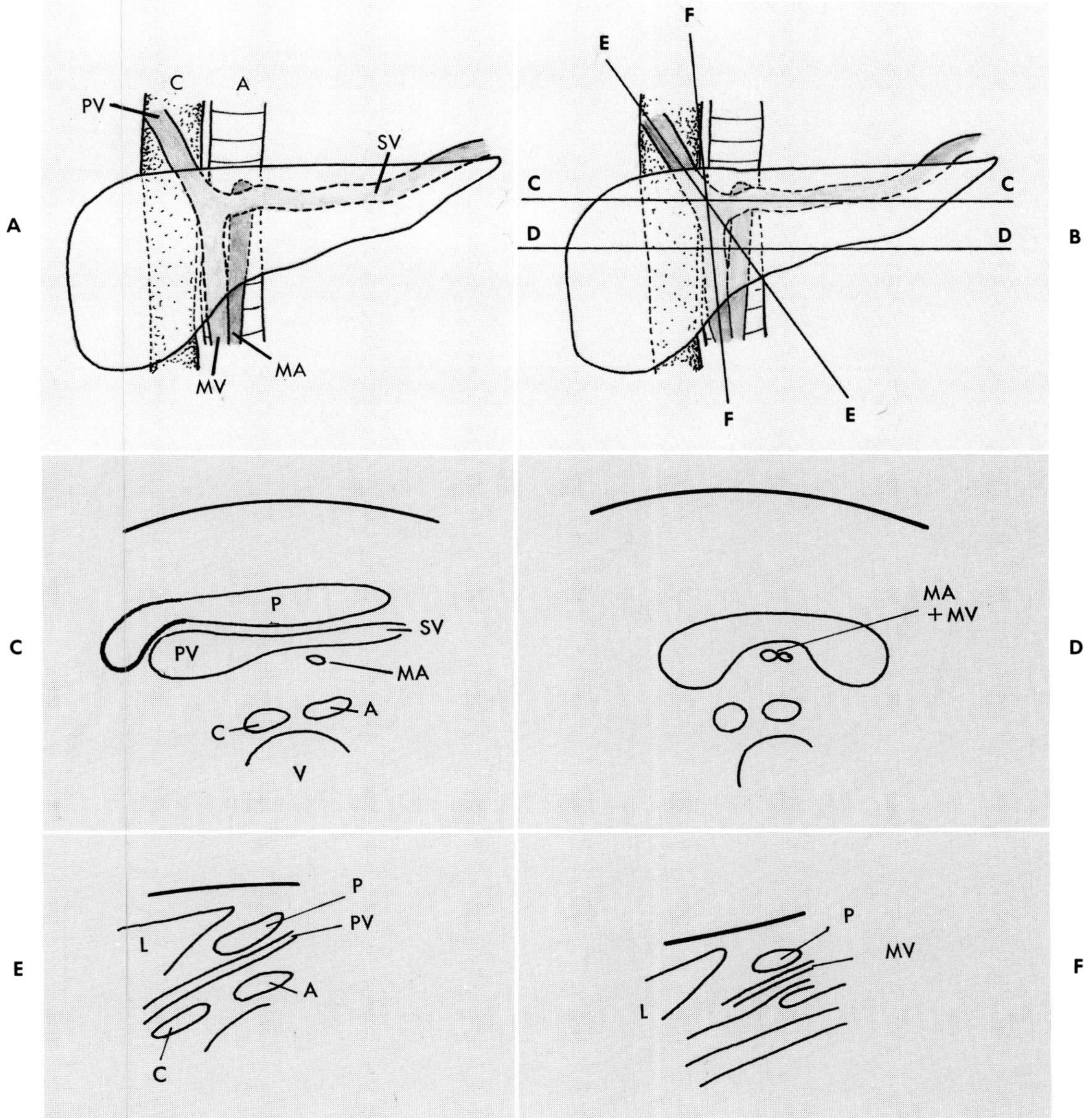

Fig. 18-4. Vascular relations of pancreas. **A,** Schematic drawing of anatomical relations of pancreas with portal system—portal vein *(PV)*, splenic vein *(SV)*, and superior mesenteric vein *(MV)*—and with vena cava *(C)*, aorta *(A)*, and its branch, superior mesenteric artery *(MA)*. **B,** Different scanning planes (*C* to *F*). **C,** Scanning plane passing through splenic vein and splenoportal junction. Pancreas *(P)* appears in front of splenic vein and splenoportal junction. Behind splenic vein is seen transverse section of superior mesenteric artery, origin of which is rather high. Behind these vessels, transverse sections of aorta and vena cava are displayed. *V*, vertebral body. **D,** More caudal section. At this level, both sections of mesenteric artery and vein are shown in close contact with pancreatic neck, just in front of large vessels. **E,** Oblique scan of right upper quadrant, passing sagittally through portal vein. Oblique section of pancreas is shown in front of mesenteric-portal junction. *L*, liver. **F,** Sagittal scan passing through mesenteric vein and mesenteric-portal junction. Sagittal section of pancreas is displayed in front of mesenteric vein.

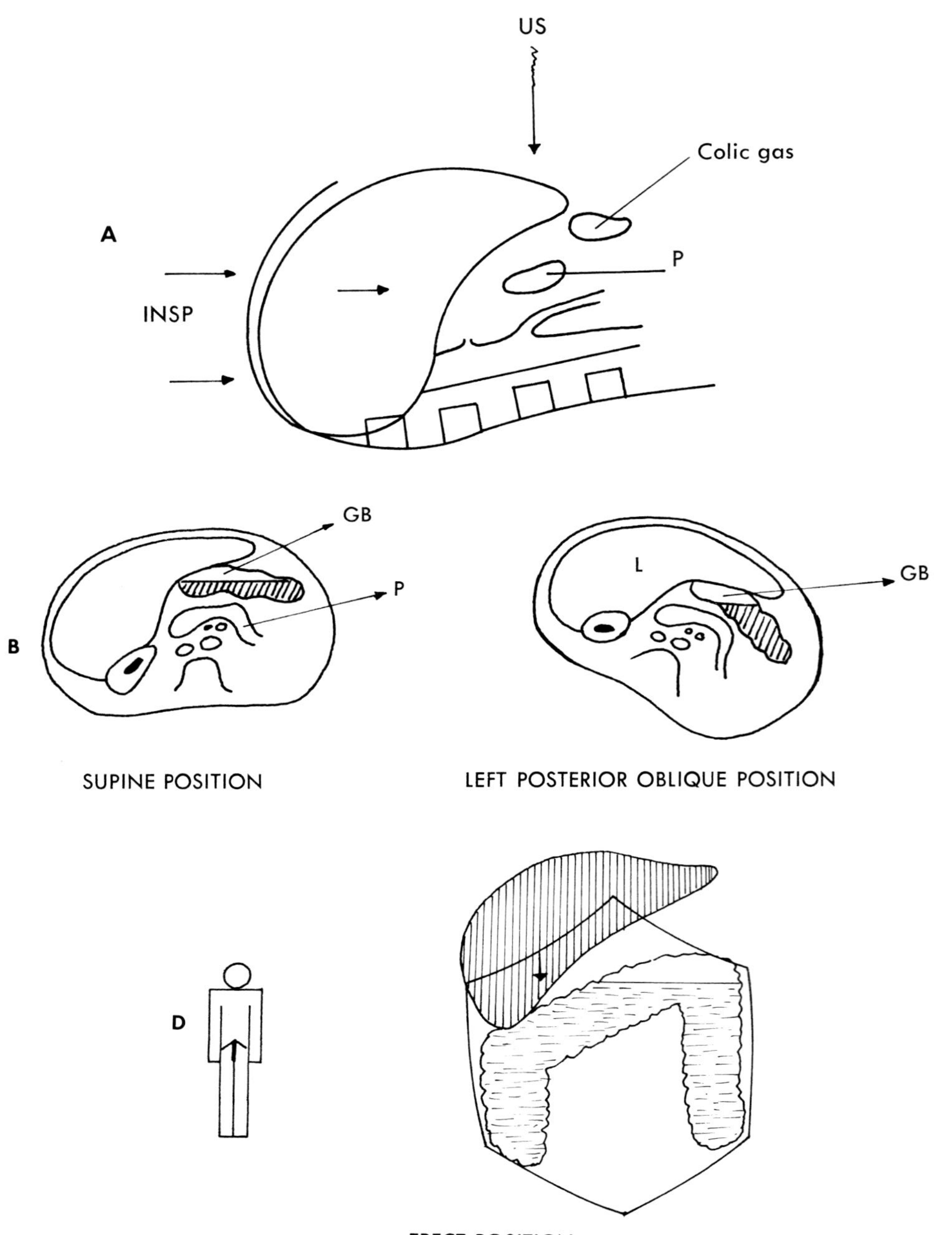

Fig. 18-5. Different artifices used to obtain better pancreatic images. **A,** Deep suspended inspiration *(INSP).* Liver moves downward and displaces gas-filled colon. *P,* pancreas; *US,* ultrasound. **B,** With patient in supine position, gas bubble *(GB)* can partially fill stomach or colon in front of pancreas *(P).* **C,** With patient in posterior left oblique position, gas bubble migrates toward right colonic flexure. Posterior right oblique position may also be used. *L,* liver. **D,** With patient in erect position, downward displacement of liver is increased, and colonic gas migrates toward flexures.

this vein runs along the superior aspect of the pancreatic body and then along its posterior aspect, a scan displaying the splenic vein will show pancreatic tissue just in front of the vein, but the pancreas will also be displayed on more caudal parallel scans. (See Fig. 18-4, *C* and *D*.)

Superior mesenteric artery and vein. Parallel scans made caudal to the splenic vein necessarily pass across the superior mesenteric artery and vein (Fig. 18-4, *D*), the transverse sections of which constitute one of the landmarks in the transverse examination. Sagittal scans performed along the mesenteric vein, as well as other scans, with slight obliquity, show the entire mesenteric and portal venous axis. A sagittal scan showing the mesenteric and portal venous axis also contains the pancreatic head or neck in sagittal section. (See Fig. 18-4, *E* and *F*.)

Vena cava and aorta. Sagittal scans passing through the vena cava include the pancreatic head, whereas aortic sagittal scans pass through the pancreatic neck. The left renal vein, as well as the left renal artery, is often displayed between the aorta and the pancreas. (See Chapter 4.)

Other anatomical relations. Other anatomical relations play a part in the ultrasonic examination of the pancreas. The duodenum and the stomach are closely related to the pancreas. Those belonging to Schammai's school propose asking the patient to drink, so as to fill up the stomach, displace air, and use the intragastric fluid as a transmitting agent, in the same way as the filled bladder is used to examine the uterus. On the other hand, the followers of Hillel prefer to examine only a fasting patient, so as to avoid confusing a piece of sirloin steak, a morsel of gefilte fish, or peanuts with a pancreatic tumor. Even though fasting is better, my associates and I endeavor to examine our patients even if their stomachs are not empty. However, if we find an abnormal pancreatic image, we think it good practice to check that image later with the stomach empty. This problem will be discussed further, along with the differential diagnosis of pancreatic diseases (Chapter 25).

Transverse colon. The transverse colon has a more distant relation to the pancreas. However, colonic gas may constitute an obstacle to the transmission of the ultrasonic beam. The less developed the left hepatic lobe, the more important the colonic obstacle. Therefore, in patients whose left hepatic lobe is especially small, it is necessary to use various artifices. (See Fig. 18-5.) The first of these is to resort to deep suspended inspiration. The second is positional change; that is, the patient is placed in the posterior left oblique position to cause the colonic gas to migrate toward the right colonic flexure, at some distance from the pancreas. Finally, one of the best ways to displace colonic gas and cause the left hepatic lobe to move downward is to examine the patient in the erect position.

CHOICE OF ULTRASONIC TECHNIQUE

Global anatomical scans are best made by contact scanning; quick transverse single-sweep scanning of the abdomen enables one to obtain high-resolution images of the pancreas, with excellent visualization of the abdominal vessels. On the other hand, the real-time technique seems better suited for sagittal scans of the vessels used as anatomical landmarks, and by its use the orientation of the gland can be perceived at once. These technical and anatomical data again show that

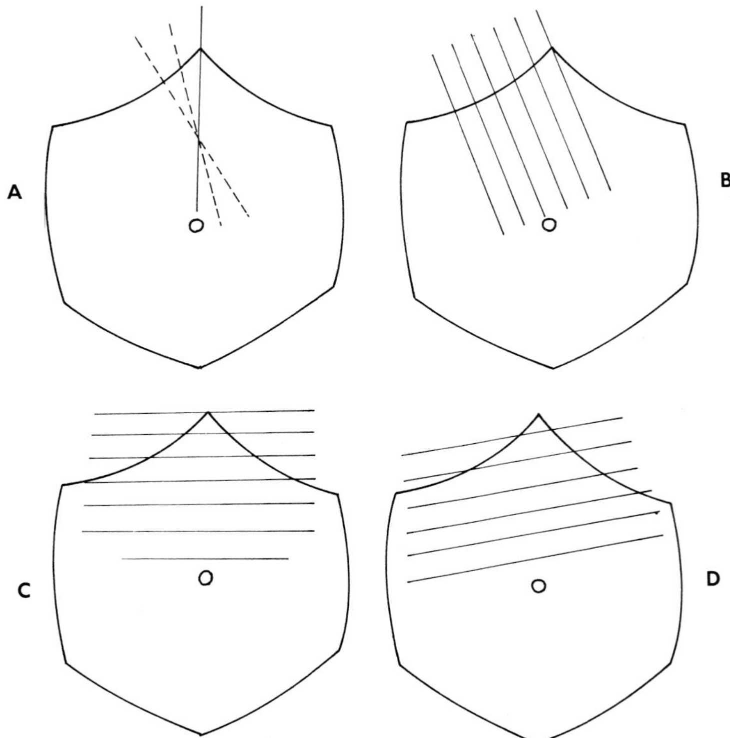

Fig. 18-6. Different scanning planes used in real-time phase of pancreatic examination.

both techniques must be combined, and following this principle led to development of the technical procedure.

PROCEDURE OF ULTRASONIC PANCREATIC EXAMINATION

The examination is begun with *real time*. The patient is recumbent. The ultrasonographer performs sagittal scans through the aorta, vena cava, and superior mesenteric vein. The orientation of the ultrasonic RTH is then slightly changed, so as to obtain oblique scans in the plane of the mesenteric-portal venous axis (Fig. 18-6, *A*). The epigastrium is then swept in sagittal scans from right to left and left to right (Fig. 18-6, *B*). This enables one to integrate mentally the morphological information in a three-dimensional way. Horizontal, transverse, and slightly oblique scans are then made, by a rocking movement of the RTH, from the xiphoid process down to the umbilicus and back, exactly as in the first step of the hepatic examination (Fig. 18-6, *B* and *C*). The use of deep suspended inspiration is useful, since it displaces the left lobe of the liver and the colon downward and distends the vena cava, facilitating the display of the pancreatic head in front of the vessel.

After this real-time step, the orientation and general shape and size of the pancreas are known. Contact scanning is then undertaken with the patient in deep sustained inspiration. Transverse scans are performed mainly by the rapid single-

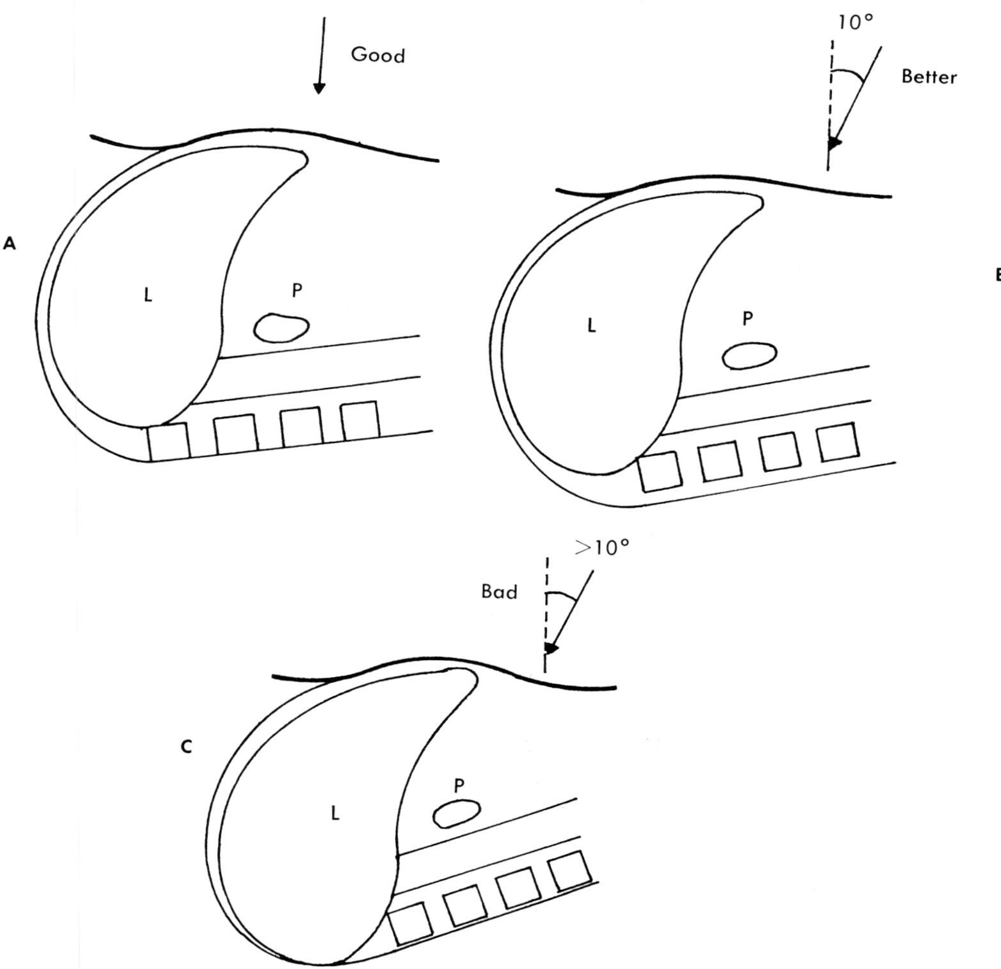

Fig. 18-7. Cranial inclination of transverse scanning plane. **A,** Scanning plane perpendicular to abdominal wall. This usually results in good images. **B,** Cranial inclination of 10 degrees. At this angle, images are usually better. **C,** Inclination over 10 degrees. Aorta is very obliquely cut. Such an inclination is unsatisfactory. *L,* liver; *P,* pancreas.

sweep technique, with the scanning angle selected from the previous real-time cuts. These more or less oblique transverse scans are made 0.5 by 0.5 cm down from the xiphoid process (Fig. 18-2, *B* and *C*). Display of the portal vein and then of the splenoportal junction zeroes in display of the pancreas itself. It is useful to incline the scanning plane somewhat cranially (Fig. 18-7), to display the upper abdomen behind the xiphoid process. Keep in mind that the pancreas lies over the great vessels, which are themselves in close contact with the spine. In the recumbent position the spine ascends caudally. Therefore too marked a cranial inclination of the scanning plane would introduce geometrical distortion. (See Fig. 18-7, *B* and *C*.) Of course, if the results are not satisfactory, the positional artifices already described must be used. Hancke and co-workers (1975) suggest using the right kidney and the spleen as references. They draw a line between the centers of these two organs to predict the level and obliquity of the pancreas. In my opinion, the simpler technique of using successive rapid parallel scans, guided by previous real-time examination, is usually quite sufficient. As already pointed out, the first part of the pancreatic examination, performed with real-time technique, results in satisfactory images in sagittal section. Therefore I only exceptionally use sagittal contact scans of the pancreatic head and body. However, to display the pancreatic tail, making sagittal contact scans of the left kidney with the patient in the prone position is absolutely necessary.

The followers of Schammai teach that the pancreatic examination is to be performed with the real-time technique only. The members of Hillel's school teach that a pancreatic examination is satisfactory only when made with contact scanning. The real-time part of the pancreatic examination lasts less than 2 minutes, whereas in a normal pancreas the contact scanning phase of the examination, thanks to the topographical information already obtained from real-time cuts, lasts only from 4 to 5 minutes. Combining both techniques usually enables one to perform a complete pancreatic examination in less than 10 minutes; in that time, hepatic, biliary, and splenic images are also obtained. Only in exceptional cases, involving stout patients, small left hepatic lobes, or abundant gastric and colonic gas, does a pancreatic examination require more time. Following are the different phases of the ultrasonic study of the pancreas:

1. Sagittal and transverse real-time scanning in suspended deep inspiration
2. Transverse parallel close-contact scans made with the patient in suspended respiration and a scanning angle determined by real-time scanning
3. Transrenal contact scans of the pancreatic tail, with patient in prone position
4. Possible additional views: sagittal and transverse real-time scans made with the patient in the erect position

Recently (Weill and associates, 1977) we tested the reliability of this technical procedure in a group of 100 normal subjects who had been referred to our department for nondigestive examinations. In this group, the ages varied from 17 to 85 years and weight from 46 to 110 kg. We obtained a satisfactory image of the pancreas in transverse section by the contact scanning technique in eighty-two of these subjects. Avoirdupois is not necessarily an obstacle. Good images can be obtained in stout patients provided the left lobe of the liver is sufficiently developed. Paradoxically, with thin patients, in whom no problem is anticipated, the examination may fail if the left lobe is small or the stomach and colon are filled with gas. In several of the eighteen patients in whom transverse contact scanning was unsuccessful, pancreatic images were nevertheless obtained with real-time sagittal scans made with the patient in the erect position. In most cases, pancreatic enlargement is seen even if the anatomical conditions are poor.

REFERENCES

Barnett, E., and Morley, P.: Abdominal echography, Borough Green, England, 1974, Butterworth & Co. (Publishers), Ltd.

Goldberg, B. B., Kotler, M. N., Ziskin, M. C., and Waxham, R. D.: Diagnostic uses of ultrasound, New York, 1975, Grune & Stratton, Inc.

Hancke, S., Holm, H. H., and Koch, F.: Ultrasonically guided fine needle biopsy of the pancreas, Surg. Gynecol. Obstet. **140:**361-364, 1975.

Hassani, N.: Ultrasonography of the abdomen, Heidelberg, Germany, 1976, Springer-Verlag.

Holm, H. H., Kristensen, J. K., Rasmussen, S. N., Pedersen, J. F., and Hancke, S.: Abdominal ultrasound, Copenhagen, 1976, Munksgaard, International Booksellers & Publishers, Ltd.

Leopold, G. R., and Asher, W. M.: Fundamentals of abdominal and pelvic ultrasonography, Philadelphia, 1975, W. B. Saunders Co.

Pietri, H., Rosello, R., Aimino, B., and Sérafino, X.: Diagnosis of small tumors of the pancreatic tail, J. Radiol. Electrol. Med. Nucl. **57:**610, 1976.

Smith, E. H., Bartrum, R. J. R., and Chang, Y. C.: Ultrasonically guided percutaneous aspiration biopsy of the pancreas, Radiology **112:**737-738, 1974.

Walls, W. J., Gonzalez, G., Martin, N. L., and Templeton, A. W.: B-scan ultrasound evaluation of the pancreas. Advantages and accuracy compared to other diagnostic techniques, Radiology **114:**127-134, 1975.

Weill, F., Becker, J. C., Kraehenbuhl, J. R., Heriot, G., and Walter, J. P.: Clinical atlas of ultrasonic radiography, Paris, 1973, Masson & Cie., Editeurs.

Weill, F., Schraub, A., Eisenscher, A., and Bourgoin, A.: Ultrasonography of the normal pancreas, Radiology **123:**417-423, 1977.

CHAPTER 19

ECHOANATOMY

ANATOMICAL LANDMARKS

Anatomical landmarks to be considered in ultrasonography of the pancreas are the vascular elements discussed as recently as the last chapter, including the *splenic vein* (Fig. 19-1), of which the anatomical relations with the pancreas will be shown in detail a little further on, and the *superior mesenteric vein,* which is located in front of the uncinate process of the pancreas, but behind the pancreatic neck. The mesenteric vein runs in an oblique left direction to merge with the splenic vein, to form the origin of the portal vein. The splenomesenteric junction is frankly retropancreatic. The surgeon has to elevate the pancreatic tissue to approach this anastomosis. The superior mesenteric artery runs parallel to the vein, usually along its left wall. Finally, the aorta and cava also are landmarks.

Superior mesenteric vessels. Sagittal scans of the mesenteric-portal axis show a sagittal section of the pancreatic neck immediately in front of the superior mesenteric vein (Figs. 19-2 and 19-10, *B*). The mesenteric-portal venous axis is a reliable landmark that we have been using for many years (Weill and coworkers, 1974). On transverse scans passing through the full width of the pancreatic tissue, the twin sections of the superior mesenteric artery and vein outline an "eyeglasses image," which lies in close contact with the posterior aspect

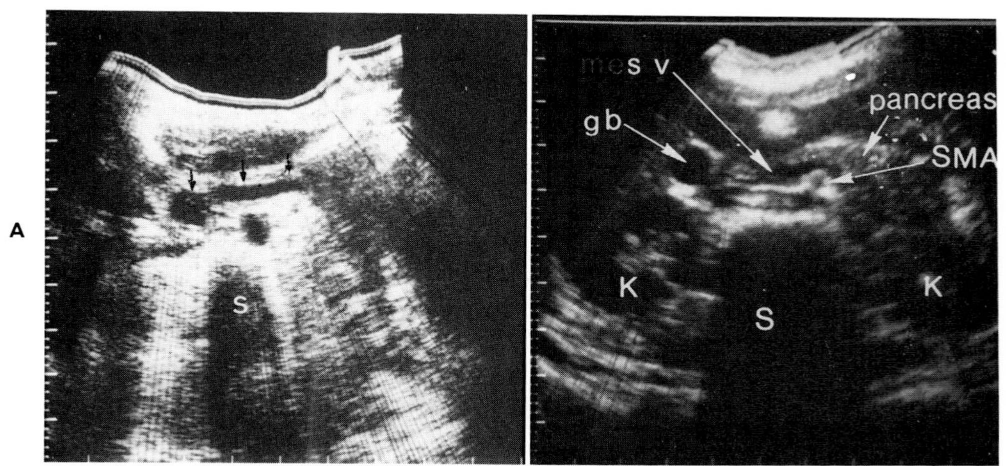

Fig. 19-1. Splenic vein, first landmark in pancreatic examination. **A,** Transverse scan of upper abdomen passing through splenic vein and splenoportal junction *(arrows).* Pancreatic head is found on more caudal scans. *S,* spine. **B,** Transverse scan. *sv,* splenic vein; *gb,* gallbladder; *SMA,* superior mesenteric artery; *K,* right and left kidneys.

of the pancreatic neck (Figs. 19-3 and 19-4). The typical eyeglasses pattern of the twin sections of the mesenteric vessels depends on the obliquity of the course of the mesenteric vein: when the latter runs vertically, parallel to the superior mesenteric artery, a transverse section displays a true eyeglasses image. If the mesenteric vein begins to change its course at a low level and to run obliquely toward the splenoportal junction, pancreatic caudal transverse scans show the sections of the two vessels at a distance from one another; more cephalic scans

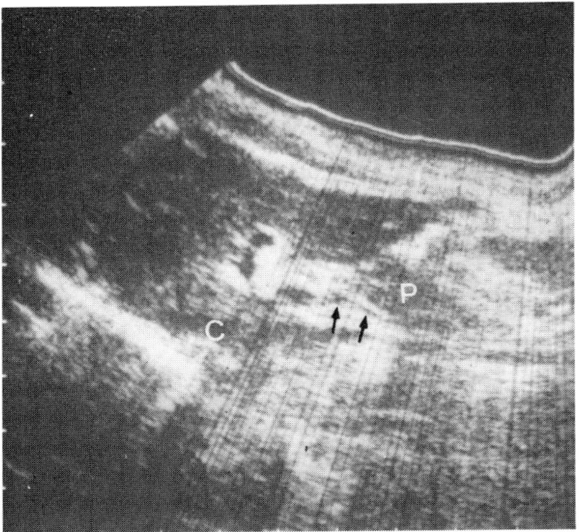

Fig. 19-2. Sagittal scan. Pancreas *(P)* is seen in front of SMV *(arrows)*. *C,* vena cava.

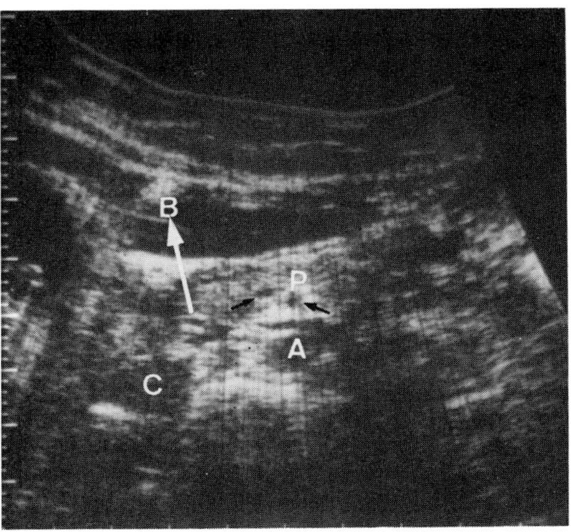

Fig. 19-3. Eyeglasses image. SMA and SMV *(arrows)* are displayed in transverse section in close contact with posterior aspect of pancreatic neck *(P)*. Their twin sections outline eyeglasses image. Immediately behind mesenteric artery is outlined transverse arterial element, which probably corresponds to origin of right renal artery. Note section of intrapancreatic common bile duct *(B)*. *C,* vena cava; *A,* aorta.

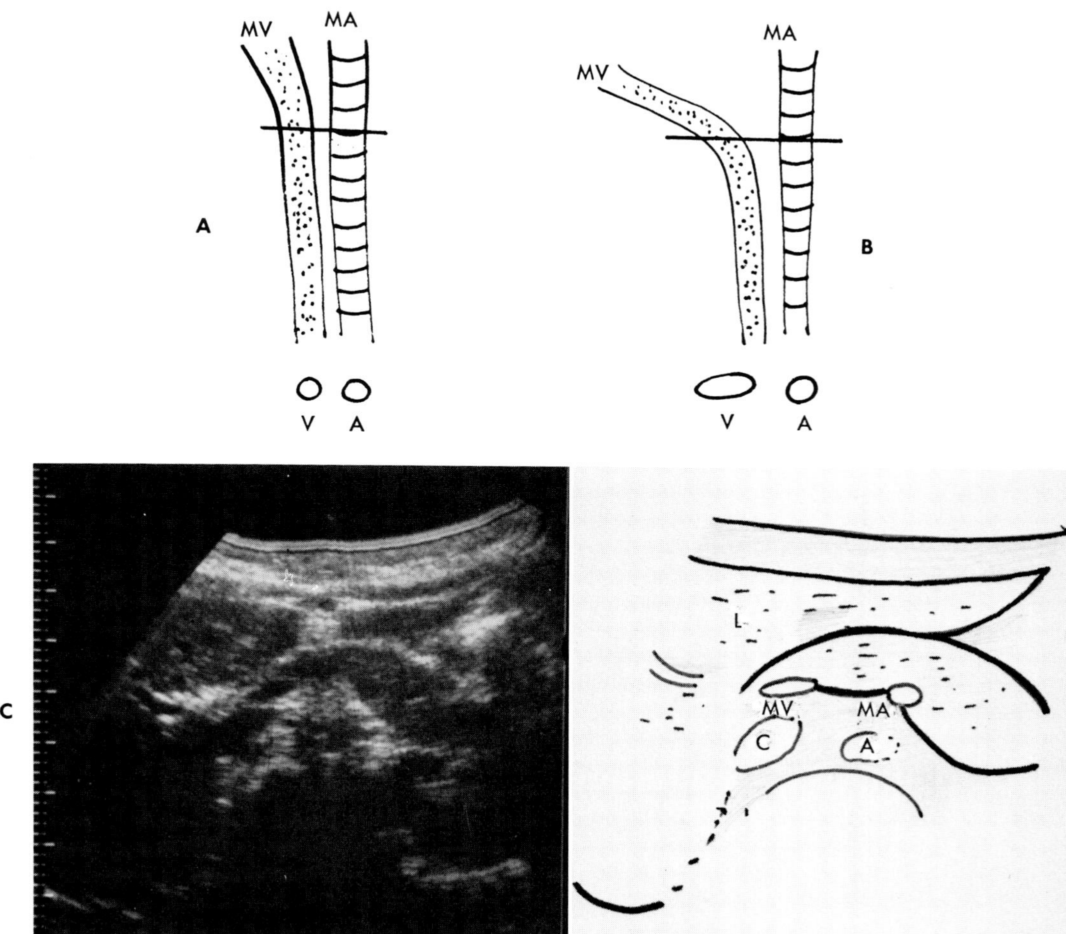

Fig. 19-4. True and distorted eyeglasses images. **A,** Superior mesenteric artery *(MA)* and superior mesenteric vein *(MV)* are parallel at level of pancreas. Their sections *(V, A)* present true eyeglasses image. **B,** Mesenteric vein running more obliquely to join low portal junction. Its section is no longer circular. **C** to **E,** Three examples of distorted eyeglasses image. *L,* liver; *C,* vena cava; *A,* aorta; *P,* pancreas; *PV,* portal vein; *LRV,* left renal vein; *N,* lymph node.

display a larger section of the vein, which is oval or racket shaped, leading to what is called a *distorted eyeglasses image.* (See Fig. 19-4.) Still more cephalic scans show the splenomesenteric-portal anastomosis itself (Fig. 19-5). This brings us back to the splenic vein itself.

Splenic vein. The splenic vein runs along the superior aspect of the pancreatic tail. It then continues farther behind the posterior aspect of the pancreas to merge with the mesenteric vein, constituting the origin of the portal vein, which is in close relation with the dorsal aspect of the pancreatic head. An enlarged splenic vein was sometimes confused with the pancreas in the course of a too rapid and superficial examination (Fig. 19-6). However, in gray scale, especially with the machines of the last generation, such a gross error has become impossible; but,

D

E

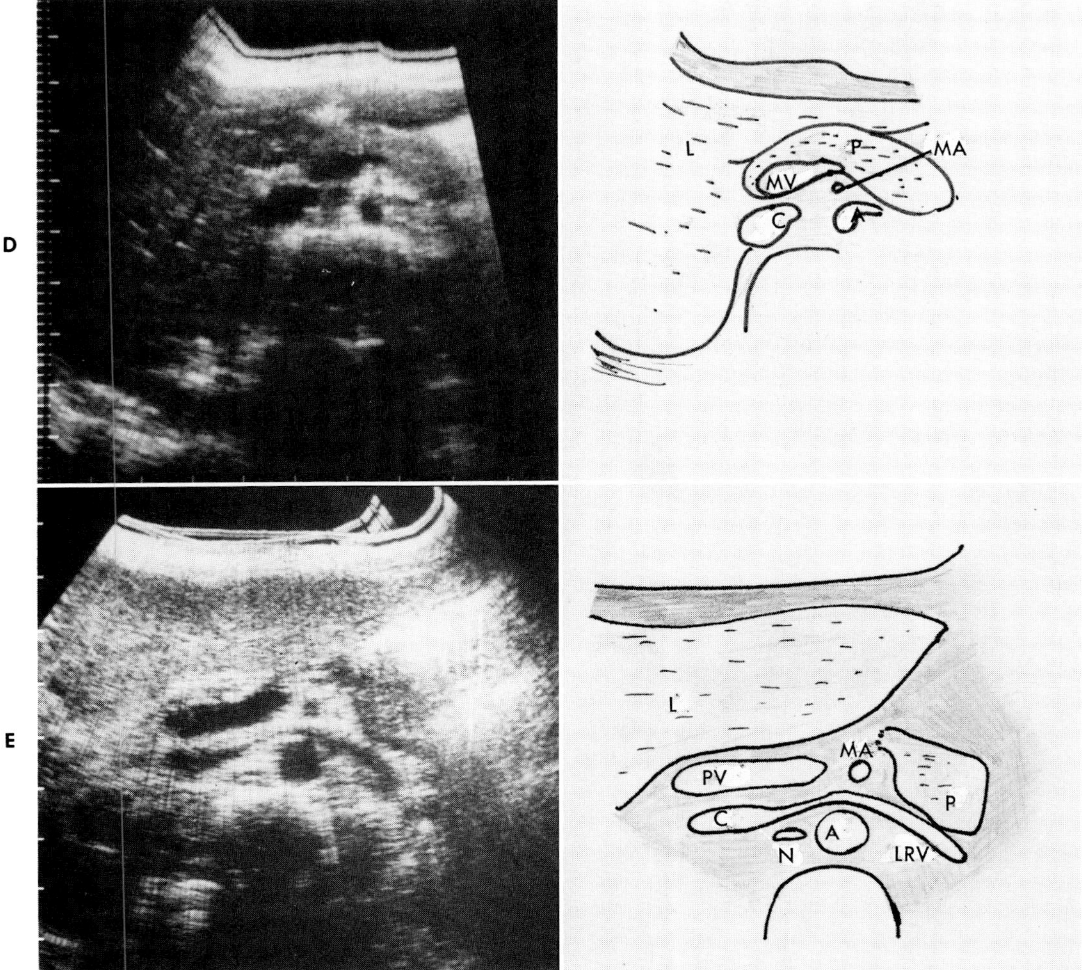

Fig. 19-4, cont'd. For legend see opposite page.

even with less advanced imaging, that error would be impossible with the help of a rational study of the vascular landmarks just reviewed. Hancke and associates (1975) pointed out the value of the display of a section of the superior mesenteric artery when a pancreas is examined by transverse scans. Since they showed us this landmark, we have used it regularly, along with the venous landmarks, in our bistable studies. In fact, the arterial landmark, if used alone, was exceptionally insufficient: the superior mesenteric artery may originate from the aorta above the level of the splenic vein. (See Fig. 19-7, *A*.) A transverse scan through the splenic vein, then, may show the mesenteric artery and not the pancreas. In front of a splenic vein in high position, there may lie no pancreatic tissue at all or only a narrow strip. (See Fig. 19-7, *A*.) On the other hand, a wide area of pancreatic

Text continued on p. 296.

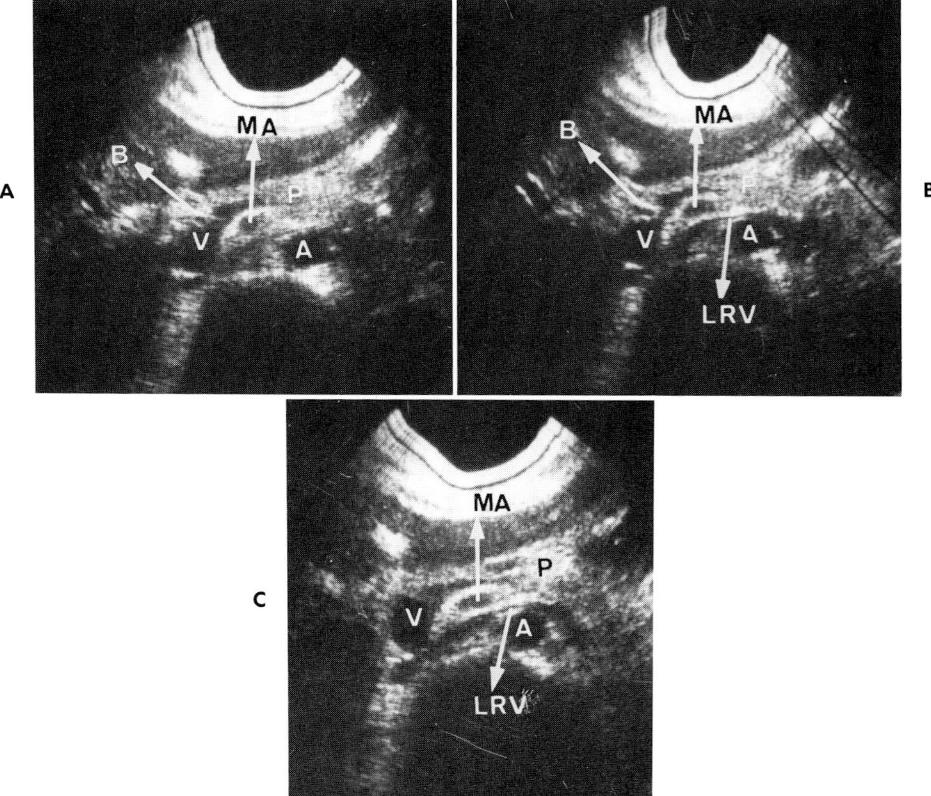

Fig. 19-5. Example of vascular relations of pancreas *(P).* Three parallel transverse scans show mesenteric artery *(MA),* portal vein, and splenoportal junction *(V),* with splenic vein appearing progressively from **A** to **C. In C,** note left renal vein *(LRV)* merging with flat vena cava. Note also transverse section of common bile duct *(B). A,* aorta.

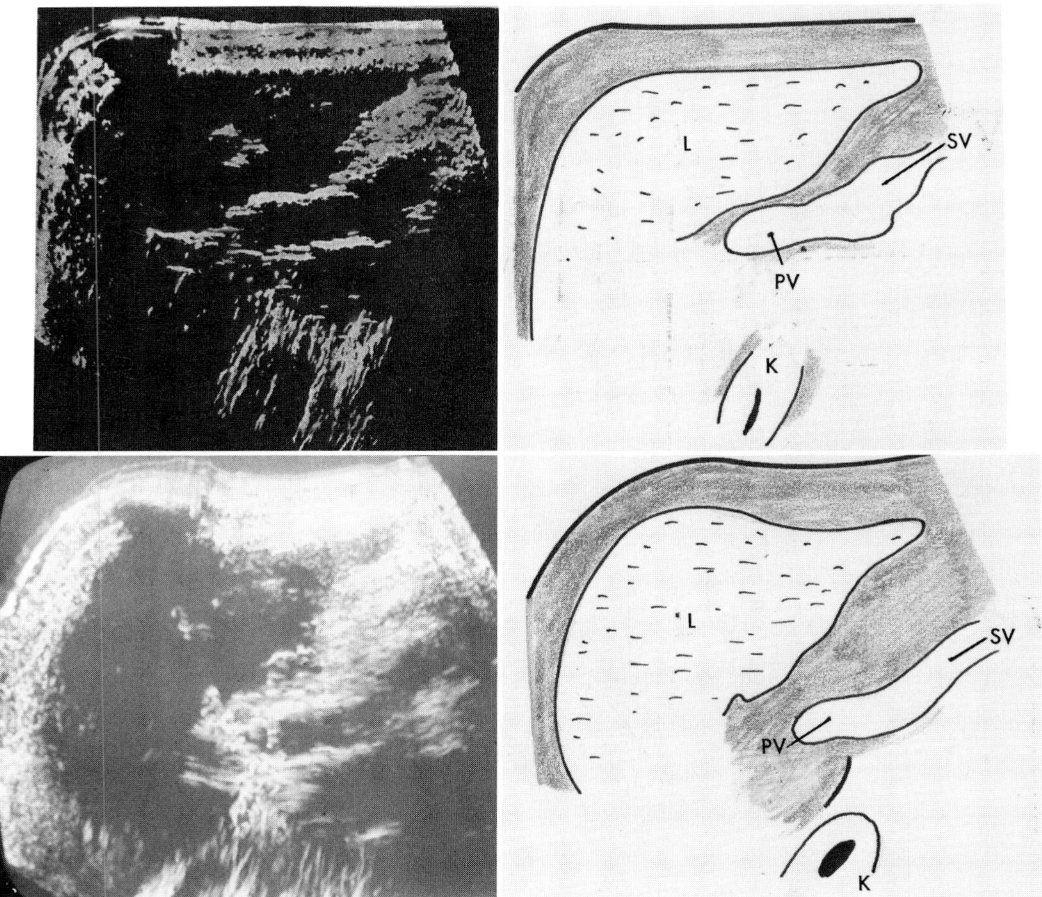

Fig. 19-6. False pancreatic image. Transverse scans and schematic drawings of upper abdomen showing enlarged splenoportal venous axis (*PV* and *SV*), which could be confused with pancreatic image. As a matter of fact, these structures extend much more to right than would pancreatic head. The search for vascular landmarks proves the image itself to be vascular. Confusion of pancreas with enlarged splenic vein has become impossible with present quality of imaging. *L,* liver; *K,* right kidney.

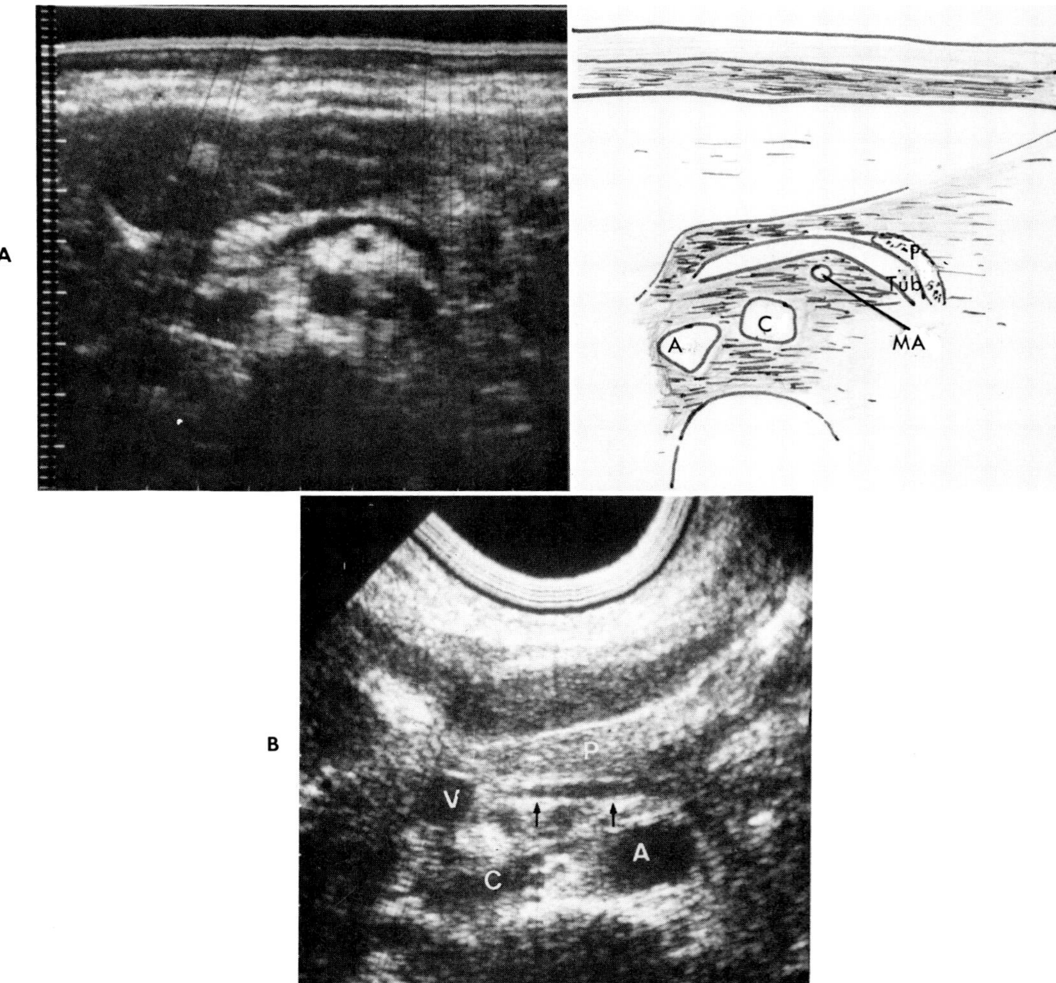

Fig. 19-7. Two types of relation of splenic vein with pancreas. **A,** Splenic vein in high position, with only thin strip of pancreatic tissue *(P)* in front of it. It was in such cases that tubular pattern of vein *(Tub)* was sometimes confused with pancreas itself in bistable imaging. Study of relation with SMA *(MA)* was then fundamental. *C,* vena cava; *A,* aorta. **B,** Splenic vein *(arrows)* in low position. There is wide section of pancreatic tissue in front of it. *V,* splenoportal junction.

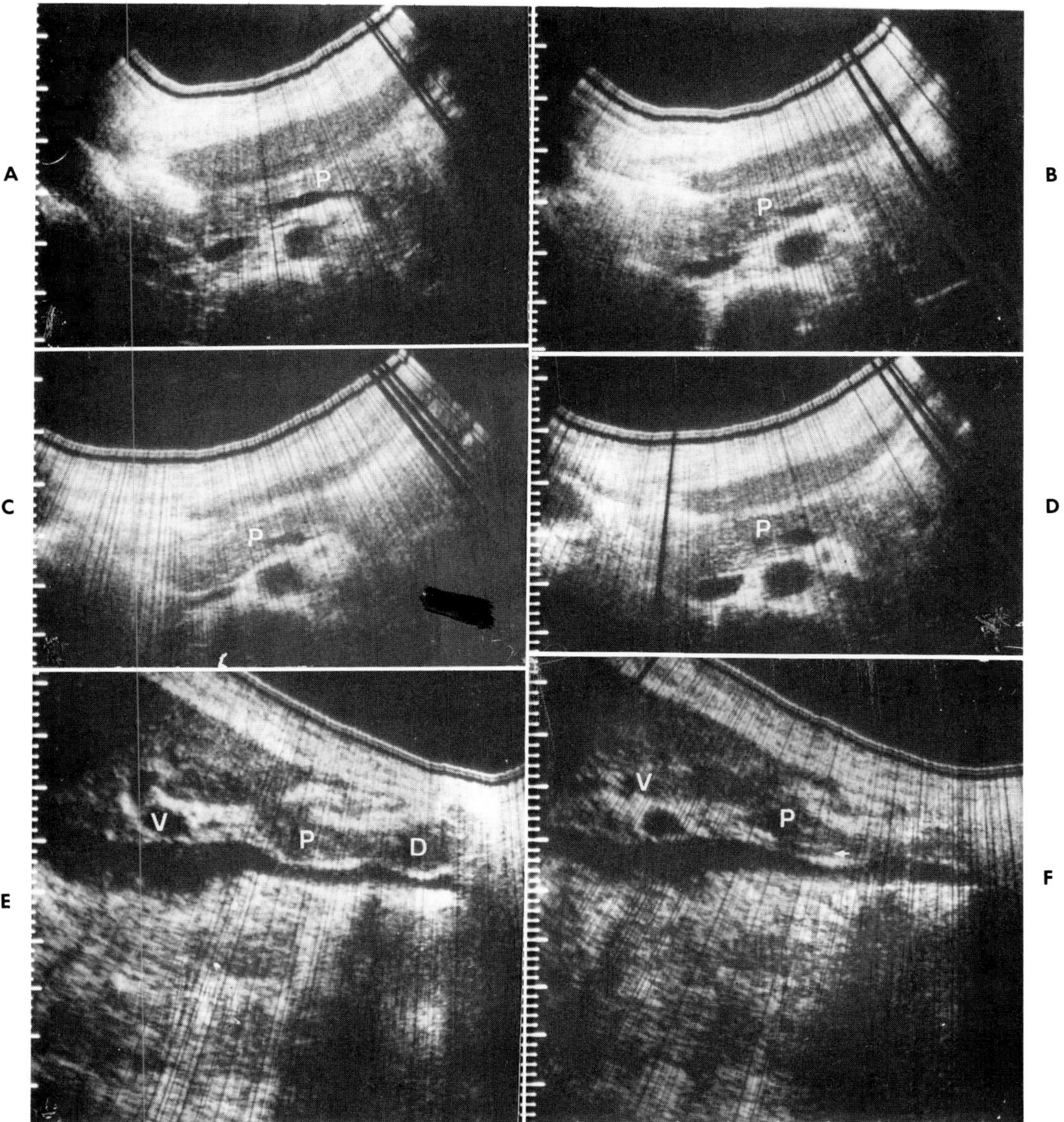

Fig. 19-8. Detailed study of vascular relations of pancreas *(P)*. **A** to **D,** Parallel transverse scans showing splenic vein and then SMV. Origin of SMA is displayed in **A** and **B.** Transverse section of SMA is shown in **C** and **D. E** and **F,** Parallel sagittal cuts. Relation of pancreatic head with SMV *(arrowhead)* is shown in **F.** In **E,** note section of third part of duodenum *(D)*. *V,* portal vein.

tissue may be found in front of a splenic vein in low position (Fig. 19-7, *B*). If vascular landmarks are used, both the mesenteric artery and the venous network must be considered (Fig. 19-8). Although the quality of present imaging, which clearly shows the pancreatic tissue, with a sharp delineation, has rendered vascular landmarks less important, they are still useful (Fig. 19-24).

LOCATION

The pancreas may be very superficially located in thin patients. While studying 130 images of normal pancreata (Weill and co-workers, 1975), we measured the distance between their anterior aspects and the skin. This distance varied from 24 to 95 mm.

SHAPE

On sagittal scans the shape of the pancreatic tissue is roughly rectangular or oval (Figs. 19-2 and 19-8, *E,* to 19-11). As sagittal sections of the pancreas are made closer to the tail of the organ, the shape tends to become more oval. This is clearly visible on sagittal posterior scans performed through the kidney. (See Fig. 19-12, *A* and *B*.)

On a global transverse scan the pancreatic head, neck, and body stretch in front of the large vessels and the twin sections of the mesenteric vessel (Fig. 19-8). The pancreatic head is more developed on its craniocaudal axis than is the neck or the body (Fig. 19-10). Therefore, although transverse scans contain the head and the body, more caudal scans contain only the head. The pancreatic head is then displayed as a parenchymal element, more or less ovoid, in relation to

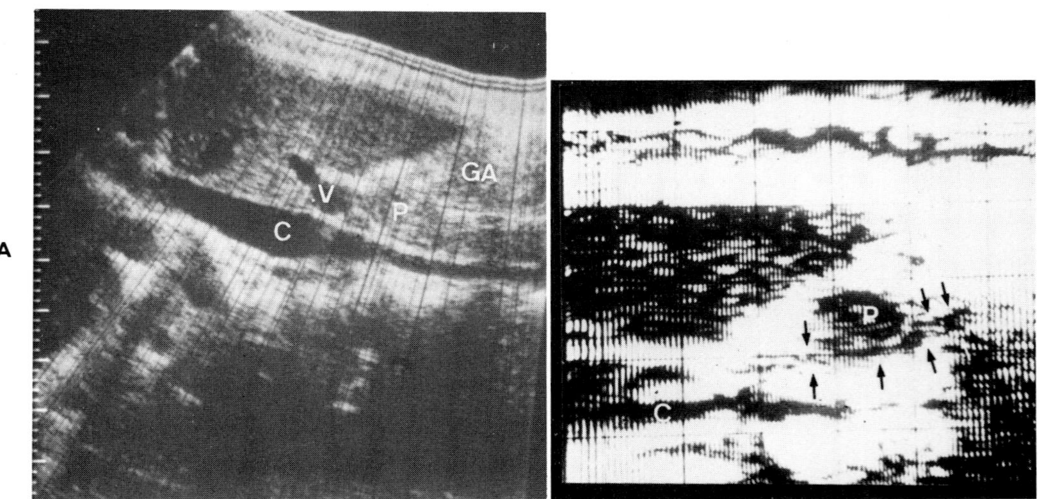

Fig. 19-9. A, Sagittal section of pancreatic head *(P)*. Above pancreas, immediately in front of vena cava *(C)*, portal vein *(V)* is displayed. Gastric antrum *(GA)* is outlined in relation to liver and pancreas. **B,** Sagittal section of pancreatic head *(P)* displaying its relation to superior mesenteric vein *(arrows)*. *C,* vena cava.

the vena cava. (See Fig. 19-13.) This pancreatic head must not be confused with a pathological mass. It is, of course, possible to build the image of the pancreas as the central element of a global section of the upper abdomen (Fig. 19-14), but to get a truly reliable pancreatic section, apnea is compulsory. Thus it is rather difficult to build a global section, since the necessary scanning time may be as much as 10 seconds. The single-sweep scanning technique can be used to build up much more precise images. That is why many of our figures display only the central epigastric area of the upper abdomen.

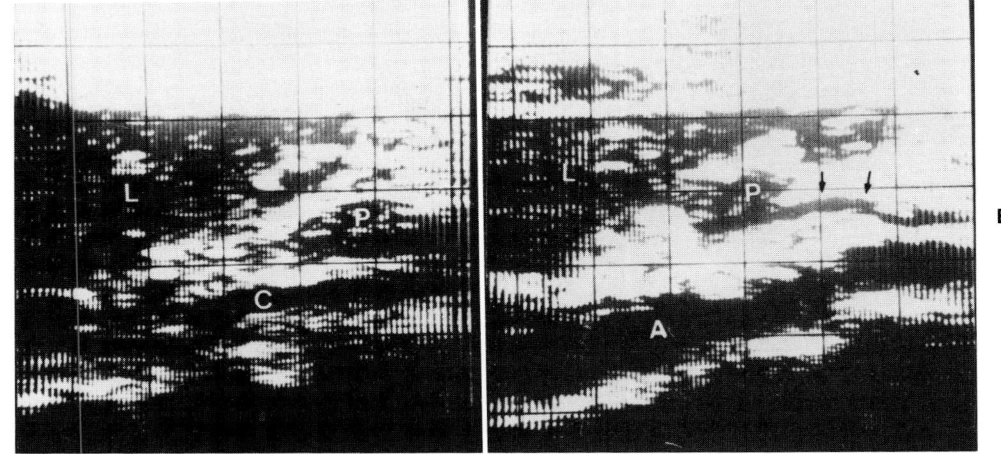

Fig. 19-10. Parallel sagittal scans of pancreas in real time. **A,** Oval shape of pancreatic head is outlined between vena cava *(C)* and right hepatic lobe *(L)*. **B,** Another scan 2 cm to left, passing through aorta *(A)*, mesenteric vein *(arrows)*, and pancreatic neck *(P)*.

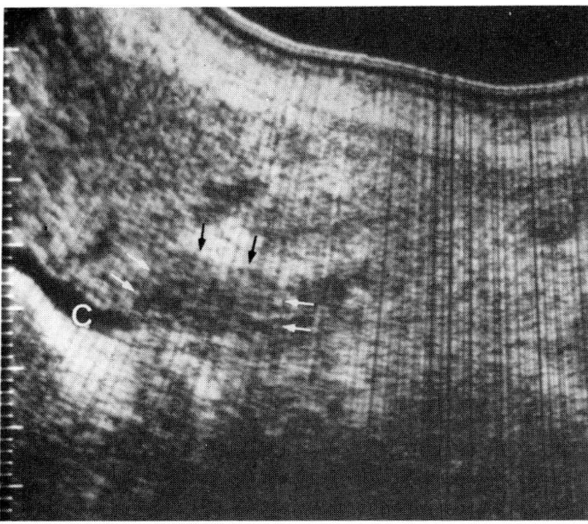

Fig. 19-11. Another sagittal section of pancreatic head *(arrows)*. Note flattening of vena cava *(C)* in absence of pancreatic head enlargement (checked during operation for right renal carcinoma). Diameter of vena cava can be reliably assessed only in real time.

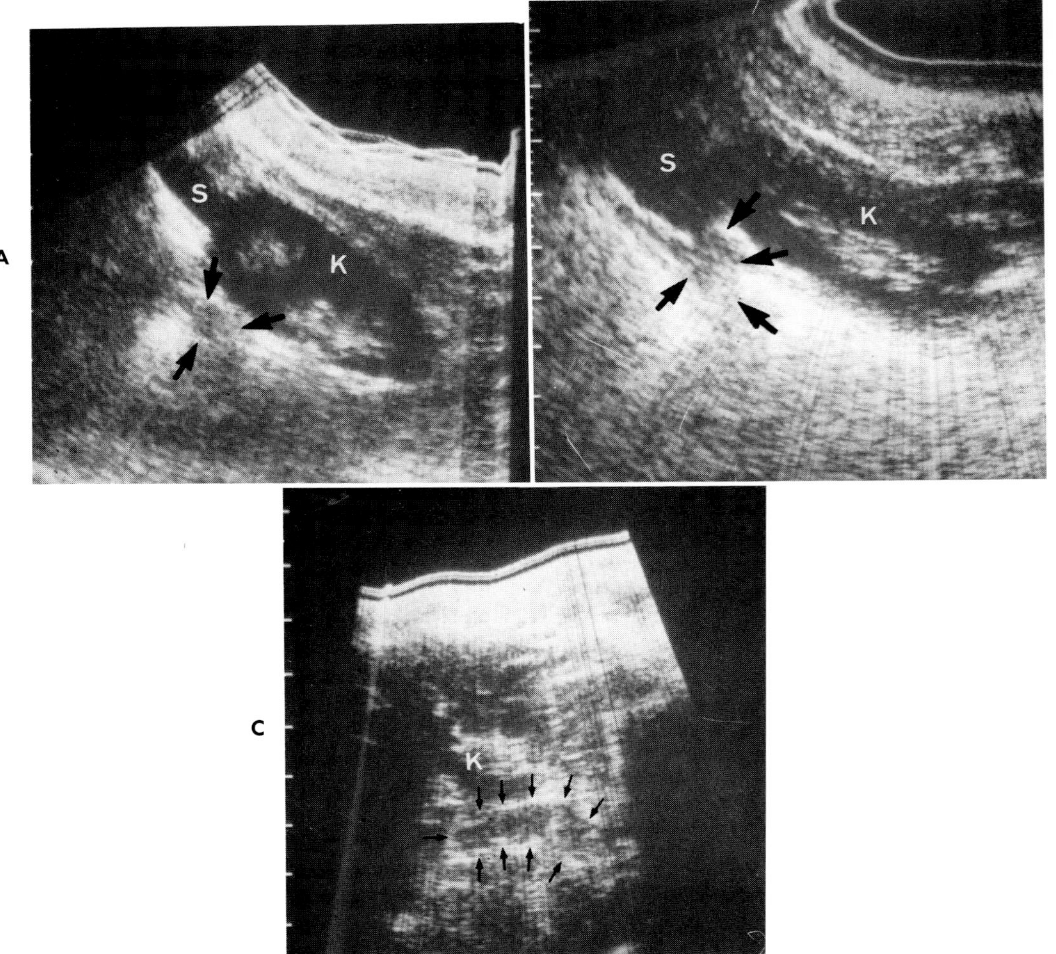

Fig. 19-12. A and **B,** Sagittal scans showing section of pancreatic tail *(arrows)* in front of upper pole of left kidney *(K)*. Pancreatic tail is in close relationship with lower pole of spleen *(S)*, as is kidney. Small spleen must not be confused with enlarged pancreatic tail. **C,** Transverse scan. Pancreatic tail *(arrows)* may be displayed on such scans. Differentiation from spleen is then easy, the more so since level of reflectivity is different in pancreas.

Our study of 130 normal ultrasonic pancreatic images showed that the shape of the pancreas follows three basic morphological types, that is, the "sausage," the "dumbbell," and the "tadpole" types (Fig. 19-15). In the sausage-type pancreas (Fig. 19-16) the neck is not well marked; the head, neck, and body are of about the same thickness. In a pancreas of the dumbbell type, the neck is thin and sharply separates the head from the body; these two are of about the same thickness (Figs. 19-14 and 19-17). In the pancreas of the tadpole type the thickness of the visible part of the gland diminishes regularly from the head to the tail (Fig. 19-18). An inverse tadpole type, with a thin pancreatic head and a progressive widening from head to neck and body (Figs. 19-4 and 19-19, *B* and *C*), is also possible. This is due to the deep impression that is sometimes produced by the

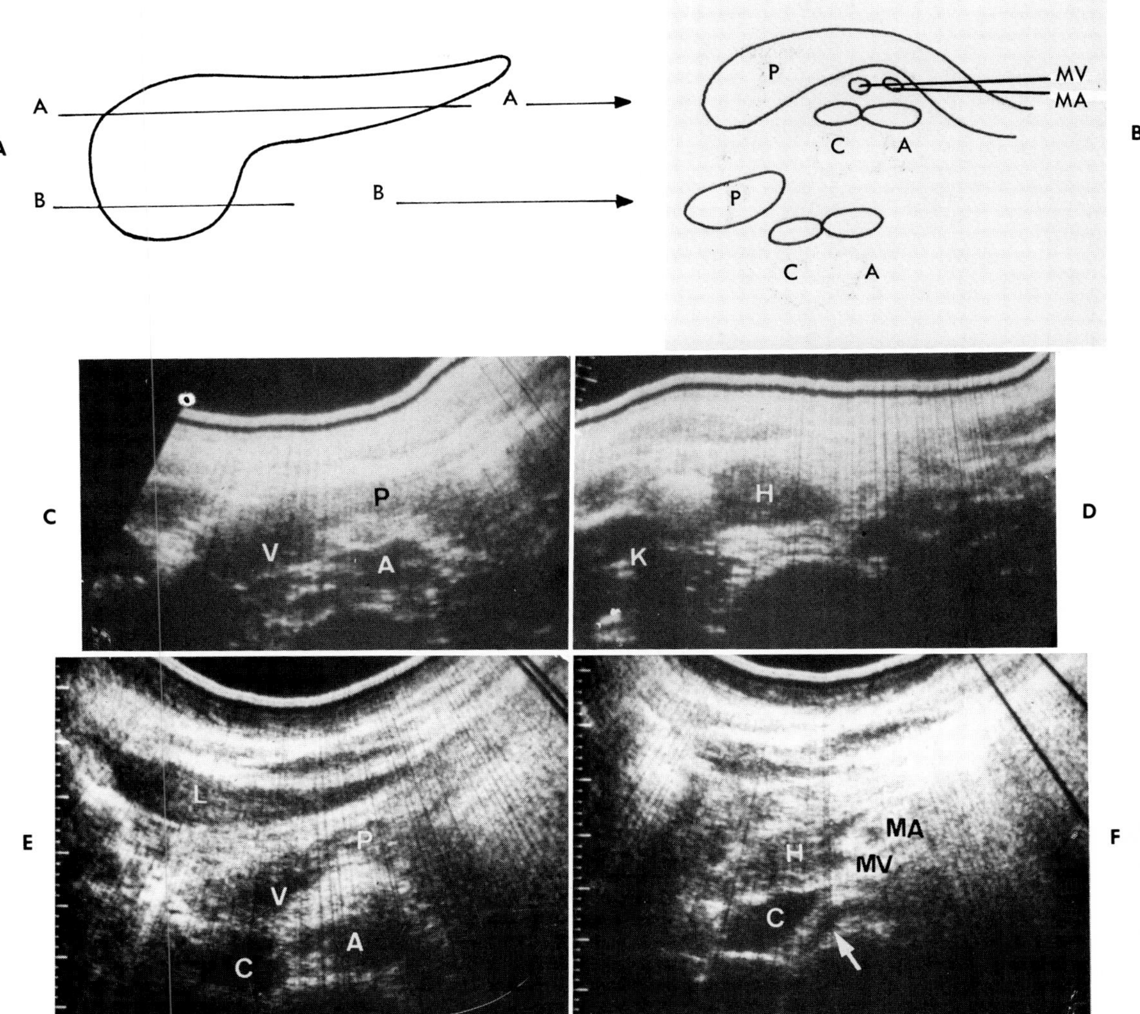

Fig. 19-13. Parallel transverse scans of pancreas. **A,** Scanning angles. Scan performed along line *AA* will display head, neck, and body of pancreas. More caudal scan performed along line *BB* will include only head of pancreas, which will appear in front of vena cava. **B,** Schematic drawing of sections. *P,* pancreas; *MV* and *MA,* mesenteric vessels; *C,* vena cava; *A,* aorta. **C** and **D,** Two parallel scans of pancreas. In **C,** global image is displayed. In **D,** which is more caudal, only head *(H)* is shown. *V,* splenoportal junction; *K,* right kidney. **E** and **F,** Another example of parallel scans. **F** passes through pancreatic head *(H)* only. *P,* pancreas; *L,* liver; *V,* portal vein; *MV* and *MA,* mesenteric vein and artery; *C,* vena cava; *A,* aorta; *arrow,* right renal artery.

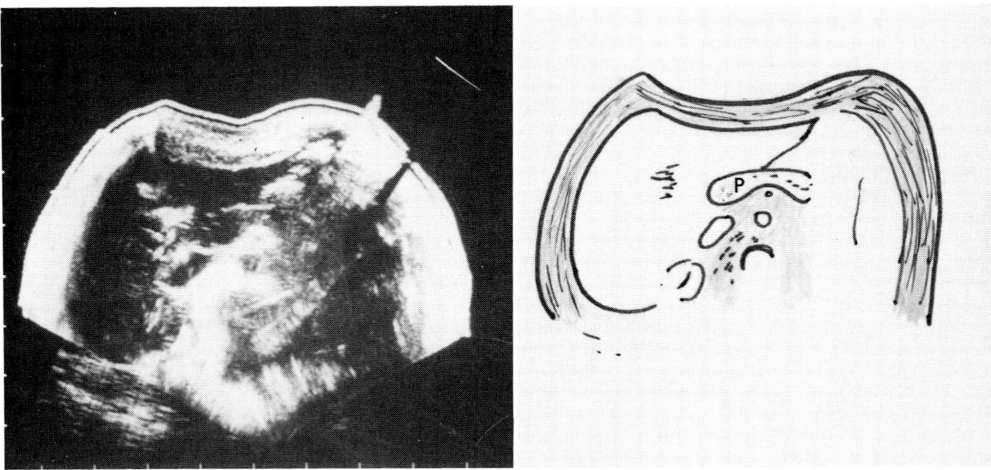

Fig. 19-14. Global transverse section of upper abdomen, displaying pancreas *(P)*. Note poor quality of image in left upper quadrant, due to colonic gas.

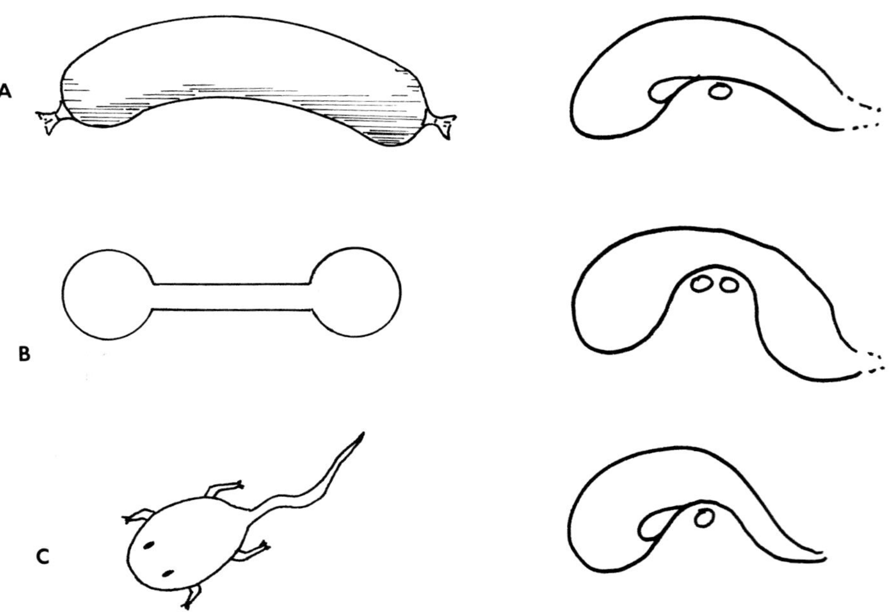

Fig. 19-15. Schematic representation of different types of pancreatic shapes. **A,** Sausage type. **B,** Dumbbell type. **C,** Tadpole type. Inverse tadpole type should be added.

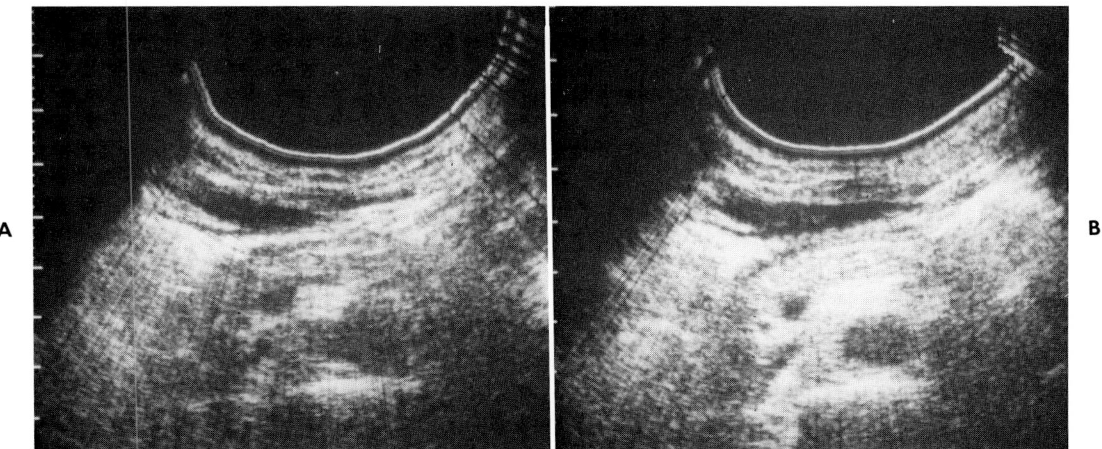

Fig. 19-16. Two examples of sausage-type pancreas. In **B,** note thin sonolucent strip, probably due to retroperitoneal fat, delineating anterior aspect of pancreas.

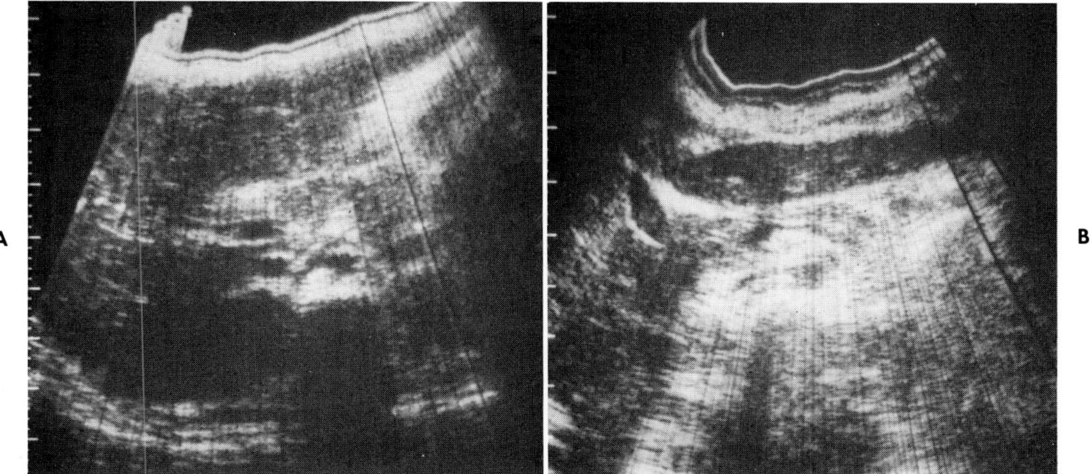

Fig. 19-17. Two examples of dumbbell-type pancreas. In **B,** note transverse section of common bile duct.

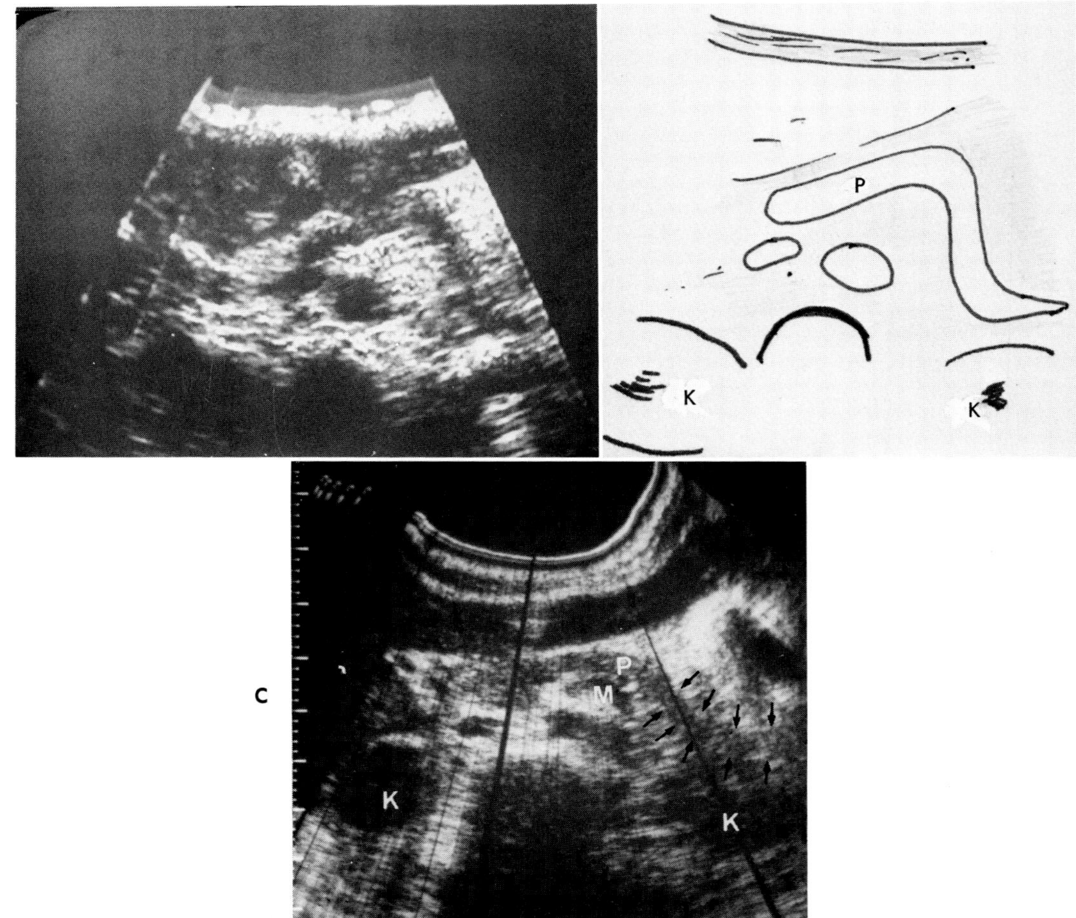

Fig. 19-18. Two examples of tadpole-type pancreas. **A** and **B,** Transverse section and schematic drawing. *P,* pancreas; *K,* kidney. **C,** Tail is outlined by *arrows. M,* SMA.

portal junction and trunk in the posterior aspect of the pancreatic head (Figs. 19-1 and 19-5). Rarely the anterior aspect of the pancreatic head may seem to bulge slightly forward; actually, such a relief corresponds to the section of the descending portion of the duodenum (Fig. 19-24, *A* and *B*). In our group of 130 normal pancreatic images, we found that 24% were sausage types, 34% dumbbell types, and 42% tadpole types.

The thin strip of the pancreatic tail is usually not displayed on transverse scans by the anterior approach because of colonic gas. That is why we emphasize the necessity for a posterior scan across the left kidney. (See Fig. 19-12.) Nevertheless, a caudal mass usually appears even through an anterior approach. The relatively easy display of the pancreatic tail, even if not enlarged, is a true advantage of computerized axial tomography over ultrasonography—or perhaps was until the recent development of new ultrasonic machines.

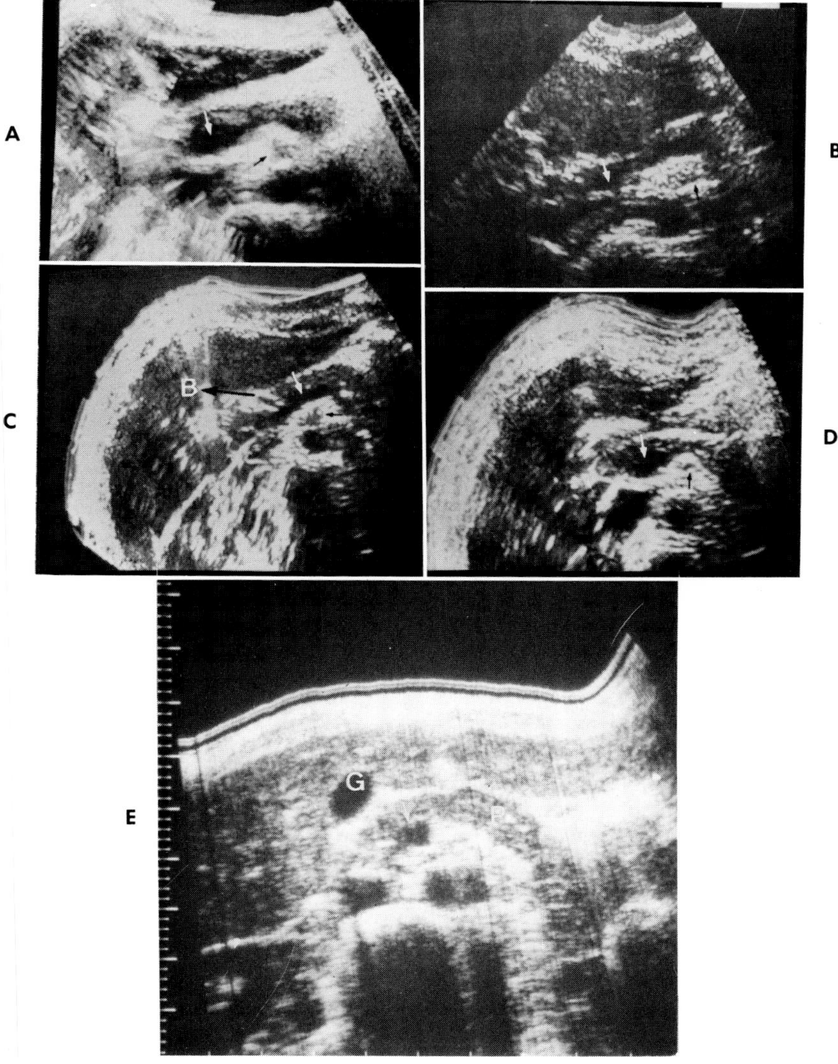

Fig. 19-19. Five normal pancreata in transverse section. **B, C,** and **E** are examples of inverted tadpole types. *Black arrows,* mesenteric artery; *white arrows,* splenoportal junction and splenic vein; *B,* section of intrapancreatic common bile duct.

SIZE

The size of the pancreas is variable. In our series of 130 normal pancreatic images, we measured the thickness of the different parts of the gland: head, neck, and corporeal-caudate area. The measurements were performed along axes perpendicular to the anterior pancreatic contour (Fig. 19-20). It was possible to measure the thickness of the head and neck in all 130 cases. However, in only fifty-five was the corporeal-caudate region sharply outlined. The results of these measurements are shown in Table 19-1 and Fig. 19-21.

Table 19-1. Pancreas thickness on transverse scans

	Minimal thickness (mm)	*Mean thickness (mm)*	*Maximal thickness (mm)*
Head (130 measurements)	11	17	30
Neck (130 measurements)	4	10	21
Corporeal-caudate area (55 measurements)	7	17	28 (32)

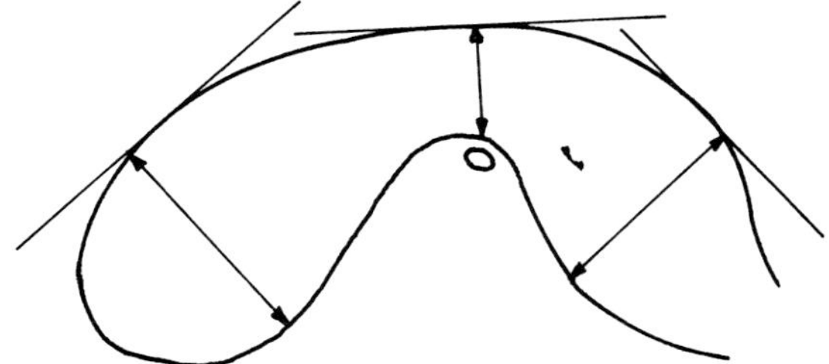

Fig. 19-20. Measurement of pancreatic thickness.

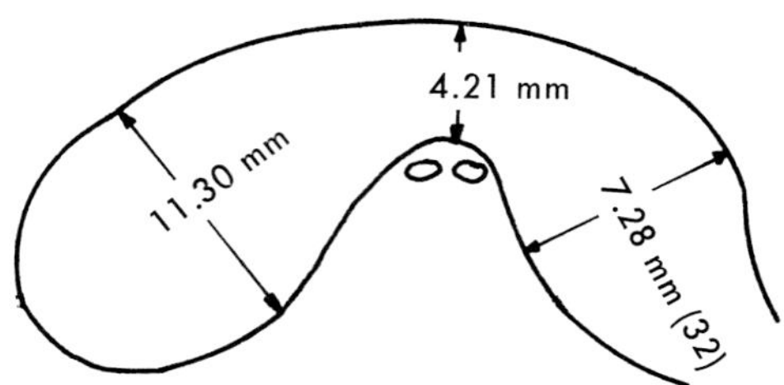

Fig. 19-21. Variations in thickness of normal pancreas.

These figures are well above those given by Laval-Jeantet and associates (1976) and slightly above those given by Haber and associates (1976). In a few dumb-bell-type pancreata we found a corporeal-caudate area thicker by 2 mm than the corresponding head. Since the maximal thickness of the head in our study was 30 mm, normal corporeal-caudate areas reaching a thickness of 32 mm are possible. This is also the case in pancreata of the inverse tadpole type. Whatever the morphological type and size of the pancreas, there is one other fundamental morphological feature, that is, the harmonious appearance of the gland as displayed on a transverse scan (Figs. 19-8 and 19-16 to 19-19). Any abnormal curvature of the contours or localized enlargement should be considered pathological. We did not, in our study, measure the craniocaudal dimension of the pancreatic head, since these data can be obtained from duodenography.

TISSUE ECHOPATTERN OF NORMAL PANCREAS

Transverse scans of the pancreatic head made with machines of the last generation often show a small tubular structure belonging to the intrapancreatic common bile duct (Figs. 19-3, 19-5, *A* and *B,* 19-17, *B,* and 19-19, *C*), as already seen in Chapter 15. This is not the only normal heterogeneity within the pancreatic tissue. Wirsung's duct, which will be dealt with again in Chapter 22, is indeed commonly displayed with last-generation machines. It appears as a narrow tubular element. (See Figs. 19-22 and 19-23.) The direction of the intrapancreatic common bile duct, which is either vertical or oblique, is quite different from that of Wirsung's duct. Besides, on a transverse scan the bile duct is cut along a much shorter portion than is Wirsung's duct. The two intrapancreatic canals are therefore unmistakable. However, there is another pitfall: a narrow sonolucent strip, probably representing retroperitoneal fat, is sometimes displayed along the anterior aspect

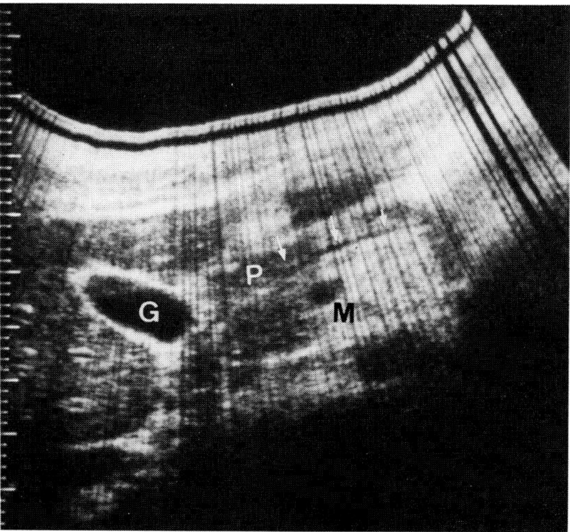

Fig. 19-22. Sagittal section of Wirsung's duct *(arrows).* Arterial element might be hypothesized in identifying that tubular structure, but its situation is too central in pancreatic head for such an assumption. *P,* pancreas; *G,* gallbladder; *M,* mesenteric vessels.

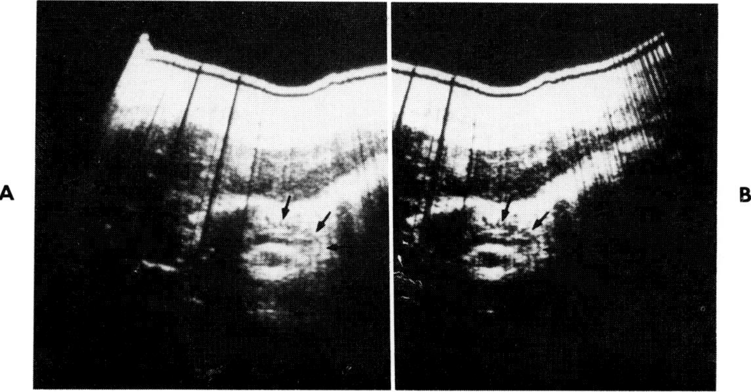

Fig. 19-23. Sagittal section of Wirsung's duct *(arrows)* in 13-year-old girl. **A,** Low-contrast imaging. **B,** Sharp contrast.

of the pancreas (Fig. 19-16); this pattern, which is anterior and not intrapancreatic, like Wirsung's duct, should not be misinterpreted. Except for this, the normal pancreatic tissue possesses a solid, homogeneous pattern. With the machines of former generations and with real time, the pancreatic tissue reflectivity used to be not very different from that of the liver: equal, slightly inferior, or, less often, slightly superior. However, with the machines of the last generation, probably because of a different dynamic range, the level of reflectivity in the pancreas is often frankly above that of the liver (e.g., Figs. 19-3, 19-5, 19-7, and 19-16). An intense level of reflectivity in the pancreas cannot therefore be considered as pathological in the absence of heterogeneity.

Another element among the criteria of normality to be taken into account is

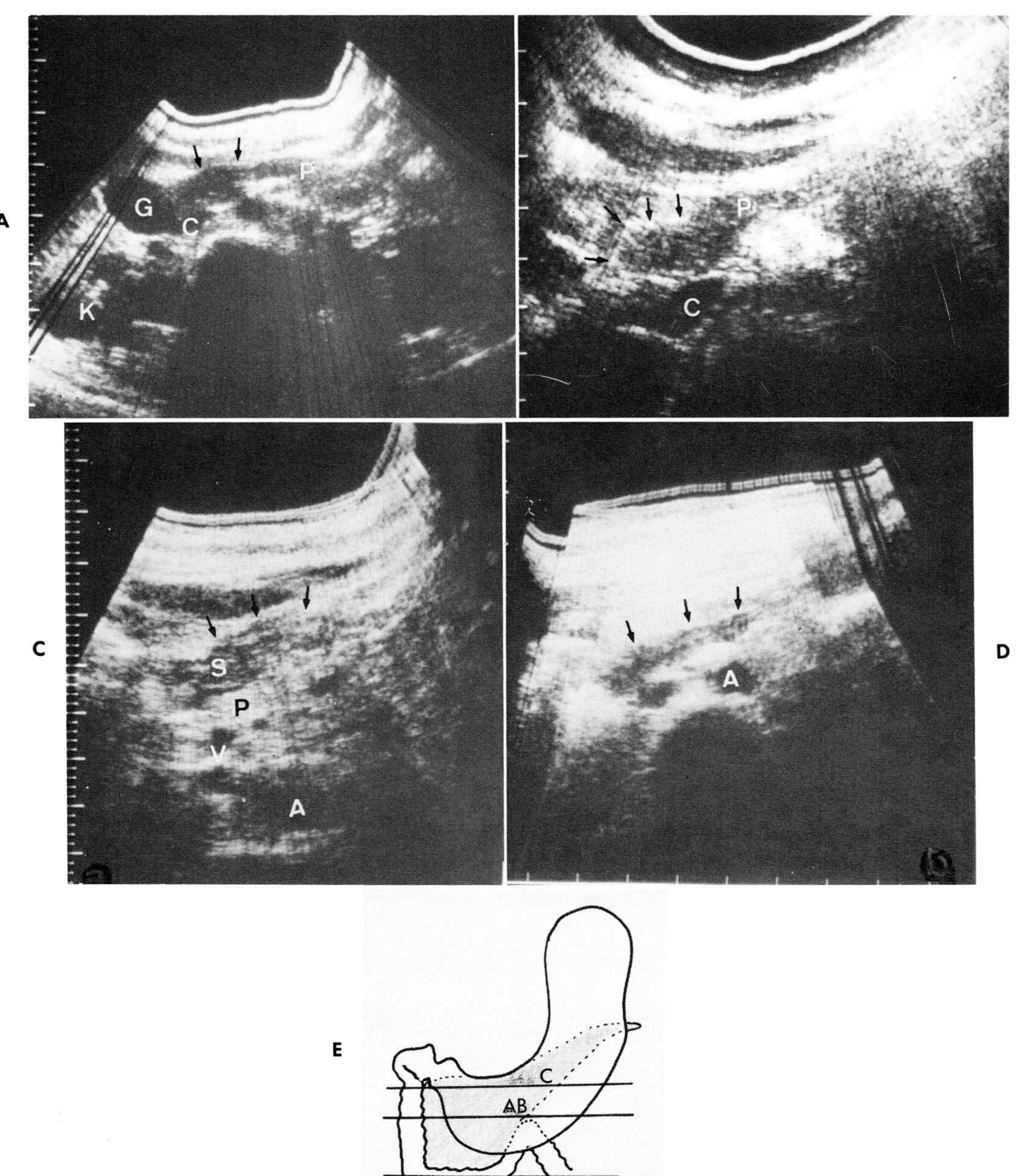

Fig. 19-24. Confusing gastric and duodenal images. **A** and **B,** Apparent enlarged pancreatic head. Actually, bulges *(arrows)* represent transverse sections of descending portion of duodenum. *P,* pancreas; *G,* gallbladder; *C,* vena cava; *K,* kidney. **C,** Apparent global section of pancreas, which in reality is stomach (*S* and *arrows*) in nonfasting patient. Pancreas is more reflective and is easily identified when vascular landmarks *(V)* are considered. *A,* aorta. **D,** False pancreatic image *(arrows),* corresponding to section of transverse portion of duodenum. **E,** Explanation of false images: scanning angles in **A** to **D.** Similar pattern may arise from transverse colon.

the condition of the vena cava and the superior mesenteric vein. Pancreatic enlargement can cause compression of the veins. If this occurs, the mesenteric vein may flatten before the vena cava does. *The absence of an image of the mesenteric vein on multiple real-time sagittal scans is a pathological feature.* The evaluation of the vena cava requires Valsalva's maneuver.

Following are the different morphological features to be evaluated in examining a pancreas ultrasonographically:

- General shape
- Harmony, sharpness, and smoothness of contours
- Thickness
- Tissue echopattern: homogeneity and level of reflectivity

PANCREATIC RELATION TO STOMACH AND DUODENUM AS A SOURCE OF PITFALLS

The stomach and duodenum (and, of course, the transverse colon, also) are often displayed on pancreatic sections, especially in nonfasting patients (Figs. 19-8, *E,* 19-9, *A,* and 19-24). They should not be misinterpreted as pancreatic tissue (or as pathological pancreatic tissue). (See Chapter 25.) An empty stomach or duodenum may appear in section as a bull's-eye image (Fig. 16-20, *C*). In case of doubt, the examination should be repeated with the patient fasting or, at least, a few hours later: a gastric or duodenal image then has another pattern, whereas a pancreatic image remains unchanged. Another important point to remember in correct identification is the study of vascular landmarks (Fig. 19-24, *C*).

REFERENCES

Barnett, E., and Morley, P.: Abdominal echography, Borough Green, England, 1974, Butterworth & Co. (Publishers), Ltd.

Goldberg, B. B., Kotler, M. N., Ziskin, M. C., and Waxham, R. D.: Diagnostic uses of ultrasound, New York, 1975, Grune & Stratton, Inc.

Haber, K., Freimanis, A. K., and Asher, M. N.: Demonstration and dimensional analysis of the normal pancreas with gray-scale echography, Am. J. Roentgenol. **126:**624-628, 1976.

Hancke, S., Holm, H. H., and Koch, F.: Ultrasonically guided percutaneous fine needle biopsy of the pancreas, Surg. Gynecol. Obstet. **140:**361-364, 1975.

Hassani, N.: Ultrasonography of the abdomen, Heidelberg, Germany, 1976, Springer-Verlag.

Laval-Jeantet, P., Gardeur, P., Tabourg, J., Monnier, J. P., and Bigot, J. M.: Anatomie échographique du pancréas normal, J. Radiol. Electrol. Med. Nucl. **57:**149-155, 1976.

Leopold, G. R., and Asher, W. M.: Fundamentals of abdominal and pelvic ultrasonography, Philadelphia, 1975, W. B. Saunders Co.

Weill, F., Aucant, D., Bourgoin, A., Eisenscher, A., and Gallinet, D.: Ultrasonic visualization of abdominal veins, Second European Congress, Munich, Germany, 1975, Abstract No. 103.

Weill, F., Aucant, D., Bourgoin, A., Eisenscher, A., and Gallinet, D.: Les repères vasculaires dans l'exploration ultrasonore du pancréas, J. Radiol. Electrol. Med. Nucl. **55:**873-876, 1974.

Weill, F., Becker, J. C., Kraehenbuhl, J. R., Heriot, G., and Walter, J. P.: Clinical atlas of ultrasonic radiography, Paris, 1973, Masson & Cie., Editeurs.

Weill, F., Schraub, A., Eisenscher, A., and Bourgoin, A.: Ultrasonography of the normal pancreas, Radiology **123:**417-423, 1977.

CHAPTER 20

ACUTE PANCREATITIS

The clinical diagnosis of acute pancreatitis is often considered but may remain unconfirmed for a long time in the absence of emergency ultrasonography. Acute pancreatitis is responsible for changes in the size, shape, and echopattern of the pancreas.

SPECIAL TECHNICAL CONDITIONS

Ultrasonography in acute pancreatitis is an emergency examination, often performed on a patient with severe abdominal pain and peripheral vascular collapse. Therefore the positional artifices previously described cannot be employed, in particular the upright position. There may be early adynamic ileus, and thus more intestinal gas will be present. Moreover, a patient with acute pancreatitis is also often obese. Despite all these unfavorable circumstances, failure in the ultrasonic examination of acute pancreatitis is uncommon because of the first morphological change, the pancreatic swelling.

PANCREATIC ENLARGEMENT

Inflammatory swelling gives rise to three types of enlargement: giant, global harmonious, and partial enlargement.

Giant enlargement

Pancreatic swelling can increase the thickness of the gland three or four times. The initial shape of the pancreas disappears, and the swollen pancreas can become spherical or look like a football and have a spheroidal or ovoid section. (See Figs. 20-1 to 20-4.)

Global harmonious enlargement

In the case of global harmonious enlargement the pancreas retains its initial shape, but every part of it is enlarged. Whatever its initial morphological type, the swelling produces a sausage shape (Figs. 20-2, 20-5, 20-6, and 20-14). The thickness of the gland may reach 5 cm at the isthmus.

Partial enlargement

In the case of partial enlargement there is only a nonspecific enlargement of the pancreatic head or corporeal-caudate area, similar to the enlargement seen in pancreatic carcinoma (Figs. 20-7 to 20-10 and 20-13).

• • •

In all these types of pancreatic swelling, an associated sign may be encountered —compression of the superior mesenteric vein and the vena cava (Fig. 20-5, *D*).

Text continued on p. 316.

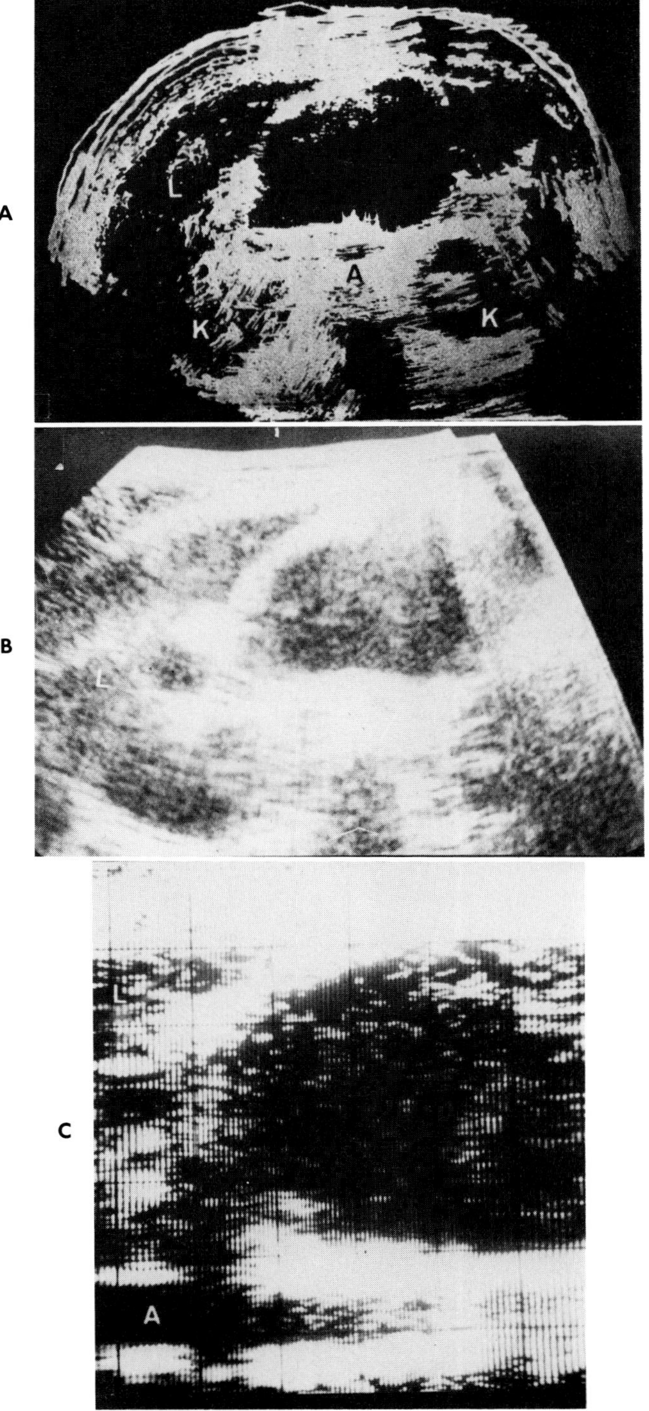

Fig. 20-1. Acute pancreatitis with giant pseudocystic swelling. **A,** Transverse scan in bistable imaging. In front of aorta *(A),* large transparent mass is outlined. *L,* liver; *K,* kidney. **B,** Transverse scan in gray scale showing, however, many echoes scattered amid this mass. **C,** Semisolid echopattern is also displayed on this sagittal real-time scan. A few days later, surgery showed swelling to have completely disappeared; thus it was due only to edema.

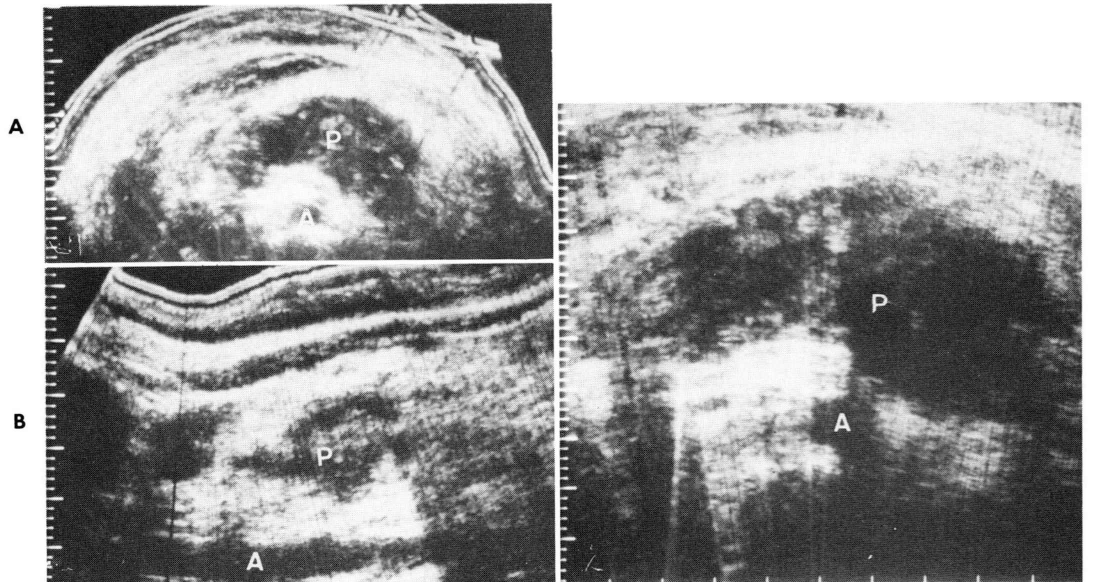

Fig. 20-2. Acute pancreatitis with giant swelling. **A,** Transverse scan showing enlarged pancreas *(P)*. *A,* aorta. **B,** Sagittal scan. **C,** Magnified parallel scan displaying sonolucent pseudocystic echopattern of enlarged pancreatic body *(P)*.

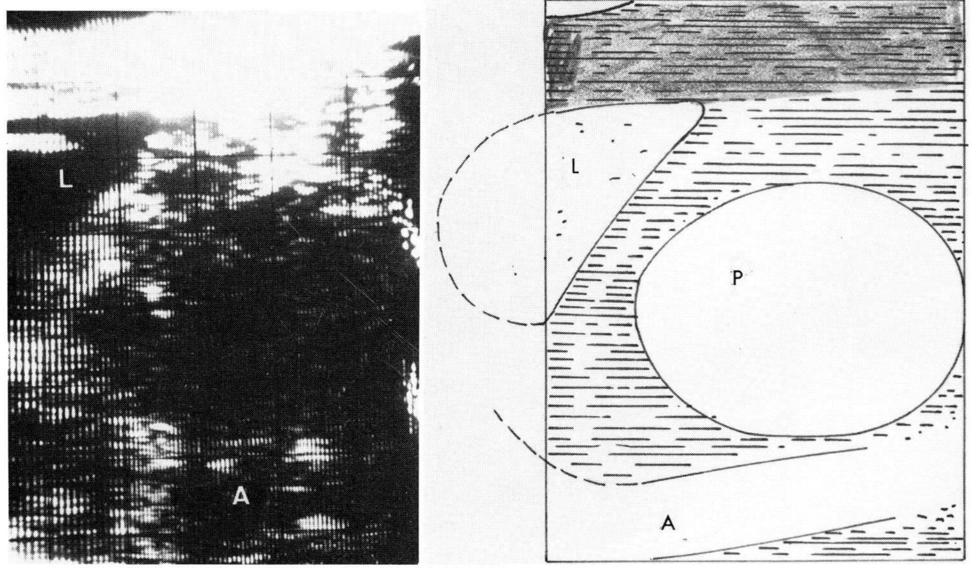

Fig. 20-3. Acute pancreatitis with giant pseudocystic swelling. This real-time sagittal scan and its schematic representation show sonolucent mass in front of aorta *(A)* and behind liver *(L)*. There are rare scattered echoes of low intensity. Posterior interface is not reinforced. This pattern is typical of pancreatic edema. *P,* pancreas.

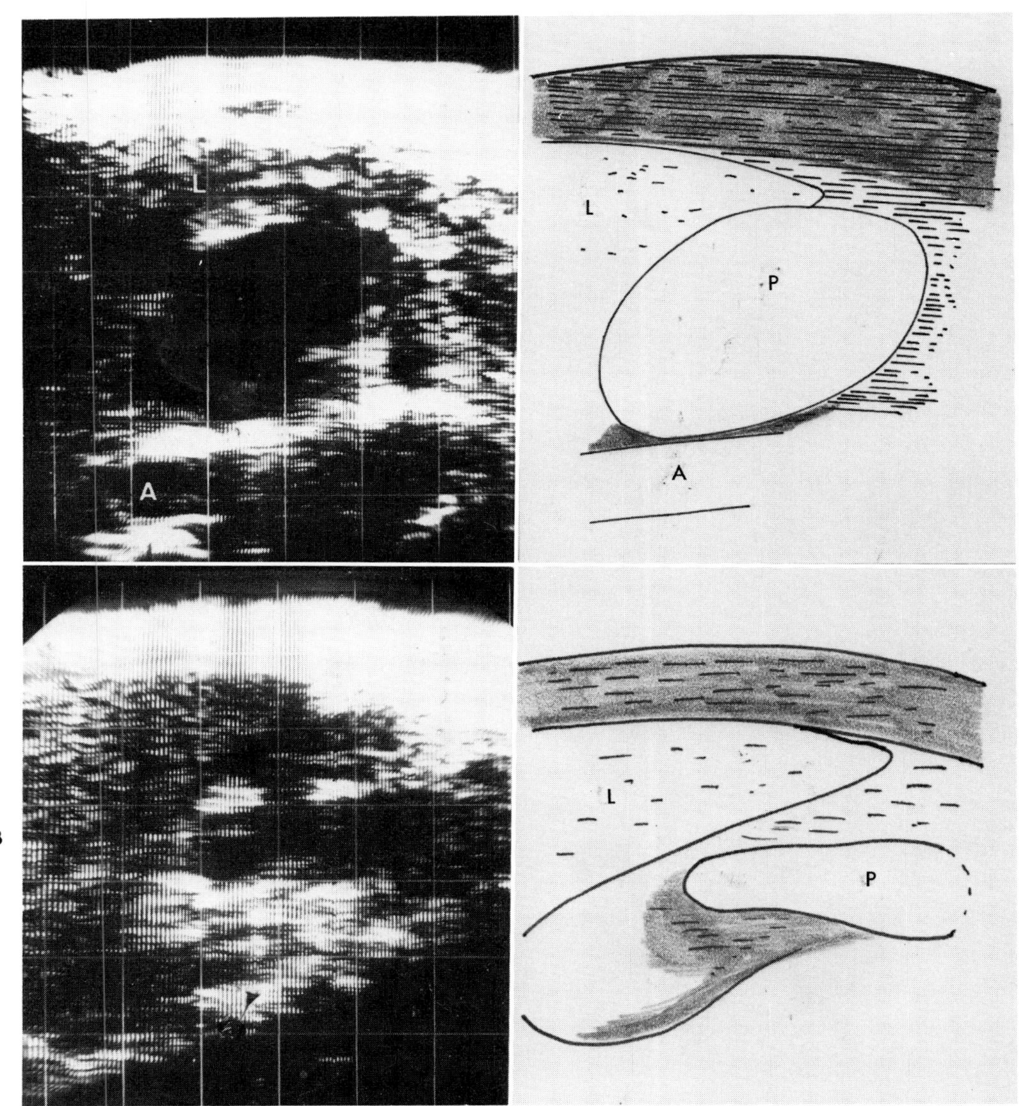

Fig. 20-4. Acute pancreatitis with giant pseudocystic swelling. **A,** Sagittal real-time scan and schematic drawing again showing rounded sonolucent mass in front of aorta *(A)* and behind liver *(L)*. There are no scattered echoes; posterior interface is sharp, as posterior wall image in true cyst would be. **B,** Two days later, mass had almost completely disappeared. *P,* pancreas.

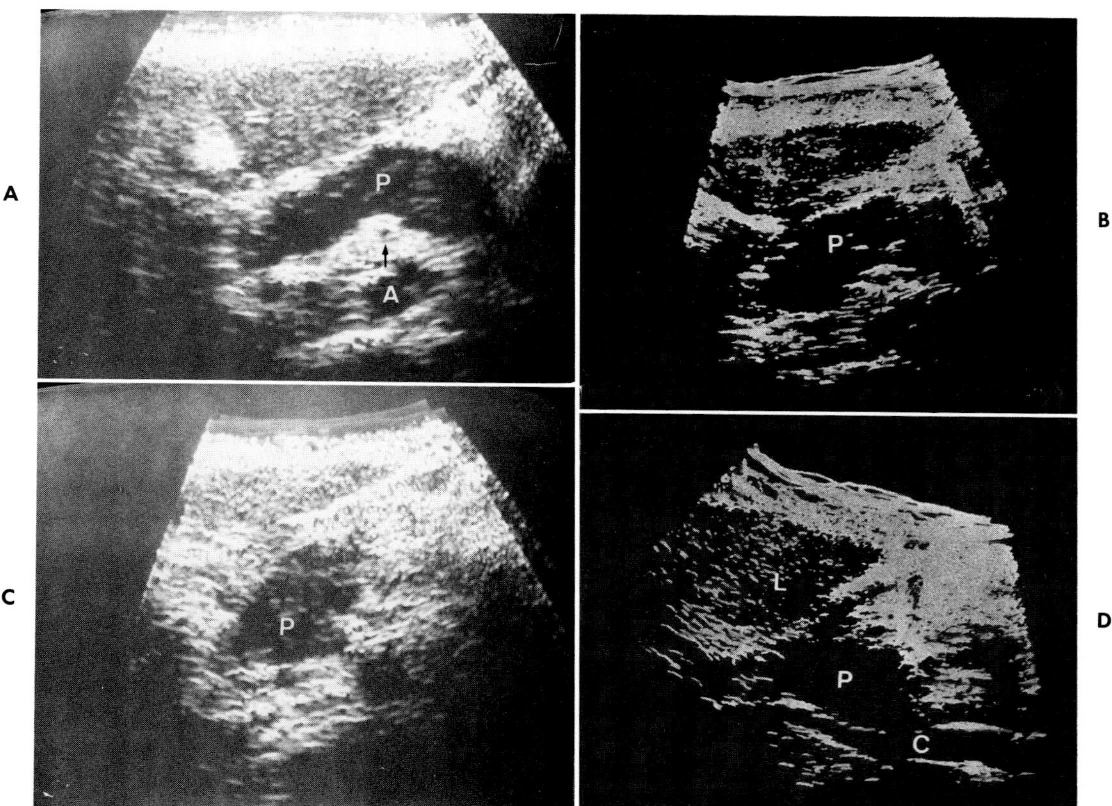

Fig. 20-5. Acute pancreatitis with global harmonious swelling. **A,** Transverse scan in gray scale showing sonolucent pancreatic tissue *(P)*. Pancreatic reflectivity is much lower than hepatic reflectivity. Isthmic and corporeal-caudate enlargements are striking. *A,* aorta; *arrow,* mesenteric vessels. **B,** Same scan in bistable imaging. **C,** Parallel, more caudal scan displaying only swollen pancreatic head *(P)*. **D,** Sagittal bistable scan showing, behind right hepatic lobe *(L)*, image of enlarged pancreatic head depressing vena cava *(C)*.

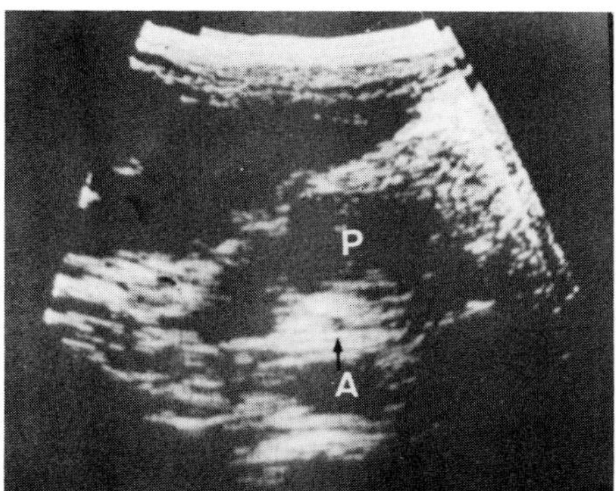

Fig. 20-6. Transverse scan showing harmonious global enlargement during hepatitis. *P,* pancreas; *A,* aorta; *arrow,* SMA.

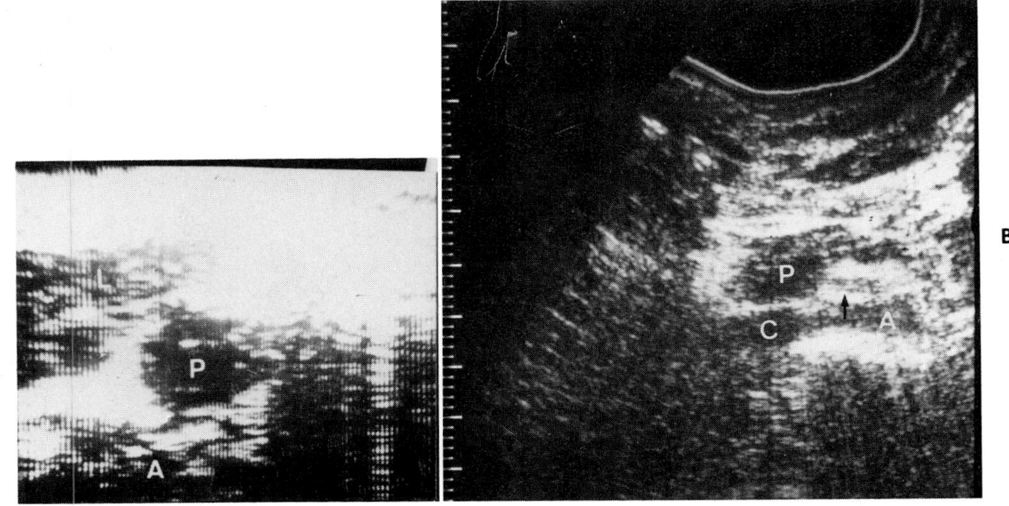

Fig. 20-7. Acute pancreatitis with partial swelling. **A,** Sagittal scan in real time showing rounded section of enlarged pancreatic head *(P)* outlined between liver *(L)* and aorta *(A)*. **B,** Transverse contact scan also showing cephalic enlargement. General shape of pancreas is distorted. Bulge in anterior aspect of neck displays polycyclic anterior outline. Area of sonolucence appears in posterior part of head. *C,* vena cava; *arrow,* mesenteric vessels; *P,* pancreas.

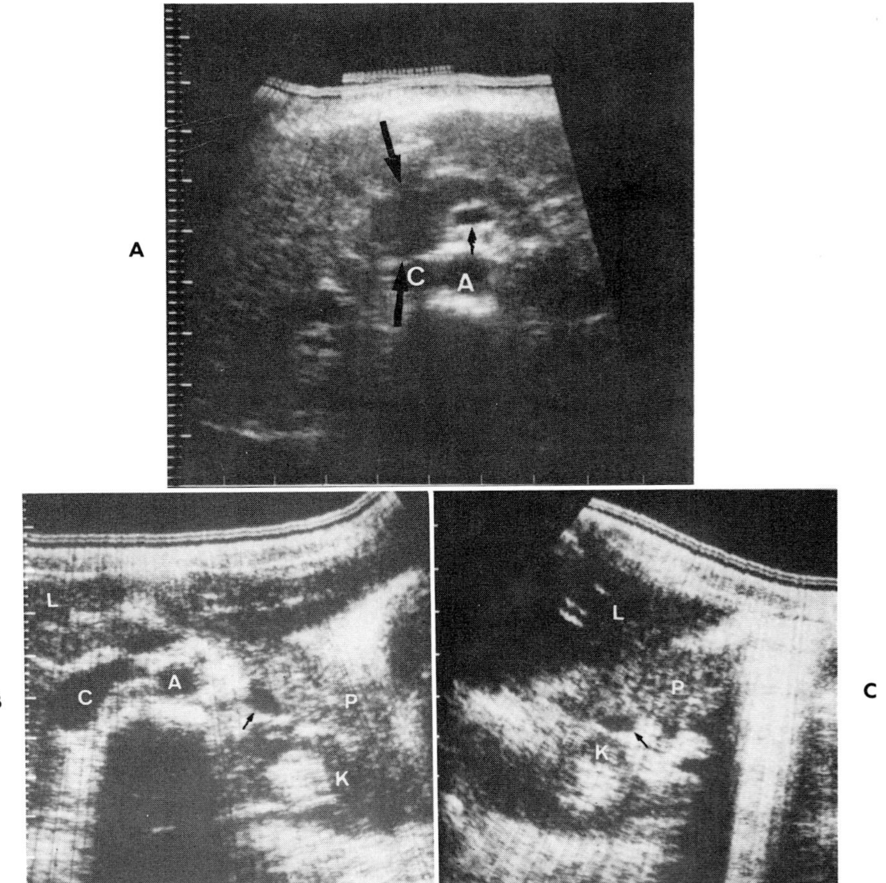

Fig. 20-8. **A,** Transverse scan in a case of acute swelling of pancreatic head. *C,* vena cava; *A,* aorta; *large arrows,* pancreas; *small arrow,* mesenteric vessels. **B** and **C,** Transverse and sagittal scans showing caudate swelling in a case of subacute recurrence on chronic reflective pancreatitis. *P,* pancreas; *K,* left kidney; *arrow,* splenic vein; *L,* liver. (**A** courtesy Dr. F. Winsberg, Montreal.)

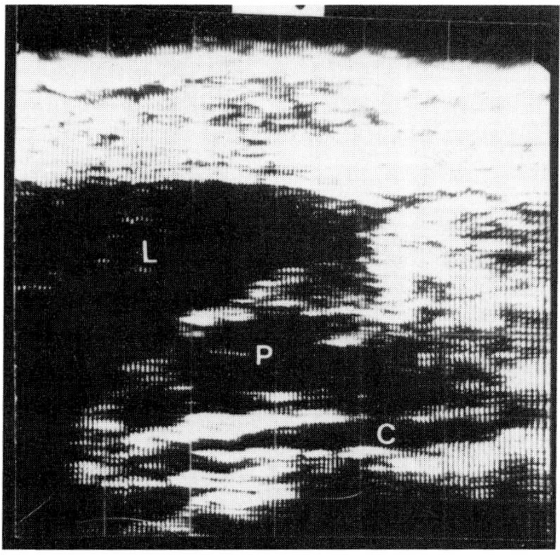

Fig. 20-9. Acute pancreatitis. This sagittal real-time scan shows head of pancreas *(P)* between liver *(L)* and vena cava *(C)*. Pancreatic head is enlarged, and its echopattern is sonolucent with rare scattered echoes. This semisolid swelling is typical of Type II.

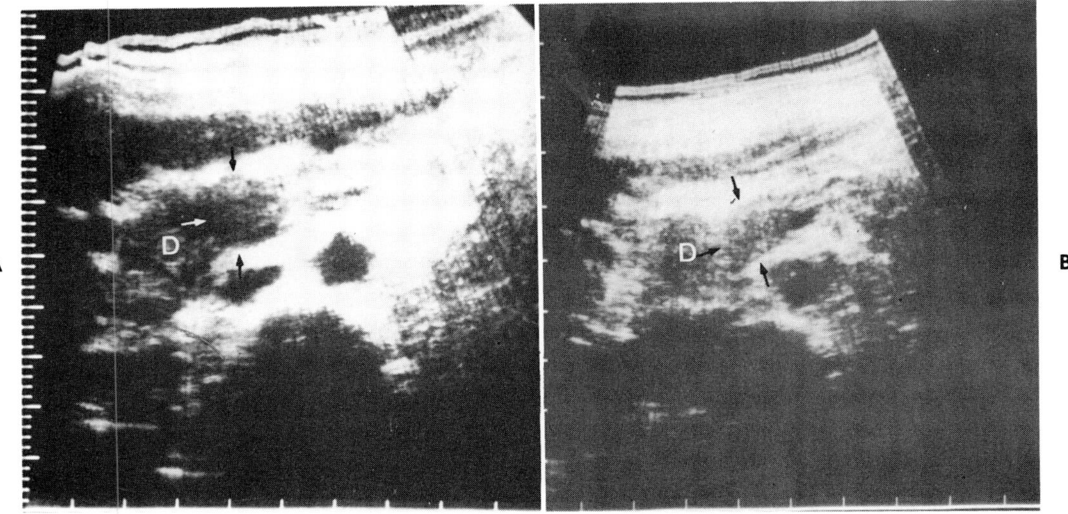

Fig. 20-10. Acute pancreatitis with partial swelling. **A,** Transverse scan showing rounded, enlarged, sonolucent pancreatic head *(arrows)*. *D,* duodenum. **B,** Follow-up 3 weeks later. Volume of pancreatic head, as well as reflectivity, is normal again.

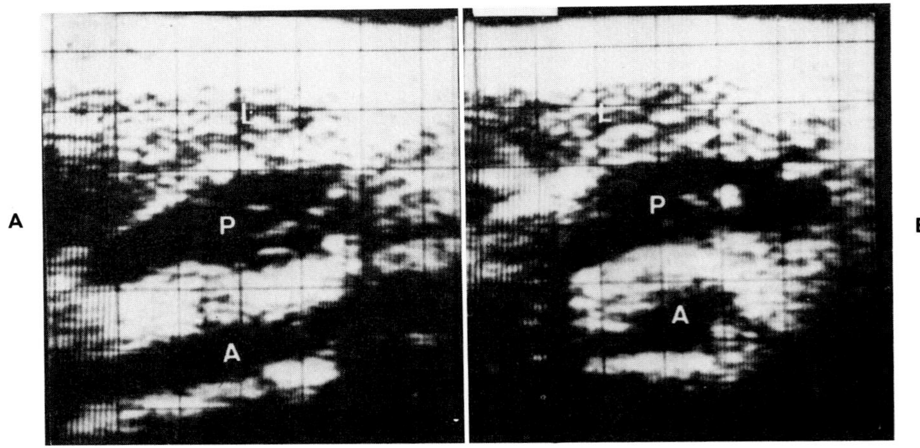

Fig. 20-11. Acute pancreatitis. **A,** Sagittal scan in real time showing enlarged pancreatic neck *(P)* of semisolid pattern (Type II) between aorta *(A)* and liver *(L)*. **B,** Transverse scan, also in real time, displaying pancreatic enlargement *(P)* involving head and neck.

CONTOURS

The contours remain well delineated and smooth. They are harmonious in a global enlargement and less harmonious in a partial enlargement, since in this type a polycyclic outline may occur (Figs. 20-9 to 20-11). When there is edema, as will be seen in dealing with the echopattern of acute pancreatitis, the posterior contour may be reinforced.

TISSUE ECHOPATTERN

In the forty-nine* (Weill and colleagues, 1976) cases of acute pancreatitis that we had the opportunity to study, we observed different types of echopatterns. In four cases the tissue echopattern was of solid type and very reflective. This was probably acute pancreatitis superimposed on chronic pancreatitis. (See Fig. 20-8, *B* and *C*.) In one case, however, this solid, reflective echopattern preceded necro-

*Now sixty.

Fig. 20-12. Necrotizing acute pancreatitis: constitution of pseudocyst. **A,** Sagittal real-time scan of right upper quadrant showing pancreatic mass *(P)* of heterogeneous pattern behind right hepatic lobe *(L)*. Scattered echoes are of higher intensity than in previous cases. **B,** New scan, made a day later, displaying increase in swelling. Echopattern is more heterogeneous. Such a rapid change of heterogeneous pattern is characteristic for necrosis. *A,* aorta. **C,** Transverse scan of abdomen, made 6 days later, showing rounded mass *(arrow)* with posterior interface reinforcement is consistent with liquid mass in front of large vessels. There are small reflective areas scatttered amid mass, which constitutes pseudocyst with floating debris. *L,* liver; *K,* kidney. **D,** Same scan in gray scale. **E,** New transverse scan of upper abdomen, made 9 days later (i.e., 2 weeks after first scan), displaying frank image of pseudocyst. Volume of collection has increased. **F,** Sagittal scan, made at same moment, showing low extension of pseudocyst in front of vena cava *(C)*.

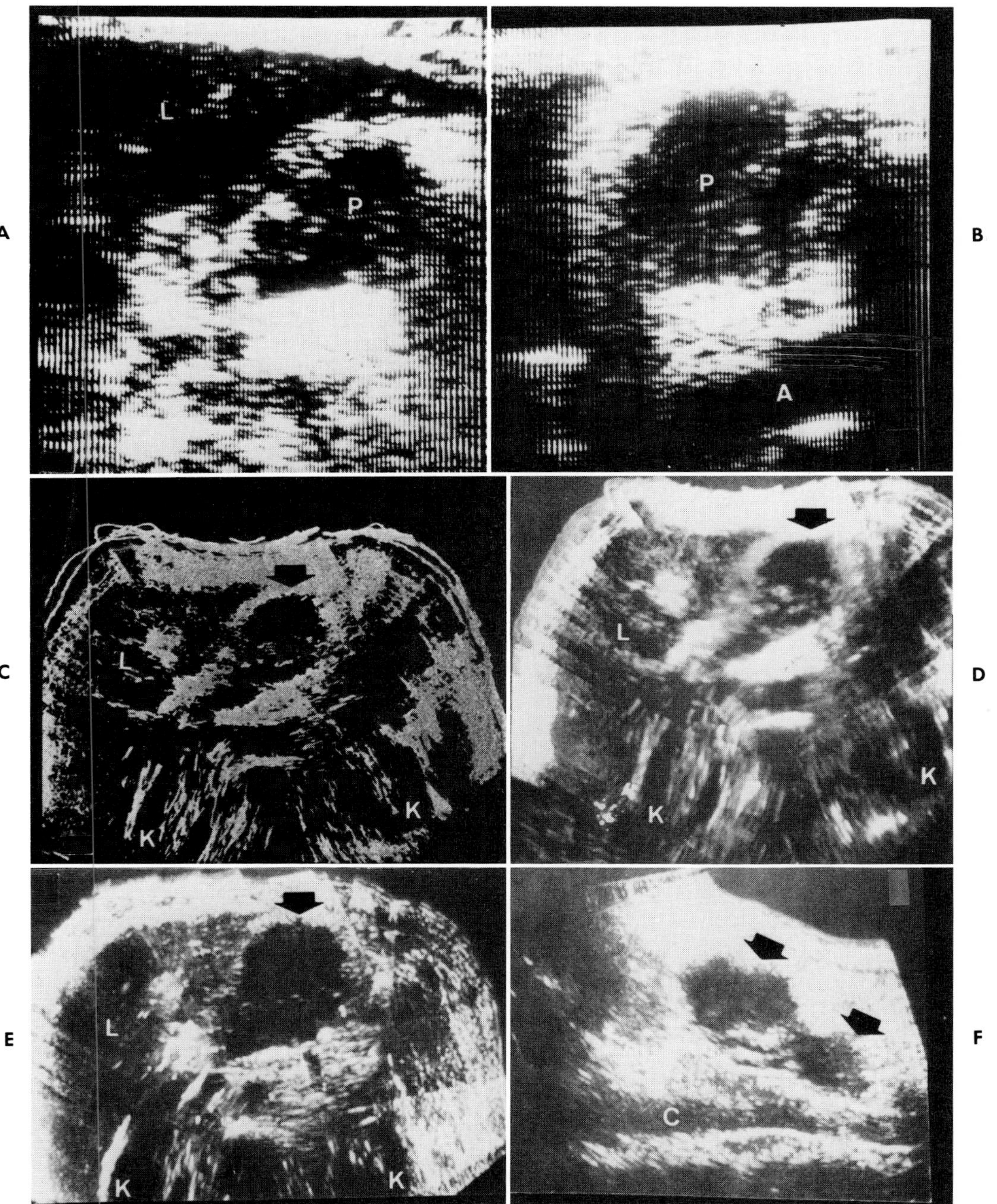

Fig. 20-12. For legend see opposite page.

sis. In all other cases the echopattern was basically sonolucent and belonged to three different types:

1. The first type (Type I) possesses a pseudoliquid echopattern without tissue echoes or with rare, scattered echoes (Figs. 20-1 to 20-4). This type of echopattern, described by Sokoloff and co-workers (1974), can mimic a pseudocyst, particularly since the posterior contour may appear frankly reinforced (Fig. 20-4). The most important consideration in such cases is their evolution, which is absolutely different from that of a pseudocyst. This type belongs to edema.

2. The second type of echopattern in acute pancreatitis (Type II) is also sonolucent, with scattered tissue echoes of low intensity, more or less grouped, and giving rise to a typical semisolid pattern (Figs. 20-5, 20-9 to 20-11, and 20-14). Confusion with a pseudocyst is not likely with this type of echopattern.

3. The third type of echopattern in acute pancreatitis (Type III) is much more heterogeneous. Liquid, semisolid, and solid areas are combined. This constellation requires one to suspect a necrotizing process. (See Figs. 20-12 and 20-16.)

In the sixty cases of sonolucent acute pancreatitis that we studied, Type II was by far the most frequent, with a rate of roughly 60%. Types I and III amounted to about 20% each.

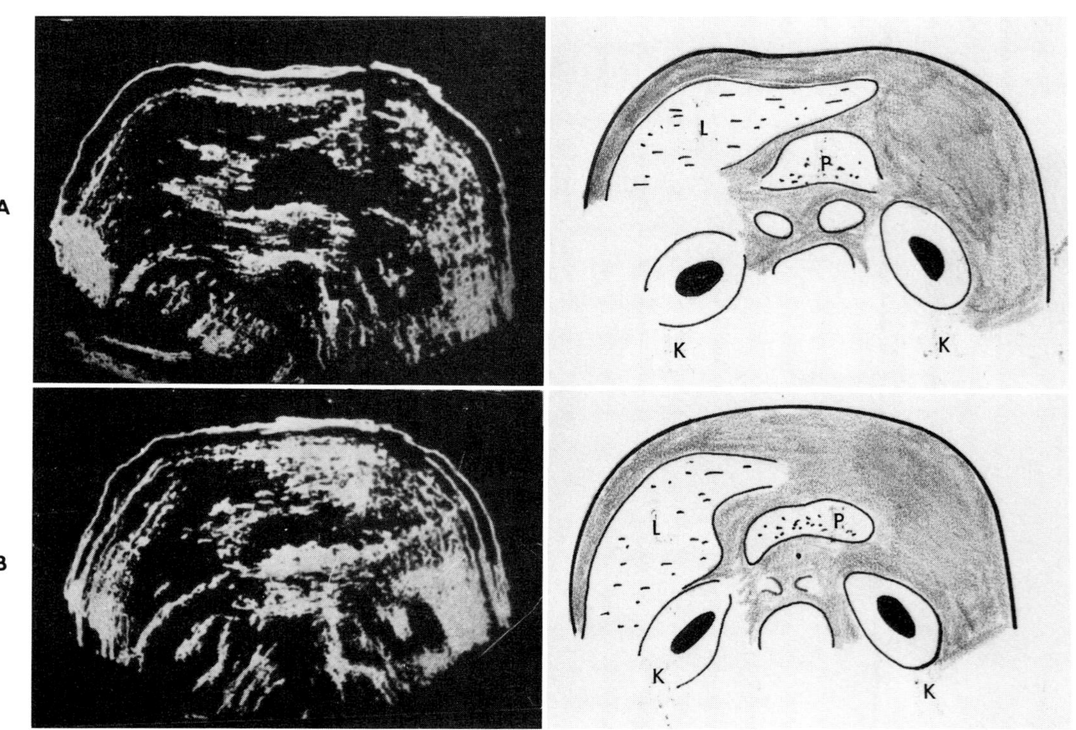

Fig. 20-13. Evolution of acute pancreatitis. **A,** Transverse scan and schematic drawing of upper abdomen showing important swelling of pancreas *(P)* between liver *(L)* and the large vessels. *K,* kidney. **B,** Identical scan and schematic representation taken 3 days later displaying important decrease in pancreatic volume.

Last, an *associated sign* to remember is the possible finding of a small amount of ascites or a pleural effusion.

EVOLUTION

In cases in which the diagnosis of acute pancreatitis does not lead to immediate surgery, it is of utmost importance to follow up the pancreatic changes by daily ultrasonic examinations. There are different modalities of evolution:

1. First, there may be a decrease in the swelling. The enlarged pancreas changes back to its normal shape and size. The most marked swellings (i.e., the giant type) decrease the most rapidly. Such a decrease, which is a sign of favorable evolution, also corroborates retrospectively the diagnosis of acute pancreatitis. (See Figs. 20-1, 20-4, 20-13, and 20-14.) Such corroboration is not without clinical interest, since in acute pancreatitis the biological abnormalities may be delayed. The decrease in swelling is accompanied by the return to normal diameter of the vena cava and the superior mesenteric vein (Fig. 20-14).

2. Less commonly, successive examinations show the opposite evolution. Usually, in the first hours of the acute stage, edema is already present. Exceptionally the swelling may be delayed, and the first examination then shows a pancreas of normal size. In such cases, successive ultrasonograms show the progressive swelling of the pancreas. (See Fig. 20-15.)

3. Another pattern of evolution occurs with necrosis. This pattern includes a Type III echopattern, as well as rapid change at successive examinations. If the clinical features do not directly lead to surgery, it is possible to observe the formation of a pseudocyst (Figs. 20-12 and 20-16). This process will be studied again in Chapter 21.

Following are the ultrasonic signs of acute pancreatitis:

Contours
- Homogeneous and regular
- Well delineated
- Smooth

Swelling
- Global giant
- Global harmonious
- Partial

Tissue echopattern
- Pseudoliquid (Type I)
- Semisolid (Type II)
- Heterogeneous (Type III)
- Solid and reflective (exceptional)

Incidental sign: Compression of vena cava and mesenteric vein

Following are the possible modalities of evolution:

Decrease of swelling
Progressive swelling
Acute necrosis
Progressive necrosis with formation of a pseudocyst

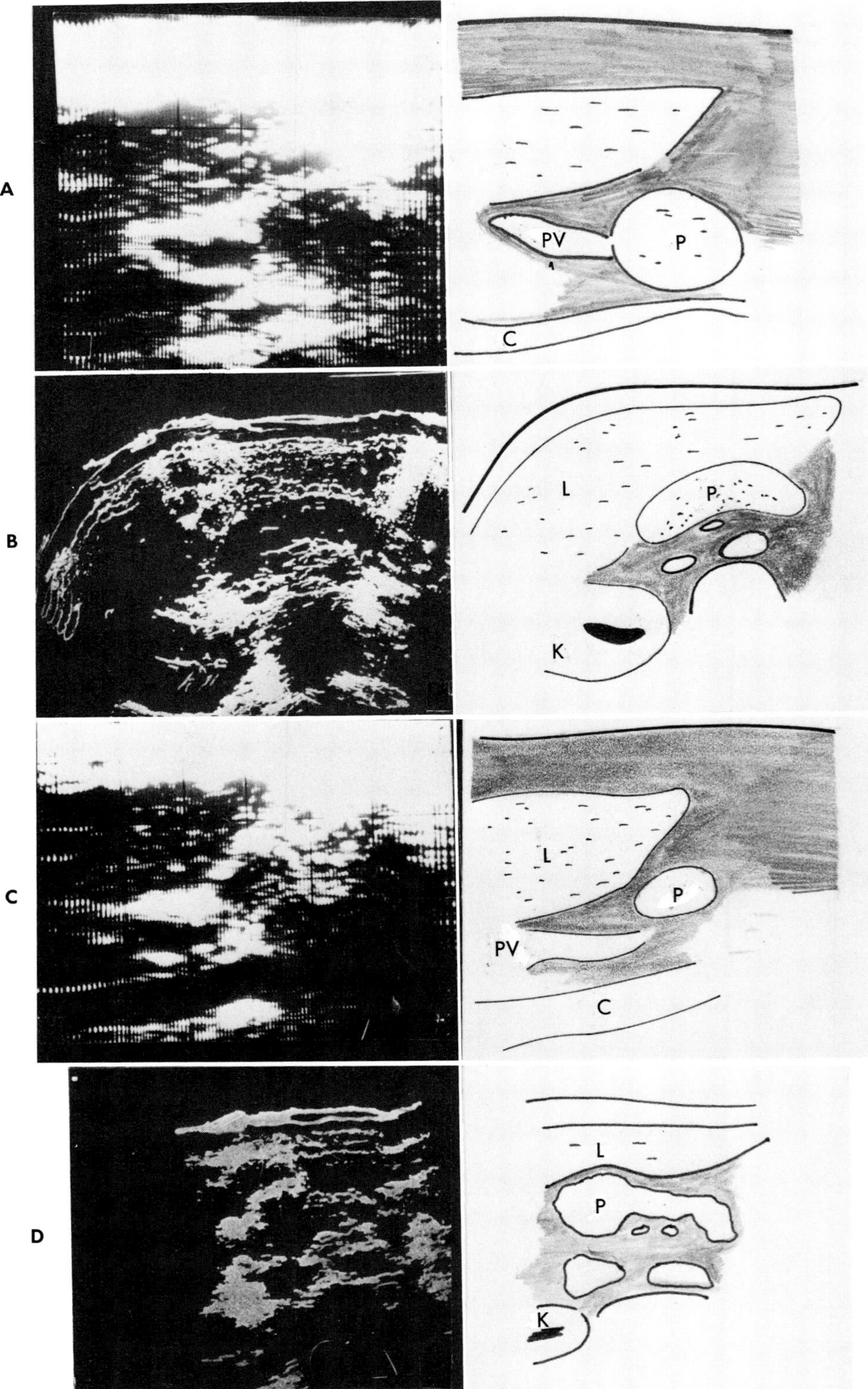

Fig. 20-14. For legend see opposite page.

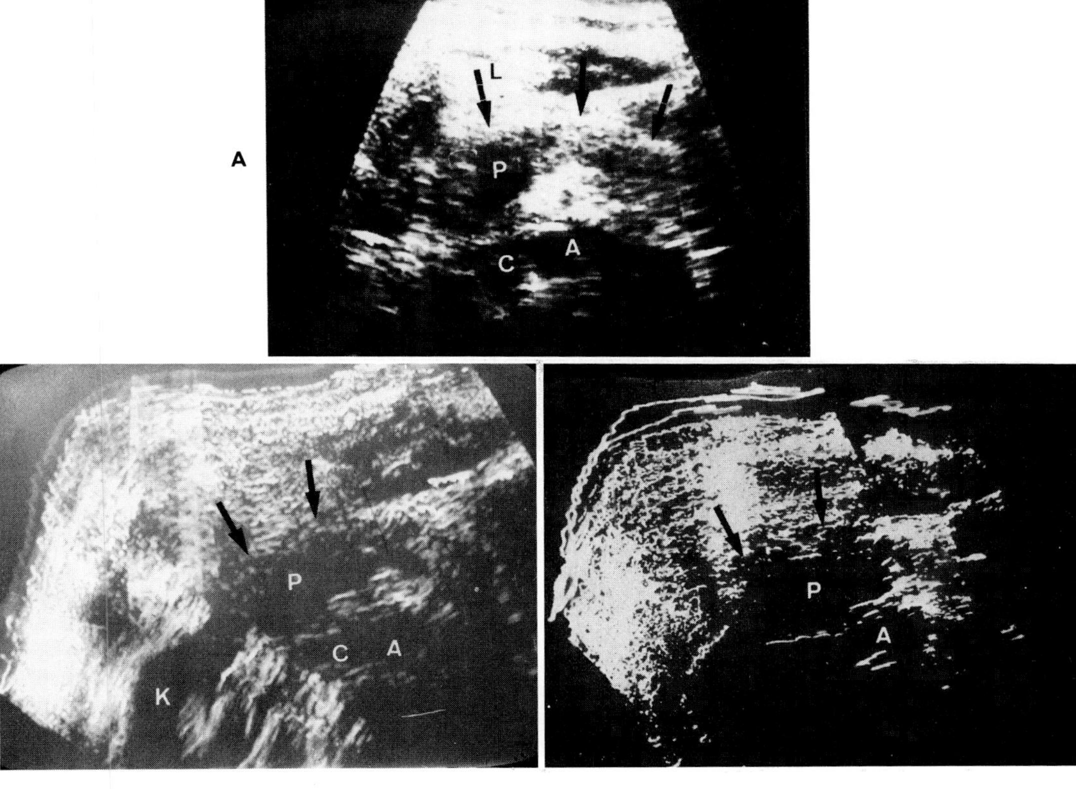

Fig. 20-15. Acute pancreatitis with progressive swelling. **A,** Transverse scan made during acute crisis showing pancreas *(P)* of normal shape and size *(arrows).* **B,** Twenty-four hours later, head of pancreas *(P)* was swollen. **C,** Forty-eight hours later, there was marked enlargement of pancreatic head. *A,* aorta; *C,* vena cava; *L,* liver; *K,* kidney.

Fig. 20-14. Acute pancreatitis: evolution. **A,** Sagittal real-time scan and schematic drawing showing semisolid pancreatic mass *(P)* of Type II in front of vena cava *(C),* below portal vein *(PV),* and behind liver. **B,** Transverse scan made at same moment and schematic drawing showing global harmonious swelling of pancreas *(P). L,* liver; *K,* kidney. **C,** Four days later, real-time sagittal scan, absolutely identical to that in **A,** as shown by vena cava and portal vein images, and schematic drawing displaying decrease in volume of pancreatic head *(P).* **D,** Transverse scan made at same moment and schematic drawing also showing decrease in pancreatic volume when compared to scan in **B.** Pancreatic contours are now irregular, and pancreatic head remains partly swollen. Vena cava and mesenteric vein, which were flattened in **B,** again show normal diameter in **C** and **D.**

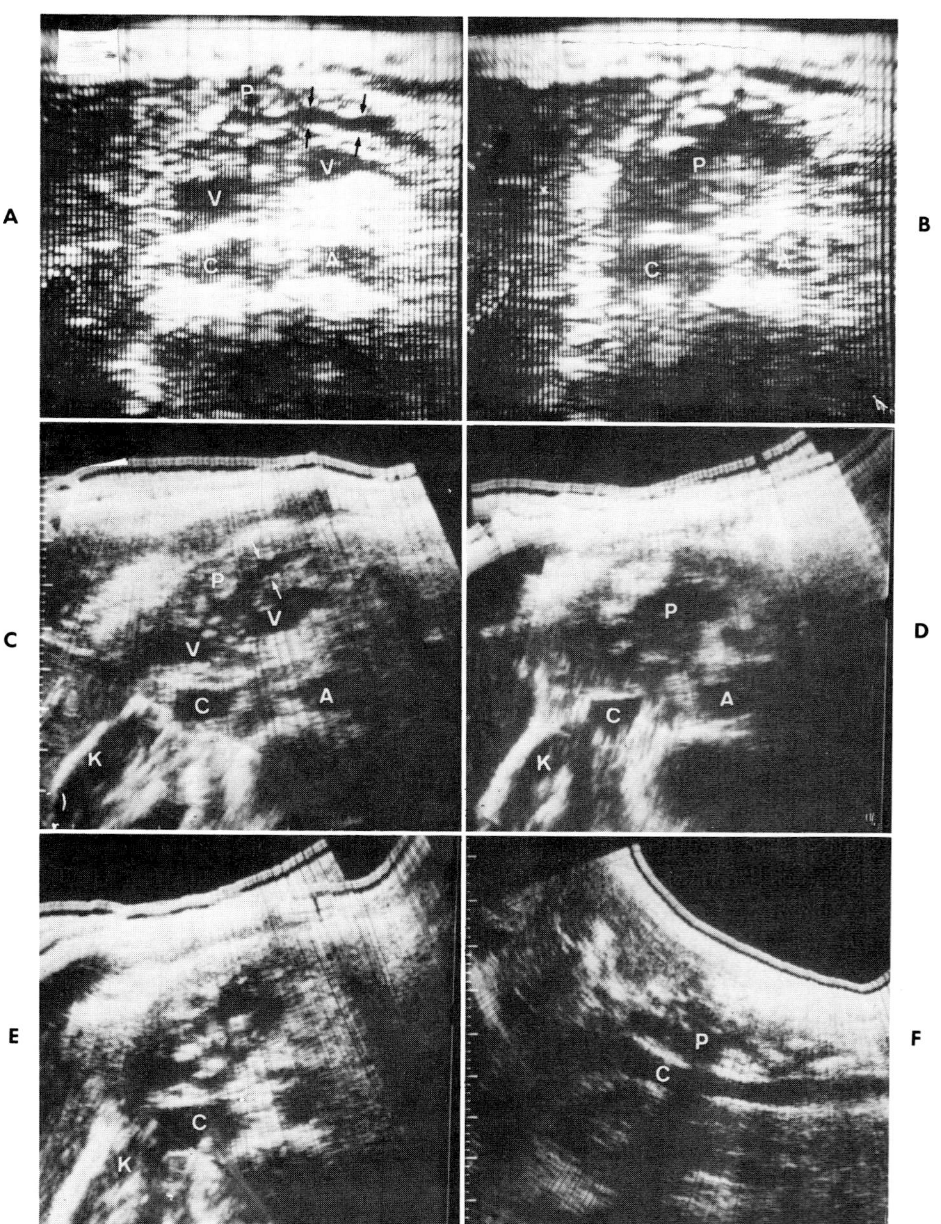

Fig. 20-16. Acute pancreatitis developed on chronic pancreatitis. **A,** Transverse real-time scan showing heterogeneous reflective pattern typical of chronic inflammation in pancreas *(P)*. Wirsung's duct *(arrows)* is enlarged. *V*, portal vein and splenic vein; *C*, cava; *A*, aorta. **B,** Parallel, more caudal scan showing pancreatic enlargement with sonolucent area. **C,** Follow-up 6 days later displaying image identical to that of **A.** *K*, kidney. **D,** However, parallel, more caudal scan, as in **B,** now shows area of necrosis in center of pancreas. **E,** More caudal scan displaying area of necrosis with reflective debris. **F,** Sagittal scan dealing with vena cava.

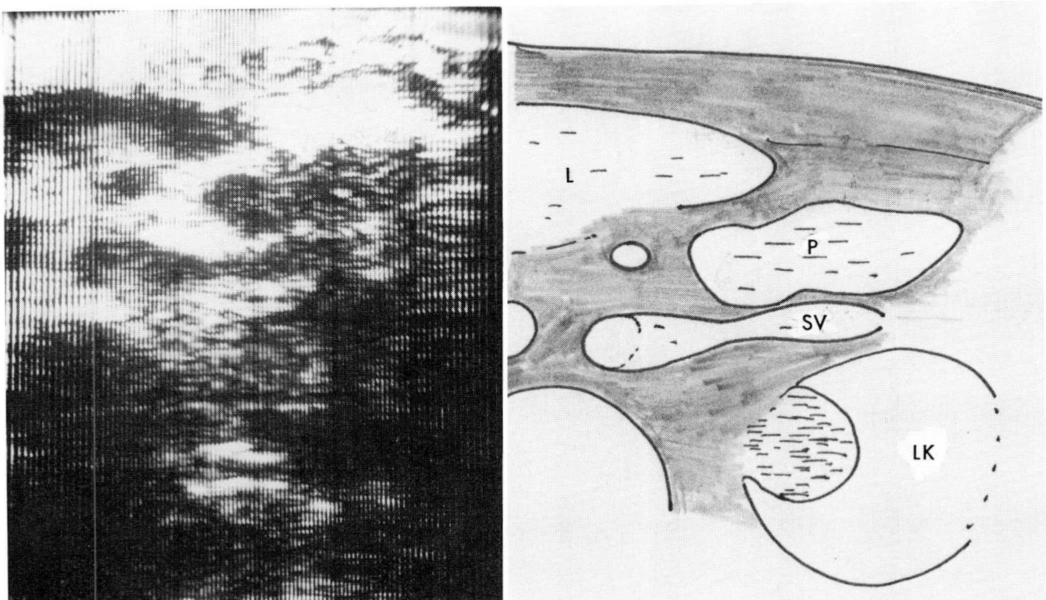

Fig. 20-17. Subacute pancreatitis of tail remaining after cephalic pancreatectomy. In front of left kidney *(LK)* and splenic vein *(SV)*, enlarged tail *(P)* is outlined. *L*, liver.

These different morphological features and evolutionary modalities permit one to distinguish different ultrasonic types of acute pancreatitis:

1. *Acute edematous pancreatitis,* with considerable swelling, but rapid detumescence, often within a few days. Aside from primary edematous pancreatitis, we have also encountered such pancreatic swellings in hepatitis and other infectious conditions, such as septicemia. This was also reported by Rabsch and Rettenmaier (1975). Are these enlargements really acute pancreatitis? In most cases, there were no specific biological abnormalities and, of course, no surgical proof. However, such enlargements, followed by a return to normal size and shape, are consistent with true inflammation of the pancreas (Fig. 20-13).

2. *Acute pancreatitis with semisolid echopattern.* This type shows less edema and a slower decrease in the swelling.

3. *Acute necrotizing pancreatitis.* The necrosis may be immediate and rapidly evolutive. In other cases the necrotizing process is slower, with progressive constitution of pseudocysts.

Three peculiar forms are still to be considered. The first involves the occurrence of an *acute episode in chronic pancreatitis.* The signs of chronic pancreatitis will be presented in Chapter 22. In cases of acute recurrence, these chronic features tend to be hidden by acute signs, quite similar to those of acute primary pancreatitis. (See Fig. 20-16.) On the other hand, in a subacute recurrence, edema may be absent. The only abnormal sign then is swelling. (See Fig. 20-8, *B* and *C*.)

The second particular form is the occurrence of *acute pancreatitis in a partly resected pancreas.* After cephalic pancreatectomy, the remaining pancreatic tail

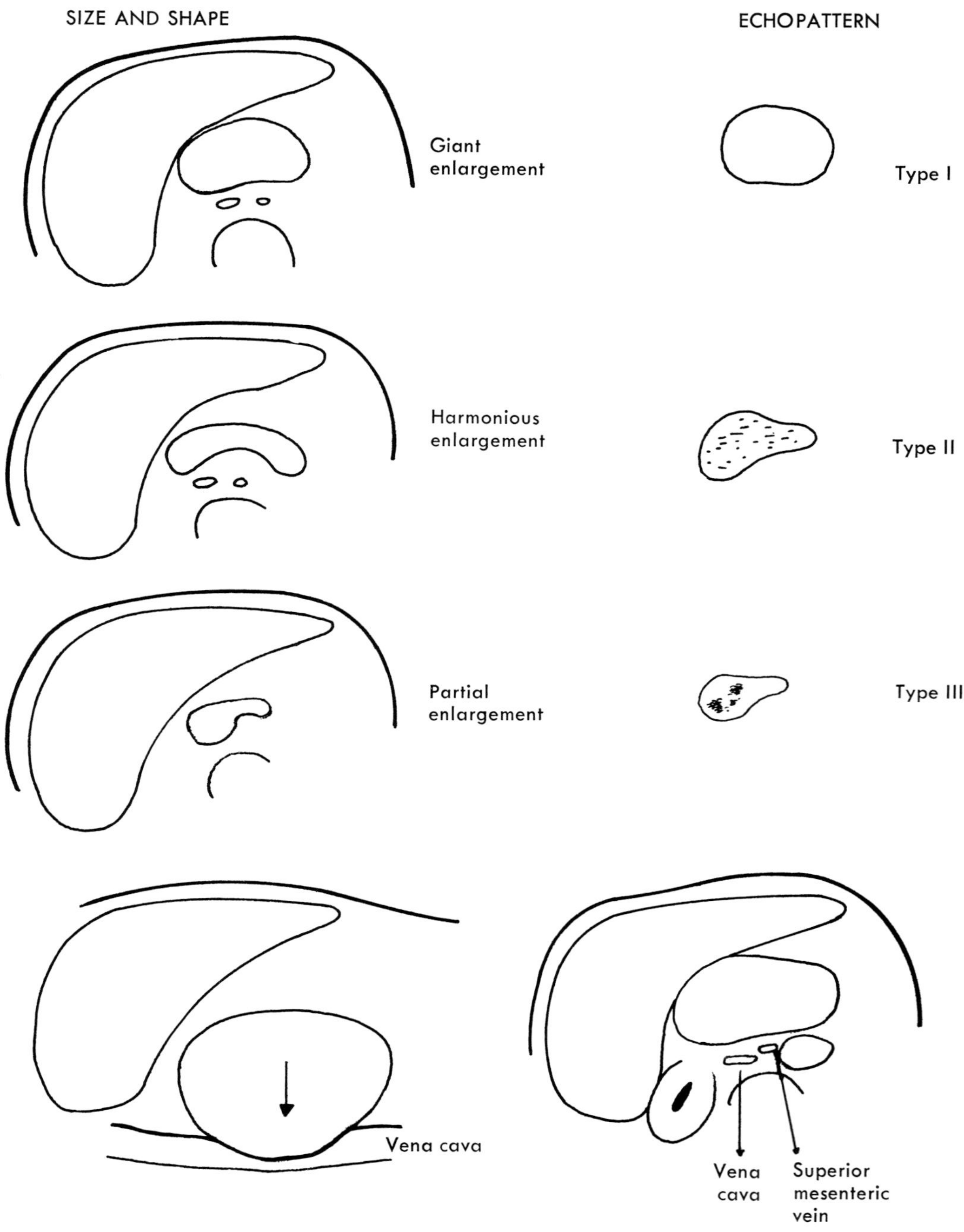

Fig. 20-18. Schematic representation of morphological anomalies in acute pancreatitis.

may become easily visible owing to inflammatory enlargement. (See Fig. 20-17.)

Third, when developing on a heterotopic islet of the pancreas, as in the duodenal wall, an acute pancreatitis may give rise to heterotopic sonolucent images. A duodenal wall hematoma is illustrated in Fig. 25-15.

The ultrasonic echopattern of *abscesses* is the same as that of necrotizing acute pancreatitis.

A last point: in cases of acute pancreatitis, one must, of course, carefully examine the biliary tract for cholelithiasis.

RELIABILITY

In our series of sixty cases of acute pancreatitis we made only two false-positive and two false-negative diagnoses. Such errors should become rare, now that the technology has improved. Our results indicate that ultrasonography should be the basic examination procedure in acute pancreatitis. In necrotic pancreatitis, if the patient is not operated on at once, angiography in search of a pseudoaneurysm is carried out after a few days.

In Chapters 24 and 25 the different steps in the differential diagnosis of pancreatic abnormalities (Fig. 20-18) will be systematically reviewed.

REFERENCES

Barnett, E., and Morley, P.: Abdominal echography, Borough Green, England, 1974, Butterworth & Co. (Publishers), Ltd.

Doust, B. D., and Pearce, J. D.: Gray-scale ultrasonic properties of the normal and inflamed pancreas, Radiology **120:**653-657, 1976.

Duncan, J. G., Imrie, C. W., and Blumgart, L. H.: Proceedings: ultrasound in the management of acute pancreatitis, Br. J. Radiol. **49:**731, 1976.

Goldberg, B. B., Kotler, M. N., Ziskin, M. C., and Waxham, R. D.: Diagnostic uses of ultrasound, New York, 1975, Grune & Stratton, Inc.

Hassani, N.: Ultrasonography of the abdomen, Heidelberg, Germany, 1976, Springer-Verlag.

Holm, H. H., Kristensen, J. K., Rasmussen, S. N., Pedersen, J. F., and Hancke, S.: Abdominal ultrasound, Copenhagen, 1976, Munksgaard, International Booksellers & Publishers, Ltd.

Leopold, G. R., and Asher, W. M.: Fundamentals of abdominal and pelvic ultrasonography, Philadelphia, 1975, W. B. Saunders Co.

Rabsch, U., and Rettenmaier, G.: Sonographically found asymptomatic enlargement of the pancreas in viral hepatitis and pneumonia, Second Congress of European Ultrasonics in Medicine, Abstract No. 100, Erlangen, Germany, 1975, Junge & Sohn.

Sokoloff, J., Gosink, B., Leopold, G. R., and Forsythe, J. R.: Pitfalls in the echographic evaluation of pancreatic disease, J. Clin. Ultrasound **2:**321-326, 1974.

Warshaw, A. L.: Inflammatory masses following acute pancreatitis. Phlegmon, pseudocysts, and abscess, Surg. Clin. North Am. **54:**621-636, 1974.

Weill, F., Becker, J. C., Kraehenbuhl, J. R., Heriot, G., and Walter, J. P.: Clinical atlas of ultrasonic radiography, Paris, 1973, Masson & Cie., Editeurs.

Weill, F., Bourgoin, A., Eisenscher, A., and Gillet, M.: Aspects ultrasonores des pancréatites aiguës. Etude de 49 patients examinés en temps réel et avec échelle des gris, Arch. Fr. Mal. App. Dig. **65:**443-454, 1976.

CHAPTER 21

PSEUDOCYSTS

TYPICAL PSEUDOCYSTS

The diagnosis of pseudocysts was one of the first applications of pancreatic ultrasonography. Their images are absolutely classic (Leopold, 1972): their pattern is typically liquid, with an echo-free area and a sharp reinforcement of the posterior wall image (Figs. 21-1 to 21-6). They may develop in any part of the pancreas. The possibility of pseudocysts of the tail, which may be masked by anterior colonic gas, requires the systematic use of a posterior approach through the left kidney (Fig. 21-4). In exceptional cases, pseudocysts may be multiple (Fig. 21-5, *A* and *B*). Their size is extremely variable. The smallest have a diameter of 2 to 3 cm (Fig. 21-1), whereas some may occupy a large part of the upper abdomen (Figs. 21-5, *C* and *D,* and 21-6). Such large pseudocysts are, of course, readily visible on x-ray films of the abdomen, since they produce displacements of the gas-filled stomach and bowel, and their diagnosis on barium series is almost unquestionable; but the early diagnosis of a pseudocyst, during its formation, is an original contribution of ultrasonography. It is not possible on an ultrasonogram to differentiate hydropancreatosis, that is, a cystic dilatation of the pancreatic canal network proximal to an obstruction, from an ordinary pseudocyst of necrotic origin.

Pseudocystic images are too well known to require detailed description, but

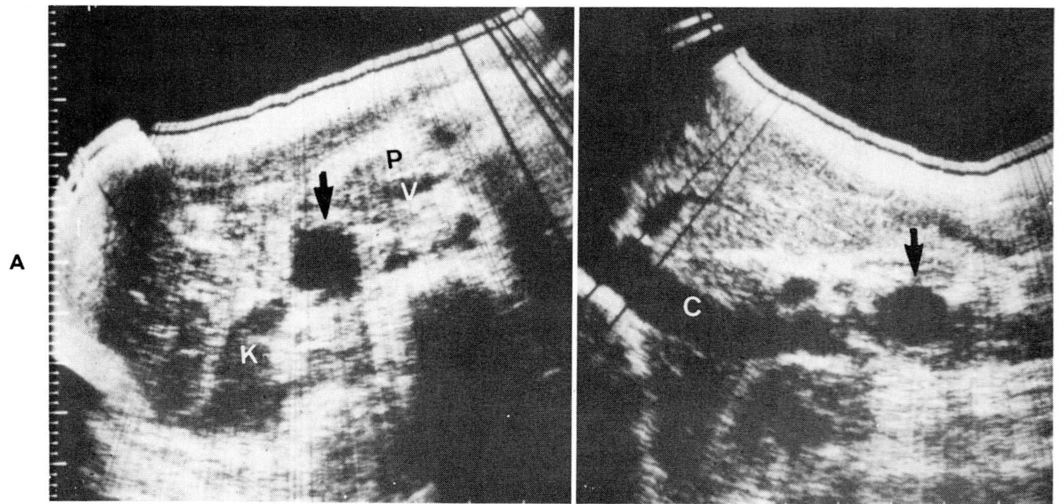

Fig. 21-1. Small cephalic pseudocyst *(arrows).* **A,** Transverse scan. *P,* pancreatic body; *V,* splenic vein; *K,* kidney. **B,** Sagittal scan. *C,* cava.

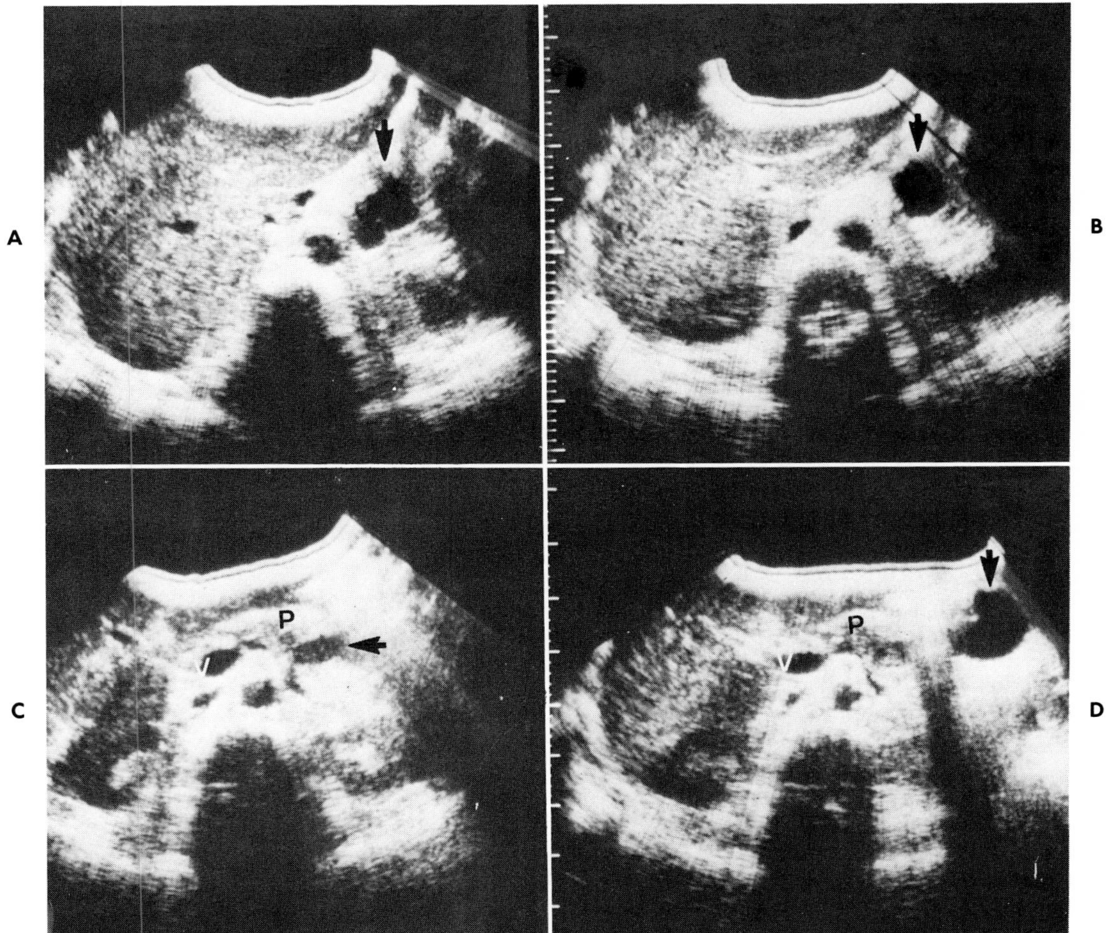

Fig. 21-2. Pseudocyst of pancreatic tail. **A,** Transverse scan of upper abdomen showing left polycyclic liquid collection *(arrow)*. **B,** Collection displayed again on parallel, more caudal scan. **C,** Parallel scan dealing with pancreas *(P)* shows relation between collection and pancreatic tail. *V,* portal vein. **D,** Last parallel scan showing extension of pseudocyst in left upper quadrant.

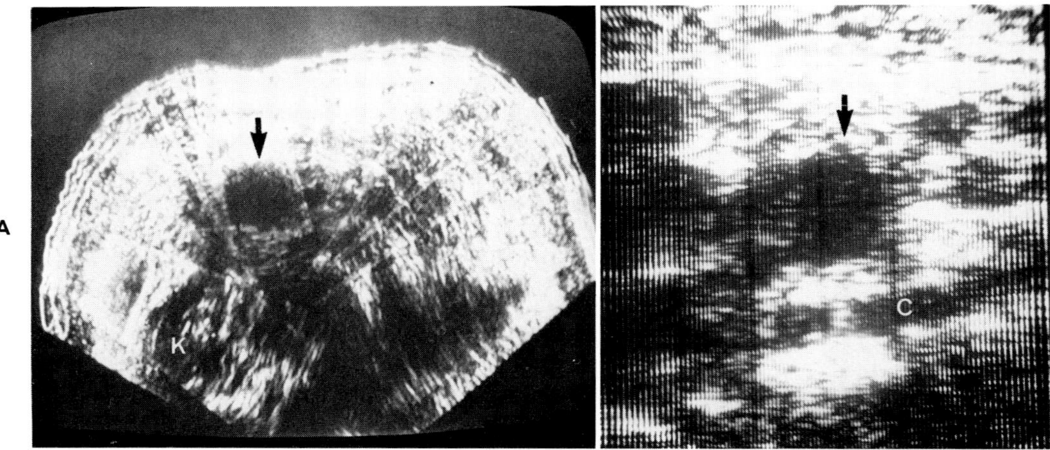

Fig. 21-3. Pseudocyst of pancreatic head discovered 2 months after onset of acute pain in upper abdomen. **A,** Horizontal scan showing rounded liquid collection *(arrow)* in front of vena cava. Posterior wall image is not very sharply delineated. *K,* kidney. **B,** Sagittal scan in real time displaying pseudocyst *(arrow)* in front of vena cava *(C)*.

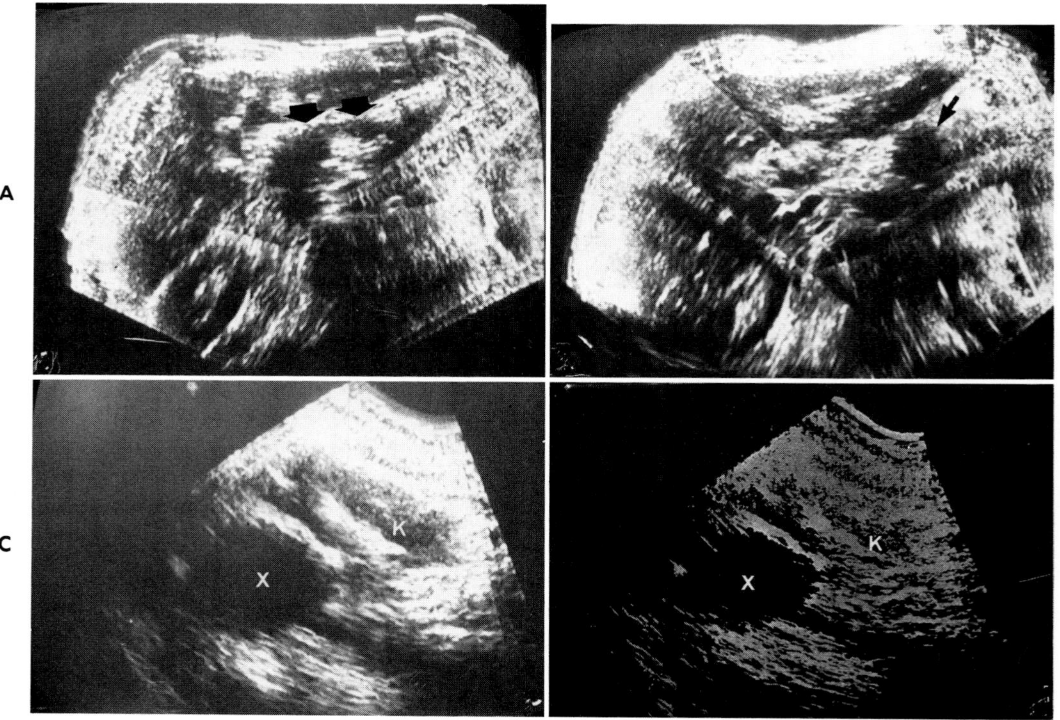

Fig. 21-4. Pseudocyst of pancreatic tail. **A,** Transverse scan showing pancreatic head and neck *(arrows)* of normal size and shape. **B,** Parallel scan, 2 cm more caudal, displaying sonolucent rounded area *(arrow)* close to left kidney. **C** and **D,** Posterior sagittal scans through left kidney showing collection *(X)* in close contact with upper pole of kidney *(K)*. Pseudocyst disappeared in 2 months without treatment.

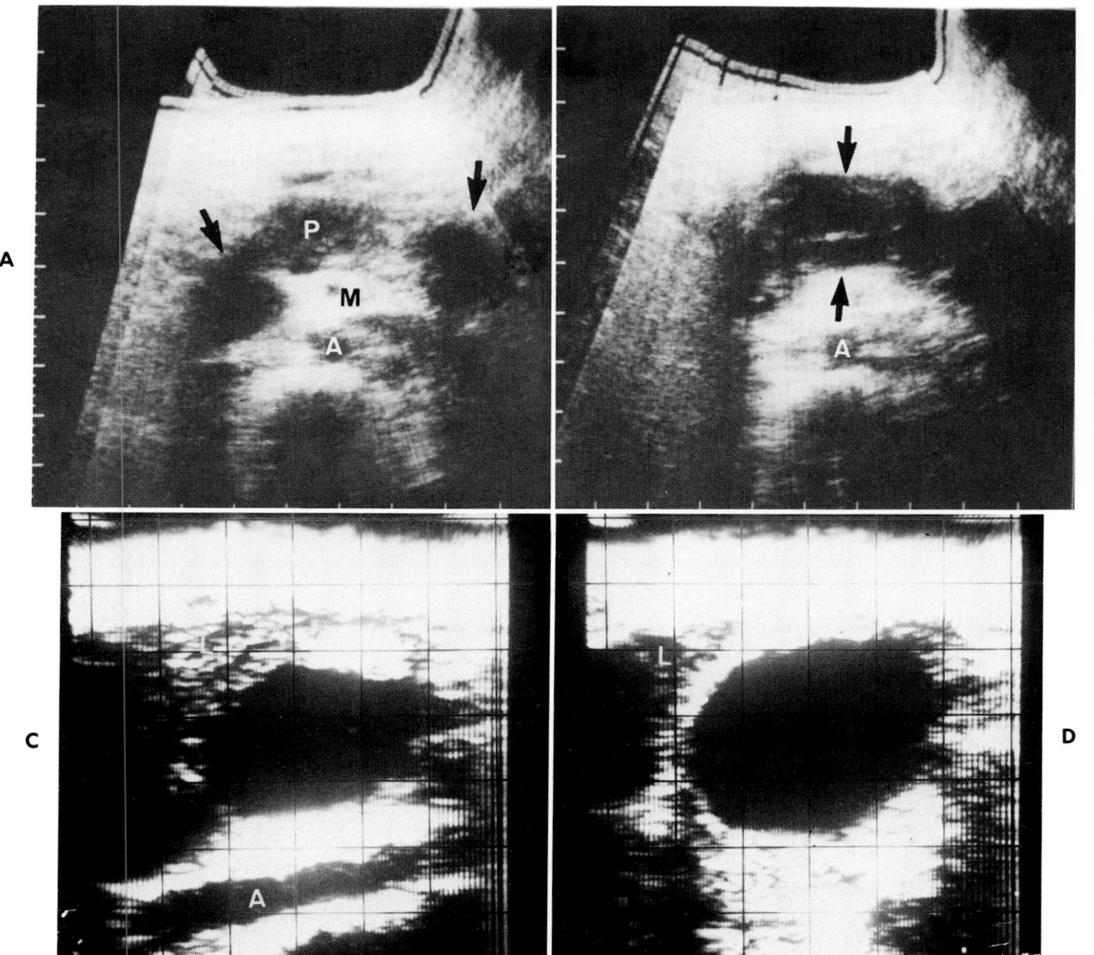

Fig. 21-5. A and **B,** Multiple pseudocysts. Patient was examined 3 weeks after initial acute crisis. **A,** Two separate pseudocysts *(arrows)* are displayed in head and tail of pancreas *(P)*. *M,* SMA; *A,* aorta. **B,** Parallel, more caudal scan showing two adjacent central pseudocysts. **C** and **D,** Typical large pseudocyst of pancreatic body. **C,** Sagittal scan. **D,** Transverse scan. *L,* liver.

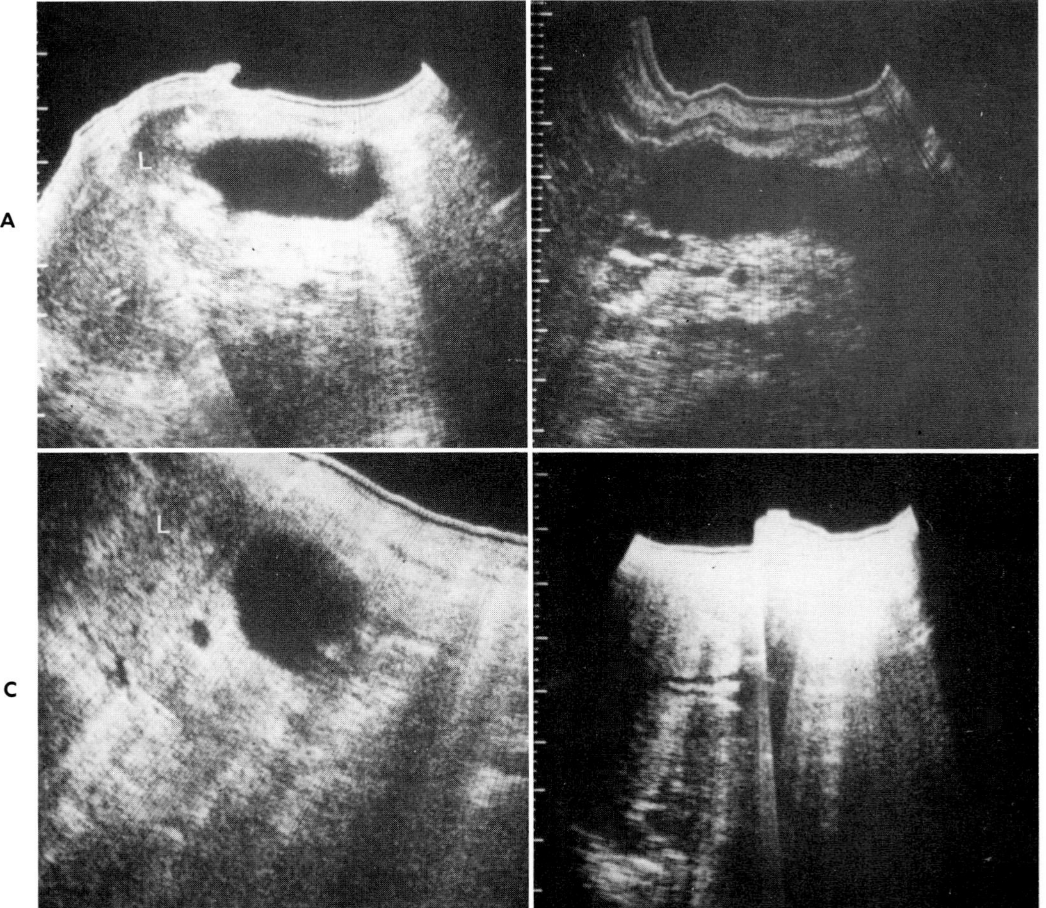

Fig. 21-6. Giant vanishing pseudocyst. Patient had abdominal pain. Palpation showed distended epigastrium. **A,** Transverse scan showing large fluid collection. **B,** Same scan with lower gain. **C,** Sagittal scan displaying extension of liquid collection, which is in contact with right hepatic lobe. Simple distention of stomach is ruled out by ordinary x-ray film of abdomen showing normal gastric air bubble. Diagnosis was giant pseudocyst of pancreas. **D,** Follow-up examination a day later, prior to surgery, which was already planned, shows total disappearance of collection. Since condition of patient improved, a barium study was performed: it showed pouch communicating with stomach, into which pseudocyst had spontaneously evacuated. *L,* liver.

the contribution of ultrasonography to the study of the development of pseudocysts and their follow-up is much more interesting.

FORMATION AND EVOLUTION

An example of the formation of a pseudocyst has been presented in the preceding chapter (Figs. 20-12 and 20-16). Now, although most pseudocysts are discovered already formed, the regular follow-up of patients suffering from acute pancreatitis permits one to observe the development of necrosis (Figs. 21-7 to 21-9). Often, in early scans the collection has an ambiguous lucent pattern with-

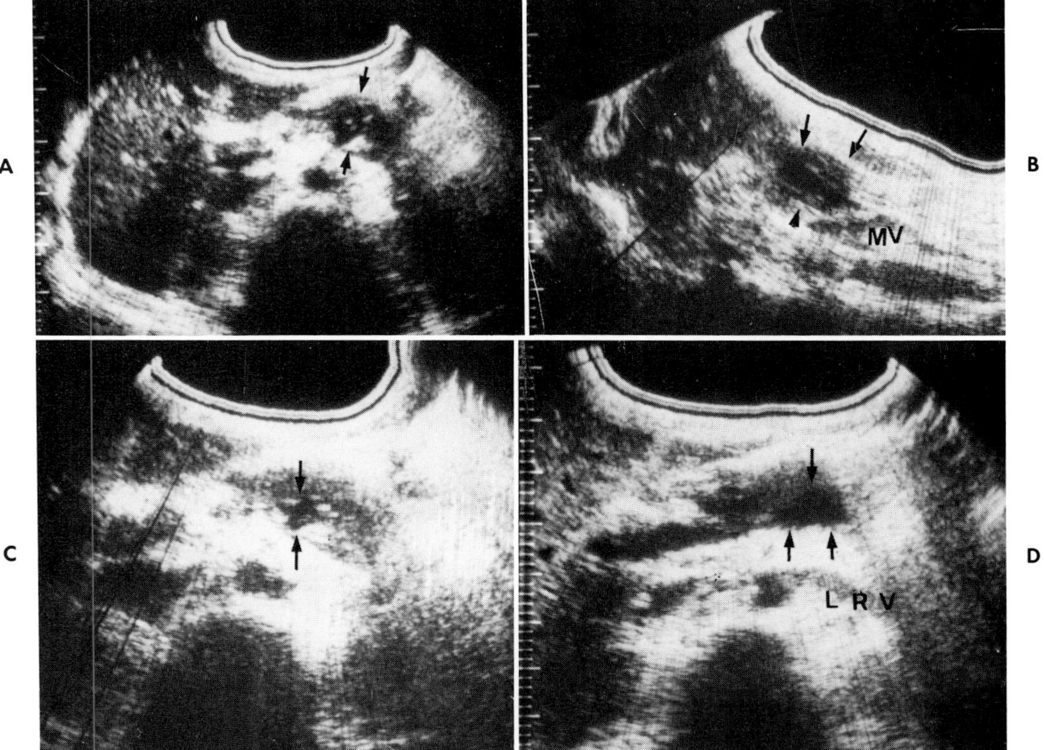

Fig. 21-7. Development of pseudocyst. Patient, already operated on for chronic pancreatitis, was referred for recurrence of abdominal pain. **A,** Transverse scan of upper abdomen showing swollen, heterogeneous pancreatic body *(arrows)*. *MV,* superior mesenteric vein. **B,** Swollen pancreas appearing on sagittal section, in front of superior mesenteric vein. **C,** Another transverse scan showing small liquid collection *(arrows)*. **D,** Extension of collection *(arrows)* outlined on parallel, more caudal scan. Reflective nodules are scattered in swollen pancreatic tissue adjacent to collection; signs of chronic pancreatitis are thus associated with signs of acute recurrence (pancreatic swelling) and of necrosis. *LRV,* left renal vein.

out reinforcement of the posterior wall image. Tissue debris floats in the necrotized area, giving rise to a semisolid pattern (Fig. 21-9, *A* and *B*). Later, this debris accumulates in the lower part of the cyst or undergoes liquefaction. The liquid pattern of the pseudocyst then becomes more characteristic (Fig. 21-9, *C*). Some cysts disappear spontaneously without surgical drainage, an evolution well known to surgeons (Bradley and Clements, 1974). The disappearance of pseudocysts may be gradual. It may also be rapid because of a spontaneous evacuation in a perforated viscus (Fig. 21-6).

ATYPICAL PSEUDOCYSTS

The atypical pseudocyst presents one of the most misleading aspects in the ultrasonic diagnosis of pseudocysts—a diagnosis that seems so easy at first glance. Some pseudocysts may extend into locations so unusual that the diagnosis of pseudo-

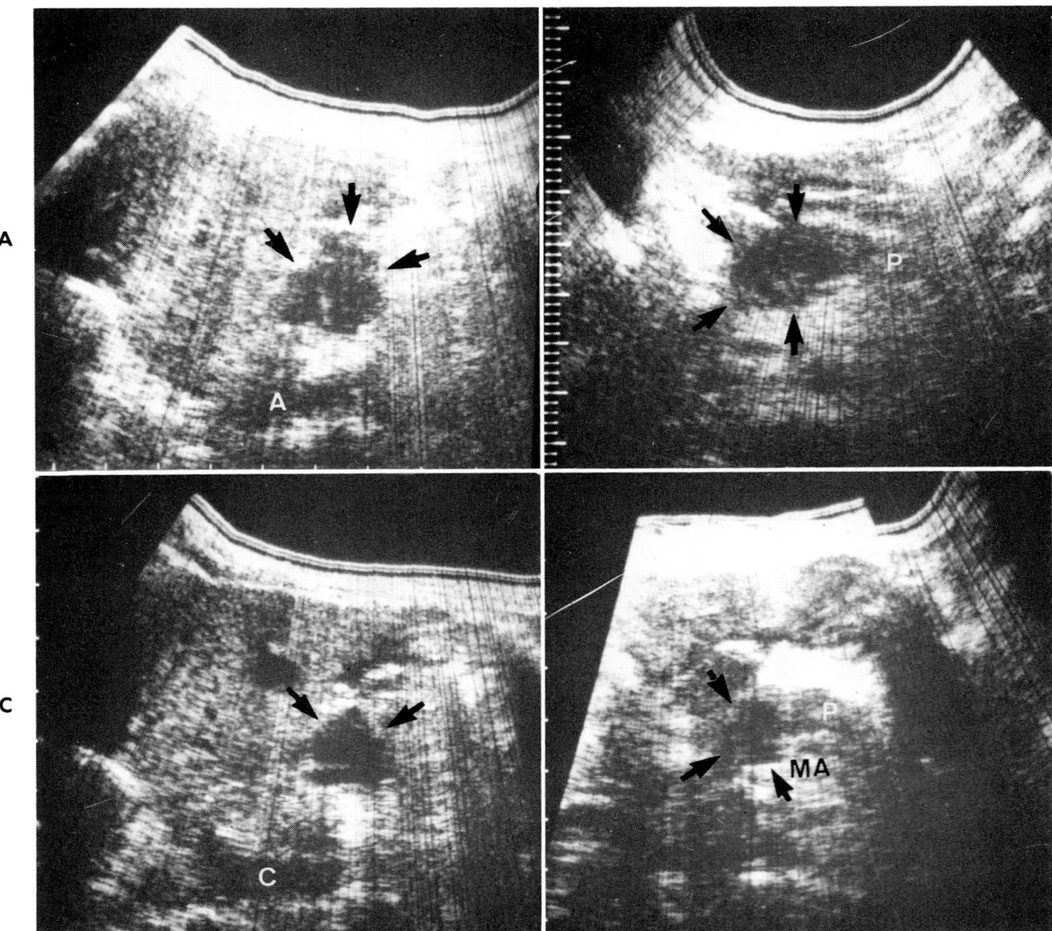

Fig. 21-8. Developing pseudocyst. **A,** Sagittal scan made during acute abdominal crisis shows, in front of aorta *(A),* enlarged pancreas *(arrows),* with polycyclic contours and heterogeneous tissue echopattern, due to acute pancreatitis. **B,** Transverse scan also showing enlarged pancreatic head *(arrows)* adjacent to normal tissue of pancreatic body *(P).* **C,** Follow-up sagittal scan, made 4 days later, shows decrease in size of pancreas; echopattern is now of liquid type. *C,* vena cava. **D,** Transverse scan showing liquid collection inside pancreatic head. Interface with normal part of pancreas is more sharply delineated. Mesenteric vessels, which were flattened, are visualized again. *MA,* SMA.

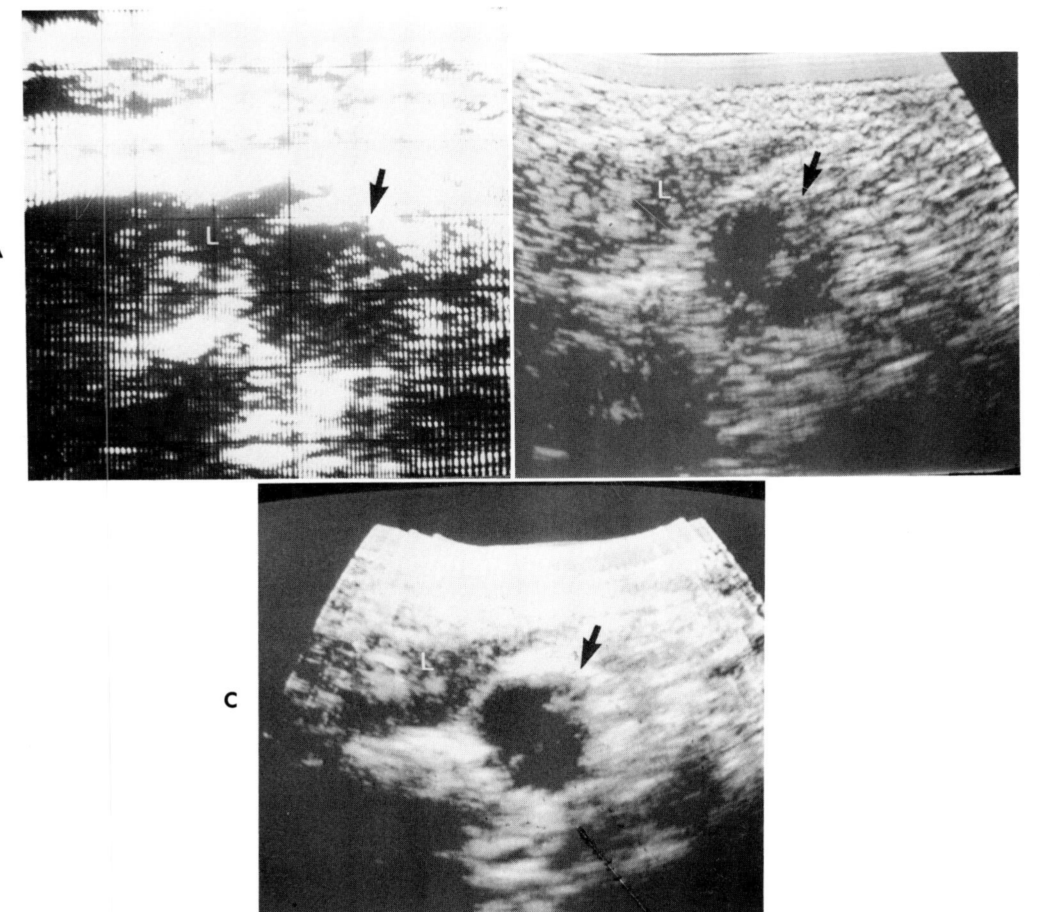

Fig. 21-9. Development of pseudocyst. **A,** Patient had undergone cholecystectomy 2 days previously. Transverse real-time scan taken during acute abdominal crisis shows sonolucent rounded mass *(arrow)* belonging to enlarged pancreatic head. Echopattern is heterogeneous. *L,* liver. **B,** New scan, made a month later by another technique (contact scanning), displays exactly same image. Echopattern has become more liquid, but small reflective areas of solid type persist. **C,** After another month, frank image of pseudocyst was displayed. It disappeared spontaneously 6 months later.

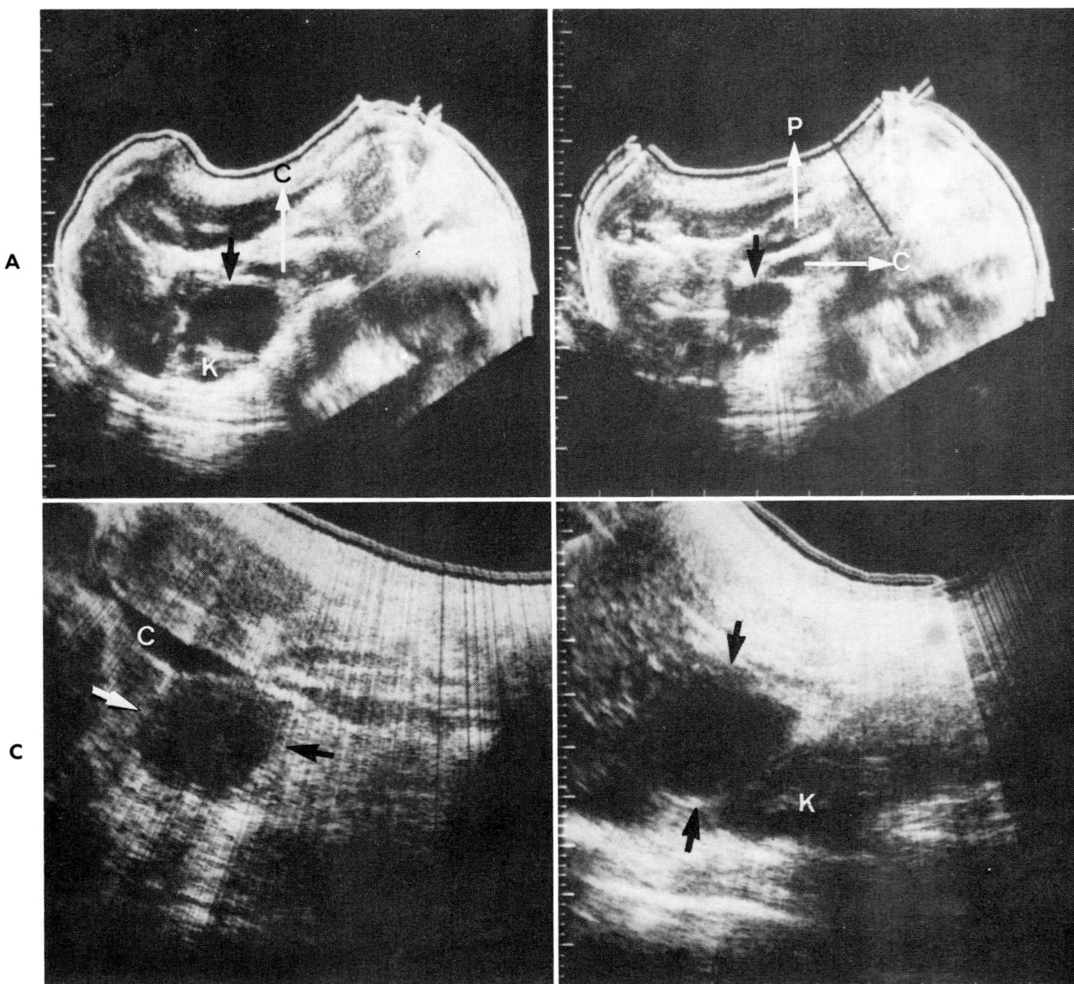

Fig. 21-10. Atypical location of pseudocyst. **A,** Transverse scan showing liquid collection *(black arrow)* between cava *(C)* and kidney *(K)*. **B,** Parallel, more caudal scan displaying pancreas *(P)*, having no evident relation with collection. **C,** Sagittal scan showing extension of collection behind vena cava. **D,** Parallel, more lateral scan showing collection to be extrarenal. Follow-up examination 6 weeks later showed spontaneous important decrease in size of pseudocyst. After another 6 weeks, disappearance was complete.

cyst is not even considered, such as that in the case presented in Fig. 14-4 of a pseudocyst that had penetrated under the hepatic capsule, mimicking a subcapsular hematoma. Some pseudocysts may migrate along the mesentery or the great vessels toward the pelvis (Fig. 20-12). Other pseudocysts may migrate toward the right side, beyond the normal limits of the pancreatic head (Fig. 21-10). Some may even penetrate into the liver tissue (Lafortune, 1977). One cannot, therefore, exclude the diagnosis of pseudocyst by the location of the collection.

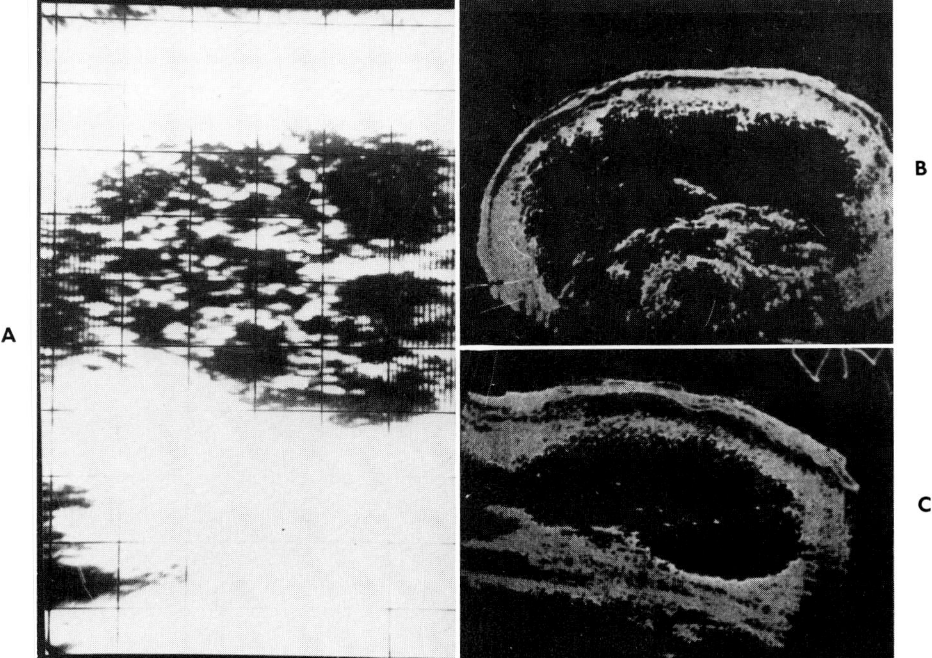

Fig. 21-11. Atypical pseudocyst. There is huge abdominal mass of multilocular pattern. **A,** Sagittal scan in real time. **B,** Transverse contact scan showing lateral extension of mass. **C,** Sagittal section showing craniocaudal extension of mass.

The most atypical pseudocyst that I ever encountered was a large abdominal mass, well marginated and of multilocular echopattern (Fig. 21-11). Its shape and echopattern suggested an ovarian cyst, although the mass did not extend to the true pelvis. Angiography did not show any specifically distorted abdominal or pelvic artery. There was no abnormal vascularization. The surgeon found it easy to resect this well-marginated mass, which had no specific topographical character or anatomical appearance. After resection he saw a small posterior bleeding area, but palpation of the pancreatic region disclosed nothing remarkable. The diagnosis remained doubtful. Two days later the young woman suddenly collapsed and died. The pathological diagnosis was necrotizing pancreatitis. The abdominal mass, then, had been the equivalent of a pseudocyst.

As a matter of fact, pseudocyst of the pancreas is one of the most deceptive of pathological entities. Since they may develop almost anywhere, they must be considered in the differential diagnosis of any abdominal collection.

Subacute and chronic pancreatitis may be associated with ascites, as well as atypical pseudocysts. In some cases, the presence of ascites is the only sign of pancreatic disease (Gouerou and colleagues, 1976). Other fluid collections in the pleural and even pericardial spaces are sometimes seen. The coexistence of such fluid collections with pseudocysts is a reliable associated sign.

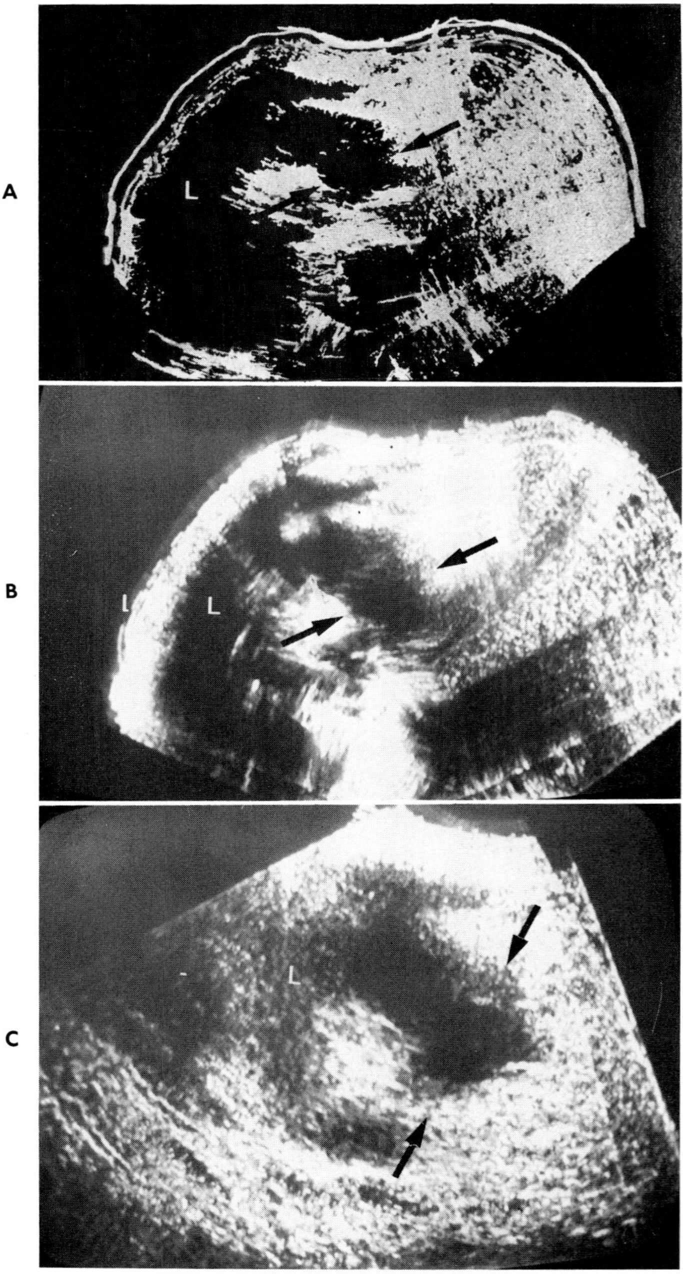

Fig. 21-12. Traumatic pancreatic hematoma. **A** and **B,** Transverse scans. Pancreatic head is enlarged and sonolucent *(arrows). L,* liver. **C,** Sagittal section. Arrows point to enlarged pancreatic head.

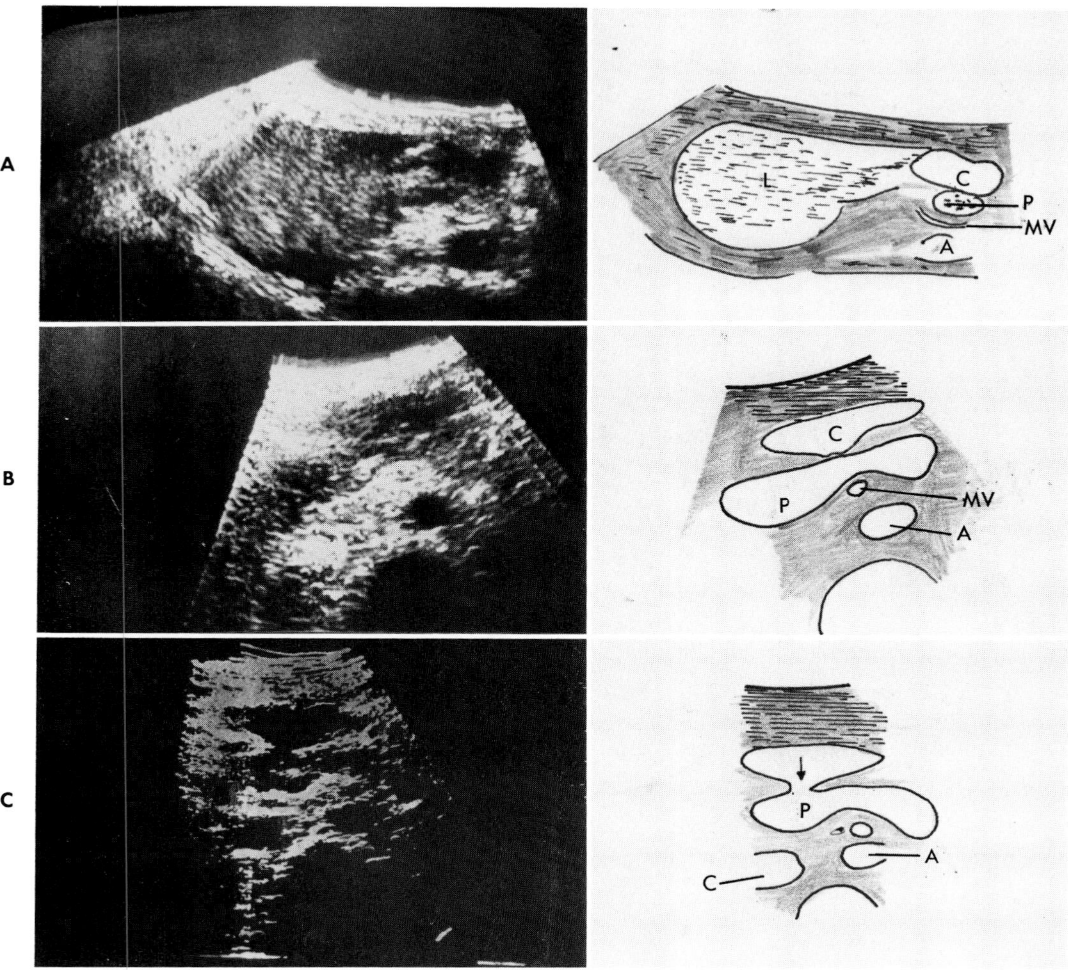

Fig. 21-13. Traumatic pancreatic hematoma. Four weeks after blunt abdominal trauma, patient complained of abdominal pain. Amylasemia was increased. **A,** Sagittal scan and schematic representation showing poorly marginated collection *(C)* in close contact with liver *(L)*. *MV,* mesenteric vein; *P,* pancreas; *A,* aorta. **B,** Transverse scan and its schematic representation outlining collection, which is rather superficially located. Collection is in close contact with anterior aspect of pancreas. **C,** Another scan, in bistable imaging, and schematic representation, displaying close relation of collection to anterior aspect of pancreatic head. This collection belongs to traumatic hematoma in lesser omental sac.

RELIABILITY

The reliability of ultrasonography in the diagnosis of pseudocysts is excellent, replacing barium studies and angiography, which display only indirect signs. With retrograde pancreatography one can opacify some pseudocysts, but there is no justification for this sophisticated and possibly aggressive procedure in the diagnosis of pseudocysts. Pancreatography is more useful in the diagnosis of Wirsung's duct stenosis. Computed axial tomography shows the liquid images of the pseudo-

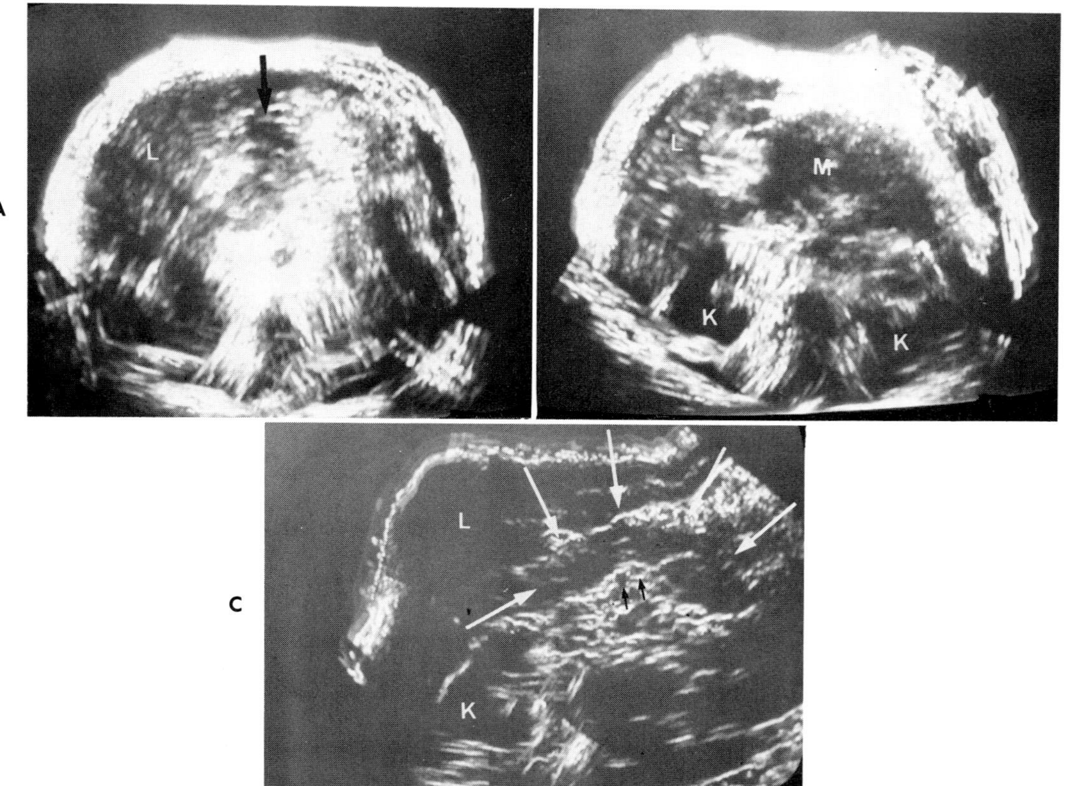

Fig. 21-14. Posttraumatic hematoma in hemophilic 7-year-old boy. **A,** Transverse scan at level of xiphoid process showing uncommonly thick abdomen for boy of that age. There is small sonolucent area *(arrow)* behind liver *(L)*. **B,** Two days later, mass *(M)* of semisolid type was outlined in front of large vessels. *K,* kidneys. **C,** Four days later, mass had disappeared, its image replaced by image of enlarged pancreas *(white arrows)*. This evolution shows that mass was pancreatic from outset. Since this condition improved, this boy was, of course, not operated on. *Small black arrows,* mesenteric vessels.

cysts much less sharply than does ultrasonography. It would be a waste to use this expensive and irradiating procedure for this type of diagnosis. Sometimes the possibility of using ultrasonography in the diagnosis of so-called early pseudocysts has been stressed. As a matter of fact, the study of developing pseudocysts shows that most of them possess their definite size almost from the beginning of the necrotizing process—a size that is usually rather large.

DIFFERENTIAL DIAGNOSIS

Not all liquid abdominal collections that are deeply located belong to pancreatic pseudocysts. The problems of differential diagnosis and its pitfalls will be examined in Chapter 25.

This chapter would be incomplete without mention of *traumatic pancreatic hematomas.* In these lesions there is a sonolucent pancreatic enlargement similar to the swelling of acute pancreatitis, as well as liquid areas similar to those of pseudocysts (Kratochwil and co-workers, 1973). (See Figs. 21-12 to 21-14.) If no surgery is necessary, the progressive resorption of the hematoma may be followed (Fig. 21-14).

REFERENCES

Barnett, E., and Morley, P.: Abdominal echography, Borough Green, England, 1974, Butterworth & Co. (Publishers), Ltd.

Bradley, E. L., and Clements, J. L.: Implications of diagnostic ultrasound in the surgical management of pancreatic pseudocysts, Am. J. Surg. **127:**164-173, 1974.

Goldberg, B. B., Kotler, M. N., Ziskin, M. C., and Waxham, R. D.: Diagnostic uses of ultrasound, New York, 1975, Grune & Stratton, Inc.

Gouerou, H., Cerf, M., Benhamou, G., Leymarios, J., and Debray, C.: Les ascites des pancréatites sub-aiguës et chroniques. Étude de 14 cas, Arch. Fr. Mal. App. Dig. **65:**433-442, 1976.

Hassani, N.: Ultrasonography of the abdomen, Heidelberg, Germany, 1976, Springer-Verlag.

Holm, H. H., Kristensen, J. K., Rasmussen, S. N., Pedersen, J. F., and Hancke, S.: Abdominal ultrasound, Copenhagen, 1976, Munksgaard, International Booksellers & Publishers, Ltd.

Kratochwil, A., Rosenmayer, F., and Howawietz, L.: Diagnosis of a traumatic pancreas cyst by means of ultrasound, Ultrasound Med. Biol. **1:**49-52, 1973.

Lafortune, M.: Personal communication, 1977.

Leopold, G. R.: Pancreatic echography: a new dimension in the diagnosis of pseudocyst, Radiology **104:**365-369, 1972.

Leopold, G. R., and Asher, W. M.: Fundamentals of abdominal and pelvic ultrasonography, Philadelphia, 1975, W. B. Saunders Co.

Weill, F., Becker, J. C., Kraehenbuhl, J. R., Heriot, G., and Walter, J. P.: Clinical atlas of ultrasonic radiography, Paris, 1973, Masson & Cie., Editeurs.

CHAPTER 22

CHRONIC PANCREATITIS

with the collaboration of **ALBERT EISENSCHER, M.D.**

Chronic quiescent pancreatitis without pseudocysts produces changes in the contours, the tissue echopattern, and, to a lesser degree, the size of the gland. A particularly difficult diagnostic problem arises in the case of acute pancreatitis superimposed on chronic pancreatitis.

ECHOPATTERN CHANGES

Change in echopatterns is, in our opinion, the most important feature of the ultrasonic diagnosis of chronic pancreatitis and consists of a frankly increased tissue reflectivity (Weill and associates, 1975) either throughout the pancreas or limited to small areas. The increase in reflectivity is particularly obvious in calcific pancreatitis. It may also be encountered in noncalcific pancreatitis and is then probably due to fibrosis. By and large, such an increase in reflectivity gives rise to a tissue echopattern of solid type that is heterogeneous; areas of intense reflec-

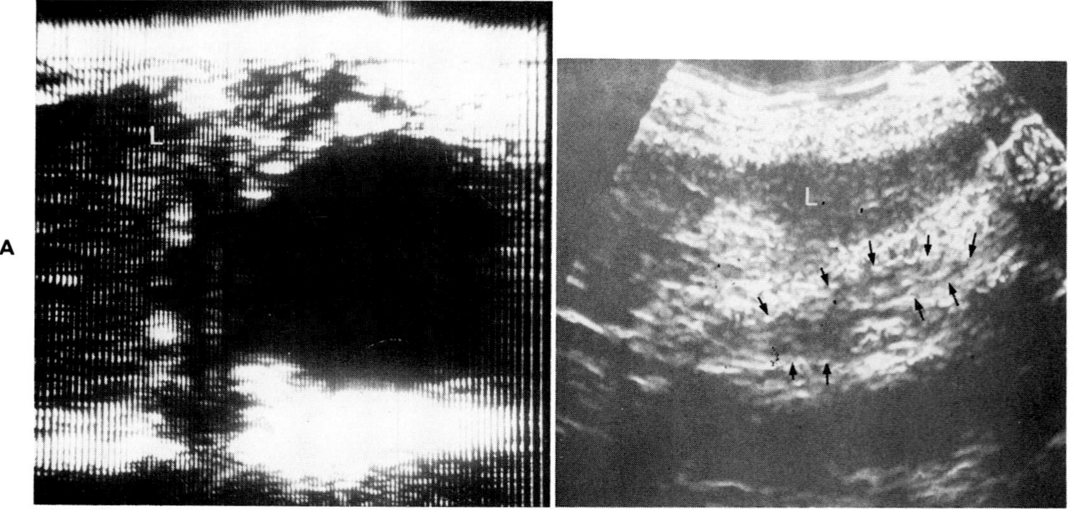

Fig. 22-1. Development of chronic pancreatitis. **A,** Sagittal scan of right upper quadrant showing large fluid collection of pseudocyst behind liver *(L)*. **B,** Transverse scan, made a month after surgery, displaying pancreatic tissue *(arrows)* behind liver. There is neither fluid nor swelling. Size and shape of pancreas are normal, but echopattern is heterogeneous.

tivity, irregular shape, and variable size are scattered in the pancreatic tissue. (See Figs. 22-1 to 22-9.) Because of these echopattern changes and perhaps the disappearance of peripancreatic fat, as CT scan studies show, the pancreatic tissue is less sharply outlined and less well differentiated from surrounding tissues, so that it may be much more difficult to show the pancreas on transverse sections (Figs. 22-4 to 22-7). On sagittal scans the superior mesenteric vein may be depressed or displaced (Figs. 22-4 and 22-9).

In our experience, a sonolucent echopattern is exceptional in quiescent chronic pancreatitis. In such cases, probably a superimposed acute or subacute process is involved. (See Fig. 22-11.)

Text continued on p. 345.

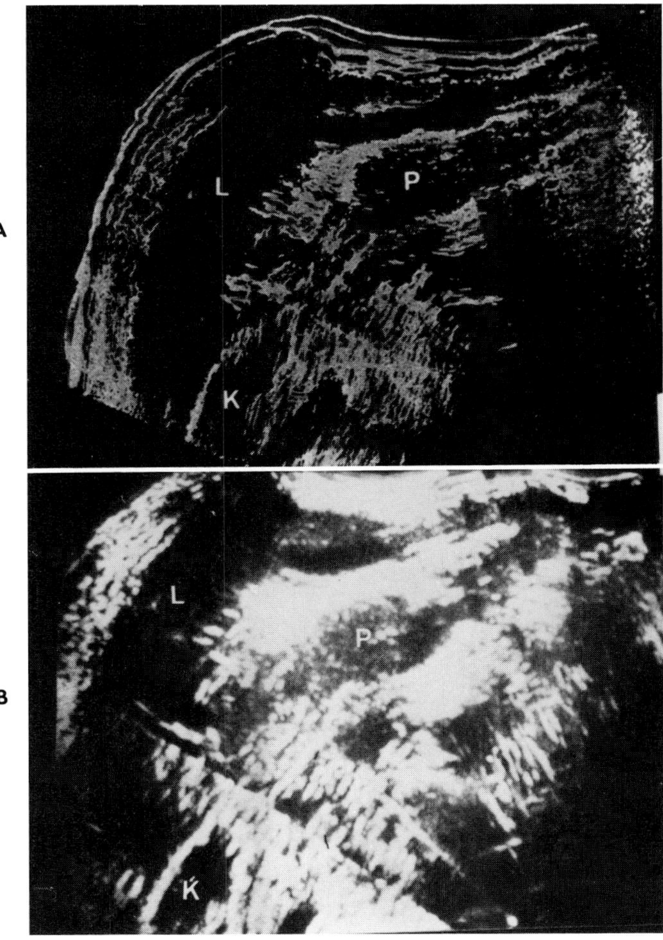

Fig. 22-2. Chronic pancreatitis. **A,** Transverse scan of upper abdomen displaying enlarged head of pancreas *(P)* behind liver *(L)*. Pancreatic contours are slightly irregular. **B,** Gray scale display showing echopattern to be heterogeneous, with small scattered nodules. *K,* kidney.

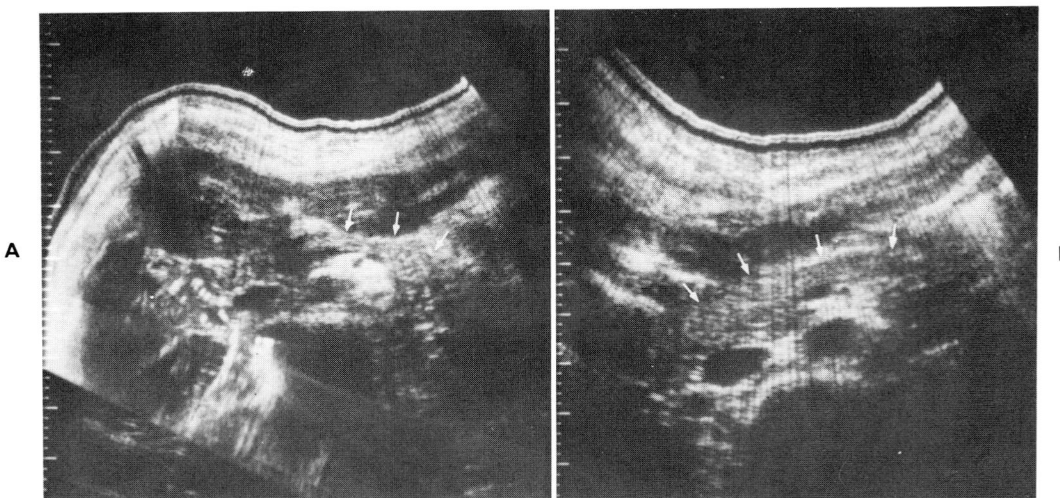

Fig. 22-3. Normal pancreas. Two parallel scans show homogeneous echopattern and regular contours of normal gland *(arrows)*. **A,** Pancreatic neck. **B,** Pancreatic head. Note splenic vein, SMA, and, on **B,** right renal artery behind vena cava.

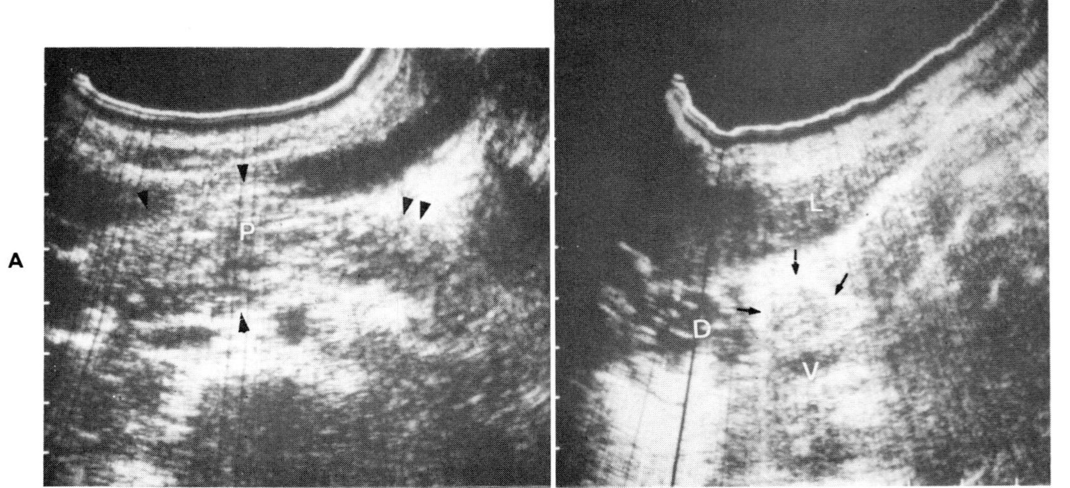

Fig. 22-4. Chronic pancreatitis. **A,** Transverse scan of pancreas (*arrowheads* and *P*) showing reflective micronodular tissue echopattern. Anterior contour of pancreatic body (*double arrowheads*) is irregular. Pancreatic head is enlarged and extends to right. This type of image demands follow-up examination to eliminate duodenal section. Note flattened vena cava and splenoportal junction. **B,** Cephalic nodule of chronic pancreatitis *(arrows)*. *V,* splenoportal junction; *D,* duodenum; *L,* liver.

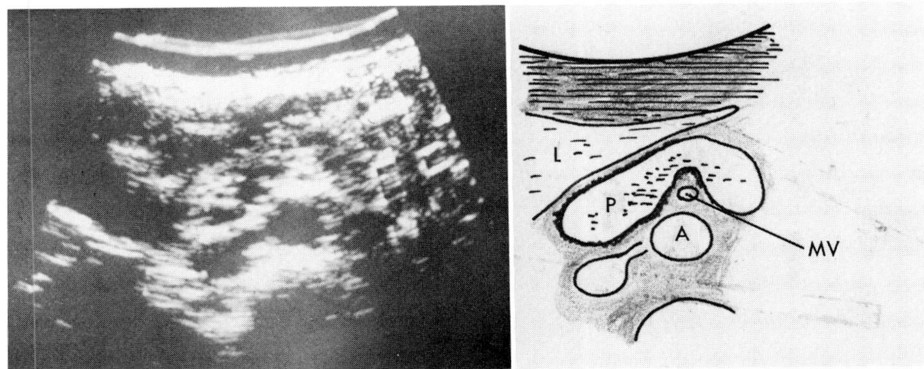

Fig. 22-5. Chronic pancreatitis. Pancreas *(P)* is of normal size; its contours are spiky. There are many small areas of intense reflectivity scattered amid glandular tissue. General reflectivity of pancreas is much higher than that of neighboring liver tissue *(L)*. *A,* aorta; *MV,* mesenteric vessels.

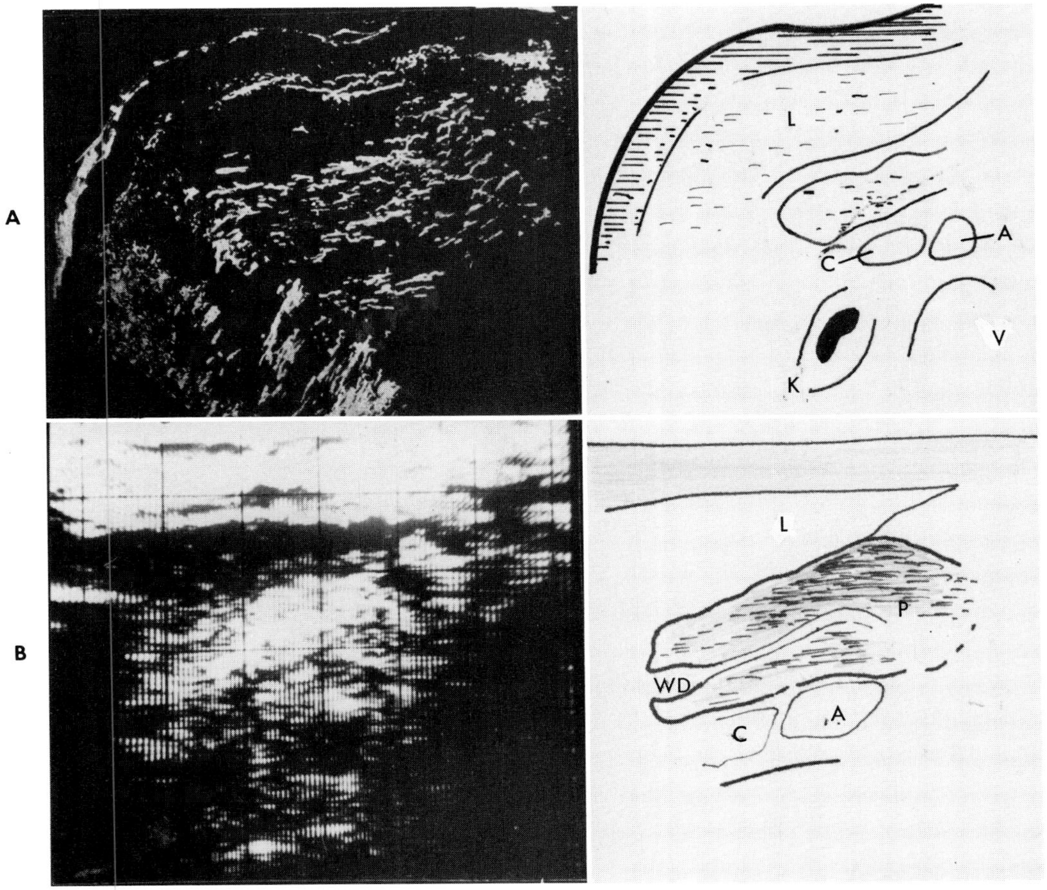

A

B

Fig. 22-6. Chronic pancreatitis. **A,** Bistable transverse scan and schematic representation showing enlarged pancreatic head with irregular contours. **B,** Real-time, slightly more axial scan and its schematic representation displaying unusually reflective tissue echopattern. There is tubular element belonging to Wirsung's duct *(WD)*, which is irregular in diameter. *L,* liver; *C,* vena cava; *A,* aorta; *P,* pancreatic head; *K,* kidney; *V,* vertebral body.

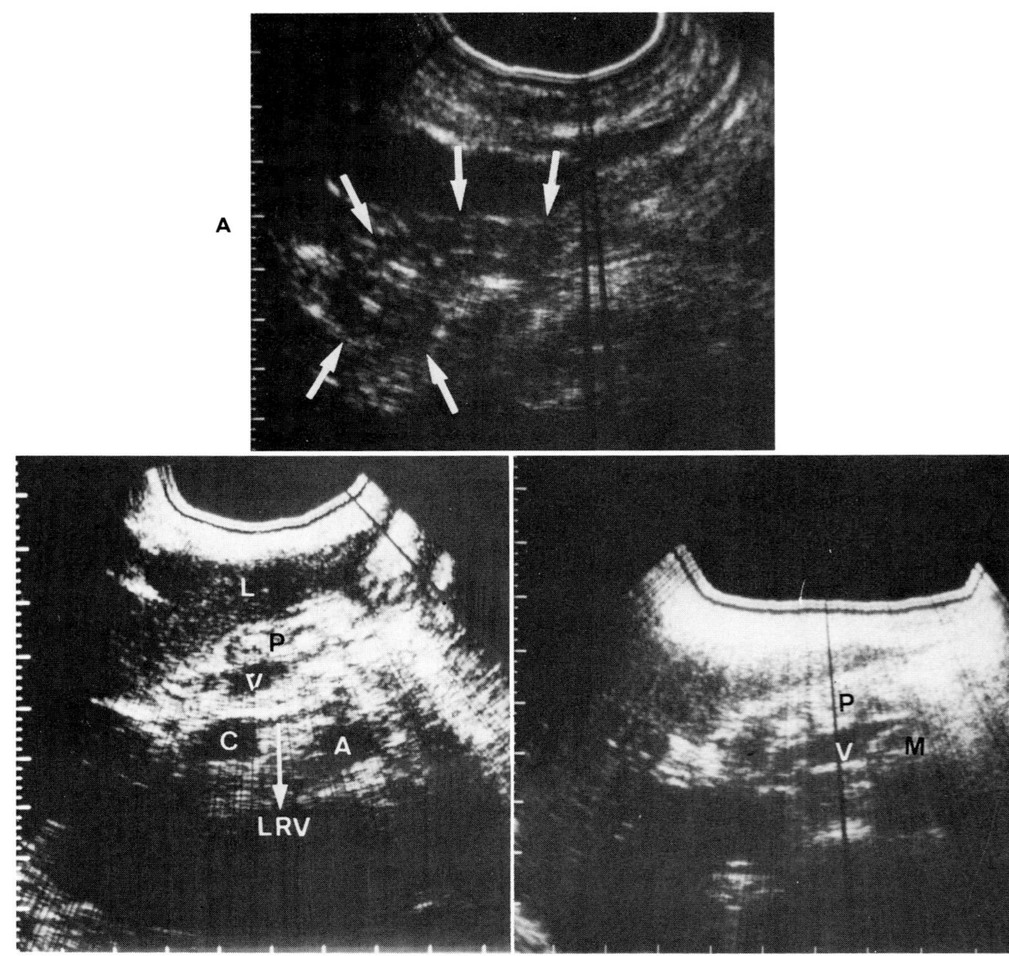

Fig. 22-7. Chronic pancreatitis. **A,** High-contrast transverse scan of pancreatic head *(arrows)* displaying several reflective nodules. Anterior and right cephalic contours are irregular. **B,** Transverse scan showing strongly reflective, heterogeneous pancreas *(P)* with irregular contours. *L,* liver; *C,* vena cava; *LRV,* left renal vein; *A,* aorta; *V,* splenoportal junction. Plain film of abdomen showed typical calcifications; there are, however, no acoustic shadows. **C,** Identical pancreatic pattern in patient operated on several years before for cholelithiasis with chronic pancreatitis. *M,* SMA.

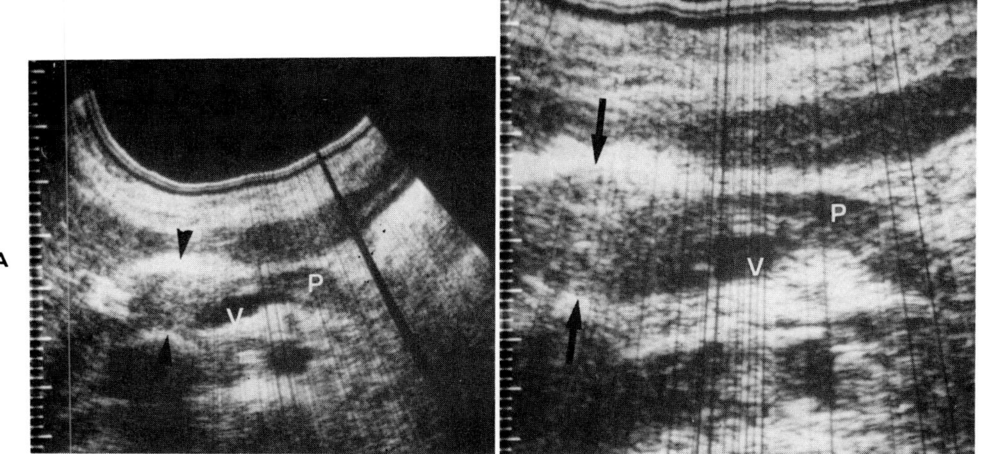

Fig. 22-8. Chronic pancreatitis. These two transverse scans show enlarged pancreatic head *(arrows).* Its anterior contour bulges forward. Tissular echopattern is more reflective in this area than in pancreatic neck or body *(P).* As already stated, such an image demands follow-up examination, to eliminate duodenal image. Note, in **B,** image of Wirsung's duct. *V,* portal vein and splenic junction.

CONTOUR CHANGES

In quiescent chronic pancreatitis the pancreatic contours, in roughly 70% of cases, are irregular, if not spiky (Figs. 22-2, 22-5 to 22-7, *A,* and 22-9, *B*). This irregularity is perhaps an artifact, due to the pancreatic tissue margins' not being well defined in this pathological condition. What seems to be the pancreatic outline may be only the limit of the reflective areas that are scattered throughout the glandular tissue. Fortunately, in chronic pancreatitis the pancreatic contours are quite different than they are in a carcinoma, at least in the absence of a superimposed acute inflammatory process, which causes swelling of the gland with more regular margins, as will be seen.

SIZE

In chronic pancreatitis the gland, except in subacute or acute recurrences, is at most slightly enlarged (Figs. 22-4, 22-6, and 22-8). In cases of acute inflammation, especially when the inflammatory process is long-standing, significant enlargement may occur.

Acute or subacute recurrences superimposed on chronic pancreatitis

As already mentioned in Chapter 20, such inflammatory processes as acute or subacute recurrences superimposed on chronic pancreatitis are not rare. They give rise to a sonolucent enlargement (Figs. 22-10 and 22-11, as well as Fig. 20-16) quite similar to that of a primary acute process. If the inflammation lasts several weeks, particularly if it gives rise to pain and loss of weight, it becomes impossible to differentiate such an inflammatory sonolucent enlargement from a tumoral sonolucent enlargement (Fig. 22-10). However, successive examinations

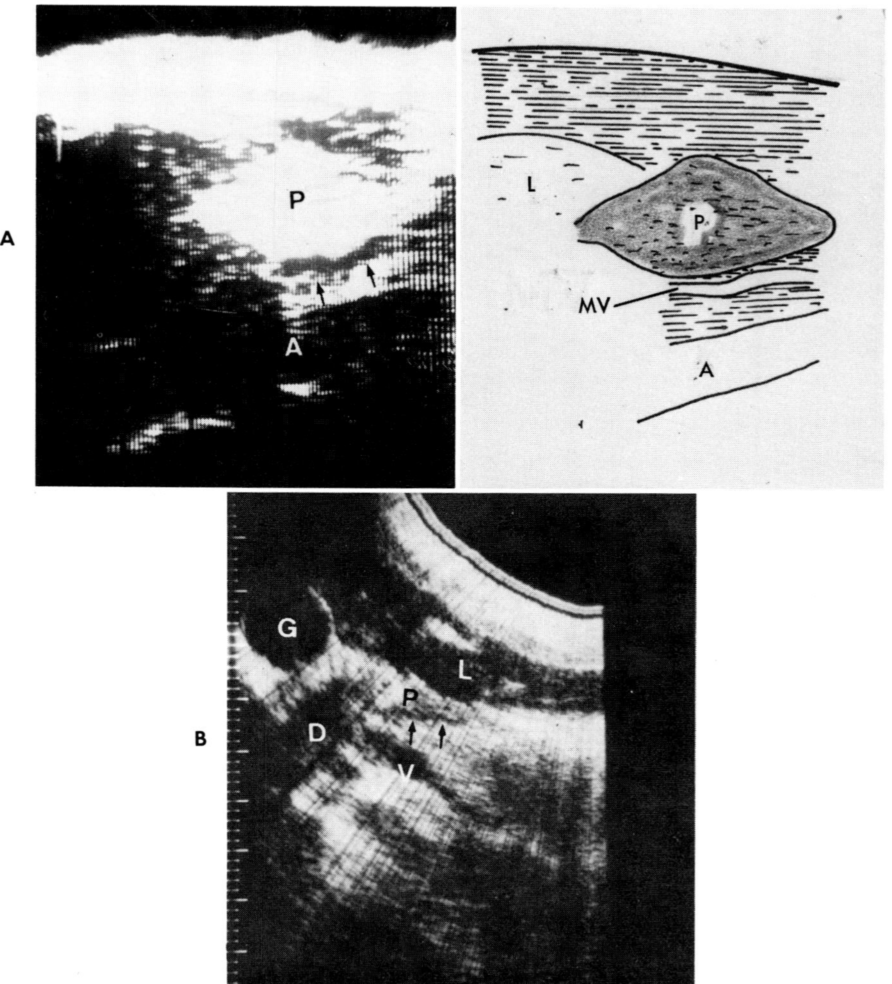

Fig. 22-9. Chronic pancreatitis. **A,** Sagittal real-time scan and schematic drawing showing, in front of slightly distorted mesenteric vein (*arrows* and *MV*), reflective nodules in pancreatic tissue *(P)*. *A,* aorta; *L,* liver. **B,** Transverse scan showing heterogeneous pancreas with reflective nodule, in front of splenoportal junction and splenic vein *(V)*. Wirsung's duct *(arrows)* is enlarged. Position of patient is oblique, to induce migration of colonic gas. Note acoustic shadow of duodenal gas *(D)*. *G,* gallbladder.

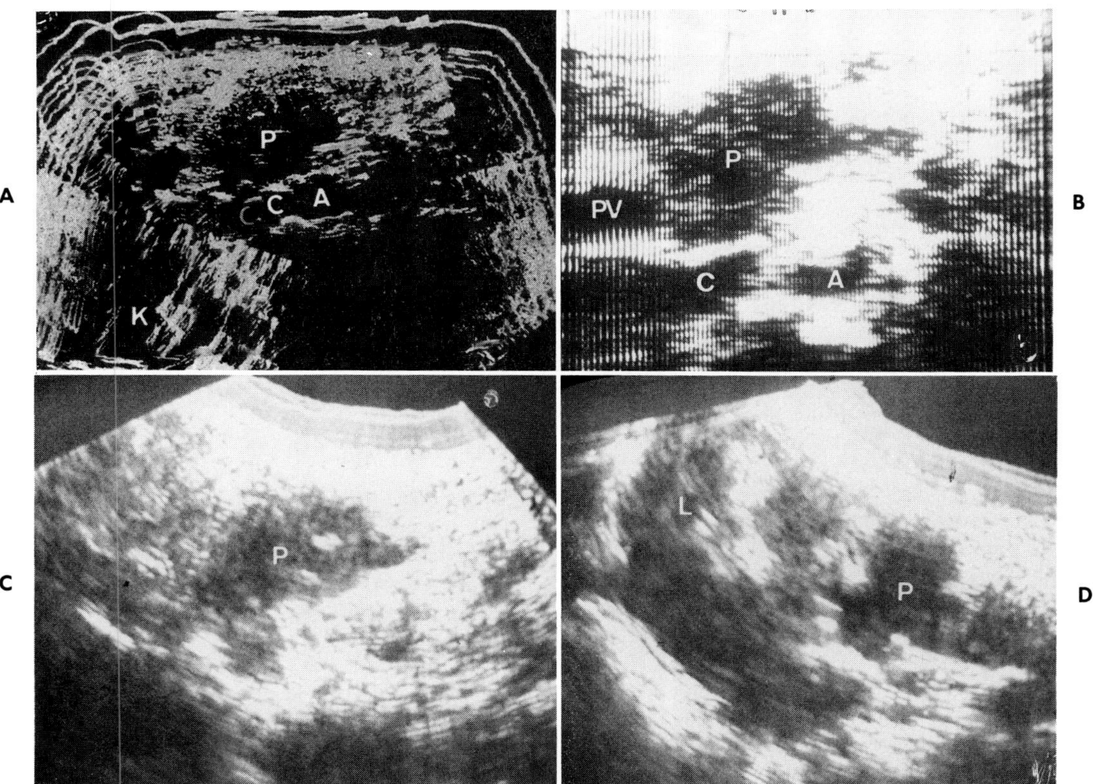

Fig. 22-10. Acute inflammatory process superimposed on chronic pancreatitis. **A,** Transverse bistable scan of upper abdomen showing sonolucent mass with polycyclic limits *(P)* in front of large vessels (*C* and *A*). *K,* right kidney. **B,** Oblique scan in real time displaying semisolid tissue echopattern. *PV,* portal vein. **C,** Gray scale display of pancreatic echopattern (*P*). **D,** Sagittal scan of swollen pancreas. *L,* liver. In such cases, ultrasonic differential diagnosis between inflammation and carcinoma is impossible.

Fig. 22-11. A, Chronic pancreatitis. Pancreatic head is of normal volume and shape *(arrows)*; contours are slightly irregular. Except for reflective nodule, tissue echopattern is sonolucent. In this case, subacute recurrence masks chronic inflammatory pattern. **B,** Transverse scan of diabetic patient complaining of abdominal pain shows sonolucent nodule *(arrows)* inside pancreas *(P),* indicating subacute recurrence. Wirsung's duct *(WD)* seems to be visible. *V,* splenoportal junction and splenic vein.

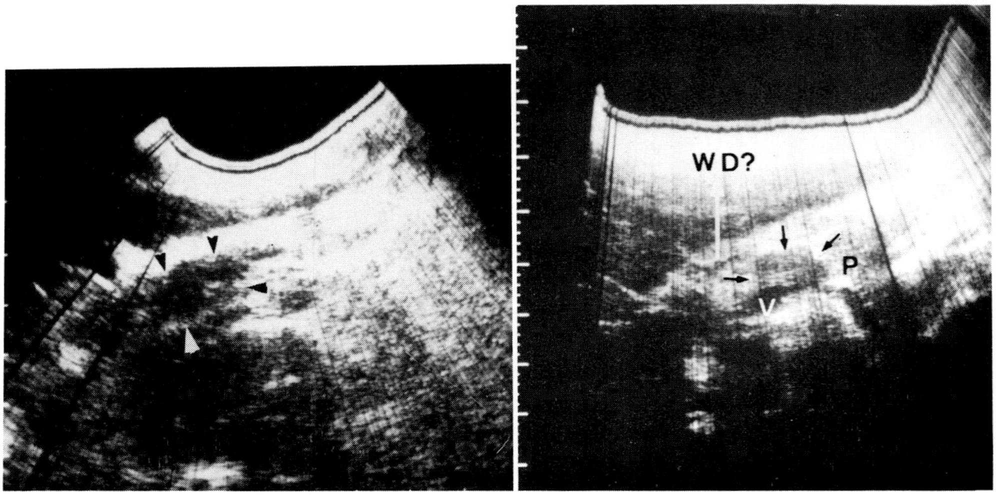

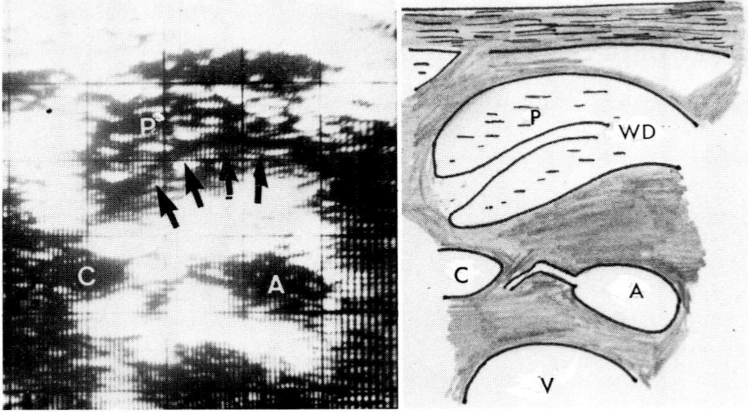

Fig. 22-12. Chronic pancreatitis. Real-time transverse scan and schematic drawing show enlarged pancreatic head *(P)* in front of large vessels (*C* and *A*). Echopattern is micronodular —typical for chronic pancreatitis. In middle of pancreatic tissue, tubular structure *(arrows)* is outlined: this is Wirsung's duct *(WD). V,* vertebral body.

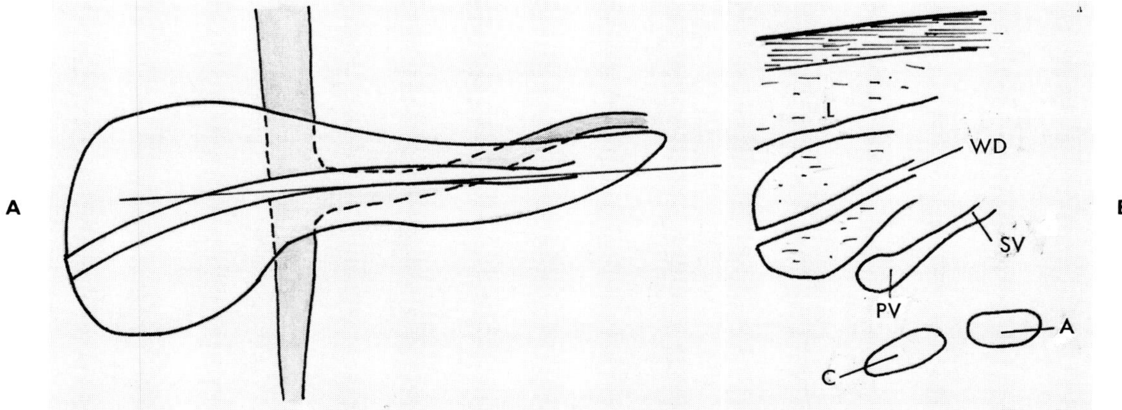

Fig. 22-13. Anatomical relations of Wirsung's duct. **A,** Schematic representation of pancreas and Wirsung's duct showing similar orientations of Wirsung's duct and splenic vein. **B,** Schematic representation of horizontal section of pancreatic head. From front to back are successively displayed liver *(L),* pancreas with Wirsung's duct *(WD),* splenic vein *(SV)* with splenoportal junction *(PV),* and, finally, great vessels *(C* and *A).* These anatomical elements are also displayed in Fig. 22-14, as well as Fig. 20-16, *A* to *C.*

may show a trend toward detumescence. This evolutive sign has a reliable value. Subacute sonolucent enlargements of inflammatory origin developing in chronic pancreatitis are probably responsible for the rare and confusing sonolucent images encountered in seemingly quiescent pancreatitis.

TUBULAR STRUCTURES—WIRSUNG'S DUCT

In chronic pancreatitis, as in other pathological conditions, pancreatic enlargement can, of course, cause compression of the *vena cava* or the *SMV* (Figs. 22-4, *A,* and 22-9). When the enlarged pancreas possesses irregular margins, these are impressed on the compressed vein.

I have already mentioned in Chapter 19 that it has become rather common to visualize *Wirsung's duct,* especially in pancreatic tissue that has an increased reflectivity (Fig. 22-12). As a matter of fact, when Dr. Eisenscher, who is fond of joking, told us that he would display Wirsung's duct, we thought he was kidding us; this was because we did not remember the excellent paper by Burger and Blauenstein (1974), in which a beautiful image of Wirsung's duct was depicted. A study of the anatomical relations of Wirsung's duct shows that the duct is on about the same level as the splenic vein and the splenoportal junction (Fig. 22-13). A transverse, slightly oblique scan of the epigastrium displays, from front to back, hepatic tissue, pancreatic tissue, Wirsung's duct, pancreatic tissue again, and, last, the splenoportal junction (Figs. 22-6, 22-8, 22-9, 22-12, 22-14, and 22-15, as well as Fig. 20-16, *A* to *C*) (Eisenscher and Weill, 1976). This possibility of displaying the image of Wirsung's duct on pancreatic sections should lead to clinical applications in chronic inflammatory conditions. It ought to be possible to outline tubular dilatations and stenoses regularly, as in Figs. 20-16, *A* to *C,* 22-12, and 22-14.

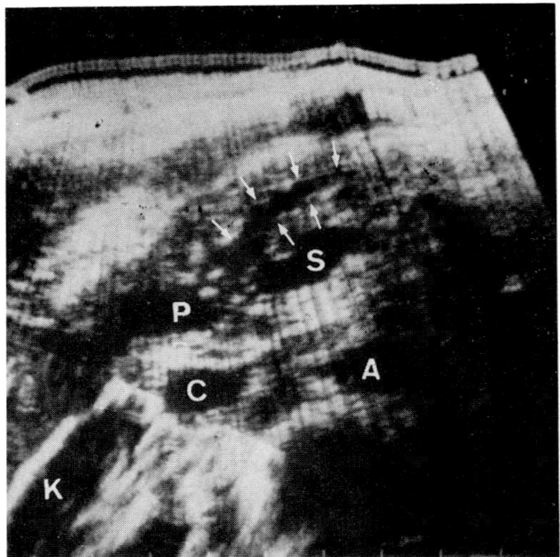

Fig. 22-14. Transverse scan of pancreas showing dilated and sinuous Wirsung's duct *(arrows)*. *P,* portal vein; *S,* splenic vein; *C,* vena cava; *A,* aorta; *K,* right kidney. (See Fig. 20-16.)

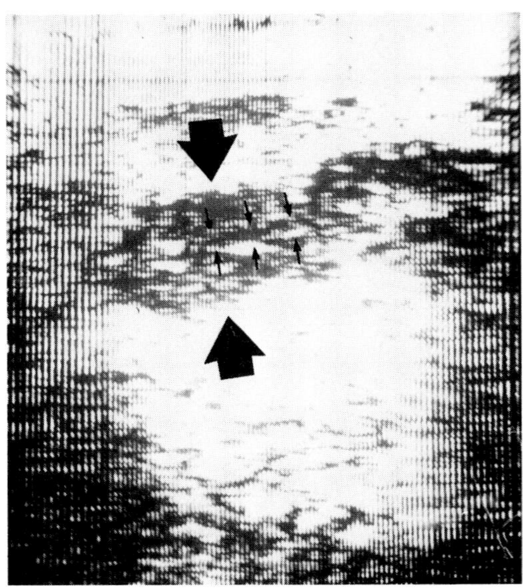

Fig. 22-15. Chronic pancreatitis: Wirsung's duct. Pancreatic head *(large arrows)* is displayed on this slightly oblique scan of epigastrium. Inside pancreatic tissue, narrow tubular structure (Wirsung's duct) is outlined *(small arrows)*.

ASSOCIATED SIGNS

One possible associated sign is a pseudocyst; another, in the case of obstructive jaundice, could be dilatation of the biliary tract (Fig. 26-21). Following and in Fig. 22-16 are presented the signs of chronic pancreatitis:

- Subnormal size
- Reflective, heterogeneous echopattern with micronodules
- Irregular, spiky contours*
- Incidental compression of the mesenteric vein and the vena cava
- Visualization of enlarged and irregular Wirsung's duct
- Pseudocyst and possible enlargement of biliary ducts

RELIABILITY

The rate of reliability in the diagnosis of quiescent chronic pancreatitis (Weill and associates, 1975) is close to 90%, frankly better than the results of associated plain radiography of the abdomen and duodenography, as well as angiography. Retrograde pancreatography ("wirsungography") is, of course, much more precise, since it consistently displays tubular lesions. This invasive procedure, however, is to be considered only if surgery is under consideration. CT scanning can display small calcifications or stones. Its value in tissue analysis when a diagnostic decision between chronic pancreatitis and carcinoma must be made is still to be

*Except in case of superimposed acute or subacute recurrence, which produces enlargement, a sonolucent echopattern, and regular contours.

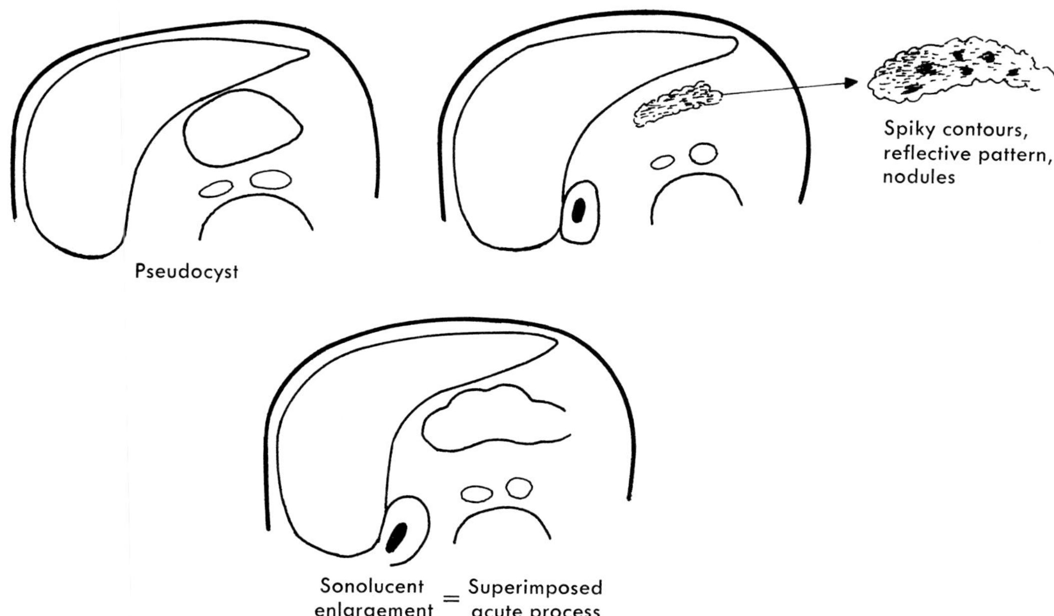

Fig. 22-16. Main ultrasonic features of chronic pancreatitis.

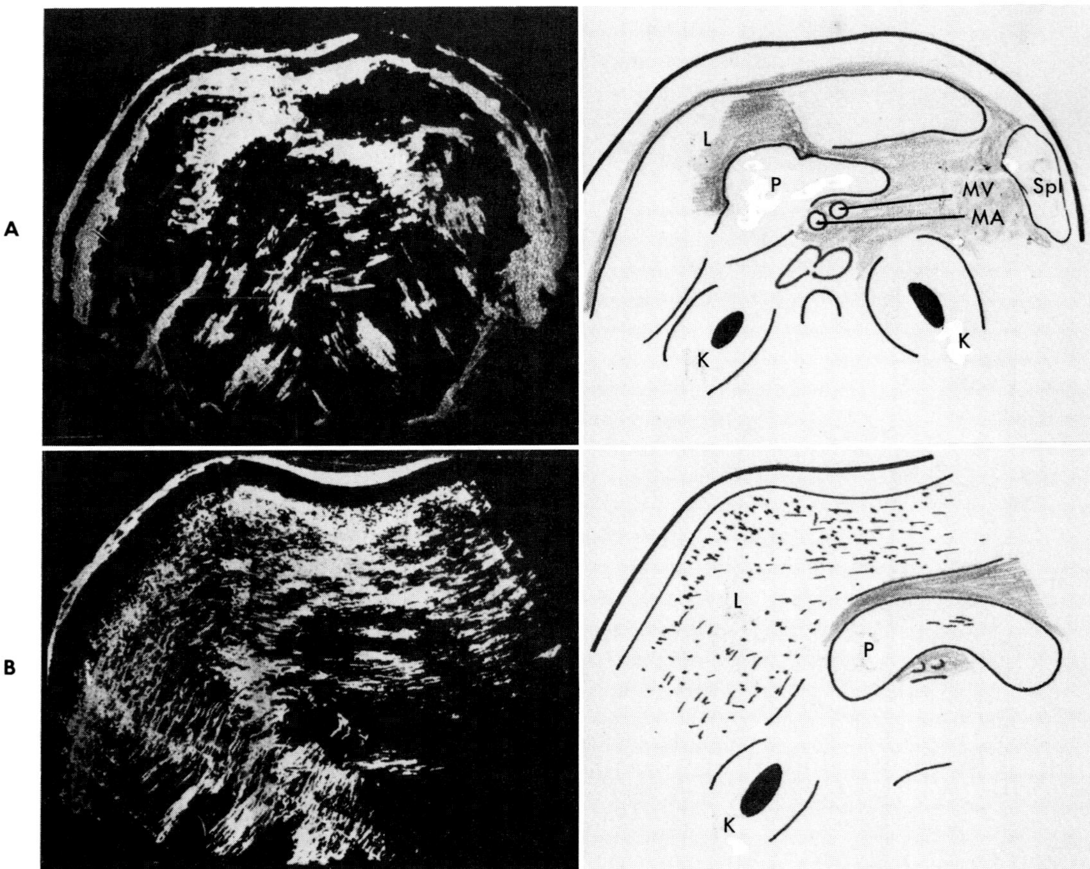

Fig. 22-17. Subacute recurrence of chronic pancreatitis. **A,** Transverse scan and schematic drawing showing large pancreatic mass (*P*). *L,* liver; *K,* kidneys; *Spl,* spleen; *MV,* mesenteric vein; *MA,* mesenteric artery. **B,** Follow-up examination 8 months later showed frank decrease in volume. Pancreatectomy, performed because of persisting pain, confirmed presence of inflammatory mass.

determined. Indeed, this is the real problem. The diagnostic difficulties arise in the presence of an enlarged pancreas with reflective nodules and sonolucent areas displayed on scans of a patient who is losing weight and complaining of abdominal pain. In such cases, an ultrasonic decision between carcinoma and subacute recurrence of chronic pancreatitis is impossible except in the presence of the following signs: marginal pseudopod-like extensions (carcinoma, Chapter 23) or global enlargement and a trend toward volume decrease (subacute recurrence, Fig. 22-17). If these signs are absent, other procedures are then helpful.

Problems of differential diagnosis will be discussed again in Chapter 24.

REFERENCES

Barnett, E., and Morley, P.: Abdominal echography, Borough Green, England, 1974, Butterworth & Co. (Publishers), Ltd.

Burger, J., and Blauenstein, V. W.: Current aspects of ultrasonic scanning of the pancreas, Am. J. Roentgenol. Radium Ther. Nucl. Med. **122:**406-412, 1974.

Eisenscher, A., and Weill, F.: Ultrasonographie du canal de Wirsung, illusion ou possibilité? Note préliminaire, paper presented at the annual meeting of the French Society for Ultrasound in Medicine and Biology, Strasbourg, France, June 28, 1976.

Goldberg, B. B., Kotler, M. N., Ziskin, M. C., and Waxham, R. D.: Diagnostic uses of ultrasound, New York, 1975, Grune & Stratton, Inc.

Hassani, N.: Ultrasonography of the abdomen, Heidelberg, Germany, 1976, Springer-Verlag.

Holm, H. H., Kristensen, J. K., Rasmussen, S. N., Pedersen, J. F., and Hancke, S.: Abdominal ultrasound, Copenhagen, 1976, Munksgaard, International Booksellers & Publishers, Ltd.

Leopold, G. R., and Asher, W. M.: Fundamentals of abdominal and pelvic ultrasonography, Philadelphia, 1975, W. B. Saunders Co.

Weill, F., Becker, J. C., Kraehenbuhl, J. R., Heriot, G., and Walter, J. P.: Clinical atlas of ultrasonic radiography, Paris, 1973, Masson & Cie., Éditeurs.

Weill, F., Bourgoin, A., Aucant, D., Eisenscher, A., and Gallinet, D.: Pancréatite chronique, cancer du pancréas, différenciation par ultrasons, Nouv. Presse Med. **4:**567-570, 1975.

Weill, F., Kraehenbuhl, J. R., Becker, J. C., Gillet, M., and Bourgoin, A.: Echotomography of the pancreas; a critical and comparative study. In Anacker, H., editor: Efficiency and limits of radiological examination of the pancreas, Stuttgart, Germany, 1975, Georg Thieme Verlag.

CHAPTER 23

PANCREATIC TUMORS

Pancreatic tumors are chiefly carcinomas, but there is no ultrasonic method of differentiating a true pancreatic carcinoma from an ampullary tumor or from a cholangiocarcinoma arising from the intrapancreatic segment of the common bile duct. More rarely, cystadenomas or islet cell tumors are encountered.

GENERAL ULTRASONIC FEATURES OF CARCINOMAS

The following data are based on the study of ninety-three pancreatic tumors with surgical proof of carcinoma.

Pancreatic enlargement

In most cases, there is partial enlargement of the head, body, or tail of the pancreas. Such partial enlargement produces loss of the harmonious character of the glandular contours and a new pancreatic shape, quite different from the basic shapes described in Chapter 19 (Figs. 23-1 to 23-8). Partial enlargement may be consistent with the presence of a rather small tumor. As was stated, the normal pancreas is no thicker than 32 mm. A cephalic thickness of 4 cm includes both the thickness of the normal glandular tissue and the tumoral tissue. The latter, then, is only 1 to 2 cm thick. (See Figs. 23-1 to 23-5 and 23-8.) Tumors of the head of the pancreas are usually fairly small, and it is ordinarily jaundice that offers the opportunity of a relatively early diagnosis. Other examples of small cephalic tumors will be given in Chapter 26. Unfortunately, the diagnosis is often made in the presence of much larger tumors. A large part of the pancreatic tissue is then swollen. (See Figs. 23-7, 23-9, 23-10, and 23-12 to 23-14.) Massive enlargement or a global harmonious enlargement such as those seen in the study of acute inflammatory processes is usually not encountered in carcinomas. There is generally no masking intestinal gas in front of the pancreatic head, so that early diagnosis is possible. At the stage in which they can be clinically suspected, tumors of the body of the pancreas are large enough to displace to the side eventually gas-filled intestinal loops. This is not the case with tumors of the tail, since in that area there are large gas collections in the colon almost constantly. In the pancreatic tail the threshold of visibility with an anterior approach is at least 3 cm in diameter (Fig. 23-12). In the search for a pancreatic tumor, as with other lesions, the systemic use of a posterior approach through the left kidney is compulsory (Fig. 23-16, *B*).

Pancreatic contours

Pancreatic contours are well defined. Rettenmaier (1973) has described localized tumoral extensions that he compared to pseudopods. Such extension images, if frequent, are, however, inconstant. (See Figs. 23-1, 23-6, *A*, 23-8, *B*, 23-

Text continued on p. 364.

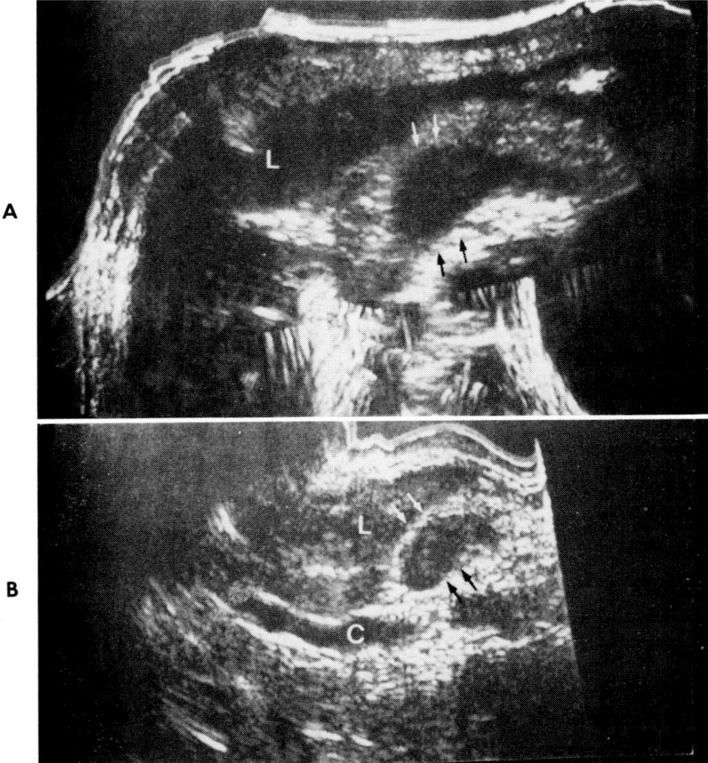

Fig. 23-1. Pancreatic cephalic tumor. **A,** Transverse scan. Head of pancreas is enlarged *(arrows)*. General shape of gland is altered, but contours remain smooth. Mass is sonolucent. Gray peripheral strip represents stomach and duodenum. *L,* liver. **B,** Sagittal scan. Note distance between tumor and vena cava *(C)*.

Fig. 23-2. Pancreatic cephalic tumor. Head of pancreas *(T)* is enlarged, and its contours are irregular, with small marginal extensions. Tissue echopattern is heterogeneous, with delineation between mass and body of pancreas *(P)*. *L,* liver; *C,* vena cava; *A,* aorta; *AS,* acoustic shadow of colonic gas.

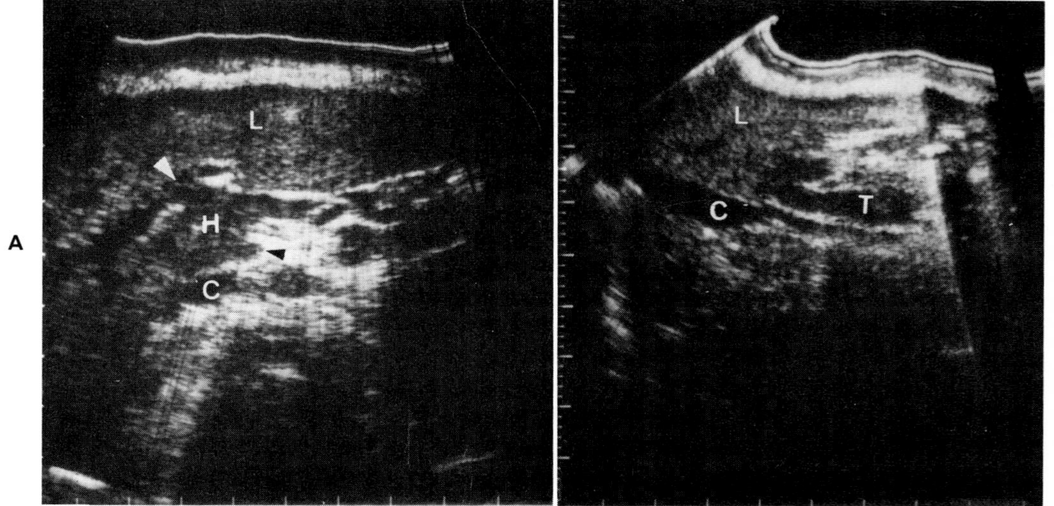

Fig. 23-3. Pancreatic carcinoma. **A,** Transverse scan displaying enlargement of pancreatic head *(H)*. There is anterolateral pseudopod-like extension *(white arrowhead)*. Small extension *(black arrowhead)* outlined in front of vena cava *(C)* seemingly belongs to normal uncinate process. *L,* liver. **B,** Sagittal scan showing pancreatic mass *(T)* with important craniocaudal extension. Behind mass, vena cava, which should be dilated because of right cardiac insufficiency, is flattened. *L,* liver.

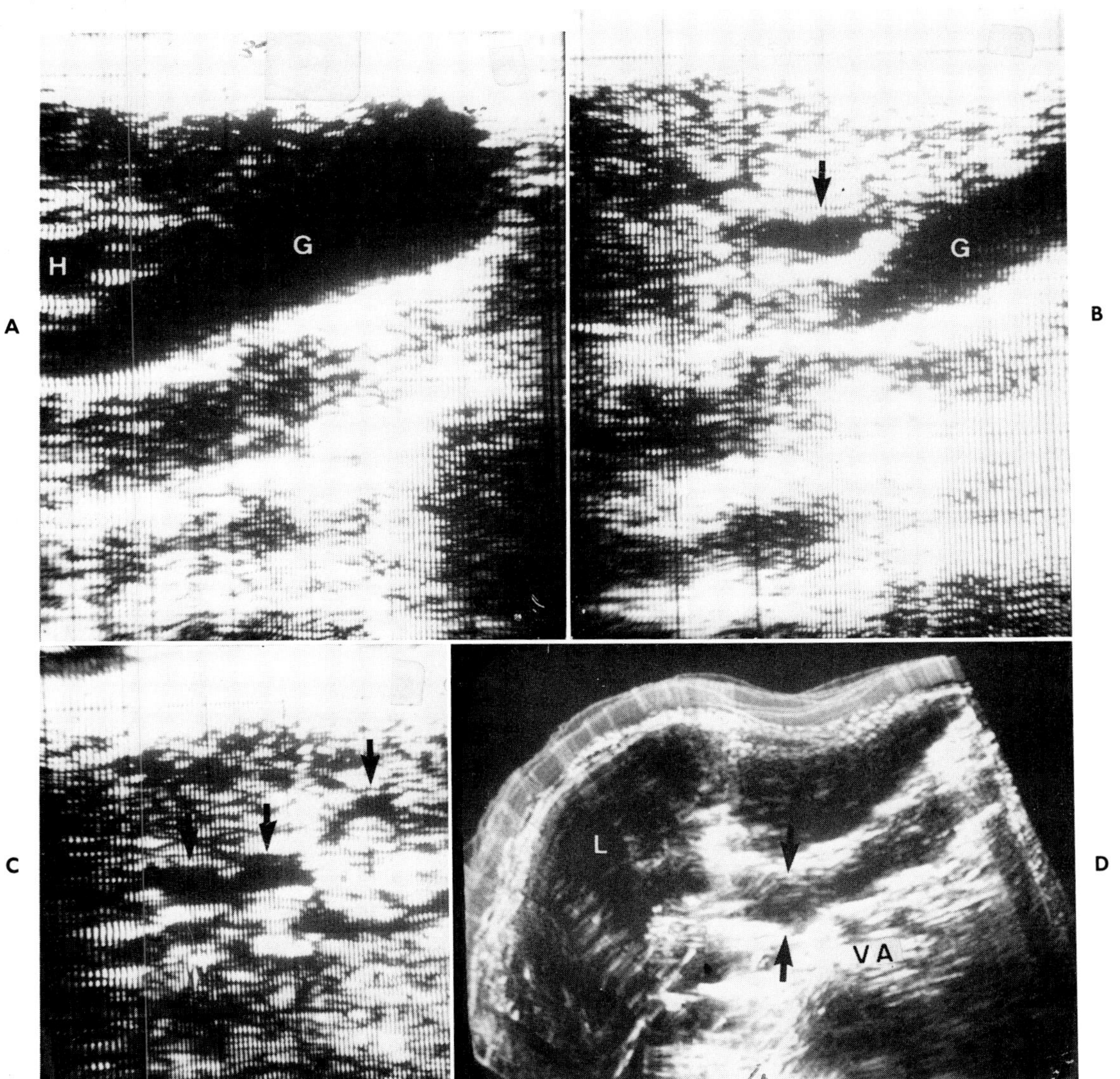

Fig. 23-4. Tumor of pancreatic head, with jaundice. **A,** Sagittal scan of right upper quadrant showing enlarged gallbladder *(G)* and common duct *(H)*. **B,** Parallel scan also displaying enlargement of biliary duct *(arrow)*. **C,** Oblique recurrent hepatic scan showing dilatation of intrahepatic biliary network *(arrows)*. **D,** Transverse scan displaying alteration of pancreatic shape, with anterior and posterior bulge at level of head *(arrows)*. Other bulges mark posterior aspect of gland. Echopattern remains sonolucent. At operation, small (2 cm in diameter) cephalic tumor corresponding to intrapancreatic cholangiocarcinoma was found, with neighboring inflammatory changes explaining body enlargement. *L,* liver; *VA,* mesenteric artery and vein.

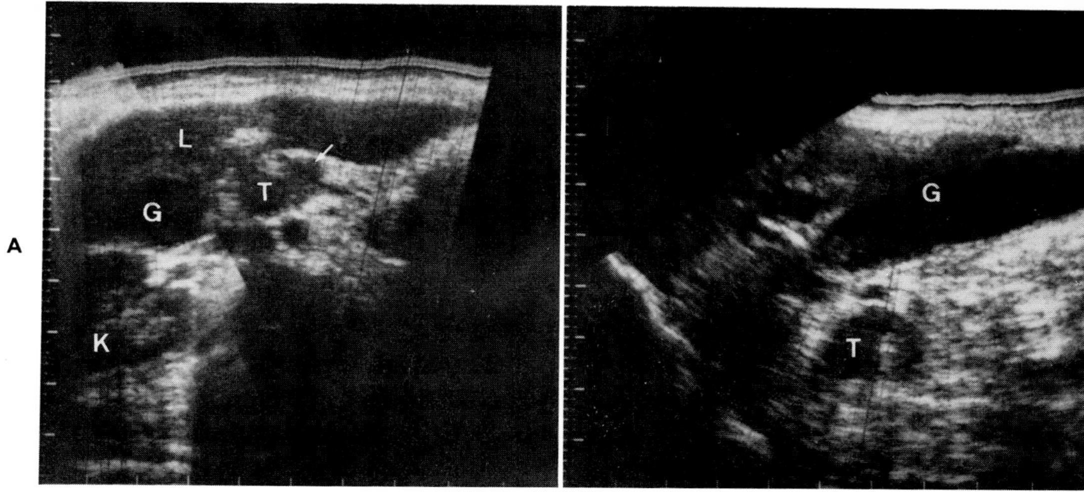

Fig. 23-5. Tumor of pancreatic head. **A,** Transverse scan of upper abdomen showing oval sonolucent mass *(T)* between liver *(L)* and large vessels. Pseudopod-like bulge *(arrow)* is outlined on its left aspect. *G,* gallbladder; *K,* kidney. **B,** Sagittal scan displaying tumor. Gallbladder and hilar bile duct are dilated. Note shotgun sign (Chapter 26). (Courtesy Dr. F. Winsberg, Montreal.)

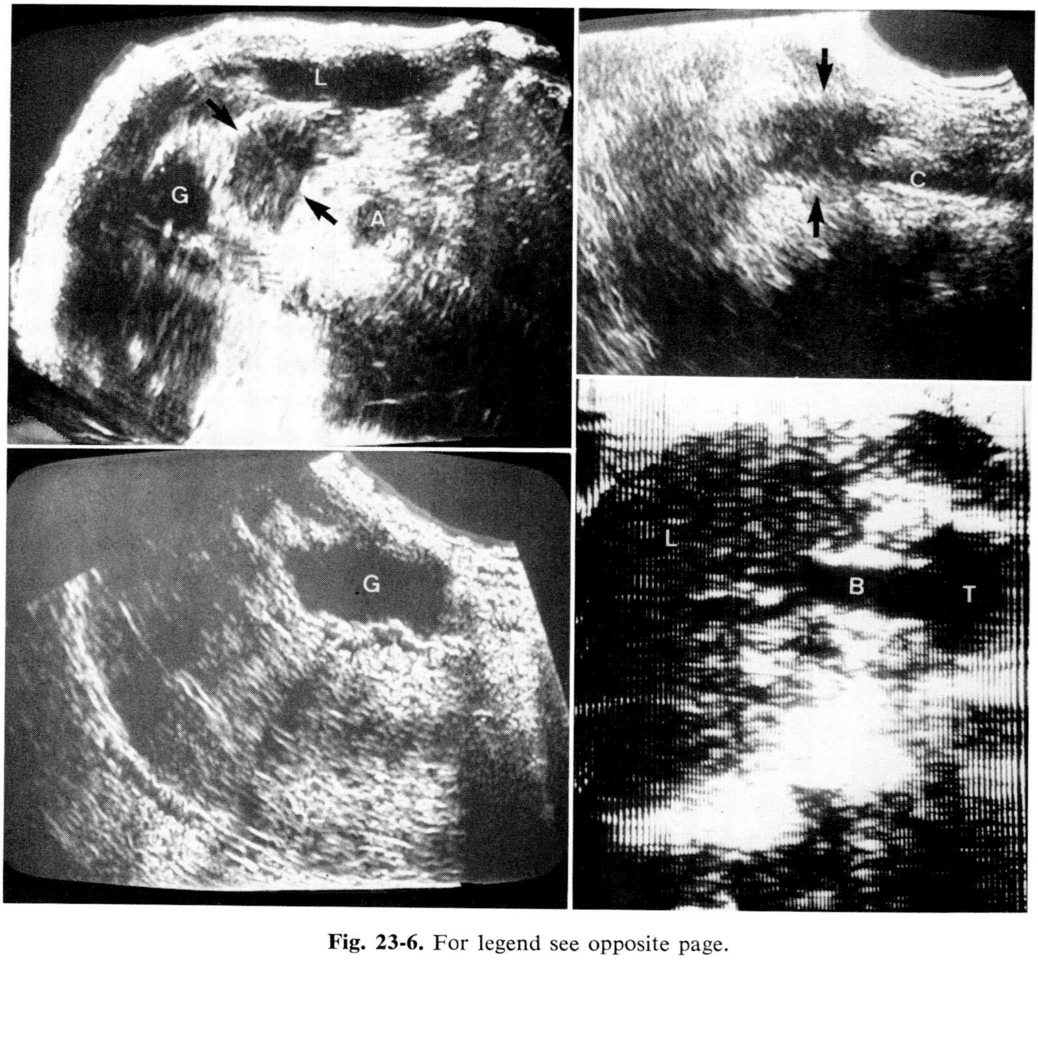

Fig. 23-6. For legend see opposite page.

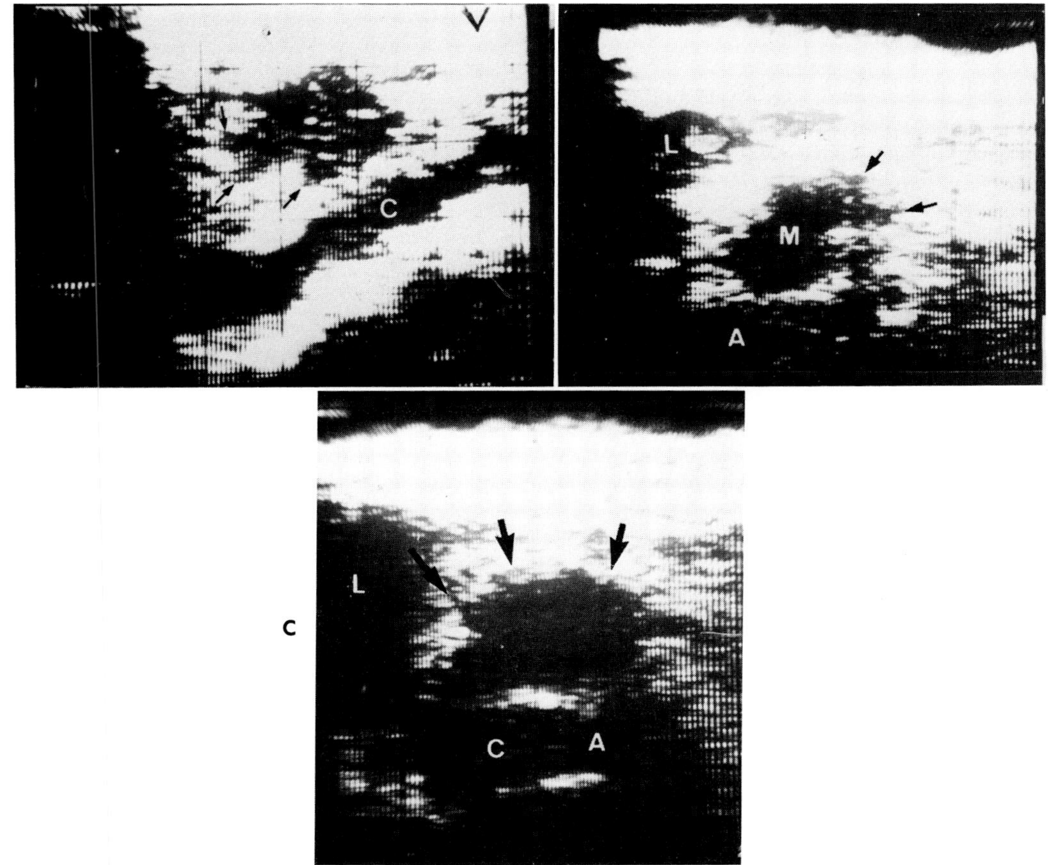

Fig. 23-7. Three carcinomas (real-time study). In these examples, tumoral echopattern is typically sonolucent. **A,** Carcinoma of pancreatic head. This sagittal scan shows multiple pseudopod-like extensions *(arrows)*. *C,* vena cava. **B,** Carcinoma of pancreatic body. Sagittal scan also displays pseudopod-like extensions *(arrows)*. *L,* liver; *A,* aorta; *M,* mass. **C,** Carcinoma of pancreatic neck and body. Anterior contours are irregular, with beginning pseudopod-like extensions.

Fig. 23-6. Pancreatic tumor with jaundice. **A,** Transverse scan of upper abdomen showing reflective mass *(arrows)* behind liver *(L)*. Dilated gallbladder *(G)* lies in close contact with mass. *A,* aorta. **B,** Sagittal scan showing tumoral mass *(arrows)* in front of vena cava *(C)*, with indistinct delineation. **C,** Parallel scan through right upper quadrant displaying enlarged gallbladder. **D,** Intercostal scan showing dilated main bile duct *(B)* and its branches above tumor *(T)*.

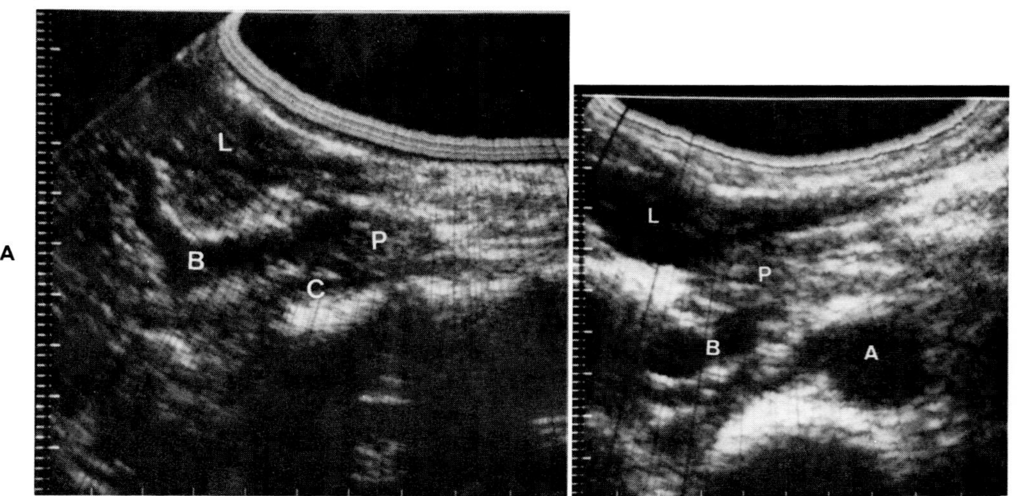

Fig. 23-8. Small tumor of pancreatic head. **A,** Sagittal scan showing small pancreatic mass *(P)* in close contact with distal segment of dilated main bile duct *(B)*. Its contours are regular; nevertheless, small caudal extension is seen in front of vena cava. Level of reflectivity is unusually high. Vena cava is flattened. *L,* liver; *C,* vena cava. **B,** Transverse scan also displaying mass. Note narrowing of intratumoral bile duct *(B)*. *A,* aorta.

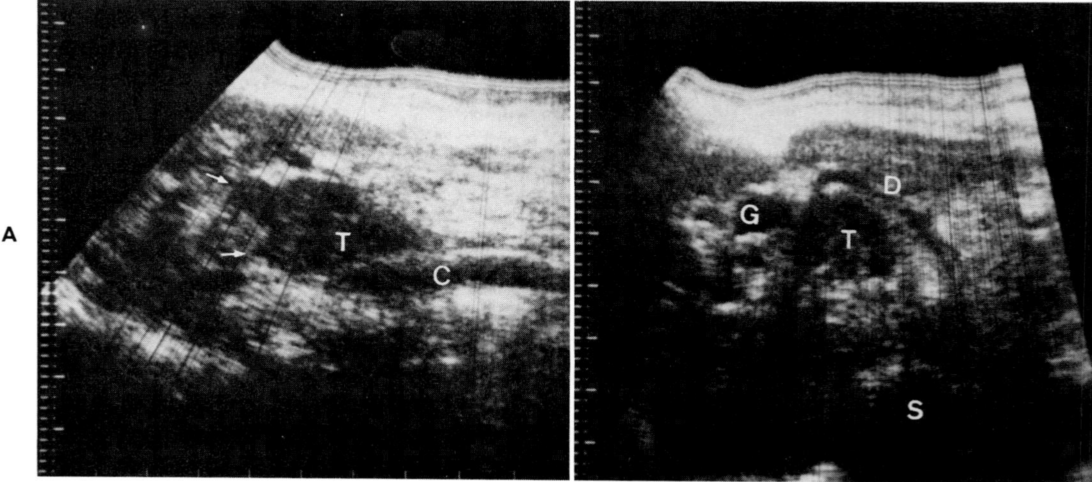

Fig. 23-9. Carcinoma of pancreatic head. **A,** Sagittal scan displaying several pseudopod-like extensions *(arrows)*. Vena cava *(C)* is flattened by mass *(T)*. **B,** Transverse scan showing large sonolucent cephalic mass in close relation to gallbladder *(G)*. Sonotransparent strip *(D)* running along its anterior aspect likely belongs to duodenum and gastric antrum. *S,* spine. (Courtesy Dr. M. Graham, Montreal.)

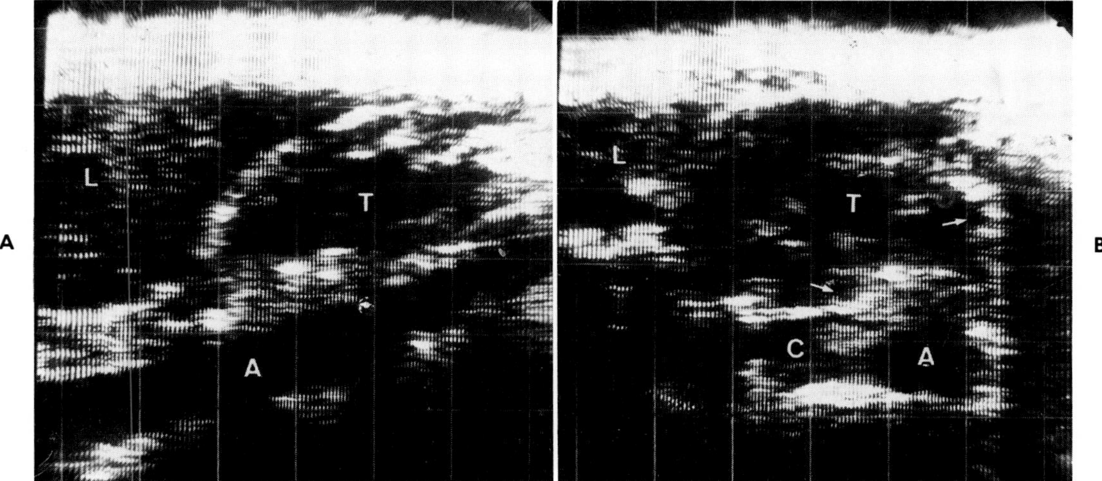

Fig. 23-10. Large tumoral mass. **A,** Sagittal scan. **B,** Transverse scan showing pseudopod-like extensions *(arrows).* Reflective areas in liver *(L)* indicate presence of metastatic deposits. *T,* tumor; *A,* aorta; *C,* vena cava.

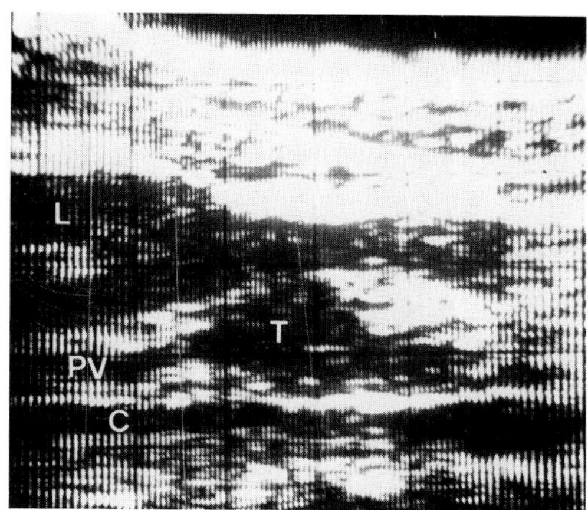

Fig. 23-11. Carcinoma of pancreatic head. Contours are smooth. Mass *(T)* flattens vena cava *(C)*. *L,* liver; *PV,* portal vein.

Fig. 23-12. Tumors of pancreatic body and tail. **A,** Transverse scan displaying tumoral mass *(T)* and neighboring normal pancreatic tissue *(P)*. Splenic vein *(V)* section is interrupted at level of tumor; this was also shown by celiac angiography. Note pseudopod-like extensions *(arrows)*. *A,* aorta. **B,** Another transverse scan displaying large, rounded, sonolucent tumoral mass on left side, representing tumor of pancreatic tail *(arrows)*. *L,* liver; *K,* kidney. (**B** courtesy Dr. F. Winsberg, Montreal.)

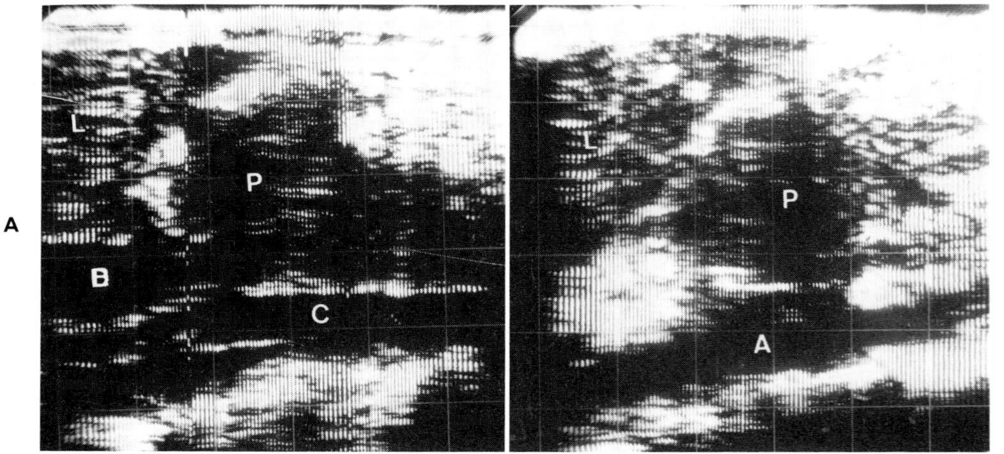

Fig. 23-13. Sonolucent echopattern of pancreatic carcinoma. **A,** Sagittal scan through vena cava (*C*) showing, between liver (*L*) and vein, greatly enlarged pancreatic head (*P*) of sonolucent echopattern with pseudopod-like extensions. Note enlarged common bile duct *(B)*. **B,** Parallel scan at level of aorta again showing section of pancreatic tumor with its sonolucent echopattern. Tumoral tissue is less reflective than liver tissue. *A,* aorta.

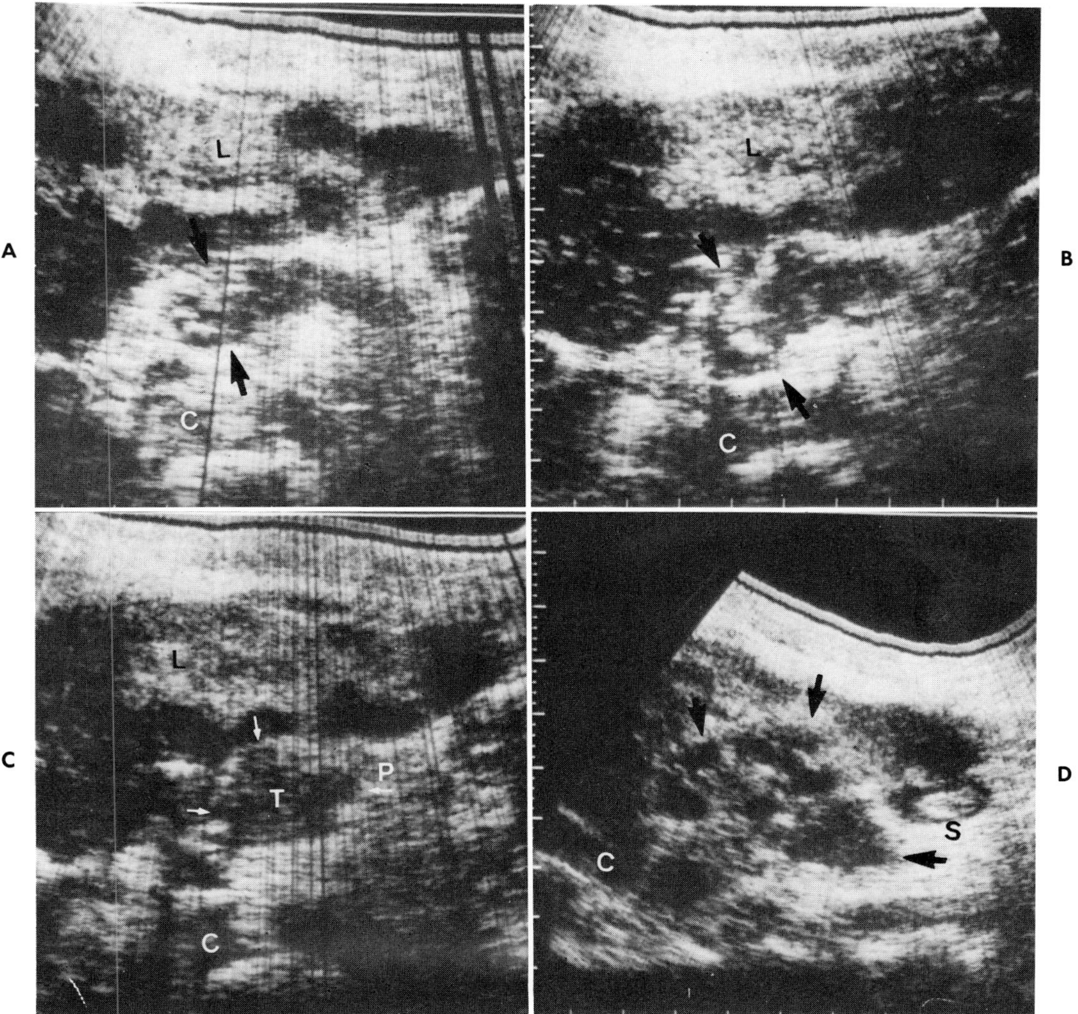

Fig. 23-14. Pancreatic carcinoma. **A,** Transverse scan at level of xiphoid displaying pancreas *(arrows)* behind liver *(L),* in which metastatic deposits are scattered. Pancreatic head is slightly enlarged, with reflective nodules consistent with chronic pancreatitis. *C,* vena cava. **B,** More caudal parallel scan showing frankly enlarged pancreatic head. There are still a few reflective nodules, but most of pancreatic tissue is sonolucent. There are several pseudopod-like extensions. **C,** More caudal scan displaying usual sonolucent pattern of tumor *(T)* and sharp extensions *(arrows).* Echopattern of tumor is less reflective than that of normal pancreatic tissue *(P).* **D,** Sagittal scan. Note flattening of vena cava. Ill-defined limit between tumor and vessel indicates vascular involvement. Note also bull's-eye ovoid structure *(S)* representing sagittal section of stomach.

11, and 23-12, *B*.) Nevertheless, the general pattern of pancreatic contours in cases involving tumors is more bumpy and irregular than in an acute inflammatory process, but not so irregular and spiky as in chronic pancreatitis (Chapter 22). Examples of well-delineated, slightly irregular contours are illustrated in Figs. 23-1, *B,* 23-3, *B,* and 23-4, *D*. Pseudopod-like images are shown in Figs. 23-2, 23-3, *A,* 23-5, *A,* 23-7, 23-9, *A,* 23-10, and 23-12, *A,* to 23-14. Contours remain rather smooth in the cases illustrated in Figs. 23-1, 23-4, and 23-8.

Pancreatic tumoral echopattern

Almost constantly, as in eighty-seven of ninety-three cases, the echopattern of the carcinoma is sonolucent, of semisolid type, that is, with a few scattered echoes. Such a tissue echopattern is similar to the Type II echopattern of acute pancreatitis. (See Figs. 23-1 to 23-5, 23-7 to 23-13, and 23-14, *C* and *D*.) With the machines of the third generation it is now possible to clearly differentiate the tumoral tissues from the neighboring normal pancreatic tissue (Figs. 23-2, 23-12, *A,* and 23-14, *C*). Possible neighboring inflammatory changes (Fig. 23-4, *D*) must be remembered. We saw only six carcinomas (roughly 5%) with a frank solid echopattern: of these, three were solid homogeneous (Figs. 23-6, *A,* and 23-8); in the three others, reflective areas and nodules were associated with large sonolucent areas (Fig. 23-14). As mentioned in Chapter 22, this pattern is similar to that of chronic pancreatitis with subacute recurrence except for possible pseudopod-like extensions. The usual pattern of pancreatic tumors is illustrated in Fig. 23-15.

Associated signs

Associated signs may include the following:

1. *Compression of the vena cava* (Figs. 23-3, *B,* 23-6, 23-8, 23-9, and 23-14, *D*) *and the superior mesenteric vein.* As a matter of fact, the mesenteric vein is usually so flattened that it is not visible. Ill-defined limits between the posterior aspect of the tumor and the anterior wall of the vena cava indicate posterior extension with caval involvement (Figs. 23-6, *B,* 23-8, *A,* and 23-14, *D*). Real-time analysis of the relations between the tumor and the vena cava is more precise;

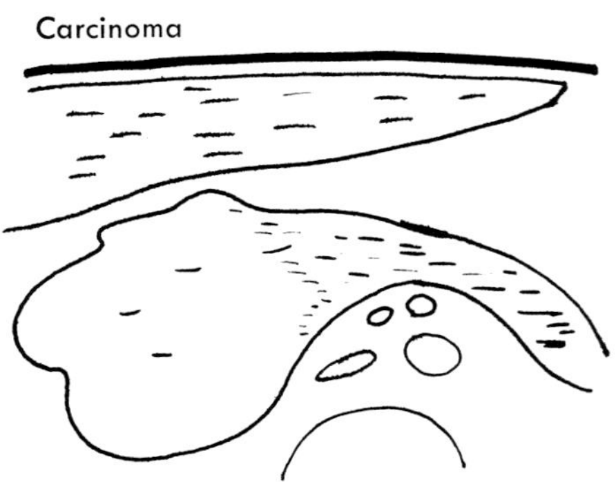

Fig. 23-15. Schematic representation of pancreatic cephalic carcinoma.

use of contrasted cavography, however, remains necessary to confirm ultrasonic indications of venous involvement.

2. *Dilatation of the biliary tract above the tumor* (Figs. 23-4, 23-6, 23-8, 23-11, and 23-13). This will also be shown in Chapter 26.
3. *Possible hepatic metastases* (Figs. 23-10 and 23-14).
4. *Rare ascites.*

• • •

Following are the main ultrasonic signs of pancreatic carcinoma:

- Partial enlargement
- Polycyclic, rather regular contours (with possible pseudopod-like extensions)
- Sonolucent echopattern of semisolid type
- Associated signs
  Vena cava and superior mesenteric vein compression
  Possible dilatation of the biliary tract
  Possible hepatic metastases

RARE TUMORS

When the islet cell tumor secretes hormones, it gives rise to a precise functional symptomatology while it is still of small size. Any radiologist practicing angiography knows how small this type of tumor can be. A diameter of 0.5 cm is not rare. The ultrasonic display of such a tumor is difficult and can be expected only when the tumor reaches a diameter of 2 cm. Nonsecreting islet cell tumors

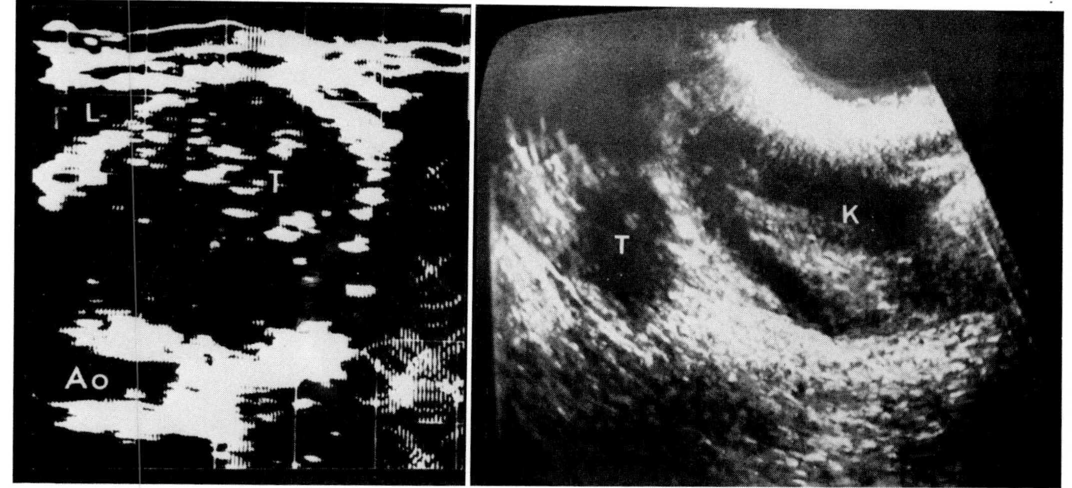

Fig. 23-16. Nonsecreting islet cell tumors. **A,** Sagittal scan showing, between liver *(L)* and aorta *(A),* large rounded tumor *(T)* of generally sonolucent echopattern with a few reflective scattered spots. **B,** Smaller islet cell tumor of pancreatic tail displayed by posterior, transrenal approach. Sonolucent area above kidney and tumor belongs to spleen. *K,* left kidney. (**A** from Weill, F., Becker, J. C., Kraehenbuhl, J. R., Heriot, G., and Walter, J. P.: Clinical atlas of ultrasonic radiography, Paris, 1973, Masson & Cie., Editeurs.)

are clinically silent until their volume is large enough to give rise to functional disturbances by compression. They are then much more accessible to ultrasonography. The two islet cell tumors that I have seen had a rounded section. The echopattern was heterogeneous in one case (Fig. 23-16, *A*) and of semisolid type in the other (Fig. 23-16, *B*).

Cystadenomas

Cystadenomas have a different pattern, depending on the extent of their cystic elements. If the tumoral cyst has a diameter of several centimeters, the cystadenoma has the appearance of a liquid collection and may be confused with a pseudocyst in the absence of intracystic tumoral vegetations (Weill and colleagues, 1973) (Fig. 23-17). Its appearance is quite different when the cyst is small. This circumstance gives rise to a common physical phenomenon encountered in hydatidiform moles, in echinococcal cysts filled with daughter cysts, and even in some polycystic kidneys. Each wall of the small cystic elements gives rise to its own ultrasonic reflection, so that finally the global echopattern is of solid type (honeycomb pattern) (Wolson and Walls, 1976). (See Figs. 23-18 to 23-20.) Certain cystadenomas may reach a large volume. As is often the case, the larger the tumoral volume, the more easily it is displayed and the more difficult is the assessment of its origin. Frankly solid areas may also be encountered in cystadenomas.

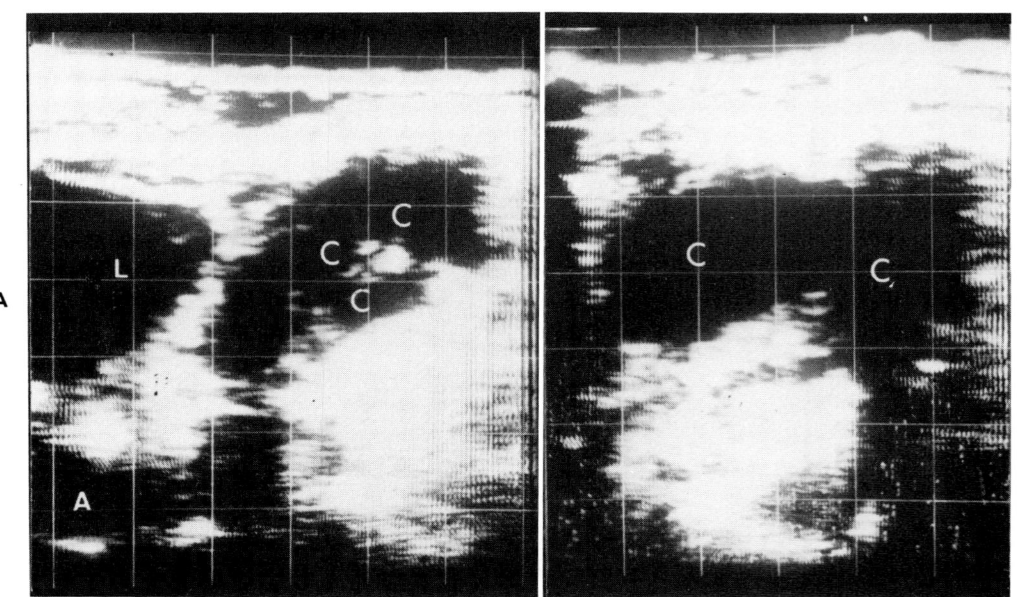

Fig. 23-17. Cystadenoma of cystic type displayed on old real-time scans. **A,** Sagittal scan through aorta showing cystic mass below liver *(L)*. Actually, cystic mass is multilocular. *A,* aorta. **B,** Transverse scan also displaying two cystic areas *(C)*. (From Weill, F., Becker, J. C., Kraehenbuhl, J. R., Heriot, G., and Walter, J. P.: Clinical atlas of ultrasonic radiography, Paris, 1973, Masson & Cie., Editeurs.)

AFTER SURGERY

The pancreatic tail remaining after cephalic pancreatectomy can be displayed by either a posterior or anterior approach (Fig. 23-21, as well as Fig. 20-17).

RELIABILITY

By and large, the rate of reliability in the diagnosis of pancreatic tumors studied in a large series is close to 90% (Weill and co-workers, 1975; Weill and co-workers, 1973). However, all deeply located masses of the upper abdomen are not of pancreatic origin. In Chapter 25 the possible cause of some false-positive diagnoses will be discussed. Most false-negative diagnoses are made in the case of small tumors in patients whose ultrasonic approach is difficult because of a small left hepatic lobe or gas-filled intestines. They may also occur in small tumors of the pancreatic tail. We believe that, if an ultrasonic examination of the pancreas is unsatisfactory or incomplete, one should turn to computerized axial tomography

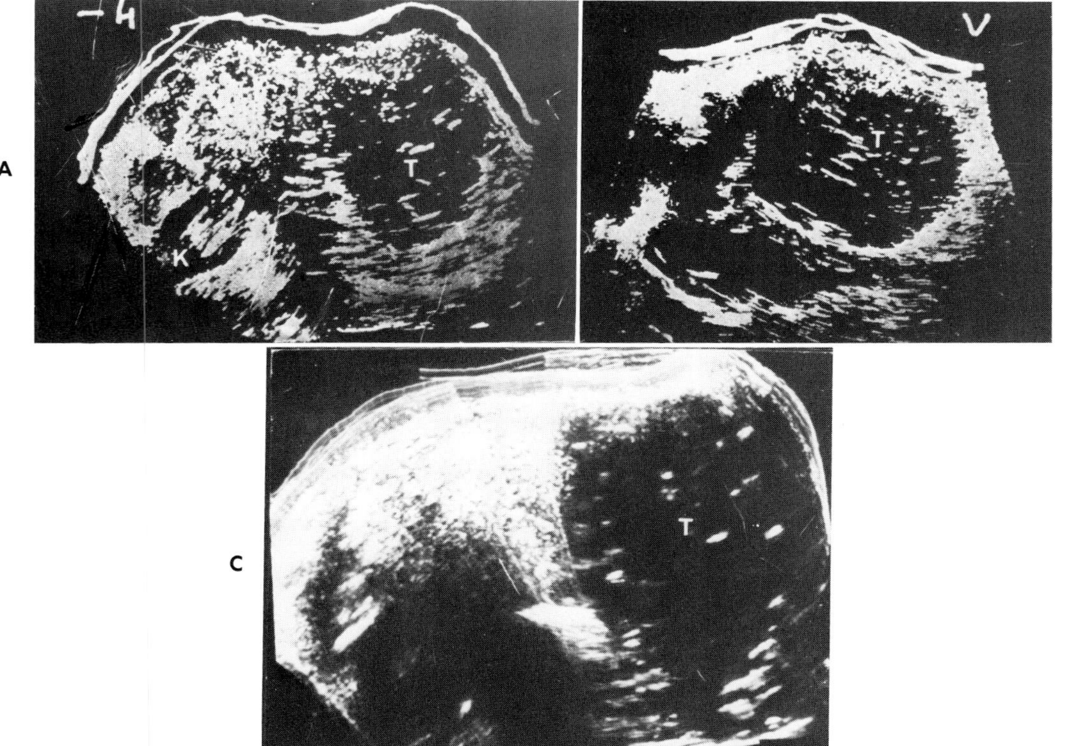

Fig. 23-18. Cystadenoma of reflective type. In this case, small cysts give rise to honeycomb pattern. **A,** Transverse scan of upper abdomen showing large tumor *(T)* occupying left flank. *K,* right kidney. **B,** Sagittal scan of tumor. **C,** Another transverse scan. Tumor was located very low but was nevertheless cystadenoma of pancreatic tail.

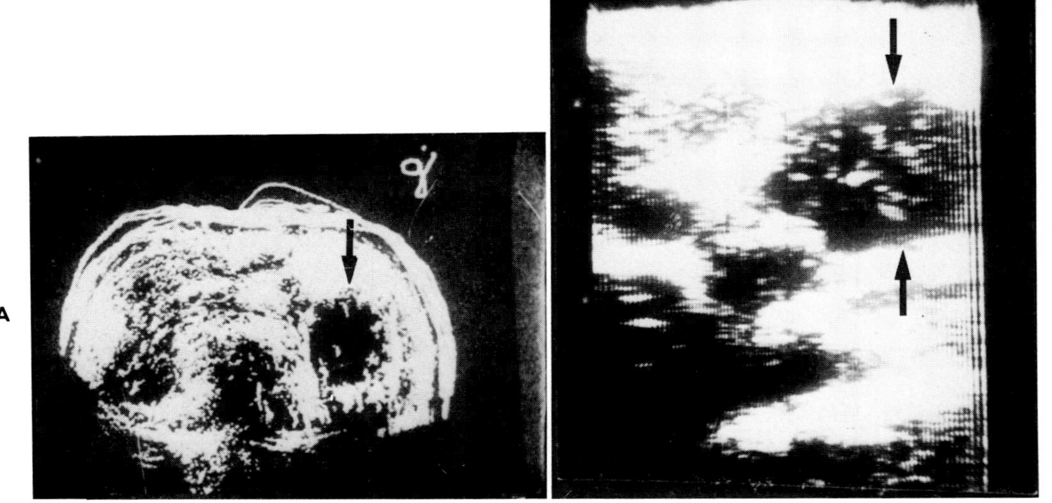

Fig. 23-19. Cystadenoma with small cysts. **A,** Transverse scan of upper abdomen displaying rounded tumor *(arrow)* of pancreatic tail. There are a few scattered intratumoral echoes. **B,** Oblique real-time scan showing typical honeycomb pattern *(arrows).*

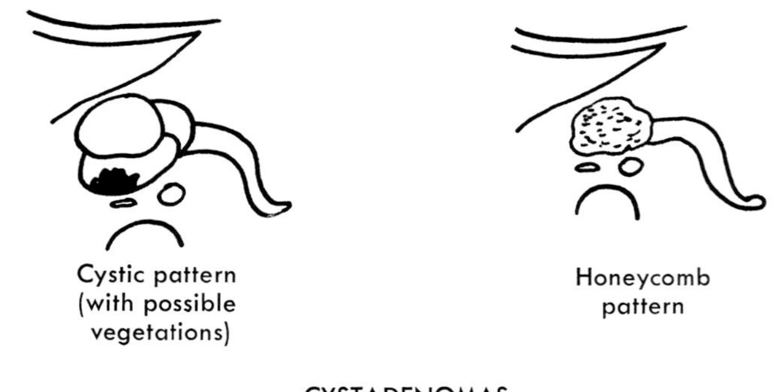

Fig. 23-20. Schematic representation of the two types of cystadenoma.

(Holm and associates, 1976; Dinn and associates, 1976; Kreel, 1976a; Kreel, 1976b; Kreel, 1977; Raskon and associates, 1976); but, of course, before using such a sophisticated procedure, conventional x-ray procedures must be added to ultrasonography. It is pointless to use ultrasound or computerized tomography to search for a small ampullary carcinoma that is readily visible on barium examination of the duodenum.

We do not consider pancreatic scintigraphy to be a reliable procedure. As for angiography, it is performed in our department only as a preoperative step, rather than a diagnostic tool, with the exception of the search for a secreting islet cell tumor. Retrograde pancreatography is used only as a preoperative step with chronic pancreatitis.

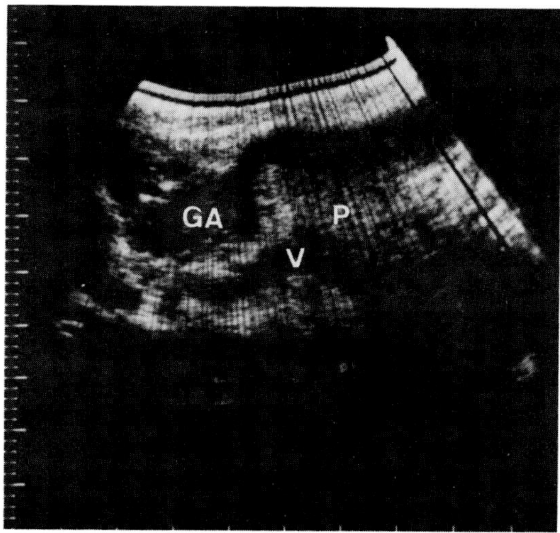

Fig. 23-21. Cephalic pancreatectomy. Gastric antrum *(GA)* has taken place of pancreatic head. *P,* remaining pancreatic body; *V,* splenic vein.

REFERENCES

Barnett, E., and Morley, P.: Abdominal echography, Borough Green, England, 1974, Butterworth & Co. (Publishers), Ltd.

Dinn, W. M., Bryan, P. J., Kieffer, S. A., Grossman, Z. D., and Winston, B.: Patterns of hepatic pathology in B-mode gray scale scanning and computerized tomography, World Federation of Ultrasound in Medicine and Biology, San Francisco, 1976, Abstract No. 538.

Engelhardt, G., and Blauenstein, U. W.: Ultraschall diagnostic von Tumoren der Pancreas Gebiet, Med. Hyg. **29:**118-122, 1971.

Goldberg, B. B., Kotler, M. N., Ziskin, M. C., and Waxham, R. D.: Diagnostic uses of ultrasound, New York, 1975, Grune & Stratton, Inc.

Hassani, N.: Ultrasonography of the abdomen, Heidelberg, Germany, 1976, Springer-Verlag.

Holm, H. H., Kristensen, J. K., Rasmussen, S. N., Pedersen, J. F., and Hancke, S.: Abdominal ultrasound, Copenhagen, 1976, Munksgaard, International Booksellers & Publishers, Ltd.

Holm, H. H., Smith, E. H., and Bartrum, R. J.: Computerized tomography or ultrasound in abdominal diagnosis, World Federation of Ultrasound in Medicine and Biology, San Francisco, 1976, Abstract No. 548.

Kreel, L.: CT of the abdomen, Symposium Ultraschall, Computerisierte Tomographie des Abdomens, Bern, Switzerland, Sept. 4, 1976a.

Kreel, L.: Liver imaging with the body scanner, paper presented at the meeting of the Société Française d'Hépatologie, Strasbourg, France, 1976b.

Kreel, L.: Computerized tomography using the EMI general purpose scanner, Br. J. Radiol. **50:**2-14, 1977.

Leopold, G. R., and Asher, W. M.: Fundamentals of abdominal and pelvic ultrasonography, Philadelphia, 1975, W. B. Saunders Co.

Pietri, H., Rosello, R., Aimino, R., and Sérafino, X.: Diagnostic des petites tumeurs de la queue du pancréas, J. Radiol. Electrol. Med. Nucl. **57:**610, 1976.

Raskon, M. M., Cunningham, J. B., Vinning, P., Salter, J., and Seyer, K.: Comparative abdominal anatomy by ultrasound and computed tomography, World Federation of Ultrasound in Medicine and Biology, San Francisco, 1976, Abstract No. 598.

Rettenmaier, G.: Pankreas Diagnostik mit der Ultraschallschnittbild Methode, Dtsch. Med. Wochenschr. **98:**1973, 1975-1977. Sonography of the pancreas, Second European Congress, Abstract No. 97, Erlangen, Germany, 1975, Junge & Sohn.

Weill, F., Becker, J. C., Kraehenbuhl, J. R., Heriot, G., and Walter, J. P.: Clinical atlas of ultrasonic radiography, Paris, 1973, Masson & Cie., Éditeurs.

Weill, F., Bourgoin, A., Eisenscher, A., and Aucant, D.: Le diagnostic ultrasonore des affections pancréatiques: une tentative d'approche rationnelle fondée sur l'analyse de 260 observations contrôlées, J. Radiol. Electrol. Med. Nucl. **56:**673-683, 1975.

Weill, F., Kraehenbuhl, J. R., Becker, J. C., Gillet, M., and Bourgoin, A.: Echotomography of the pancreas; a critical and comparative study. In Anacker, H., editor: Efficiency and limits of radiological examination of the pancreas, Stuttgart, Germany, 1975, Georg Thieme Verlag.

Wolson, A. H., and Walls, W. J.: Ultrasonic characteristics of cystadenoma of the pancreas, Radiology **119:**203-205, 1976.

CHAPTER 24

ULTRASONIC SYNOPTIC STUDY OF PANCREATIC DISEASES—differential diagnosis of pancreatic diseases (exclusive of nonpancreatic lesions)

Following are the different morphological features of the pancreatic lesions presented in the previous chapters. They are also depicted in Fig. 24-1.

I. Causes and degree of pancreatic enlargement
   - A. Acute pancreatitis ++
   - B. Acute pancreatitis superimposed on chronic pancreatitis ++
   - C. Pancreatic tumor +
   - D. Chronic pancreatitis ±

II. Pancreatic contours
   - A. Acute pancreatitis: regular or polycyclic contours
   - B. Chronic pancreatitis: spiky contours
   - C. Pancreatic tumors: pseudopod-like extensions

III. Causes of increased pancreatic reflectivity with nodular echopattern
   - A. Chronic pancreatitis (usual)
   - B. Pancreatic tumors (exceptional)

IV. Causes of sonolucent enlargements
   - A. Acute pancreatitis
   - B. Subacute pancreatitis
   - C. Acute pancreatitis superimposed on chronic pancreatitis
   - D. Carcinomas

V. Causes of liquid collections
   - A. Pseudocysts and hydropancreatoses
   - B. Cystadenomas
   - C. Exceptional cases
     1. Congenital cysts
     2. Echinococcal cysts
     3. Traumatic hematomas (and abscesses)

As pointed out in Tables 24-1 and 24-2, complementary examinations may be necessary. Angiography has no specificity with regard to liquid collections. Computerized axial tomography is less demonstrative in cystic lesions than ultrasonography. With regard to liquid masses, retrograde pancreatography (wirsungography) does not seem to add useful information. In case of doubt and in countries where echinococcus disease is not endemic, ultrasonically guided puncture, as advised by

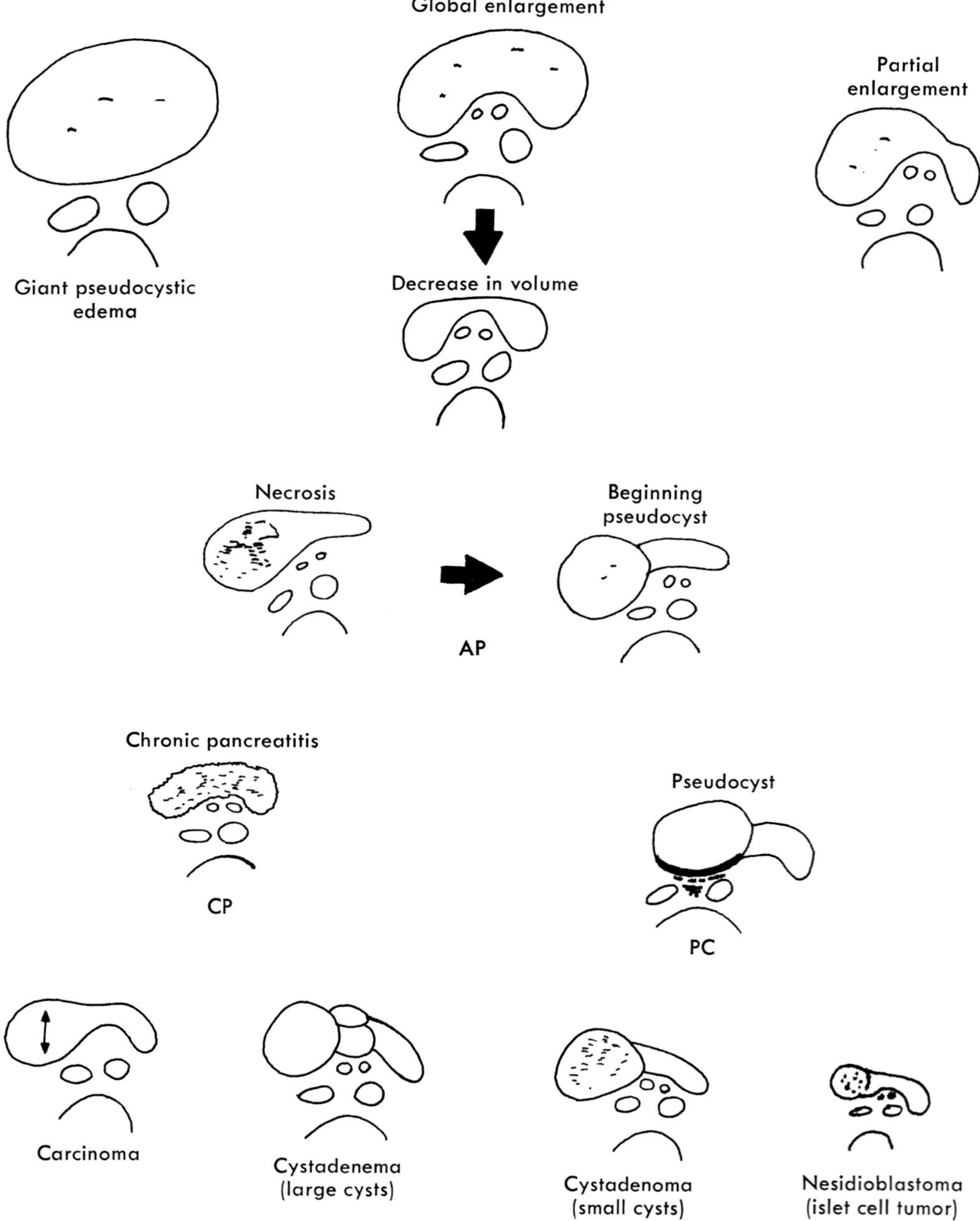

Fig. 24-1. Different morphological features of pancreatic lesions.

Table 24-1. Diagnostic policy in case of sonolucent mass

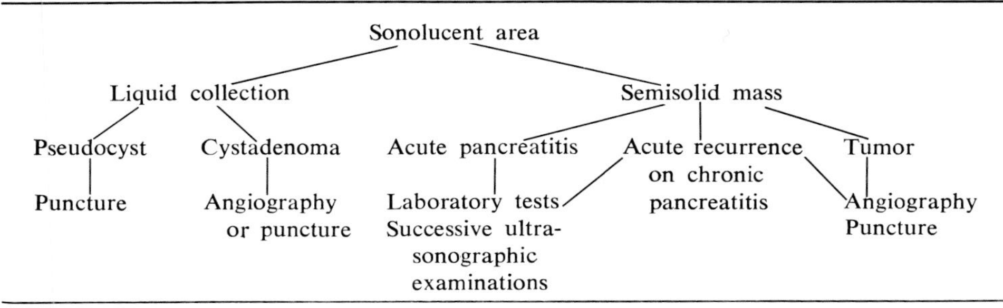

Table 24-2. Diagnostic policy in case of reflective masses

Reflective mass	
Exceptionally, carcinoma or cystadenoma	*Usually, chronic pancreatitis*
• Polycyclic contours Possible pseudopod-like extensions Possibly, significant enlargement	• Irregular, spiky contours Moderate enlargement
• Angiography Puncture	• Ultrasonic follow-up Contingently, retrograde pancreatography, puncture

the Danish school (Hancke and Heje, 1975; Holm, 1971; Holm and colleagues, 1976; Hancke and colleagues, 1975), is probably the best complementary diagnostic procedure. In my opinion, the only complementary examinations to be considered in acute pancreatitis are the laboratory tests. Except for a plain x-ray film of the abdomen, no other radiological procedure besides ultrasonography is useful. The only diagnostic problem that may arise with ultrasonic images is the differentiation between a primary acute pancreatitis and a carcinoma; but, if the ultrasonic images may be rather similar, the clinical data, the laboratory results, and above all the evolution are quite different. The problem is much more difficult in the case of acute pancreatitis superimposed on chronic pancreatitis. In such cases the laboratory tests are often uncharacteristic. Abdominal pain and loss of weight may be present in subacute inflammatory processes, as well as in carcinomas. Angiography may show signs consistent with a carcinoma when displaying arterial encasement and irregular narrowing or obstructions of small arterial structures, but even such vascular anomalies are not absolutely specific. Even the surgeon is not always able, by palpation, to differentiate a tumor from an inflammatory enlargement. This can be important, since a duodenopancreatectomy may be at stake. Retrograde pancreatography can be useful in this situation. The results of computerized axial tomography do not at present (1977) appear to be more specific than ultrasonographic images. Again, ultrasonically guided biopsy is probably the most rational diagnostic approach.

Reflective masses pose less difficult problems. As pointed out in Table 24-2, complementary examinations are usually not necessary in chronic pancreatitis, since the nodular reflective echopattern and the irregular, spiky contours are rather specific. Although certain Wirsung's duct stenoses are now displayed on ultrasonograms, retrograde pancreatography remains the principal examination in chronic pancreatitis when surgery is being considered.

This diagnostic policy, based on analysis of the different morphological features displayed by ultrasonic images, results in an ultrasonographic reliability that is close to 90% (Weill and co-workers, 1975b). However, all masses and all liquid collections in the region are not pancreatic. Before undertaking a morphological analysis of pancreatic lesions, one must be sure that the abnormal image really belongs to the pancreas. There are numerous pitfalls, which will be reviewed in the next chapter.

REFERENCES

Barnett, E., and Morley, P.: Abdominal echography, Borough Green, England, 1974, Butterworth & Co. (Publishers), Ltd.

Bourgoin, A.: L'échotomographie pancréatique; étude critique comparative, thesis, Besançon, France, 1971, University of Besançon.

Burger, J., and Blauenstein, U. W.: Current aspects of ultrasonic scanning of the pancreas, Am. J. Roentgenol. Radium Ther. Nucl. Med. **122:**406-412, 1974.

Filly, R. A., and Freimanis, A.: Echographic diagnosis of pancreatic lesions, Radiology **96:** 575-582, 1970.

Goldberg, B. B., Kotler, M. N., Ziskin, M. C., and Waxham, R. D.: Diagnostic uses of ultrasound, New York, 1975, Grune & Stratton, Inc.

Hancke, S., and Heje, L.: The diagnosis of pancreatic lesions by means of ultrasonic scanning and ultrasonically guided puncture, Second European Congress, Ultrasonics in medicine, Abstract No. 99, Erlangen, Germany, 1975, Junge & Sohn.

Hancke, S., Holm, H. H., and Koch, F.: Ultrasonically guided percutaneous fine needle biopsy of the pancreas, Surg. Gynecol. Obstet. **140:**361-364, 1975.

Hassani, N.: Ultrasonography of the abdomen, Heidelberg, Germany, 1976, Springer-Verlag.

Holm, H. H.: Ultrasonic scanning in the diagnosis of upper abdominal diseases. In Böck, T., and Ossoinig, V., editors: Ultrasonographia medica, vol. 3, Vienna, 1971, Verlag der Wiener Medizinischer Akademie.

Holm, H. H., Kristensen, J. K., Rasmussen, S. N., Pedersen, J. F., and Hancke, S.: Abdominal ultrasound, Copenhagen, 1976, Munksgaard, International Booksellers & Publishers, Ltd.

Holmes, J. H., Findley, L., and Franck, B.: Diagnosis of pancreatic diseases using ultrasound, Trans. Am. Clin. Climatol. Assoc. **85:**224-234, 1973.

Kitamura, T., Kawai, S., Nakagawa, F., Horiuchi, N., and Morrii, T.: Ultrasonic diagnosis of the pancreas, Jpn. J. Clin. Med. **31:**562-568, 1973.

Kitamura, T., Nakagawa, F., Morrii, T., and Kawai, S.: Ultrasonogram of the pancreatic cancer, Med. Ultrasound **9:**73-74, 1971.

Kobayashi, N.: Diagnosis of pancreatic diseases by ultrasound, Med. Ultrasound **9:**1-2, 1971.

Leopold, G. R.: Echographic study of the pancreas, J.A.M.A. **232:**287-289, 1975.

Leopold, G. R., and Asher, W. M.: Fundamentals of abdominal and pelvic ultrasonography, Philadelphia, 1975, W. B. Saunders Co.

Murat, J., Chinille, E., Floyrac, G., Garnier, G., Crassas, Y., Planiol, T., and Aron, E.: Echography and scintigraphy in the diagnosis of the diseases of the pancreas, Arch. Fr. Mal. App. Dig. **62:**449-463, 1973.

Rettenmaier, G.: Pankreasdiagnostik mit der Ultraschallschnittbildmethode. Pankreassonographie, Dtsch. Med. Wochenschr. **98:**1975-1977, 1973.

Rettenmaier, G.: Sonography of the pancreas; techniques of examination and results, Second European Congress, Ultrasonics in medicine, Abstract No. 97, Erlangen, Germany, 1975, Junge & Sohn.

Rettenmaier, G., and Gail, K.: Echographie pancréatique, J. Radiol. Electrol. Med. Nucl. **53:** 745-746, 1972.

Smith, E. H., Bartrum, R. J., Jr., and Chang, Y. C.: Ultrasonically guided percutaneous aspiration biopsy of the pancreas, Radiology **112:**737-738, 1974.

Sokoloff, J., Dosink, B., Leopold, J., and Forsythe, J. R.: Pitfalls in the echographic evolution of pancreatic disease, J. Clin. Ultrasound **2:**321-326, 1974.

Walls, W. J., Gonzalez, G., Martin, N. L., and Templeton, A. W.: B-scan ultrasound evaluation of the pancreas. Advantages and accuracy compared to other diagnostic techniques, Radiology **114:**127-134, 1975.

Weill, F., Bourgoin, A., Eisenscher, A., and Aucant, D.: Le diagnostic ultrasonore des affections pancréatiques: une tentative d'approche rationnelle fondée sur l'analyse de 260 observations contrôlées, J. Radiol. Electrol. Med. Nucl. **56:**673-683, 1975a.

Weill, F., Kraehenbuhl, J. R., Becker, J. C., Gillet, M., and Bourgoin, A.: Echotomography of the pancreas; a critical and comparative study. In Anacker, H., editor: Efficiency and limits of radiological examination of the pancreas, Stuttgart, Germany, 1975b, Georg Thieme Verlag.

Weill, F., Kraehenbuhl, J. R., Ricatte, J. P., Gillet, M., and Becker, J. C.: L'exploration tomo-échographique du pancréas, Presse Méd. **79:**1641-1644, 1971.

CHAPTER 25

OF HUMPS, LUMPS, AND SWAMPS: differential diagnosis of pancreatic anomalies; pitfalls; different kinds of abdominal tumors (intraperitoneal and retroperitoneal)

DIAGNOSIS AND PITFALLS OF LIQUID IMAGES

Liquid images of gastric origin

A pseudocyst-like image may belong to a stomach dilated because of pyloric stenosis (Fig. 25-1). The changes in appearance produced by positional displacement, of course, permit one to rule out a retroperitoneal collection. In fact, I have several times drawn attention to an important methodological point: the clinical examination and radiological records must be complete. A patient with pyloric stenosis should not be referred for ultrasonography in search of a pancreatic lesion without having had a barium examination.

Even in the absence of pyloric stenosis a merely full stomach may mimic a pancreatic cyst, as shown in Fig. 25-2, which displays a sonolucent structure. In fact, a close look detects, between the "mass" and the great vessels, a linear transverse image of the pancreas. The latter itself was better seen when the patient was examined a second time while fasting (Fig. 25-2, *B*). The possibility of making such an error must always be kept in mind, although it occurs only exceptionally. Before one considers an image definitely abnormal, it is advisable to repeat the examination with the patient fasting and again after refilling the stomach with tap water. Such a maneuver, alas, would be useless in the presence of the rare cystic masses due to gastric or intestinal duplication (Gorelik and colleagues, 1976) but would be useful in a case of fluid-filled duodenal diverticulum.

Liquid images of colonic origin

An intestinal loop may also mimic a pancreatic lesion, particularly a lesion of the pancreatic tail, as depicted in Fig. 25-3. Once again, it is advisable to perform a second examination a few hours later before arrival at a final diagnosis. In general, the left upper quadrant is one of the most deceptive anatomical regions when examined through the anterior approach.

Liquid images of pleural origin

Liquid images of pleural origin constitute a rather surprising source of error. Fig. 25-4 shows an image of a liquid collection occupying the whole left upper quadrant. Such an image suggests a renal or pancreatic mass. In fact, it was due to a diaphragmatic pleural effusion bulging into the abdominal cavity.

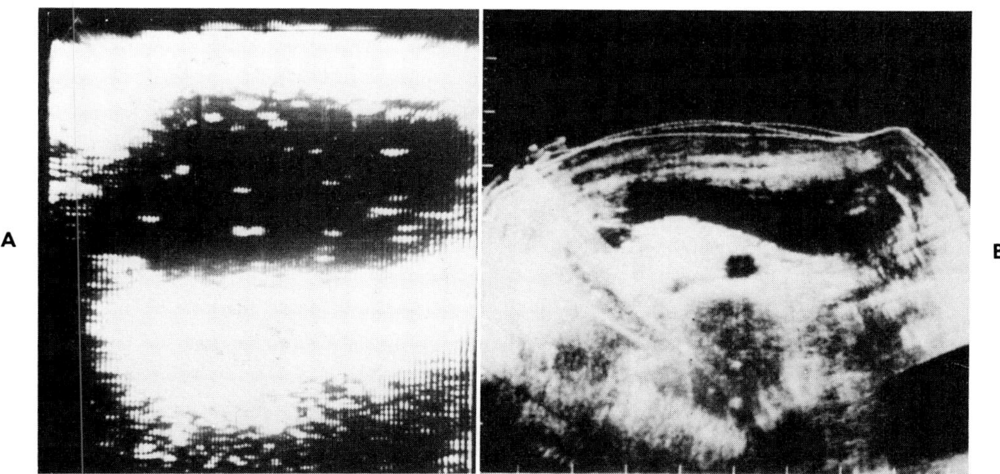

Fig. 25-1. Images of gastric origin. **A,** Real-time transverse scan. This liquid collection, with scattered, mobile echoes, represents a stomach dilated because of pyloric stenosis. **B,** Gray scale contact scan pattern in another case of pyloric stenosis. Patient was referred for supposed acute pancreatitis.

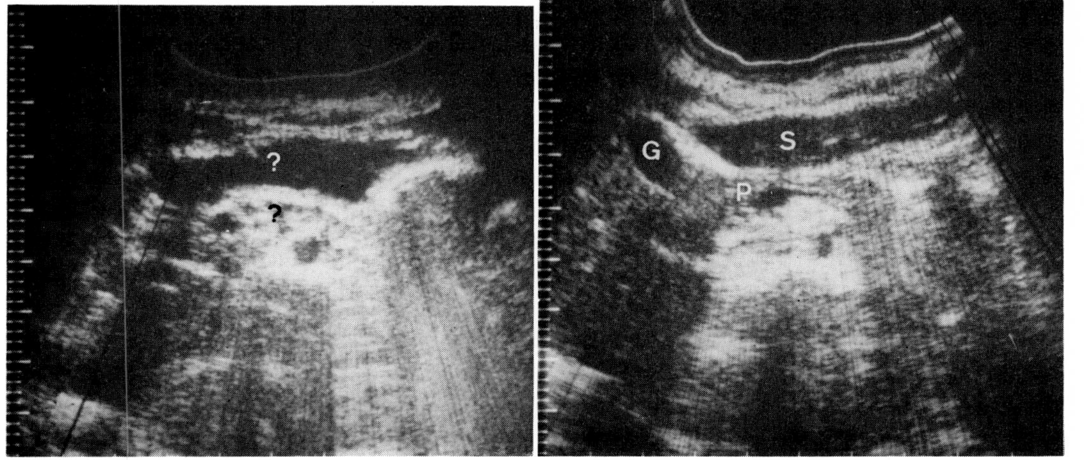

Fig. 25-2. Transverse scans and schematic drawings of epigastrium. **A,** Liquid mass in front of indistinct structure could belong to pseudocyst of pancreas. **B,** Another scan and schematic representation of now fasting patient distinctly showing pancreas *(P)* in front of splenoportal junction. Liquid mass belonged to full stomach *(S),* which is now empty. Gallbladder *(G)* is now displayed. *L,* liver.

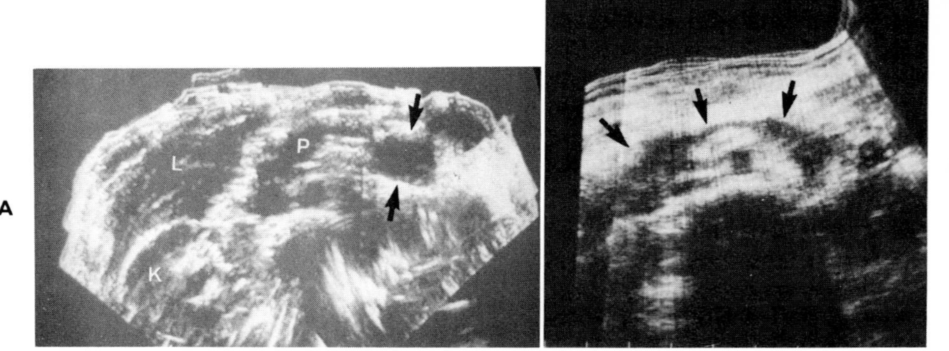

Fig. 25-3. False images of colonic origin displayed on transverse scans of upper abdomen. **A,** Pancreatic head and neck *(P)* are clearly displayed. In the corporeal-caudate region, there is sonolucent rounded area *(arrows),* which could belong to pathological process of pancreatic tail. This image had disappeared when patient was reexamined. *L,* liver; *K,* kidney. **B,** Pseudopancreatic image *(arrows)* of transverse colon.

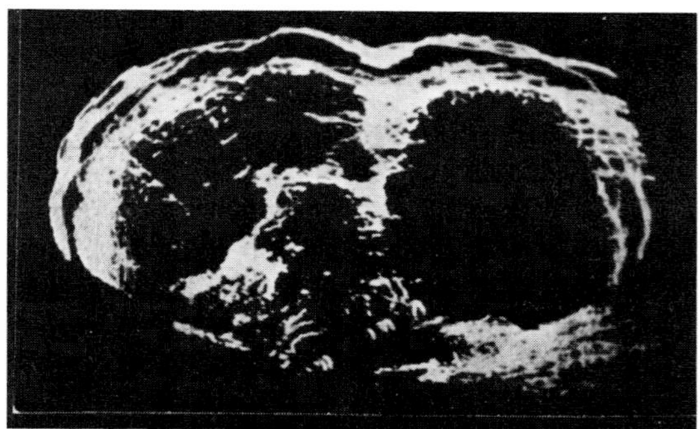

Fig. 25-4. Transverse scan of upper abdomen. There is large fluid collection in left upper quadrant. At first glance this collection was thought to belong to pseudocyst of pancreatic tail. However, sagittal scans showed it actually to represent pleural effusion, which depressed diaphragm. (Courtesy Dr. A. Eisenscher, Vesoul, France.)

Ascites

Holm and associates (1976) have pointed out that an ascitic collection in the lesser omental bursa may mimic a pancreatic pseudocyst. Loculated ascites may also suggest a pancreatic collection (Fig. 25-5).

Aortic aneurysms

Aortic aneurysms are typical deep-lying fluid masses. In fact, their more or less saccular shape, their continuity with the abdominal aorta above the dilatation (Figs. 25-6 and 25-7), and the absence of a normal aortic image in the vicinity of the mass should make the diagnosis readily apparent. Intraluminal thrombi produce a semisolid pattern that could, at first glance, lead to the consideration of other diagnoses (Fig. 25-8), but analysis of the relationships between the mass and the aorta rapidly excludes consideration of the pancreas. In cases of dissecting or ruptured aneurysm, a clinical syndrome of collapse and pain may arise and

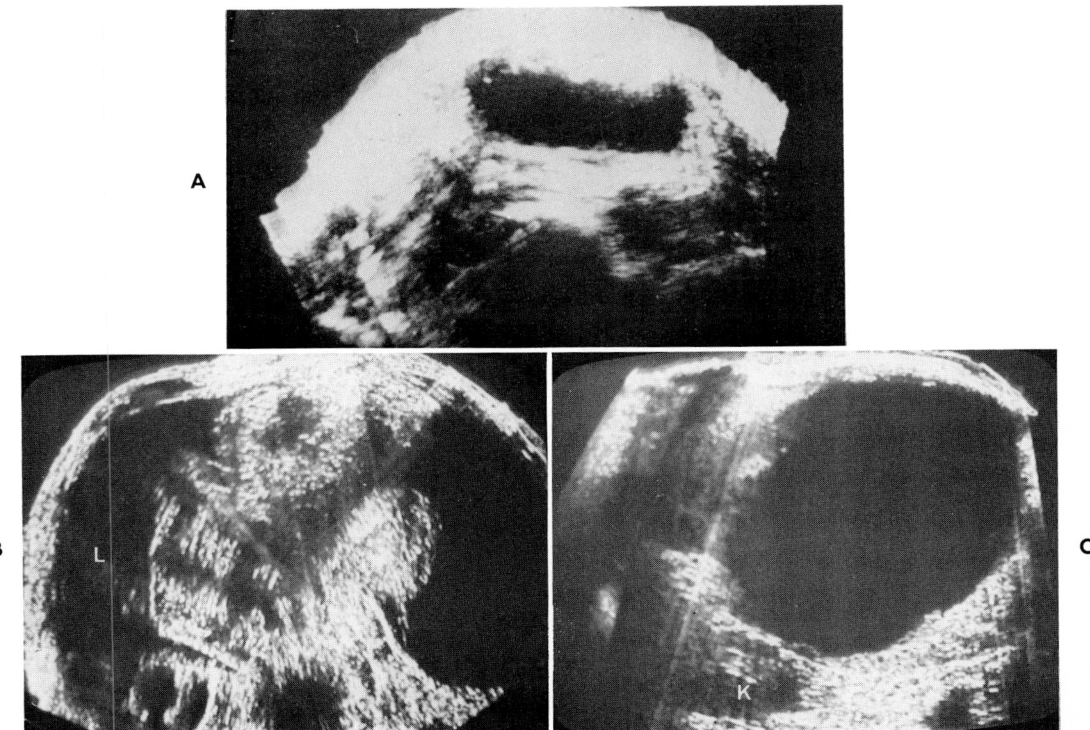

Fig. 25-5. A, Central abdominal collection representing, not pancreatic pseudocyst, but septate ascites, due to peritoneal carcinomatosis. **B** and **C,** Transverse and sagittal scans of another such liquid collection. *L,* liver; *K,* left kidney.

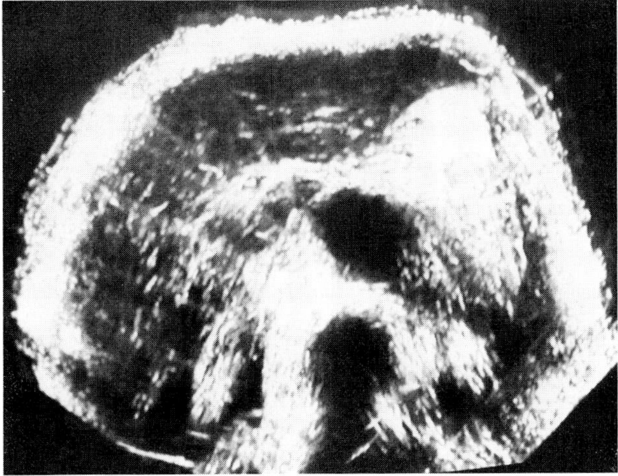

Fig. 25-6. Deep-lying transparent collection displayed on transverse scan. There is no aortic image behind collection, which therefore belongs to aortic aneurysm.

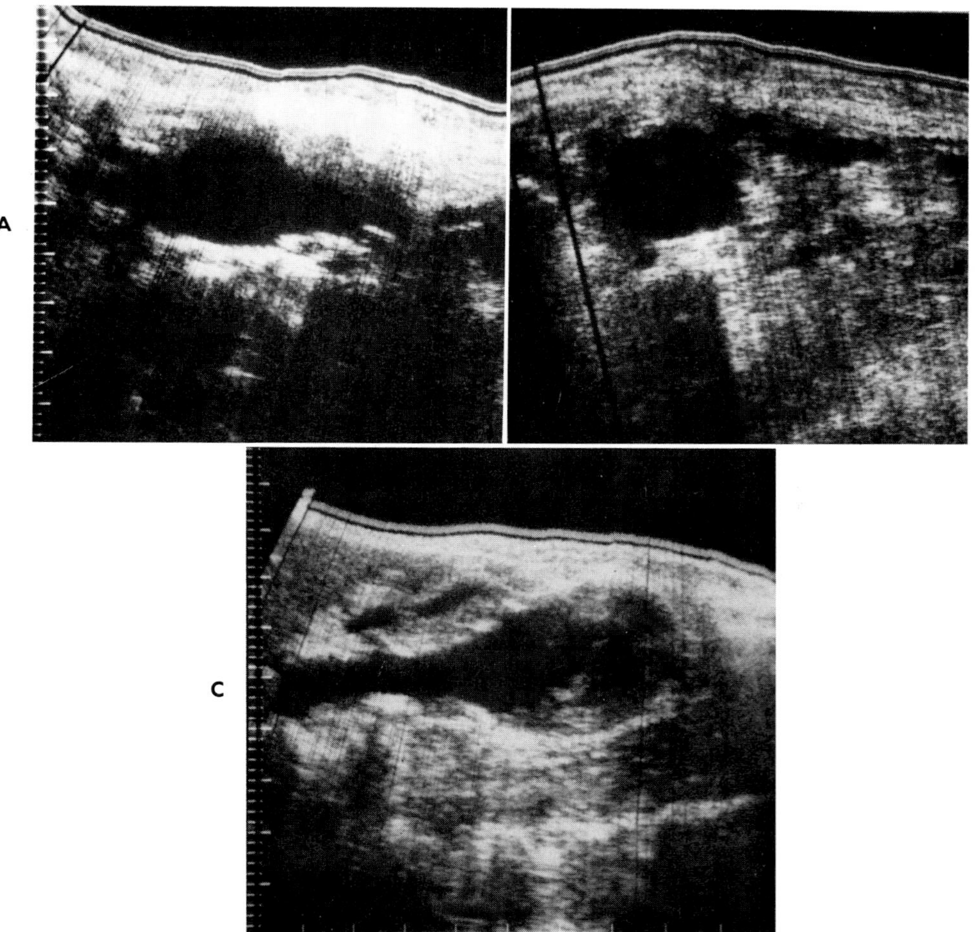

Fig. 25-7. Aortic aneurysm. **A,** Sagittal scan in real time showing junction of aorta and aneurysm. **B,** Transverse real-time scan. **C,** Another example of aortic aneurysm displayed on sagittal scan. Note thrombi in distal part of the sac. Note also anteriorly displayed mesenteric vein between liver and cranial part of sac.

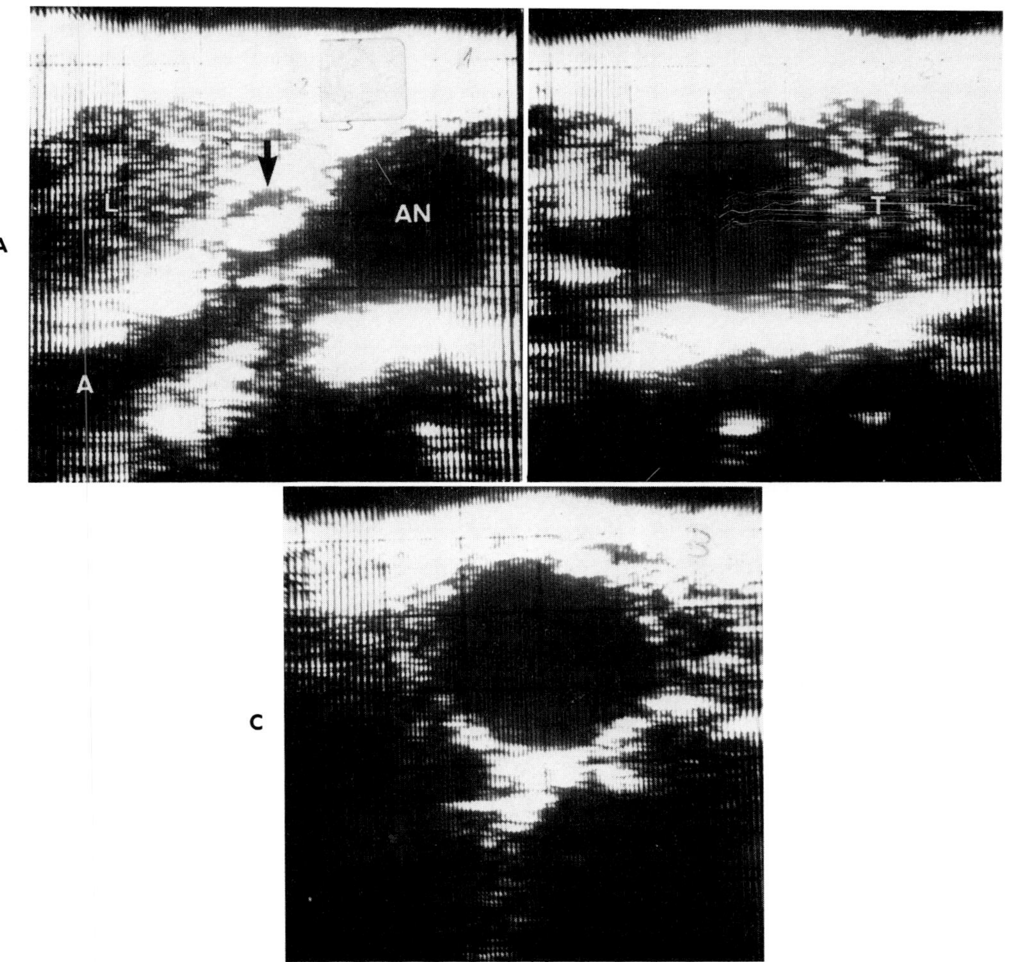

Fig. 25-8. Aneurysm of aorta. **A,** Sagittal real-time scan again showing relation of abdominal aorta *(A)* to aneurysm *(AN).* Superior mesenteric vein *(arrow),* which is seen between aneurysm and liver *(L),* is displaced forward. **B,** Parallel sagittal scan displaying solid pattern belonging to thrombi *(T)* in lower part of aneurysmal pouch. **C,** Transverse scan. Absence of normal aortic image behind mass enables one to identify it as aneurysm.

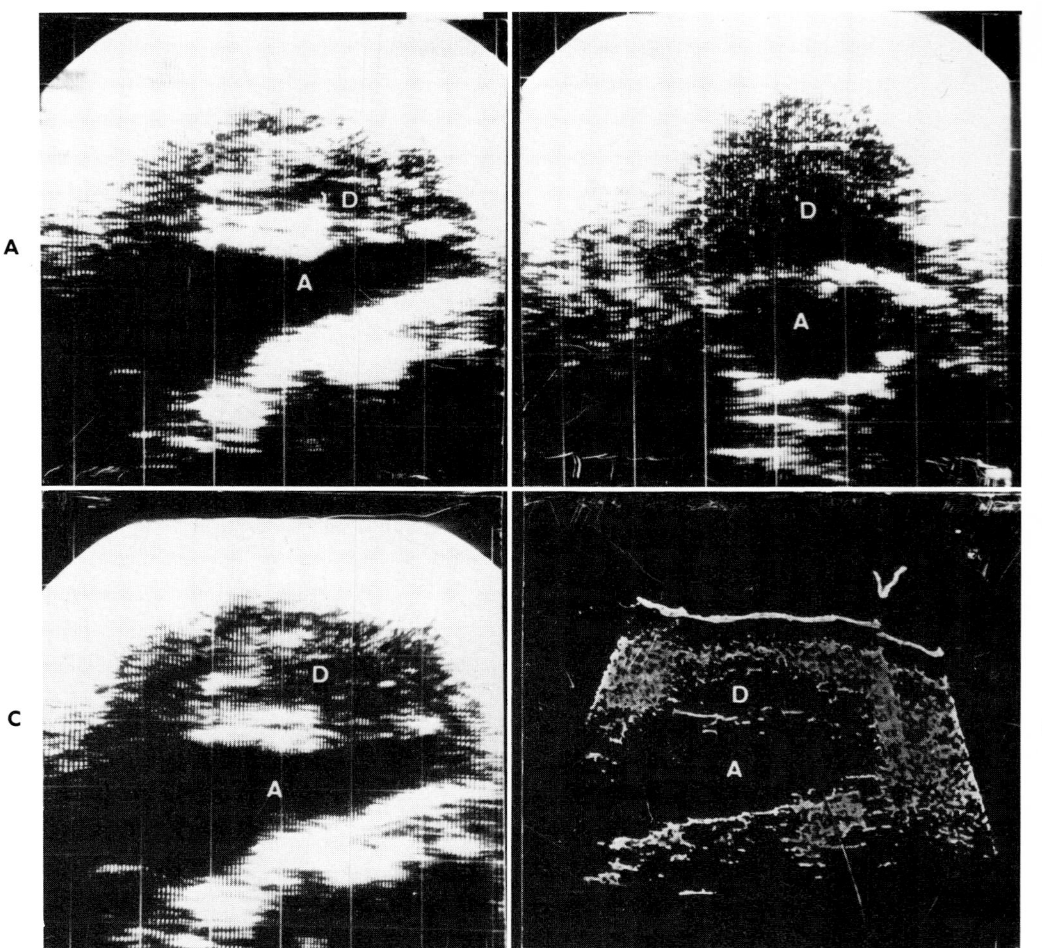

Fig. 25-9. Dissecting aneurysm of aorta. **A,** Sagittal real-time scan showing enlarged aortic lumen *(A)*. In front of this is displayed sonolucent area belonging to dissected wall *(D)*. **B,** Transverse scan in real time also displaying dissection in front of aortic main lumen. **C,** Another real-time scan better displaying semisolid pattern extending between two wall images. Surgery showed aneurysm with dissection and fissuration. **D,** Dissection is seen again, as a double wall image on a sagittal bistable scan.

suggest acute pancreatitis. Ultrasonograms show in such cases a deep-lying mass that seems to be distinct from the aorta, but such preaortic masses belong to the hematoma extending in the aortic wall in case of dissection and around the vessel in case of fissuration (Weill and colleagues, 1974; Winsberg and colleagues, 1974). Indeed, in different transverse and sagittal scans (Figs. 25-9 and 25-10), the abnormal pattern can be seen to belong to a double vascular image, not to the aorta and an adjacent lesion.

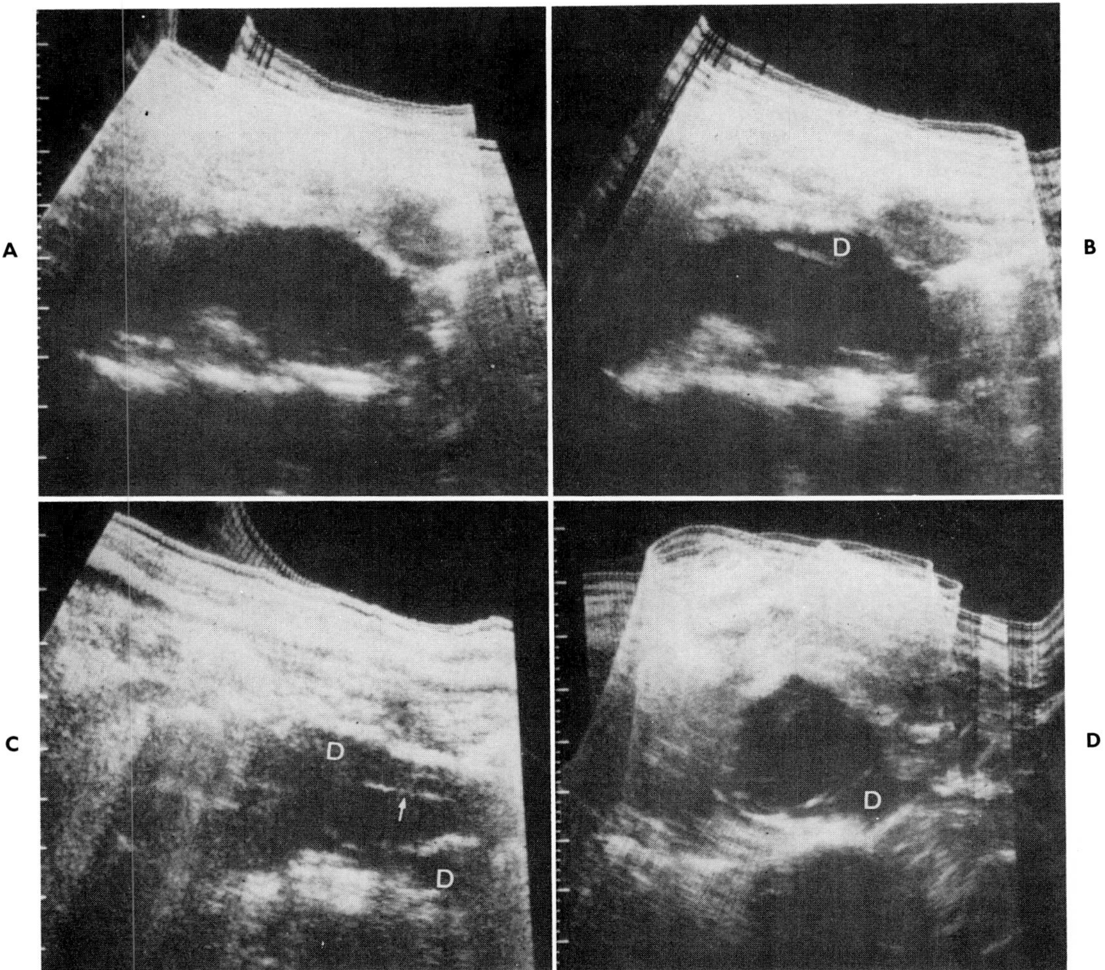

Fig. 25-10. Aortic aneurysm with dissection and beginning fissuration. **A** and **B,** Sagittal sections showing double lumen *(D)*. **C,** Parallel sagittal scan. Note systolic-diastolic undulations of intima *(arrow)*. **D,** Transverse section.

Mesenteric cysts

Mesenteric cysts arising in the root of the mesentery, in front of the left kidney, are thus very close to the pancreatic tail, so that they may mimic a pseudocyst of the tail. However, they are usually located somewhat lower than the pancreatic tail, close to the lower pole of the kidney. Moreover, their walls are often calcified, which is unusual in a pancreatic pseudocyst. (See Fig. 25-11.)

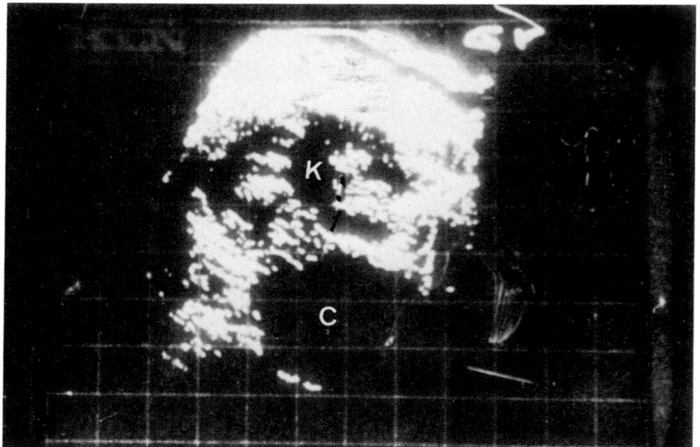

Fig. 25-11. Cyst of mesenteric insertion. Transverse posterior scan of renal region, made with patient in prone position, shows rounded area *(C),* which could be confused with pseudocyst of pancreatic tail, in front of kidney *(K).*

A

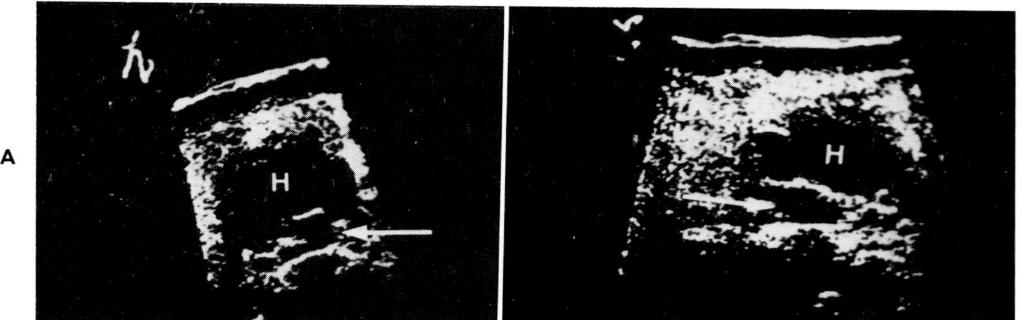

B

Fig. 25-12. Abdominal fluid collection. Patient had acute abdominal syndrome, with pain and collapse. Surgeon, in another hospital, had palpated a mass and decided to operate. He found pulsatile mass, which he believed to be consistent with diagnosis of aortic aneurysm—a lesion that he was not prepared to operate on. Patient was referred, after laparotomy, to our hospital. **A,** Transverse scan displaying abdominal collection *(H)* and normal aortic image *(arrow).* **B,** Sagittal scan again showing normal aortic image behind collection. Presence of this image rules out possibility of aneurysm—a conclusion confirmed by aortography. Second operation disclosed spontaneous hematoma of mesenteric insertion.

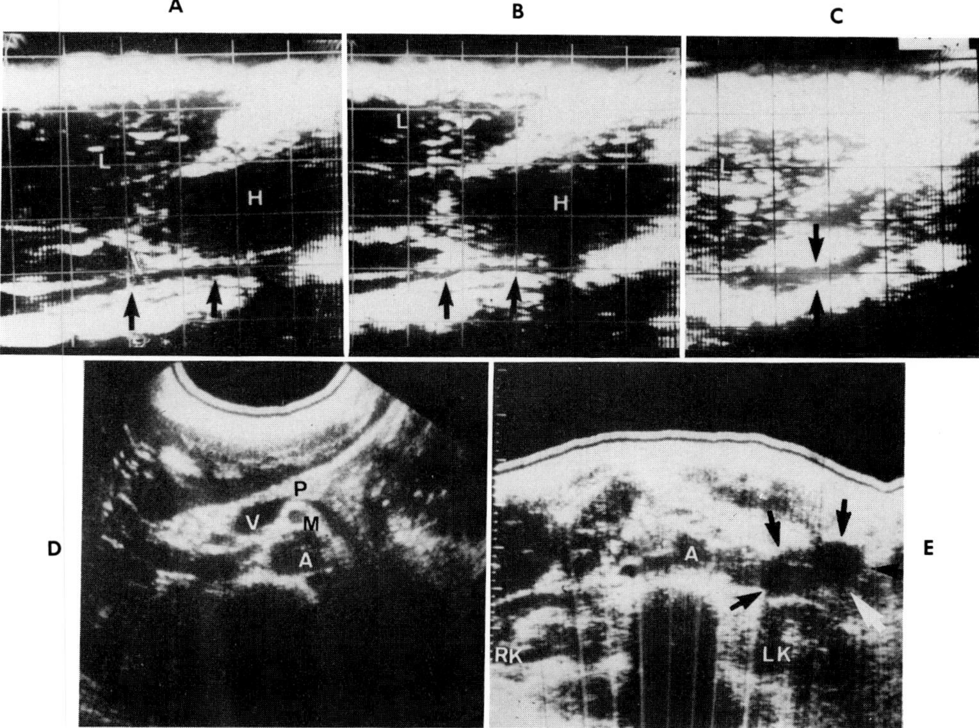

Fig. 25-13. A to **C**, Retroperitoneal hematoma in child, after surgery for traumatic rupture of right kidney. **A**, Sagittal scan passing through liver *(L)* and vena cava *(arrows)*. In front of vena cava, large hematoma *(H)* is shown. **B**, Identical scan made few days later showing no change. **C**, Identical scan made 3 weeks later showing hematoma to have disappeared. Image of vena cava is normal again. **D** and **E**, Two parallel transverse scans of patient undergoing anticoagulant therapy and complaining of diffuse abdominal pain. **D**, Normal pattern of pancreas (*P*). *V*, splenoportal junction and splenic vein; *M*, SMA; *A*, aorta. **E**, Four cm more caudal scan showing transparent area *(arrows)* corresponding to retroperitoneal hematoma in front of left kidney (*LK*). *RK*, right kidney.

Liquid images of renal origin

Anterior renal cysts always clearly relate to the kidney. They are never confused with pancreatic masses. More difficult problems arise with left adrenal cysts.

Hematomas and abscesses

Mesenteric hematomas. I have seen two deep-lying liquid collections distinct from the aorta that were due to spontaneous mesenteric hematoma (Fig. 25-12).

Retroperitoneal hematomas. Retroperitoneal hematomas may be seen after trauma or in patients undergoing anticoagulant therapy. Such hematomas developing near the great vessels may mimic a collection of pancreatic origin (Fig.

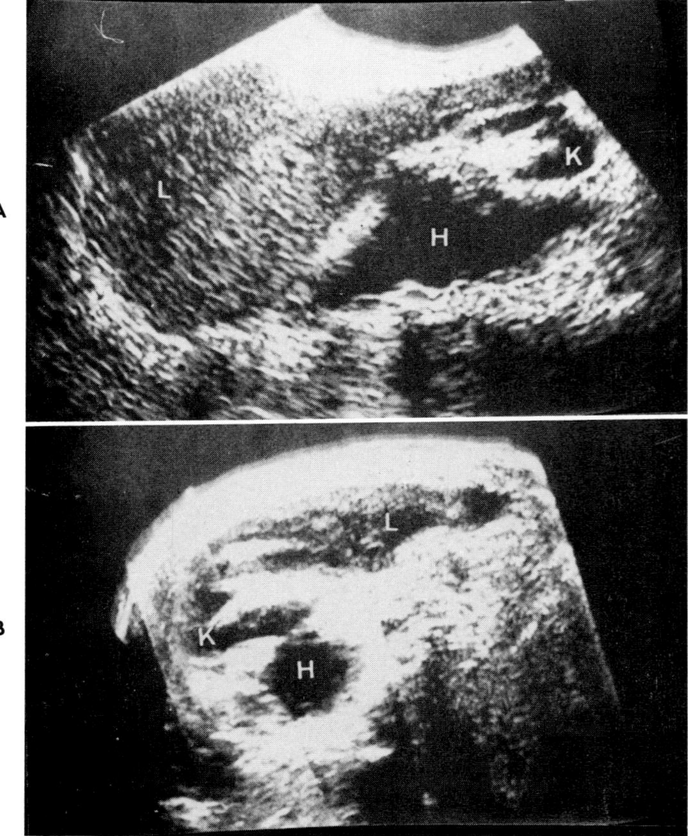

Fig. 25-14. Retroperitoneal collection. Patient under therapy for lymphoma suddenly complained of back pain. **A,** Sagittal scan of right upper quadrant showing fluid collection *(H)* between liver *(L),* right kidney *(K),* which is displaced forward, and posterior abdominal wall. **B,** Transverse scan again showing well-marginated fluid collection behind right kidney. Collection turned out to be abscess.

25-13). When they extend laterally between the posterior abdominal wall and the kidney, they are quite different from a pancreatic collection, and the differential diagnosis is then much easier. A similar problem occurs with a retroperitoneal abscess (Fig. 25-14).

Hematomas in intestinal or duodenal walls. Hematomas in the intestinal or duodenal walls may mimic pancreatic pseudocysts (Fig. 25-15). A small bowel hematoma is movable with the intestinal loop when palpated under echoscopic real-time control, but this is not the case with a duodenal hematoma. The latter is readily diagnosed by barium studies that show an imprint on the duodenal lumen. The distortions caused by the hematoma on the duodenum are quite different from those produced by a pancreatic mass. These signs are well known to radiologists and should, of course, be employed in the comprehensive evaluation of the patient. If, as often happens, the ultrasonic examination is the first abdominal examination, comparison with the GI series is compulsory.

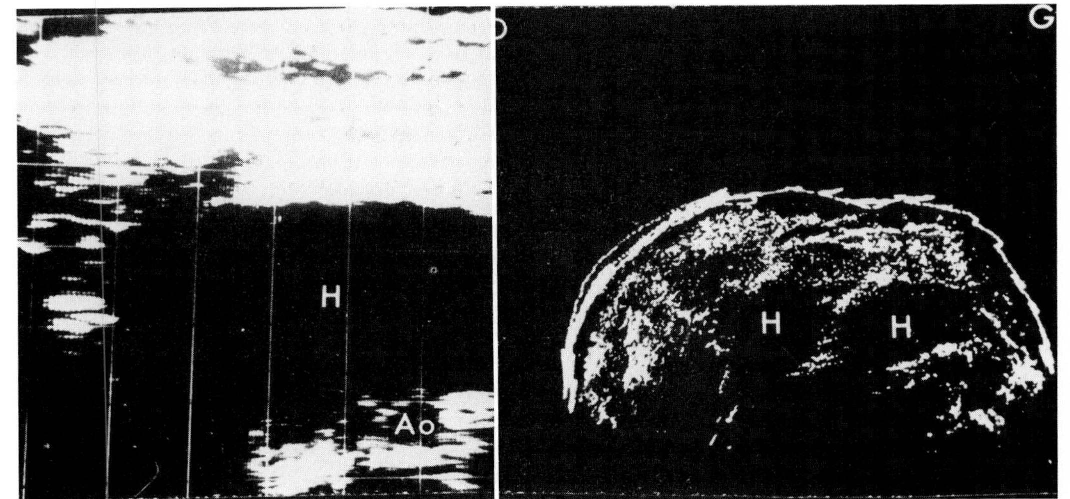

Fig. 25-15. Marginated fluid collection. **A,** Transverse scan in real time showing collection *(H)* in front of aorta *(Ao).* **B,** Transverse contact scan showing collection to be biloculate. It is hematoma in duodenal wall. (From Weill, F., Becker, J. C., Kraehenbuhl, J. R., Heriot, G., and Walter, J. P.: Clinical atlas of ultrasonic radiography, Paris, 1973, Masson & Cie., Editeurs.)

Other abdominal hematomas and abscesses. Despite the fact that such lesions do not properly belong to the differential diagnosis of pancreatic lesions, I would like to discuss briefly a few *other kinds of abdominal hematomas and abscesses.* As a matter of fact, the search for hematomas, especially in patients under anticoagulant therapy, is a daily problem. In such cases, abdominal pain or swelling is often misinterpreted as a tumoral mass. These are, first, pelvic hematomas, extending along the psoas muscle sheath. In a normal patient, transverse scans of the lower abdomen and pelvis display the oval or circular sections of the psoas muscles (Fig. 25-16) symmetrically on each side of the spine.* Occurrence of an asymmetrical pattern is consistent with the presence of a hematoma or an abscess (Figs. 25-17 and 25-18). Enlargement of the psoas muscle may also be due to psoas inflammation associated with appendicitis (Fig. 25-19). I have already described an appendiceal abscess (Fig. 14-10). Please do not jump to the conclusion that the diagnosis of appendicitis is a function of ultrasonography. Hematoma of the rectus abdominis sheath has a quite typical image (Duval and co-workers, 1975). In transverse section, this is a paramedial oval sonolucent area (Fig. 25-20). On a sagittal section the image is more elongated, so that its inferior limit is confused with the upper border of the pubis. In gray scale a semisolid pattern due to blood clots may be displayed.

Following are the *different diagnoses* to be considered when ultrasonography shows a deep-lying *collection of liquid type* before concluding that there is pancreatic enlargement.

*Rarely in a very athletic subject, there may be confusing hypertrophy of the psoas.

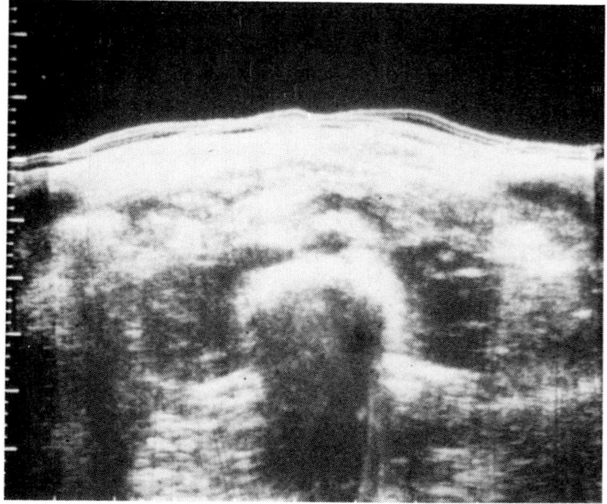

Fig. 25-16. Section images of normal psoas muscles, displayed on transverse abdominal scan. Muscles are displayed on either side of spine.

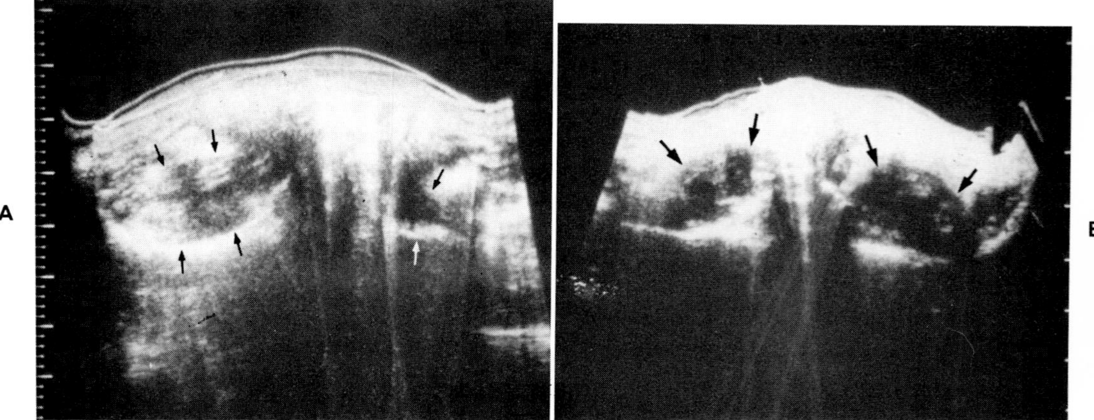

Fig. 25-17. Hematomas of psoas muscle sheath, developed under anticoagulant therapy. **A,** Enlargement of right psoas section, marked by *arrows,* as is normal left psoas. **B,** Enlargement of left psoas in another patient.

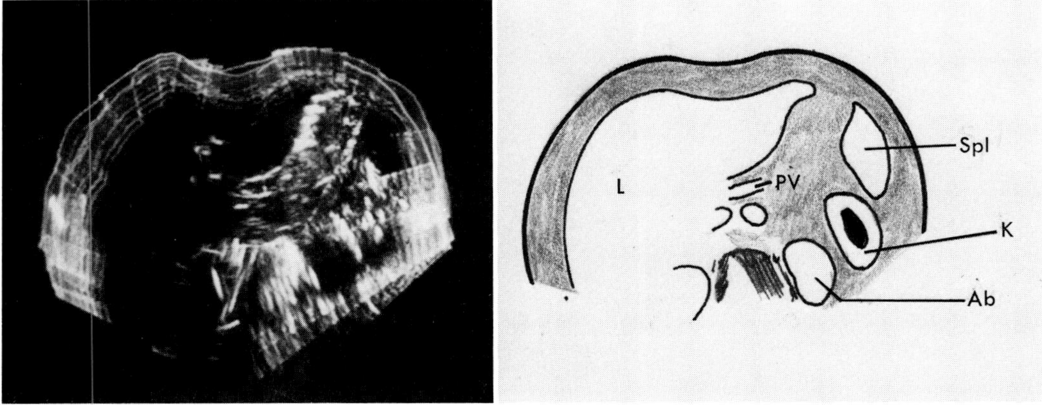

Fig. 25-18. Retroperitoneal abscess. This transverse scan and schematic drawing of upper abdomen shows, between displaced left kidney *(K)* and spine, collection *(Ab)*—tuberculous abscess, spreading along psoas sheath and originating from tuberculous spondylitis. *L,* liver; *Spl,* spleen; *PV,* portal vein.

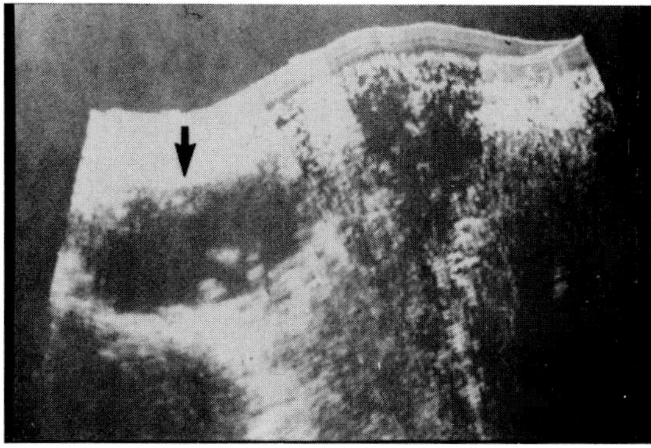

Fig. 25-19. Enlargement of section of right psoas muscle *(arrow)* in relation to appendicitis (psoitis).

- Gastric retention (and duodenal diverticulum)
- Colonic retention
- Left diaphragmatic pleural effusion
- Septate ascites
- Ascites in the omental bursa
- Aortic aneurysm
- Dissecting aortic aneurysm
- Mesenteric cyst
- Mesenteric hematoma
- Retroperitoneal hematoma or abscess and intraperitoneal abscess

DIAGNOSIS AND PITFALLS OF SOLID MASSES

As was seen in Chapter 22, there are not many other diagnoses to be considered with images of markedly increased reflectivity, such as those of chronic pan-

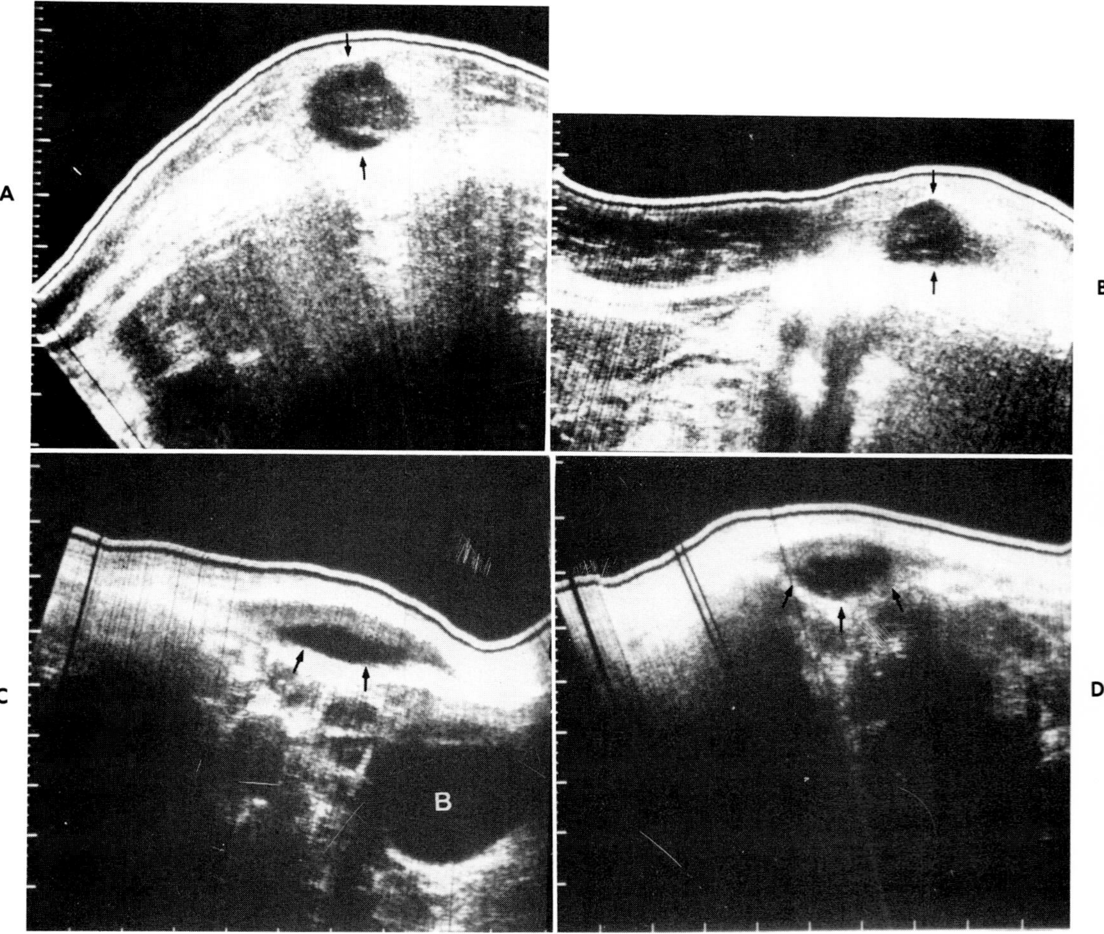

Fig. 25-20. Hematoma *(arrows)* of rectus sheath. **A,** Transverse scan. **B,** Sagittal scan. **C** and **D,** Sagittal and transverse scans in another case. *B,* bladder.

creatitis, apart from the reflective content of a full stomach. On the other hand, nothing resembles a pancreatic tumor more than an intragastric hamburger (Fig. 25-21). The followers of Schammai try to assess the specific morphological features of sauerkraut, apple pie, and pizza; Hillel's adherents advise performing a new examination on the fasting patient if in doubt. As a matter of fact, the main problem in the presence of a seemingly pancreatic solid mass is the diagnosis of other retroperitoneal masses.

Lymph nodes

Enlarged lymph nodes, the ultrasonic pattern of which was described by Asher and Freimanis in 1969, may on transverse scans give rise to a pattern similar to that of a pancreatic carcinoma (Figs. 25-22 to 25-24). Several differential criteria are to be assessed. The first is the possibility of showing the image of the pancreas distinct from the lymph nodes (Fig. 25-23). The next is identification of a much greater craniocaudal extension of the mass than would be expected in a pancreatic tumor (Fig. 25-24).

Sometimes enlarged nodes extend behind the aorta, so that it is displaced from the spine (Fig. 25-22, *A*). This appearance is absolutely typical of lymphadenopathy. It would be a gross error to confuse intra-aneurysmal marginal thrombi with periaortic lymph nodes (Fig. 25-22, *B*).

Last, an important sign is anterior displacement of the superior mesenteric vein (Weill and associates, 1975) (Figs. 25-23, *F*, 25-25, and 25-26), although the rare pancreatic tumor arising from the uncinate process may also displace the mesenteric vein forward. On the other hand, as illustrated in Fig. 25-27, comprehensive study of the upper abdomen often shows a primary tumor, the discovery of

Text continued on p. 398.

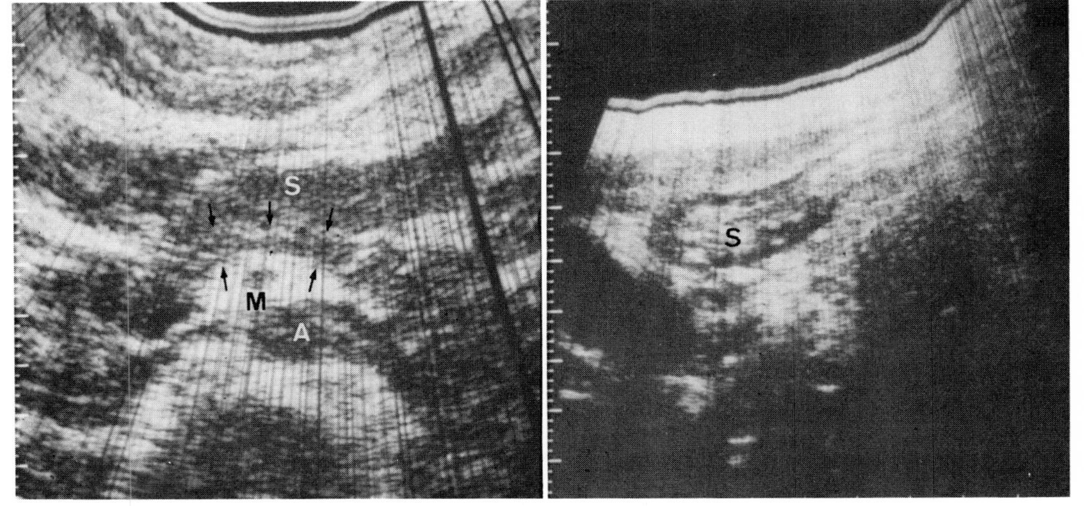

Fig. 25-21. A, At first glance, there seems to be pancreatic mass, but actually contours *(arrows)* of pancreas are outlined. Seeming pancreatic mass is instead filled stomach *(S)*. *A,* aorta; *M,* superior mesenteric artery. **B,** Another example of pseudomass of gastric origin.

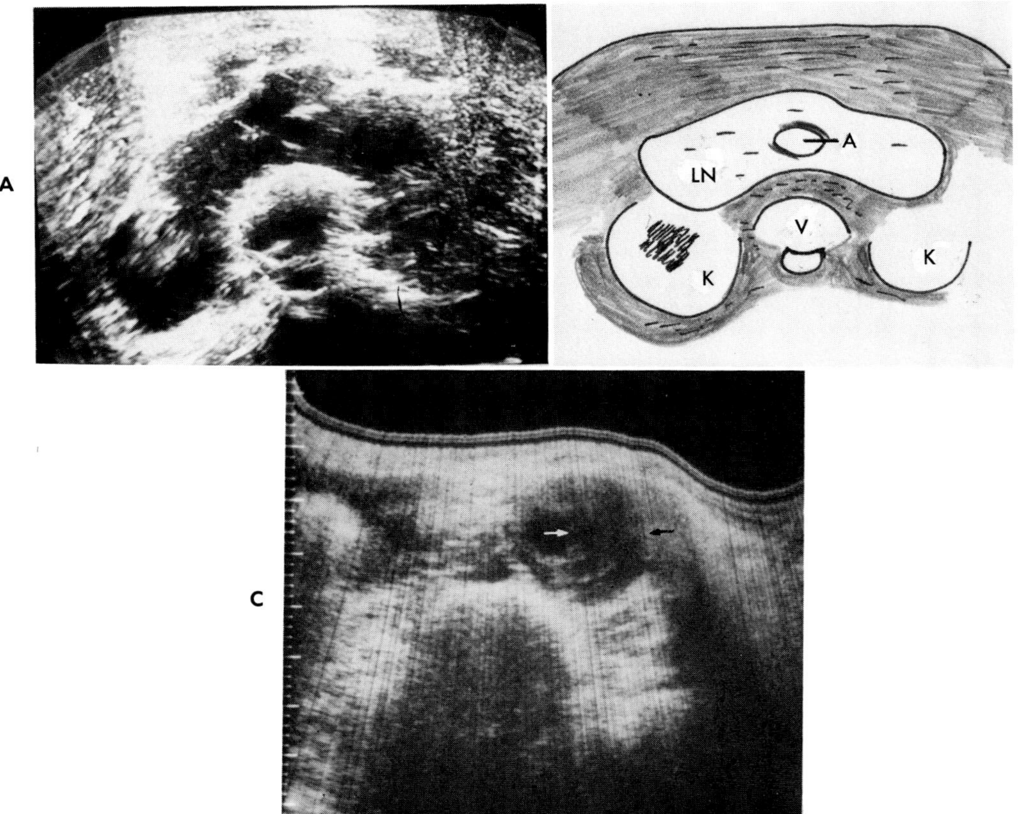

Fig. 25-22. A and **B,** Lymph nodes. Transverse scan and schematic representation show, in front of spine (*V,* vertebral body), crescent-shaped mass (*LN*) surrounding aorta (*A*). It therefore cannot represent enlarged pancreas. *K,* kidneys. **C,** Partially thrombosed aortic aneurysm displayed on transverse scan. Intra-aneurysmal marginal blood clots *(arrows)* must not be confused with periaortic lymph nodes.

Fig. 25-23. Two examples of multiple lymph nodes. **A,** Transverse scan of upper abdomen showing biloculate sonolucent mass, which could belong to tumor of body of pancreas. However, there are multiple rounded adjacent masses *(arrows)* in front of spine *(S)* and aorta *(A).* **B,** Parallel, more caudal scan also displaying multiple individual small masses, the sections of which look like bunch of grapes. **C,** Sagittal section. These multiple lymph nodes *(arrows)* are result of lymphoid leukemia. **D,** Transverse scan of upper abdomen of another patient showing several rounded masses *(arrows)* on each side of splenic vein *(S).* **E,** Parallel, slightly more caudal scan, displaying pancreas *(P)* and individual mass *(LN)* in close relation to its anterior aspect. Masses in **D** and **E** belong to metastatic lymph nodes in case of advanced gastric carcinoma. Gastric mass *(G)* is outlined between left hepatic lobe and pancreatic body. *C,* vena cava. **F,** Sagittal section. Mesenteric vein *(VM)* separates lymph nodes from gastric mass. *L,* liver.

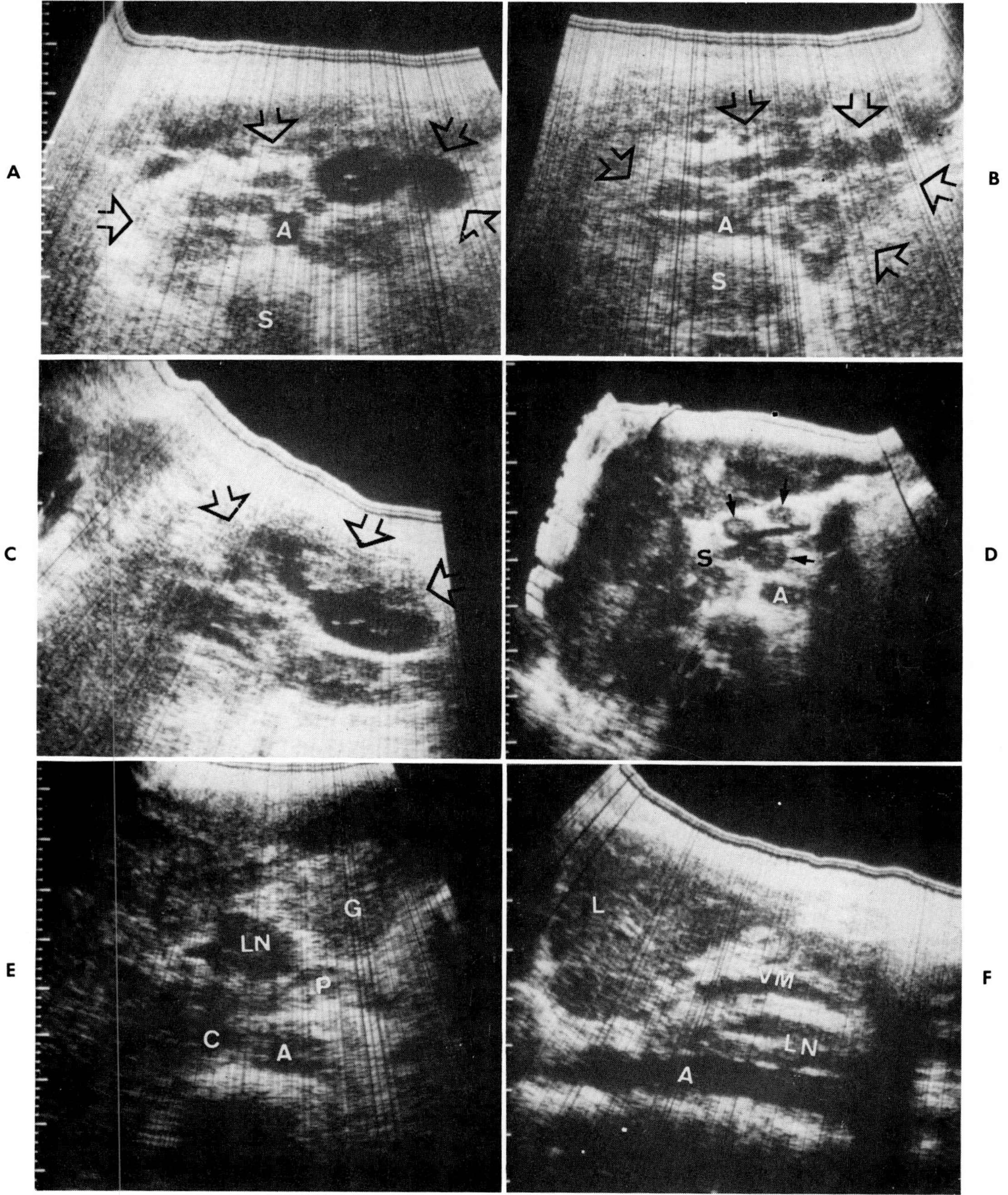

Fig. 25-23. For legend see opposite page.

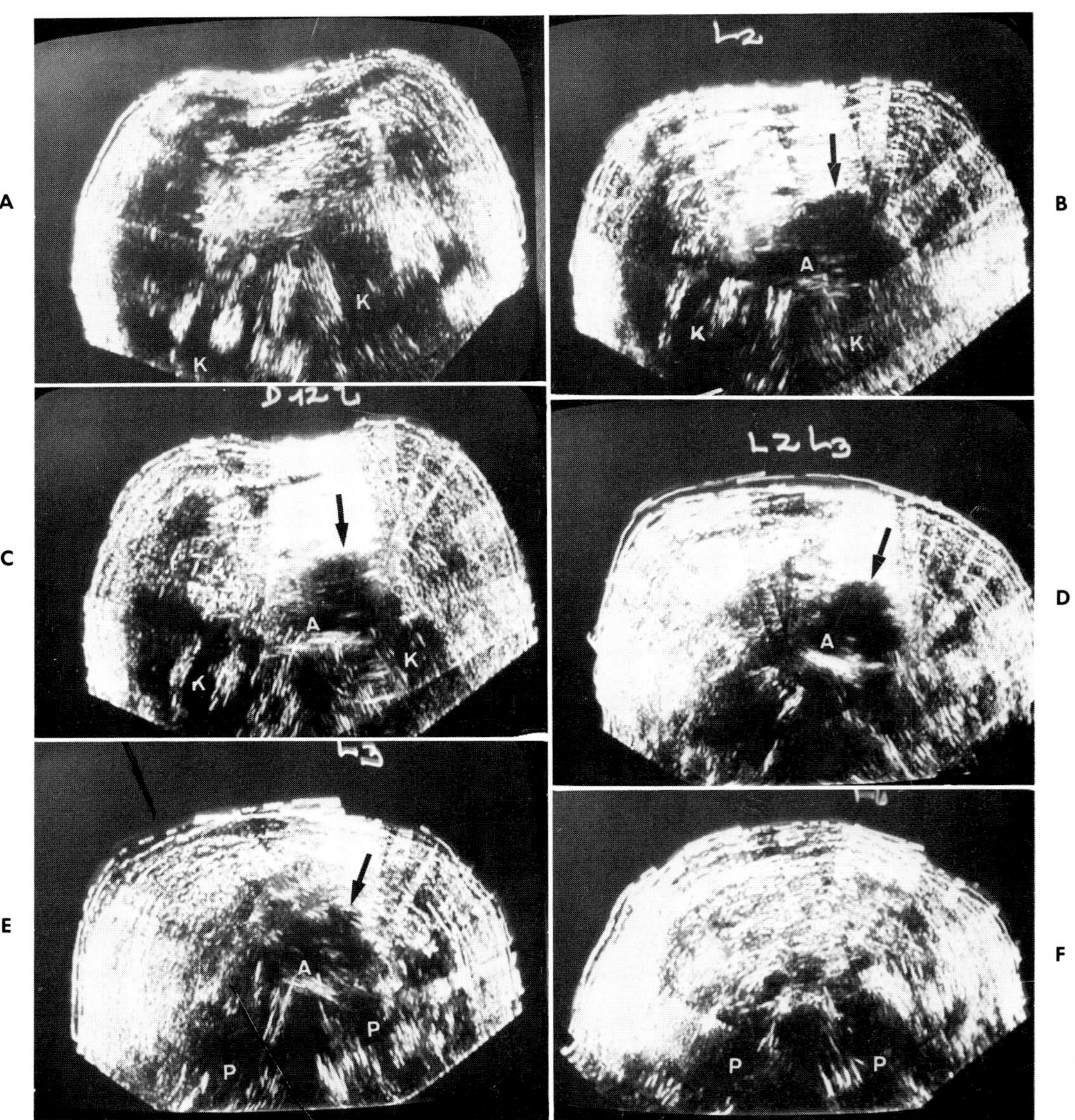

Fig. 25-24. A to **F,** Six parallel transverse scans. Of these six sections, four (from L-1 to L-3) show posterior mass *(arrows)* with polycyclic contours and sonolucent echopattern. This mass corresponds to metastatic deposits of testicular teratoma in retroperitoneal lymph nodes. *K,* right and left kidneys; *A,* aorta; *P,* psoas muscle.

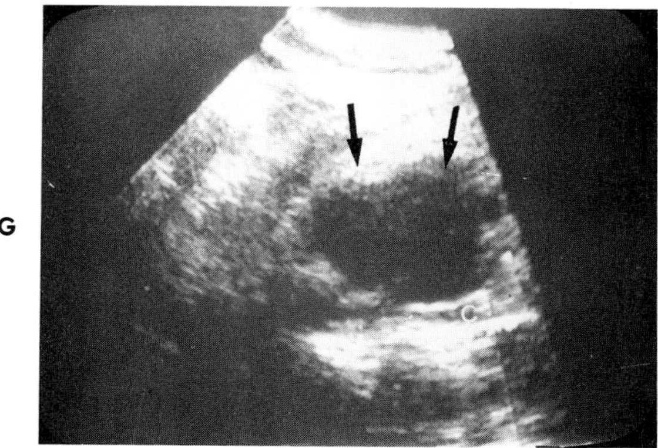

Fig. 25-24, cont'd. G, Sagittal scan. Mass flattens vena cava *(C)*. Polycyclic but smooth contours and, above all, craniocaudal extension show that mass is not pancreatic.

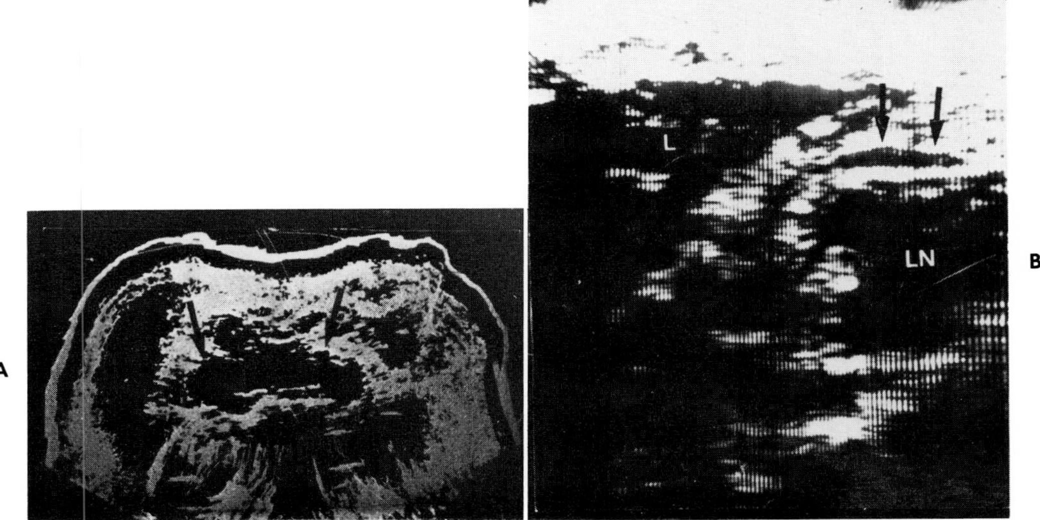

Fig. 25-25. Lymph nodes—mesenteric vein sign. **A,** Transverse scan displaying, in front of great vessels, sonolucent area *(arrows)*, shape of which is not very different from enlarged pancreas. Vena cava and aorta are flattened. **B,** Sagittal scan again showing this deep sonolucent mass *(LN)*, which pushes mesenteric vein *(arrows)* anteriorly. With possible, but rare, exception of pancreatic tumor arising from uncinate process, such forward displacement of mesenteric vein establishes diagnosis of adenopathy. *L,* liver.

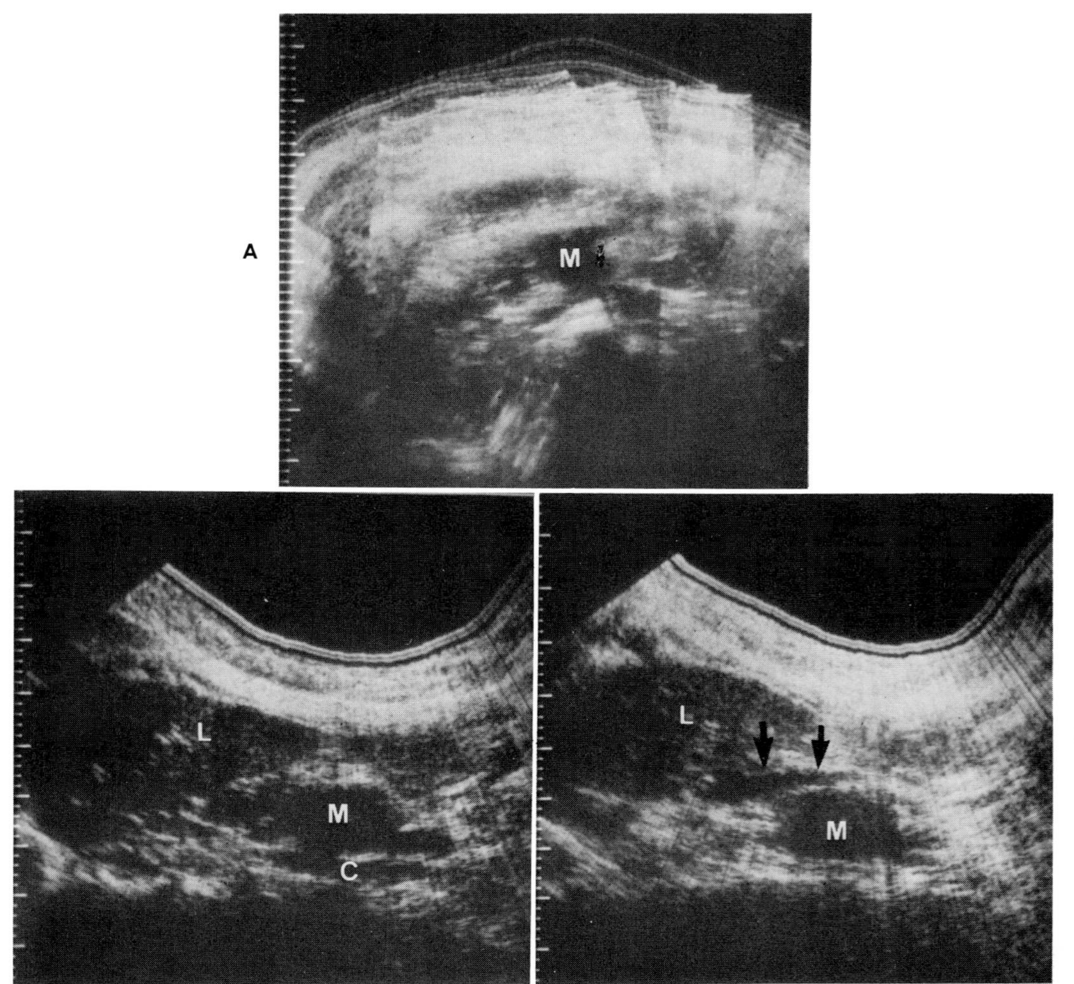

Fig. 25-26. Lymph nodes: mesenteric vein sign. **A,** Transverse scan of upper abdomen showing mass *(M)* in relation to large vessels. **B,** Sagittal scan also showing mass in front of vena cava *(C). L,* liver. **C,** Parallel scan again showing mass, which is pushing mesenteric vein *(arrows)* forward. This shows mass to be ganglionic, not pancreatic.

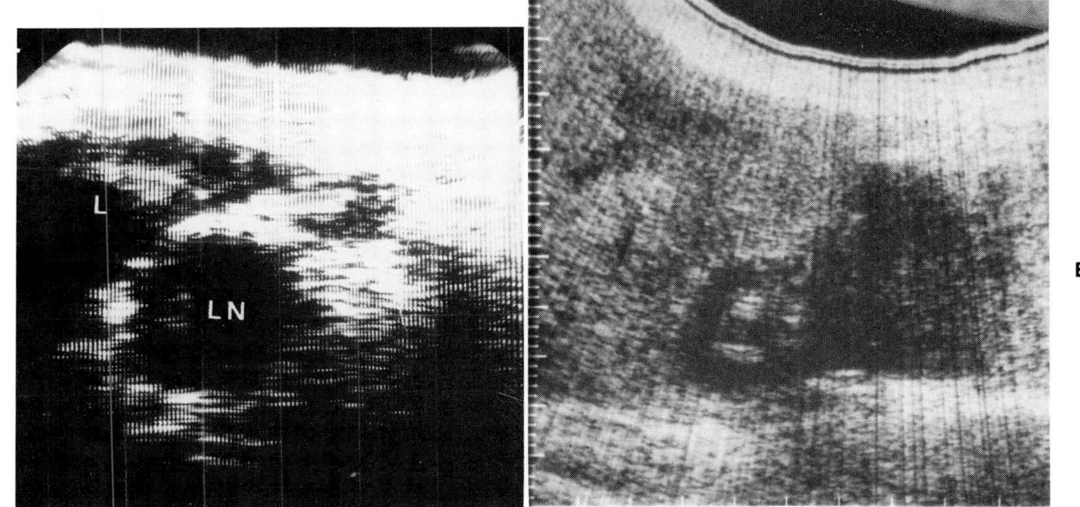

Fig. 25-27. A, Patient complained of abdominal pain. Barium enema showed small impression on inferior wall of transverse colon. Sagittal scan and schematic representation of abdomen show rounded mass *(LN)* behind liver *(L)*. Diagnosis of pancreatic carcinoma was made. It was incorrect. Situation of mesenteric vein had not been studied, and examination of upper abdomen was incomplete. **B,** Actually, there was renal carcinoma, and mass belonged to metastatic lymph node.

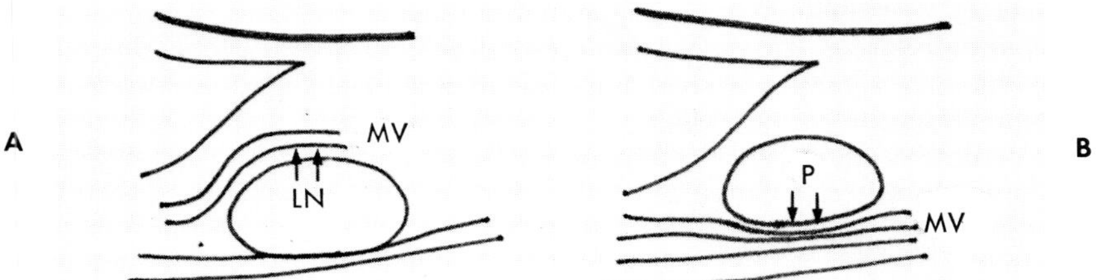

Fig. 25-28. Sign of mesenteric vein *(MV)*. **A,** Forward displacement *(arrows)* due to lymph nodes *(LN)*. **B,** Posterior displacement (compression) *(arrows)* due to pancreatic mass *(P)*.

which allows easy interpretation of retroperitoneal ganglionic metastatic deposits. Despite the rare possibility of an uncinate pancreatic tumor, this sign of the mesenteric vein should be remembered as a reliable sign. There is forward displacement of the mesenteric vein with lymph node masses and posterior displacement of this vein with pancreatic tumors (Fig. 25-28), often with such flattening of the vein that its image disappears. *Associated signs* of lymphoma, such as splenomegaly or pleural effusion, may be encountered (Fig. 25-29). However, pleural effusions may also

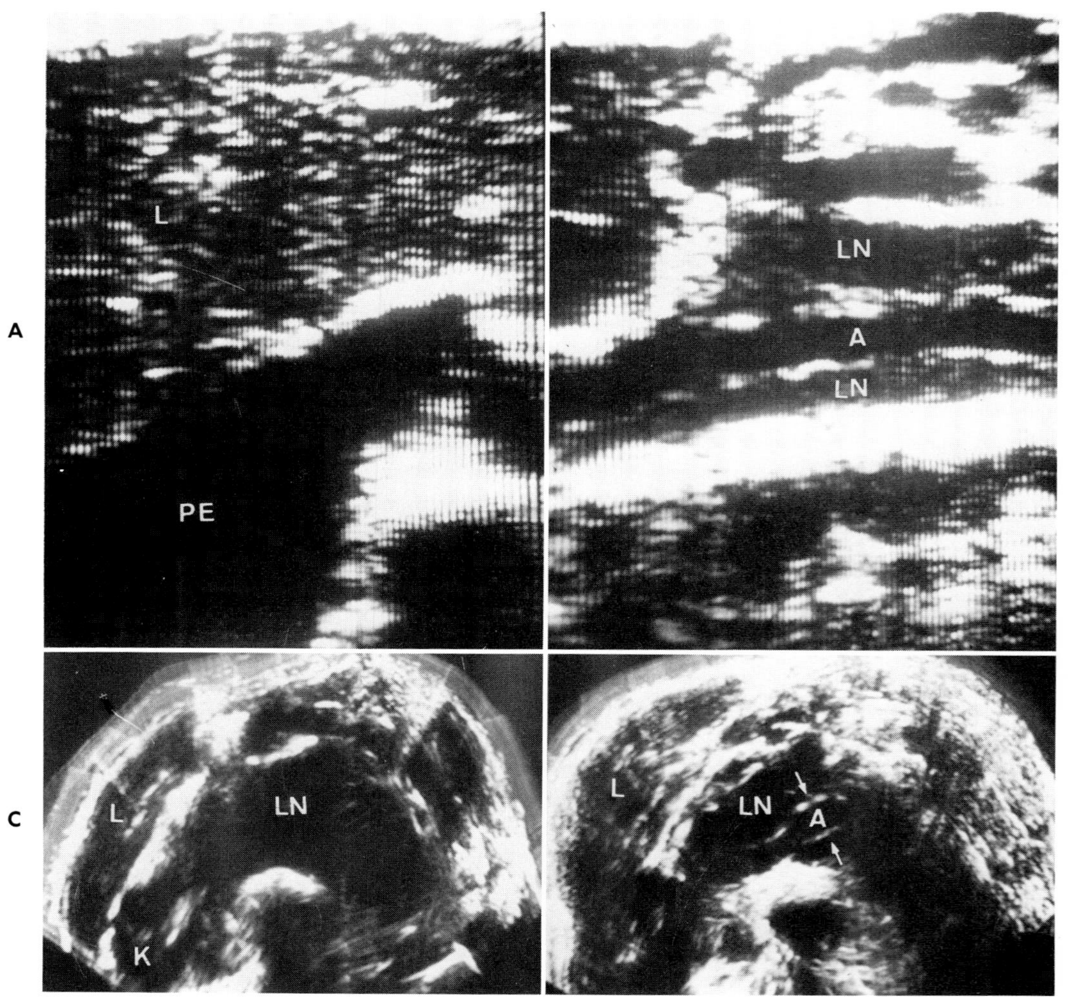

Fig. 25-29. Lymph nodes: associated signs. **A,** Oblique recurrent subcostal scan displaying heterogeneous pattern within liver *(L)*. Between posterior wall and liver, there is fluid collection belonging to pleural effusion *(PE)*. **B,** Sagittal scan of abdomen passing through aorta *(A)* displays periaortic sonolucent cuff *(LN)*. This is typical image of lymphadenopathy. **C,** Transverse scan at low-gain setting displays contours of ganglionic mass. *K,* kidney. **D,** With higher gain, image of aorta *(arrows)* appears surrounded by adenopathy.

exist in acute pancreatitis. Of course, when the great vessels are surrounded by a mass, any further diagnostic discussion is useless. As illustrated by the previous figures, the echopattern of lymph nodes is more sonolucent than that of pancreatic carcinomas. Lymph nodes may look rather like a fluid collection, but without reinforcement of the posterior interface. Moreover, a gray scale study of the echopattern with adequate dynamic range always shows scattered echoes of semisolid type.

Other retroperitoneal masses

Other retroperitoneal masses, such as *sarcomas* arising from abdominal wall or juxtapancreatic connective tissue (e.g., liposarcomas, rhabdomyosarcomas, and fibrosarcomas) may resemble pancreatic tumors (Fig. 25-30). Liposarcomas are

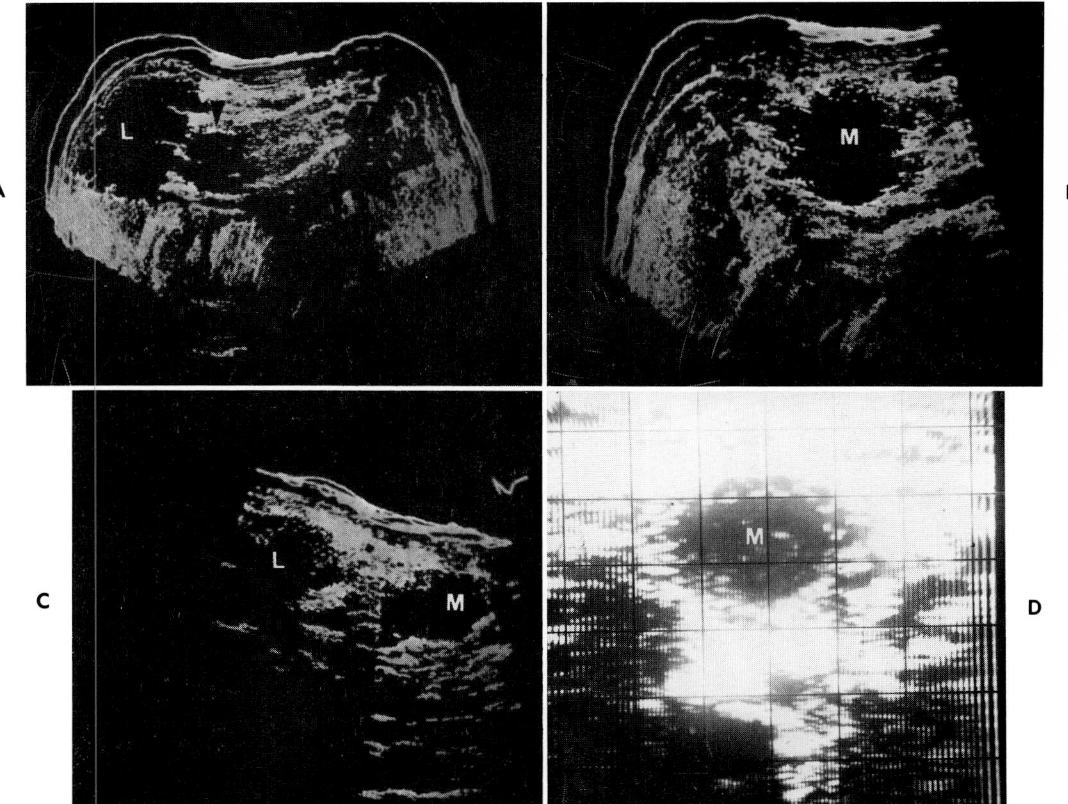

Fig. 25-30. Retroperitoneal sarcoma. Patient complained of abdominal pain and of rapid loss of weight. **A** and **B,** Two parallel transverse scans showing deep-lying rounded mass (*arrowhead* and *M*) seemingly of pancreatic head. *L,* liver. **C,** Sagittal scan displaying mass below liver. **D,** Real-time scan showing solid-type echopattern. Actually, this mass did not represent pancreatic tumor but was sarcoma arising from connective tissue of posterior aspect of omental pouch.

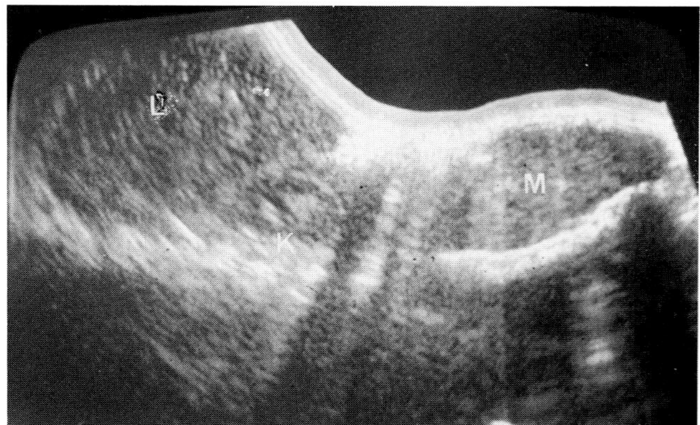

Fig. 25-31. Another example of retroperitoneal mass. This sagittal scan of abdomen, extending from diaphragm to pelvic region, displays below liver (*L*) and kidney (*K*) large mass *(M)* occupying right iliac fossa. This mass belongs to metastatic deposit of prostatic carcinoma.

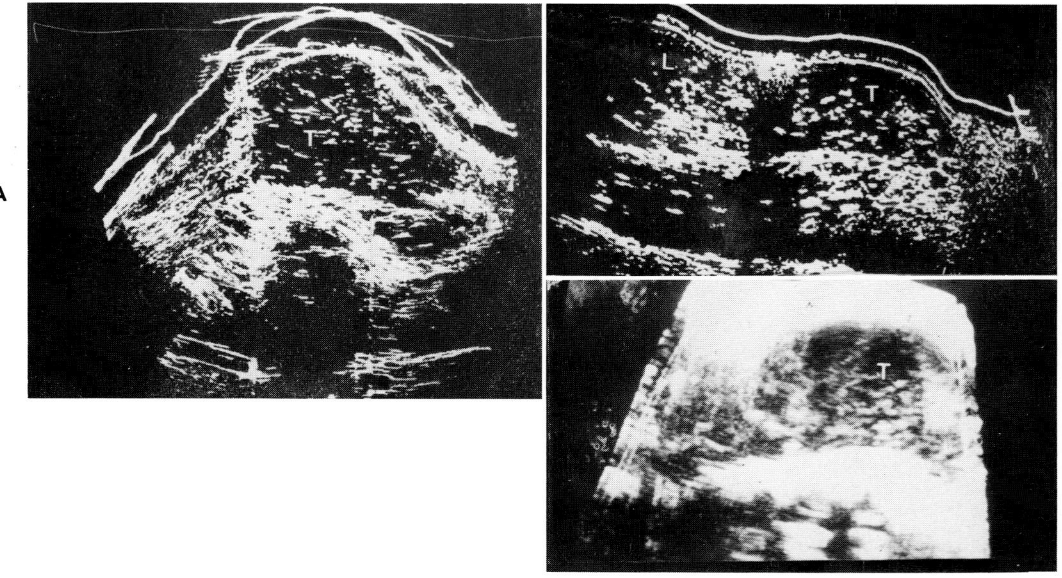

Fig. 25-32. Retroperitoneal mass—neurogenic tumor. **A,** Transverse scan of 8-year-old child displaying well-marginated tumor *(T),* of solid pattern. **B** and **C,** Sagittal scans displaying craniocaudal extension of this solid mass, which belongs to neuroblastoma. *L,* liver.

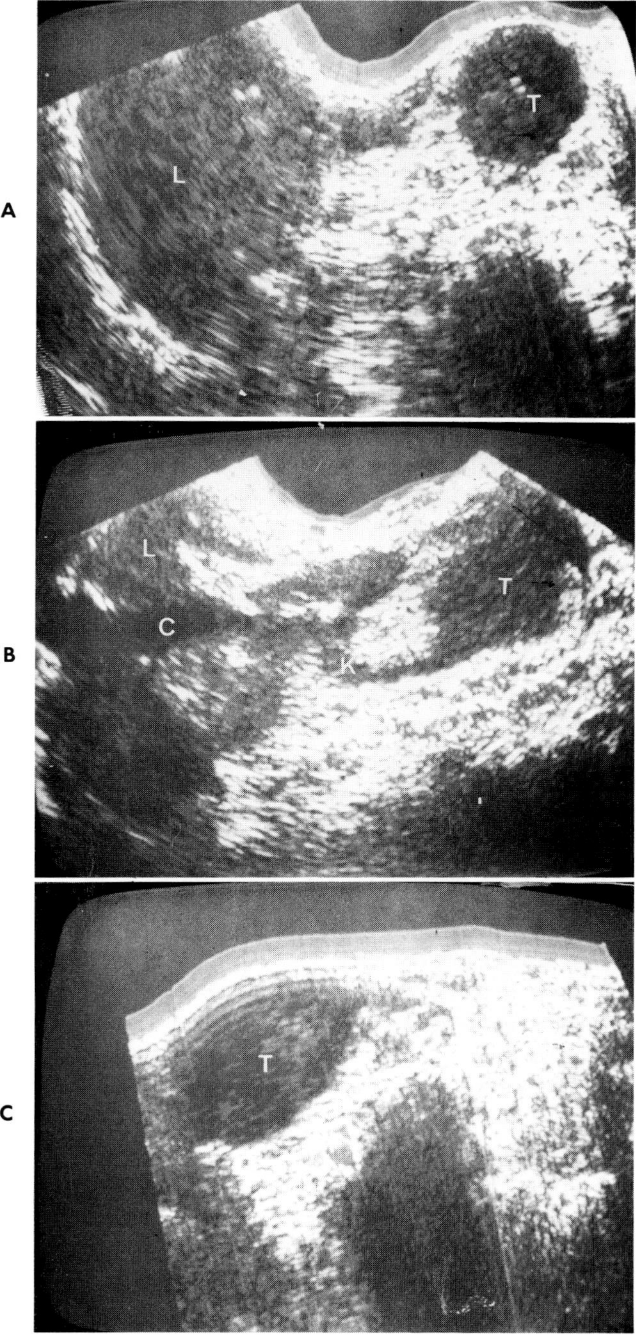

Fig. 25-33. Palpable abdominal mass—renal carcinoma. **A,** Sagittal scan through liver *(L)* displaying rounded, superficial, well-marginated, sonolucent tumor *(T).* **B,** Another, more external sagittal scan shows that tumor extends from lower pole of mobile right kidney *(K). C,* vena cava. **C,** Transverse scan of mass.

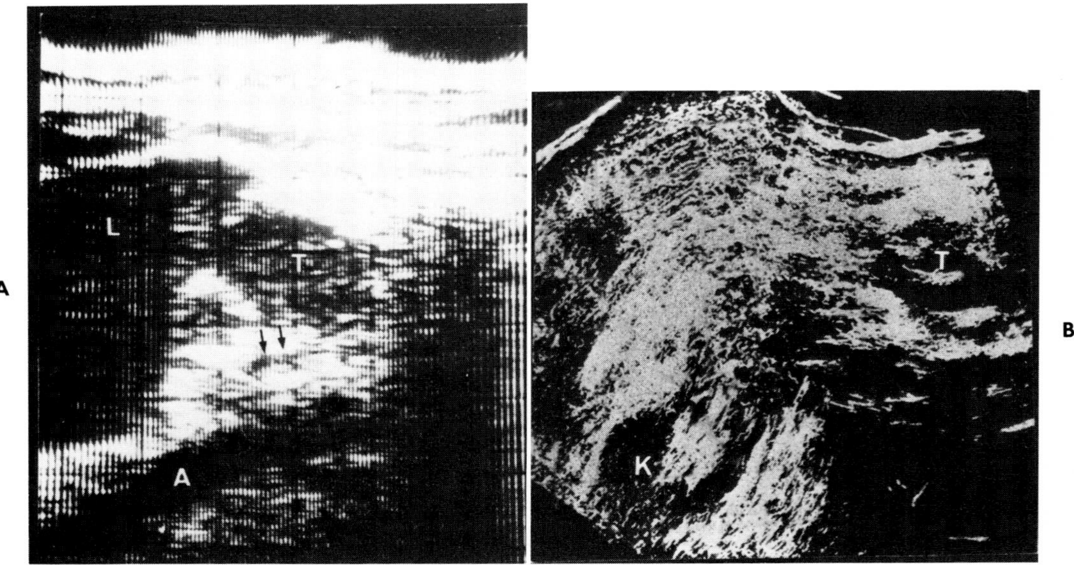

Fig. 25-34. Deep mass. **A,** Sagittal real-time scan displaying liver *(L)* and aorta *(A)* shows tumoral mass *(T)* located in front of mesenteric vein *(arrows).* **B,** Transverse scan showing tumoral mass in relation to large vessels. Mass represents gastric carcinoma.

very sonolucent. Rhabdomyosarcomas and fibrosarcomas have a more solid pattern (Figs. 28-23 and 28-25). Again, it is necessary to display, as well as possible, the exact position of the mesenteric vein, which is pushed forward, and the aorta, which may be laterally displaced. Even more than lymph nodes, sarcomas usually possess a greater craniocaudal extent than does a pancreatic tumor (Fig. 25-31). *Neurogenic tumors* are located more laterally, and their echopattern is much more reflective than the pattern of a pancreatic tumor (Fig. 25-32). When the differential diagnosis involves pancreatic tumor and a retroperitoneal tumor of other origin, other examinations such as lymphography, celiac angiography, abdominal aortography, and selective angiography of the lumbar arteries may, of course, prove necessary. The contribution of computerized axial tomography to this type of differential diagnosis seems invaluable.

Other tumors (renal, gastric, and colonic) and masses (postoperative abdominal)

An ill-matched group of intraperitoneal tumors will now be considered. A tumor may occur in a mobile kidney. Such tumors are discovered by simple palpation. Their ultrasonic identification is easy. (See Fig. 25-33.) The main problems occur in cases of gastric and colonic tumors (Holm and colleagues, 1976; Lutz and colleagues, 1973; Winsberg and colleagues, 1974). Certain gastric tumors give rise to deep sonolucent areas, the echopattern of which is quite like that of a pancreatic tumor (Figs. 25-34 and 25-35). Of course, if such an image belongs to a palpable mass, palpation under echoscopic real-time control may show mobility incompatible with a pancreatic tumor; but an infiltrative gastric mass may

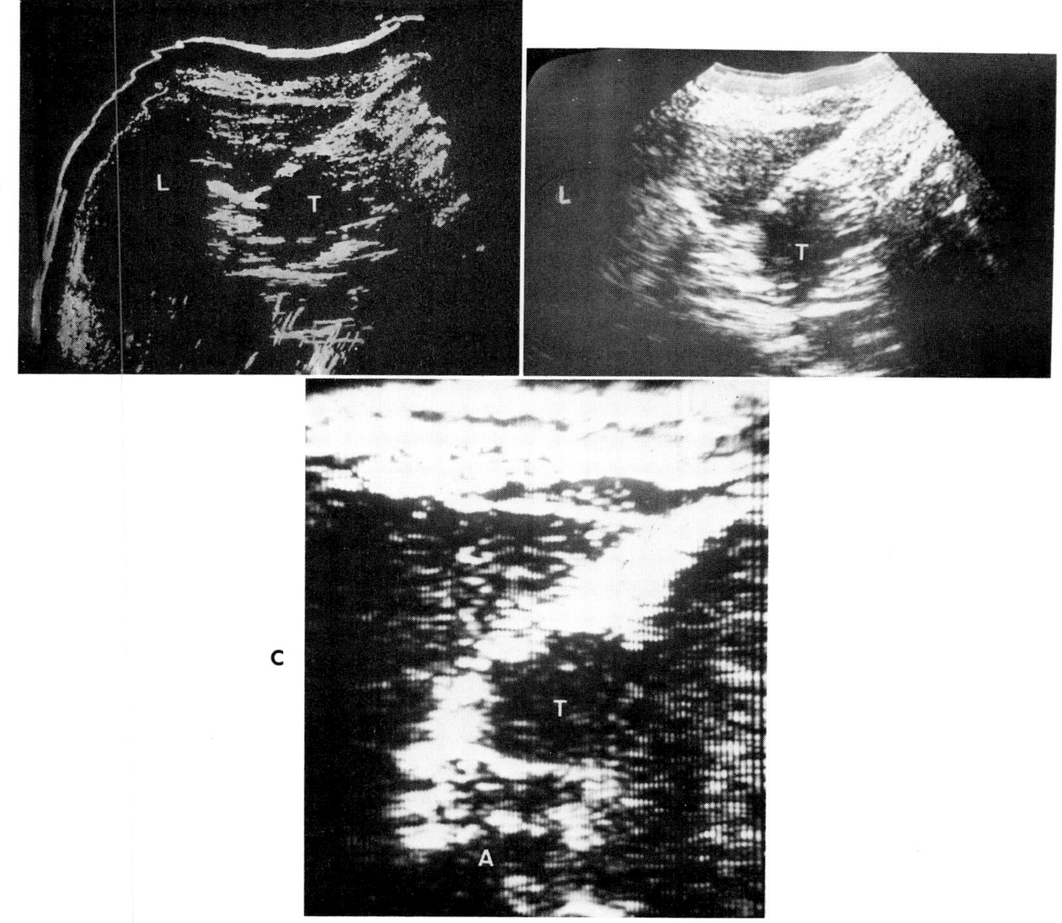

Fig. 25-35. Deep-lying mass of epigastrium. **A** and **B,** Transverse scans showing well-marginated tumor *(T)* between large vessels and liver *(L)*. **C,** Real-time sagittal scan showing tumor. Again, this is gastric carcinoma. *A,* aorta.

not move. Once again, one must remember how necessary a complete radiological record is, with ultrasonic and radiological images. A patient with a gastric tumor should take the barium examination results to the ultrasonic department or at least undergo such an examination later. A more difficult problem may arise in cases of gastric tumor with extragastric extension. Such tumors seem to be extrinsic on barium examination and even endoscopically. Ultrasonography reveals an image of a mass in the left upper quadrant; this may lead to consideration of a tumor of the pancreatic tail if the mass is not mobile. (See Fig. 25-36.) Since such tumors may be supplied by branches of the splenic artery, angiography can also be misleading. Lutz and Petzolodt (1976) described a particular pattern seen in gastric or colonic tumors, consisting of "cockade" images, with reflective central areas and sonolucent crowns (Figs. 25-37 and 25-38, *A*). However, this cockade pattern is not con-

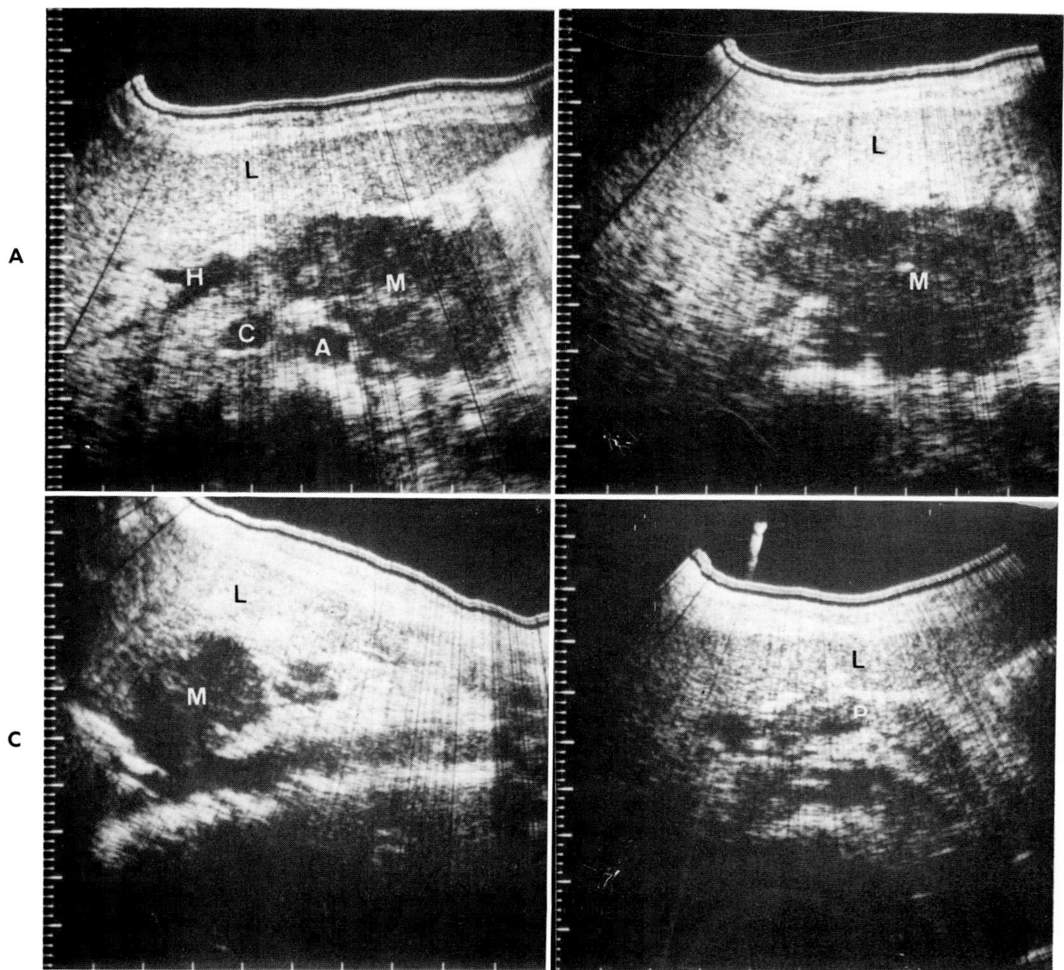

Fig. 25-36. Deep-lying mass. **A** and **B,** Parallel transverse scans of upper abdomen. *L,* liver; *M,* mass; *H,* liver hilus; *A,* aorta; *C,* vena cava. **C,** Sagittal scan. This mass could belong to pancreas. **D,** More caudal transverse scan, however, shows normal pancreas *(P).* Mass had arisen from gastric wall, probably from pancreatic islet.

stant. On the other hand, this pattern is not specific. Normal sections of the duodenum or stomach may present the same pattern (Fig. 25-38, *B*). The solid echopattern of abscesses with gas bubbles was mentioned in Chapter 14.

A last particular is illustrated by Fig. 25-39. Such material gives rise to strongly reflective masses. Textile folds may appear as linear reflections.

Quite a few possible pitfalls have now been reviewed. To get along, one needs to bear them in mind when confronted with a misleading image. These many different diagnostic possibilities are listed below, but first I would like to review two main principles of pancreatic examination policy:

1. Any pathological pancreatic image must be verified by a further examination carried out some hours later. At least one of the two examinations must be carried out with the patient fasting.

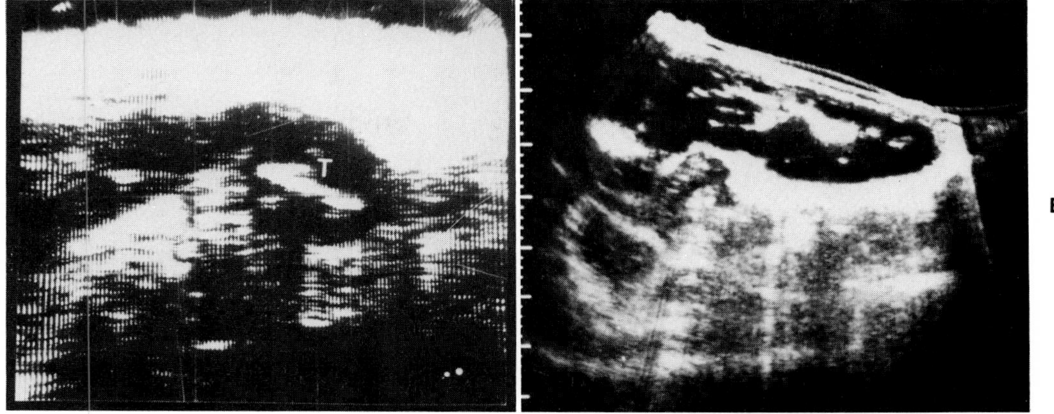

Fig. 25-37. A, Epigastric tumor *(T)* with "cockade" pattern. This is gastric carcinoma. **B,** Elongated cockade pattern. Stomach enlargement is due to Ménétrier's disease. (**B,** courtesy Dr. A. Eisenscher, Vesoul, France.)

2. The ultrasonographic data must be evaluated with all the conventional radiological results, such as x-ray films of the abdomen and barium opacification.

Following are the different diagnoses:

Retroperitoneal masses
- Aortic aneurysms
- Dissecting aneurysms of the aorta
- Retroperitoneal hematomas and abscesses
- Retroperitoneal tumors other than adenopathy
- Retroperitoneal lymph nodes

Intraperitoneal masses
- Mesenteric cysts
- Mesenteric hematomas
- Ascites in the omental bursa
- Septate ascites
- Gastric retention
- Intestinal retention
- Gastric tumors
- Colonic tumors

Liquid masses
- Aneurysms of the aorta
- Dissecting aneurysms of the aorta
- Retroperitoneal hematomas and abscesses and other abdominal abscesses
- Mesenteric hematomas
- Mesenteric cysts
- Gastric retention
- Intestinal retention

Solid masses
- Solid gastric retention

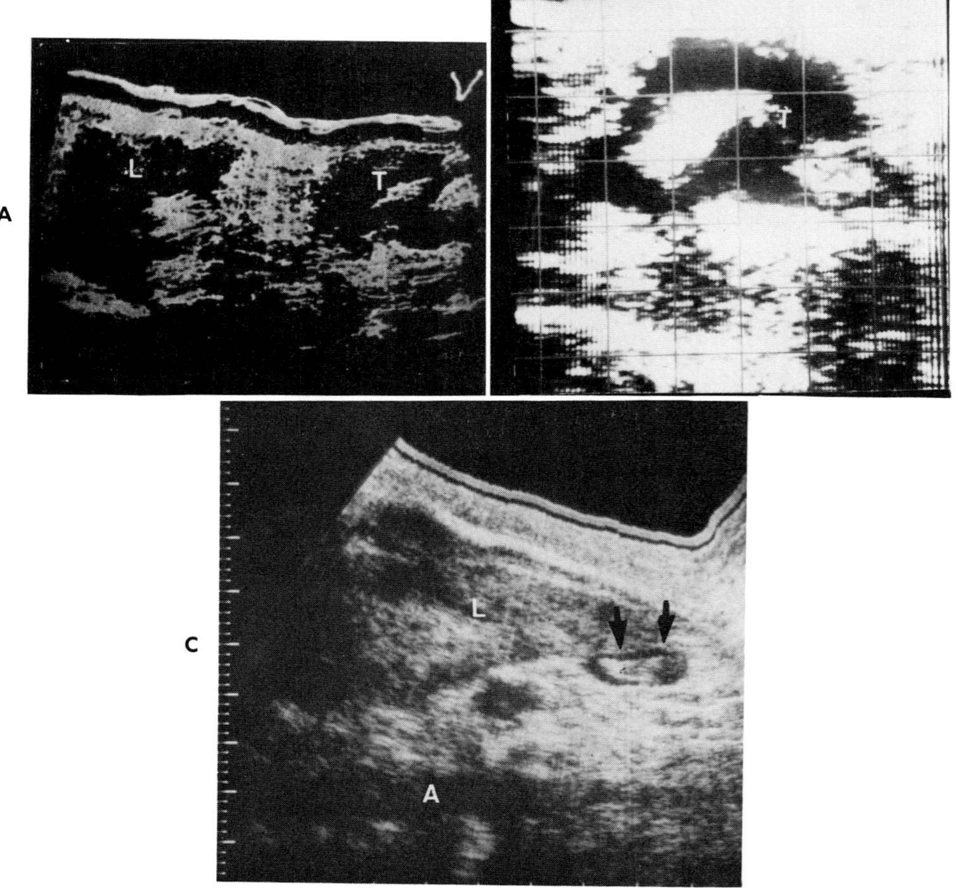

Fig. 25-38. Another example of cockade pattern in abdominal tumor. **A,** Sagittal scan. Tumor *(T)* is outlined well below liver *(L)*. **B,** Transverse scan. This is colonic carcinoma. **C,** Cockade pattern displayed on sagittal section of normal stomach *(arrows)*. *A,* aorta.

Gastric tumors
Colonic tumors
Retroperitoneal lymph nodes
Retroperitoneal tumors

Morphological features to be verified in the presence of a deep mass

Relation of the mass to the aorta and vena cava
Relation of the mass to the mesenteric vein
Relation of the mass to the kidney
Relation of the mass to the spine
Craniocaudal extension
Presence or absence of a normal pancreatic image
Associated signs such as splenomegaly and pleural effusion

Now that many different ultrasonic signs have been discussed in previous chapters, I have grouped in the following table the particular diagnostic problems arising after surgery, without listing possible preexisting anomalies (for instance, the shell sign of a calcified gallbladder).

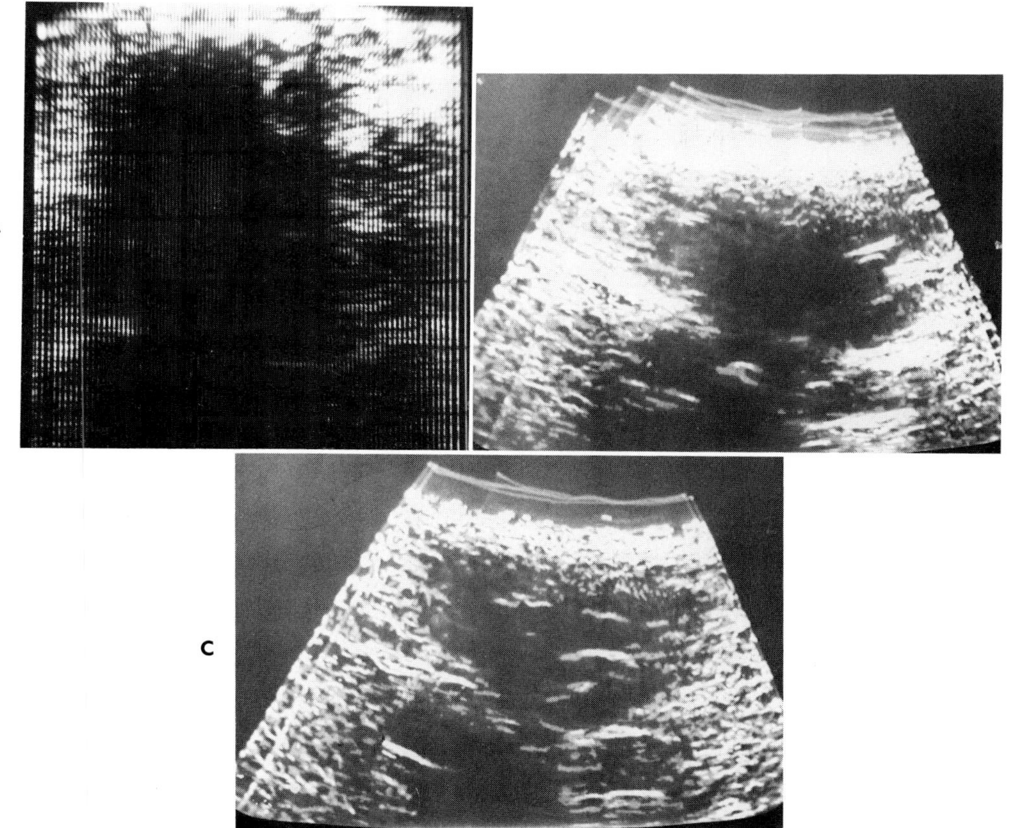

Fig. 25-39. Palpable infraumbilical mass discovered 2 months after pelvic operation. **A,** Real-time transverse scan: no transmission. **B,** Contact scan made with 1.5-MHz transducer. Mass is partially outlined, without image of its posterior interface. **C,** With 1-MHz transducer, mass is completely outlined. What is your diagnosis?*

*This mass belonged to surgical tissue left in abdomen during preceding operation. Intense reflection with acoustic shadow seems rather characteristic for textile material.

Table 25-1. Ultrasonic findings in acute postoperative abdominal problems

Shell sign	*Fluid collection*	*Areas of semisolid echopattern*	*Areas of solid echopattern*
Gas in fixed intestinal loop Surgical sponge	Fluid-filled intestinal loop Urine leakage Bile leakage Blood Collected abscess	Edematous intestinal loop Omentitis Abscess Blood with blood clots Acute pancreatitis	Conglomerate of adherent intestinal loops and omentum Abscess with gas bubbles

REFERENCES

Asher, W. M., and Freimanis, A. K.: Echographic diagnosis of retroperitoneal lymph node enlargement, Am. J. Roentgenol. Radium Ther. Nucl. Med. **105:**438-445, 1969.

Barnett, E., and Morley, P.: Abdominal echography, Borough Green, England, 1974, Butterworth & Co. (Publishers), Ltd.

Duval, J. M., and Mambrini, A.: Intérêt de l'échotomographie dans le diagnostic des hématomes de la gaine des droits, Nouv. Presse Méd. **4:**349-350, 1975.

Goldberg, B. B., Kotler, M. N., Ziskin, M. C., and Waxham, R. D.: Diagnostic uses of ultrasound, New York, 1975, Grune & Stratton, Inc.

Gorelik, I., Goldman, S. M., Minkin, S. D., Abrams, S. J., and Salik, J. O.: Gastric duplication originating from the tail of the pancreas—ultrasonically demonstrated, J. Clin. Ultrasound **4:**429-432, 1976.

Hassani, N.: Ultrasonography of the abdomen, Heidelberg, Germany, 1976, Springer-Verlag.

Holm, H. H., Kristensen, J. K., Rasmussen, S. N., Pedersen, J. F., and Hancke, S.: Abdominal ultrasound, Copenhagen, 1976, Munksgaard, International Booksellers & Publishers, Ltd.

Hsu, C.-Y., and Wolf, S. B.: Ultrasonic contrast study to identify stomach contents, World Federation of Ultrasound in Medicine and Biology, San Francisco, 1976, Abstract No. 516.

Leopold, G. R.: A review of retroperitoneal ultrasonography, J. Clin. Ultrasound **1:**82-87, 1973.

Leopold, G. R.: Ultrasonic abdominal aortography, Radiology **96:**9-14, 1970.

Leopold, G. R., and Asher, W. M.: Fundamentals of abdominal and pelvic ultrasonography, Philadelphia, 1975, W. B. Saunders Co.

Lutz, H., and Petzolodt, R.: Real time and gray scale ultrasound in the diagnosis of gastroenterological diseases, World Federation of Ultrasound in Medicine and Biology, San Francisco, 1976, Abstract No. 529.

Lutz, H., Sturm, G., and Hartwich, G.: Comparative sonographic and lymphographic investigation of retroperitoneal lymph nodes in malignant lymphomas, Verh. Dtsch. Ges. Inn. Med. **79:**507-508, 1973.

Mittelstaedt, C.: Ultrasonic diagnosis of omental cysts, Radiology **117:**673-677, 1975.

Walls, W. J.: The evaluation of malignant gastric neoplasms by ultrasonic B-scanning, Radiology **118:**159-163, 1976.

Weill, F., Aucant, D., Bourgoin, A., Eisenscher, A., and Gallinet, D.: Ultrasonic visualization of abdominal veins, Second European Congress, Ultrasonics in medicine, Abstract No. 103, Erlangen, Germany, 1975, Junge & Sohn.

Weill, F., Kraehenbuhl, J. R., Becker, J. C., Milleret, P., and Gillet, M.: Aspect tomoéchographique des dissections artérielles et des fissurations anévrismales, Nouv. Presse Méd. **2:**227-228, 1973.

Weill, F., Kraehenbuhl, J. R., Ricatte, J. P., Aucant, D., Gillet, M., and Makridis, D.: Le diagnostic ultrasonore des dissections aortiques et des fissurations anévrismales, Ann. Radiol. **17:**49-54, 1974.

Winsberg, F., Cole-Beuglet, C., and Mulder, D. S.: Continuous ultrasound "B" scanning of abdominal aortic aneurysms, Am. J. Roentgenol. Radium Ther. Nucl. Med. **121:**626-633, 1974.

CHAPTER 26

JAUNDICE

Hepatic, biliary, and pancreatic diseases have already been discussed. The ultrasonic examination of the jaundiced patient progresses in a systematic fashion. The first goal is recognition of the biliary tree dilatation: common bile duct, intrahepatic biliary network, and gallbladder dilatation. The second aim in the ultrasonic examination is to identify the exact level of obstruction and if possible the obstructive lesion. In jaundice with intrahepatic cholestasis, ultrasonography shows the extrahepatic biliary tree to be normal and may possibly indicate the presence of specific liver disease. Finally, in certain cases of intrahepatic jaundice and especially in hepatitis, the result may be no abnormal ultrasonic findings at all.

EXAMINATION PROCEDURE

As in any examination of the biliary tree, it is wise to examine the fasting patient. However, this is not absolutely compulsory, since a dilated obstructed gallbladder remains distended even after eating. In my opinion, the use of real-time technique in this situation is of utmost importance because of the flexibility and rapidity that it provides. Only with real-time precision can one make an accurate assessment of the anatomical morphology. Differentiation between the common bile duct and portal vein and between the intrahepatic biliary network and intrahepatic blood vessels requires immediate adjustment of the scanning plane to the axes of these anatomical structures. The study of the anastomosis of the hepatic veins with the vena cava, the hilar portal branches with the portal vein, and the intrahepatic biliary ducts with the common bile duct requires a rapid succession of scanning planes, which is available only with real-time examination.

IDENTIFICATION OF OBSTRUCTION

Gallbladder enlargement

Gallbladder enlargement is easy to identify by ultrasound (Figs. 26-1 to 26-4) and may even be palpable. It is, however, apparent that palpation may cause confusion of other right upper quadrant masses with a dilated gallbladder. Moreover, the presence of an enlarged gallbladder does not necessarily indicate obstruction of the common bile duct in the jaundiced patient. The difficulty of establishing normal values for the volume of the gallbladder has already been indicated (Chapter 16). The upper limit of normal is considered to be 200 ml, but the pathologically dilated gallbladder may exceed that value or, on the other hand, may never attain it. When the volume of the gallbladder is less than 200 ml, the contraction test is used for confirmation, but even this test, at least with a fatty meal, is not absolutely reliable. Rettenmaier (1975) emphasizes the value of palpation under eschoscopic real-time control, since this allows one to assess the tension of the obstructed gallbladder.

A B

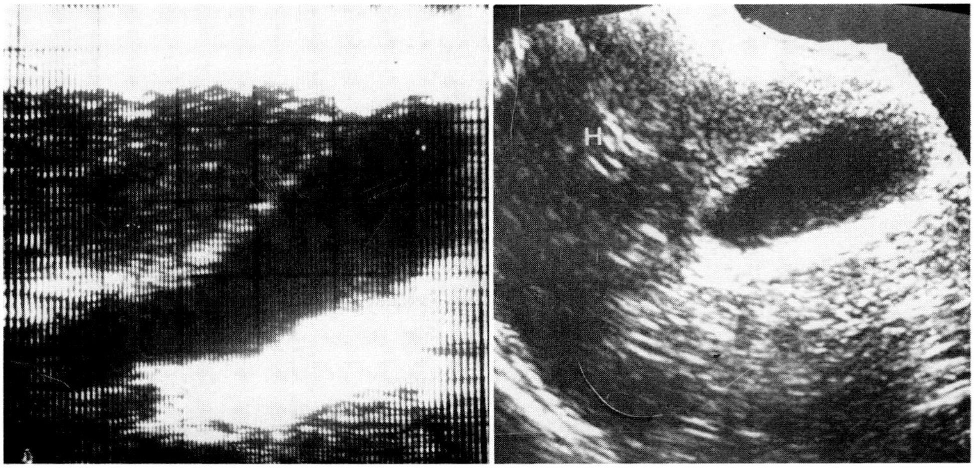

Fig. 26-1. Dilatation of gallbladder in case of obstructive jaundice. **A,** Sagittal real-time scan. **B,** Sagittal gray scale contact scan. Estimation of gallbladder volume was over 200 ml. *H,* hilar structures.

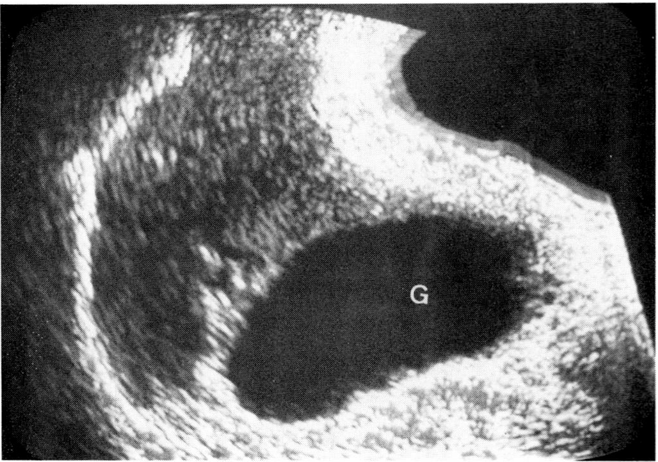

Fig. 26-2. Another example of gallbladder *(G)* dilatation with volume over 200 ml.

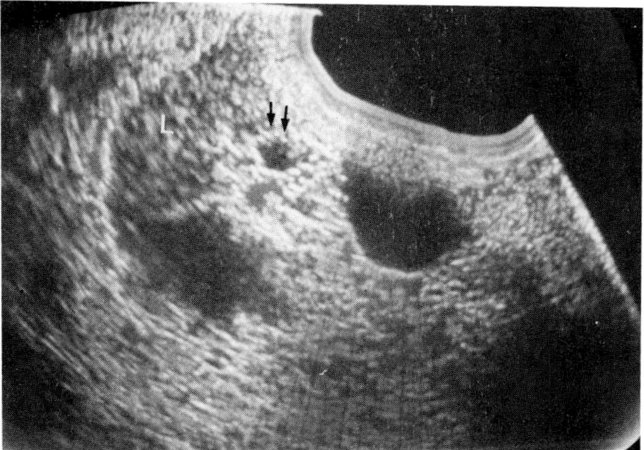

Fig. 26-3. Another example of dilated gallbladder. Size of gallbladder is to be compared to size of liver *(L)*. Note dilatation of hilar junction *(arrows)*.

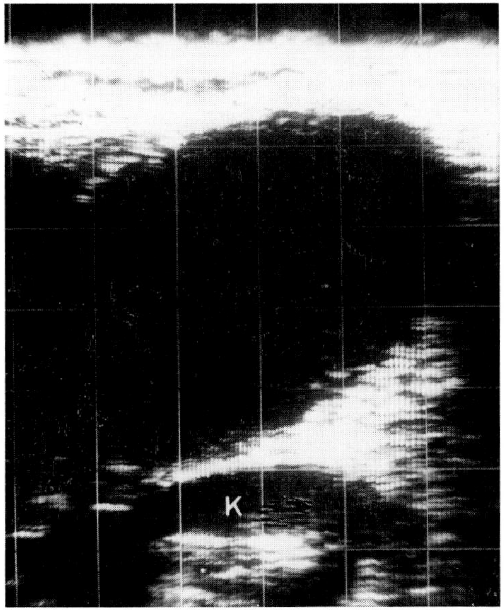

Fig. 26-4. Giant dilatation of gallbladder. Approximate volume is over 500 ml. Comparison of gallbladder with kidney section *(K)* is striking.

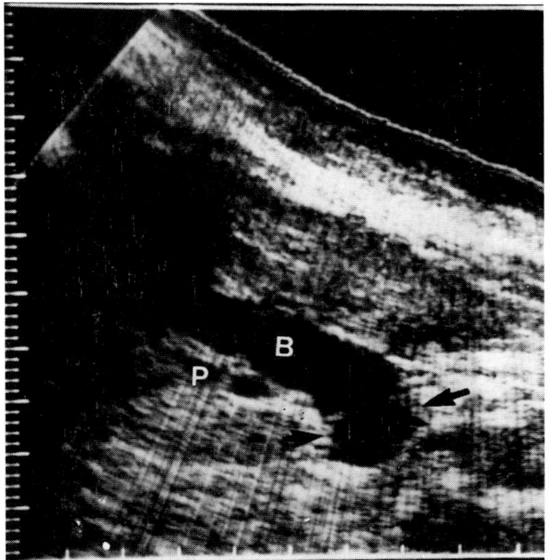

Fig. 26-5. Sagittal section of enormously dilated common bile duct *(B),* with diameter of over 2 cm. Note flattened portal vein *(P).* Lowest part of bile duct is pseudocystic *(arrows),* due to sharp bend.

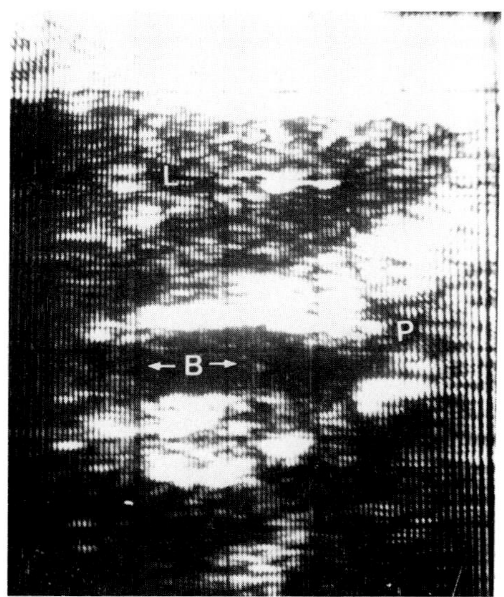

Fig. 26-6. Dilatation of main bile duct *(B).* This oblique real-time scan shows, behind liver *(L),* tubular element, diameter of which is about 1.5 cm. Small pancreatic nodule *(P)* is obstructing common bile duct.

The gallbladder examination is of course not limited solely to volumetric assessment. One must look also for stones, tumors, and other abnormalities.

Dilatation of bile duct*

It has been shown (Chapter 15) that the main bile duct becomes visible when its diameter is about 4 mm. Since in normal subjects the diameter is variable, it can be considered definitely pathological only when over 1 cm. (See Figs. 26-5 and 26-6.) A dilated bile duct can be easily identified by two objective and reliable means: one is the real-time study of tubular junctions; the other, recognition of what I call the *sign of the double-barreled gun* (or *gun sign*).

Study of tubular junctions. On a sagittal scan, it is always possible to display the superior mesenteric vein and thus to identify the mesenteric-portal axis. The sagittal section of the portal vein extends caudally through the mesenteric-portal junction. A long venous section is displayed, whereas the bile duct, which extends caudally no farther than its duodenal junction, appears in its distal part as a shorter segment (Fig. 26-7). The same observation is made on transverse scans with regard to the splenoportal axis: this venous axis appears as a long segment, extending to the left, whereas the dilated bile duct extends to the left no farther than the pancreatic head (Fig. 26-20, *D*). In addition, the junction of the main bile duct with the dilated intrahepatic ducts can be studied, as well as the junction of the portal vein with its hilar branches, if the anterior location of the biliary junction is kept in mind (Fig. 26-8)—a point that will be brought out again in discussion of the gun sign. Sagittal, oblique, transverse, oblique recurrent, and intercostal cuts are used in the real-time study of tubular junctions (Weill and associates, 1974).

Gun sign. In Chapter 15, the parallel images of the common bile duct and portal vein in the infrahepatic, as well as the hilar, region were discussed. In normal subjects the diameter of the bile duct is smaller than that of the portal vein. When dilatation occurs, the diameters of both tubular structures tend to become equal, so that the two parallel ducts resemble a double-barreled gun. (See Figs. 26-8 to 26-11.) In fact, the dilated bile duct may compress the portal vein so that the former is of larger caliber than the latter. Even then, the gun sign remains obvious. Three types of cuts are used to display the gun sign: first, in the infrahepatic area, sagittal or slightly oblique scans, adjusted to the direction of the portal axis (Figs. 26-8 to 26-11, *A*); second, in the hilar region, intercostal scans; last, transverse contact scans of the hilar region. The latter show also the two tubular elements in close contact: the biliary duct in front and the portal venous branches behind (Fig. 26-9, *B*), presenting a group of parallel lines (Figs. 26-11, *B*, 26-18, *D*, 26-19, *C*, and 26-20, *C*). More caudal transverse scans permit one to show the bile duct and the portal vein in transverse section. Two rounded images, close to each other, are then outlined. (See Figs. 26-9, *C*, and 26-11, *C*.) The rounded section of an enlarged main bile duct on a transverse scan of the right upper quadrant is often seen in the jaundiced patient (Figs. 26-17, *B*, and 26-26, *C*).

Text continued on p. 418.

*See p. 221 for definition.

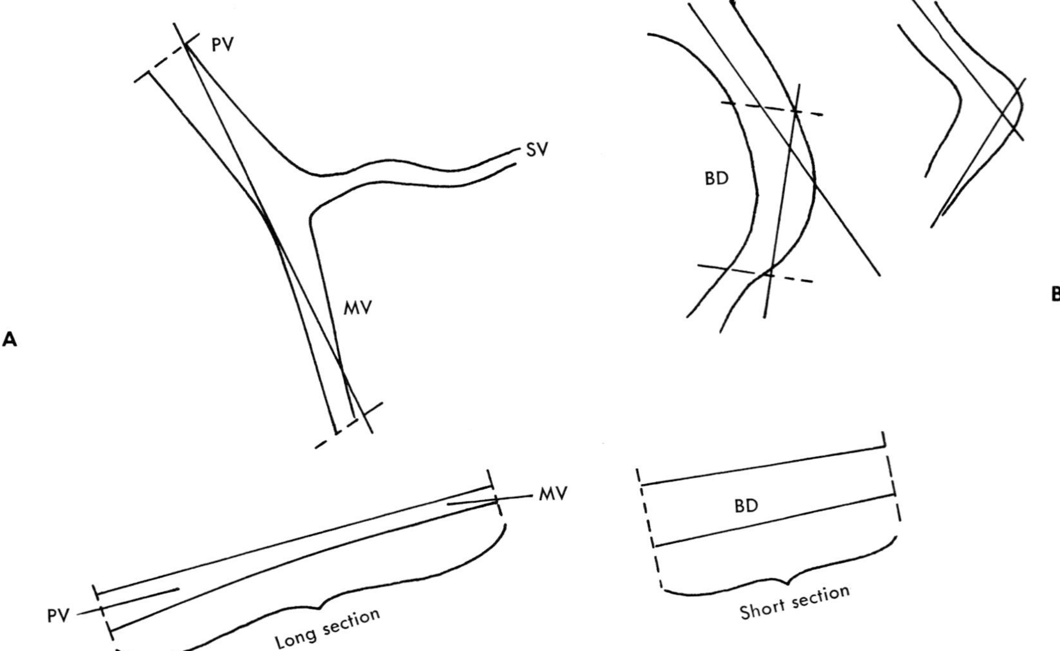

Fig. 26-7. Differences in longitudinal display of mesenteric-portal axis. **A,** Venous axis. Sagittal scan can display long venous segment. *PV,* portal vein; *SV,* splenic vein; *MV,* mesenteric vein. **B,** Main bile duct *(BD)*. Often only short segment is displayed by sagittal scan.

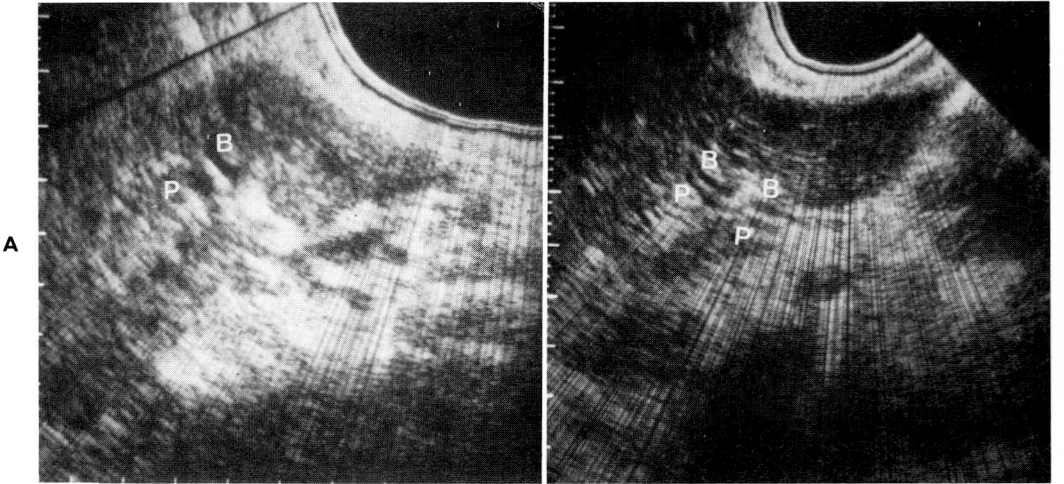

Fig. 26-8. Dilatation of hilar portion of biliary tree—hilar gun sign. **A,** Dilated biliary junction *(B)* displayed on intercostal scan in front of portal division *(P)*. Two ductal elements are parallel, like two barrels of game rifle. **B,** Another example on transverse scan of different patient.

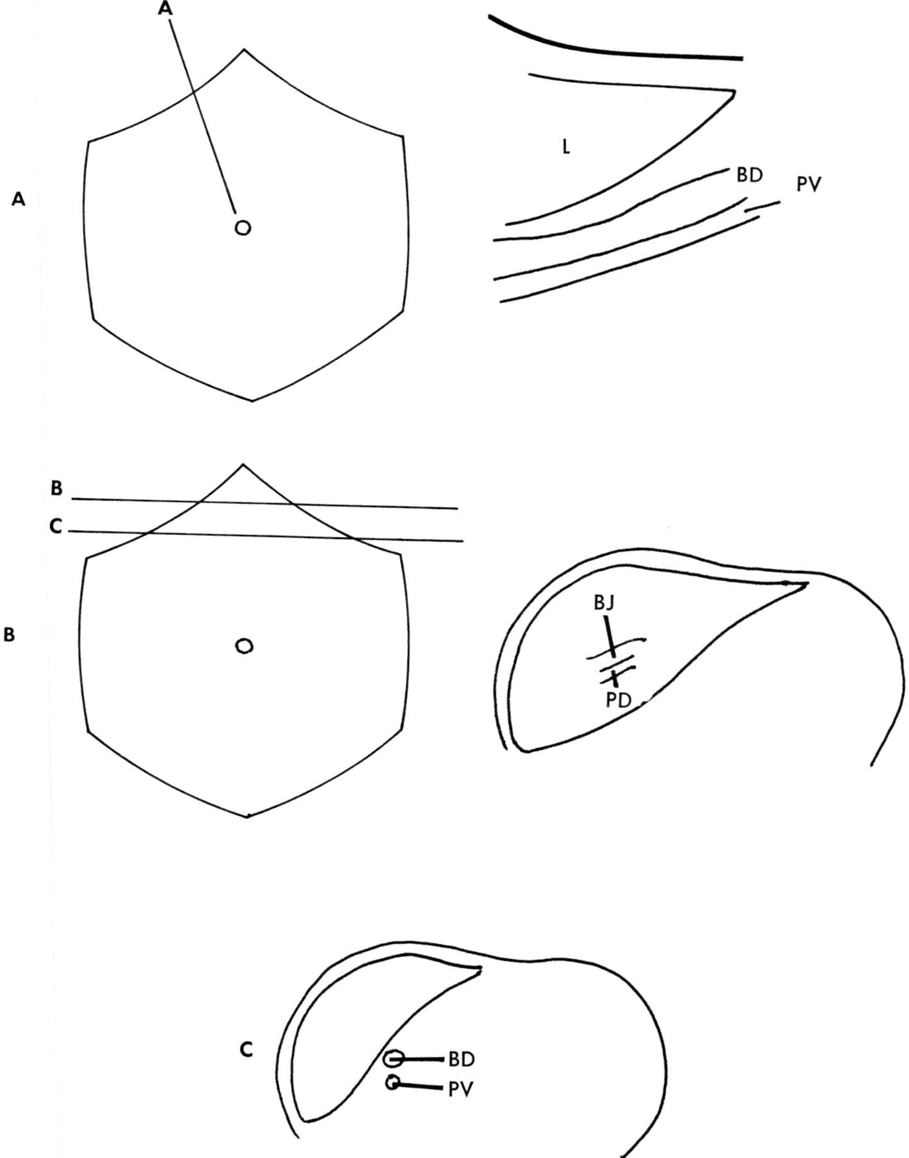

Fig. 26-9. Schematic representation of gun sign. **A,** Oblique scan of right upper quadrant will display, behind liver *(L),* coupled sagittal sections of common bile duct *(BD)* in front and portal vein *(PV)* in back. **B,** Transverse scan of hilar region displays three parallel lines delineating biliary hilar junction *(BJ)* in front and portal division *(PD)* behind. **C,** More caudal parallel scan displays twin transverse sections of common bile duct in front and portal vein behind. Image in **B** is also displayed by intercostal cuts.

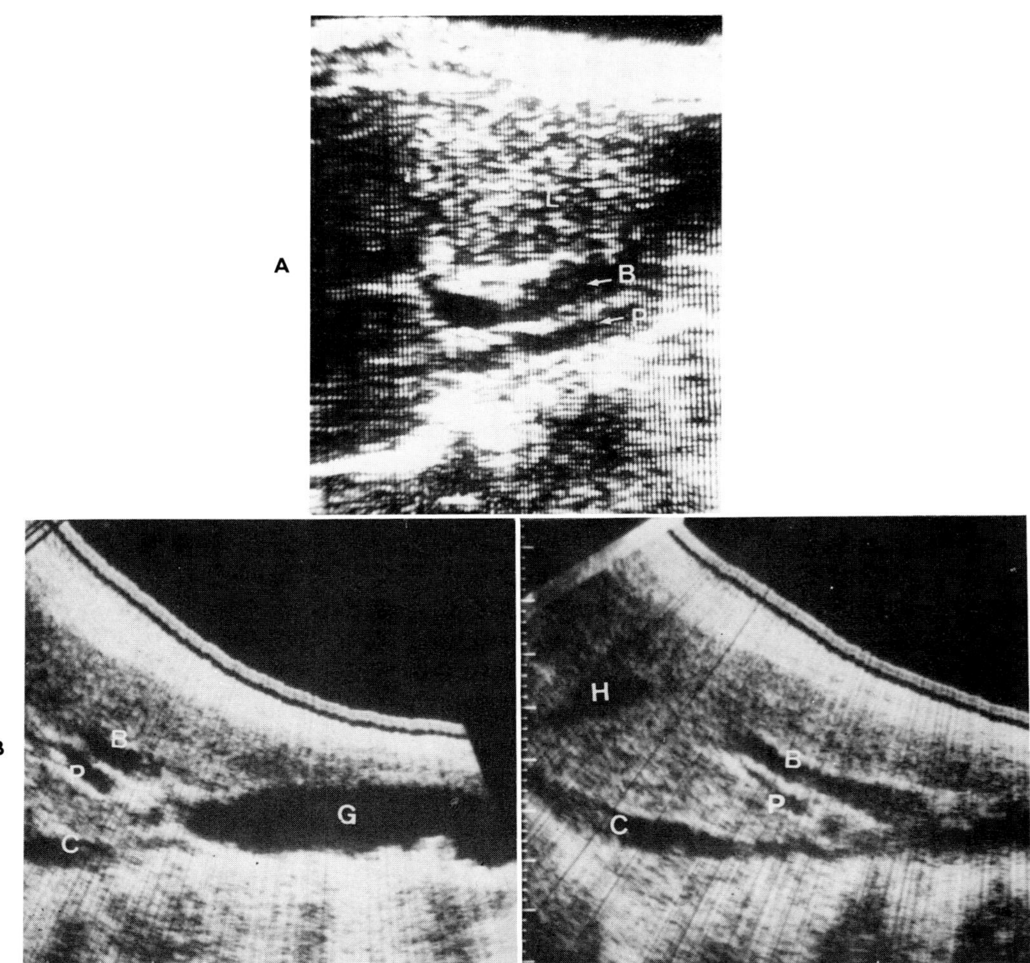

Fig. 26-10. Gun sign. **A,** Real-time intercostal scan showing bile duct *(B)* in front of portal vein *(P)*. Bile duct is wider than portal vein. Note biliary junction on left (cranial) part of bile duct. *L,* liver. **B** and **C,** Another example. **B,** In hilar area. **C,** In infrahepatic area. *G,* dilated gallbladder; *C,* vena cava; *H,* hepatic vein.

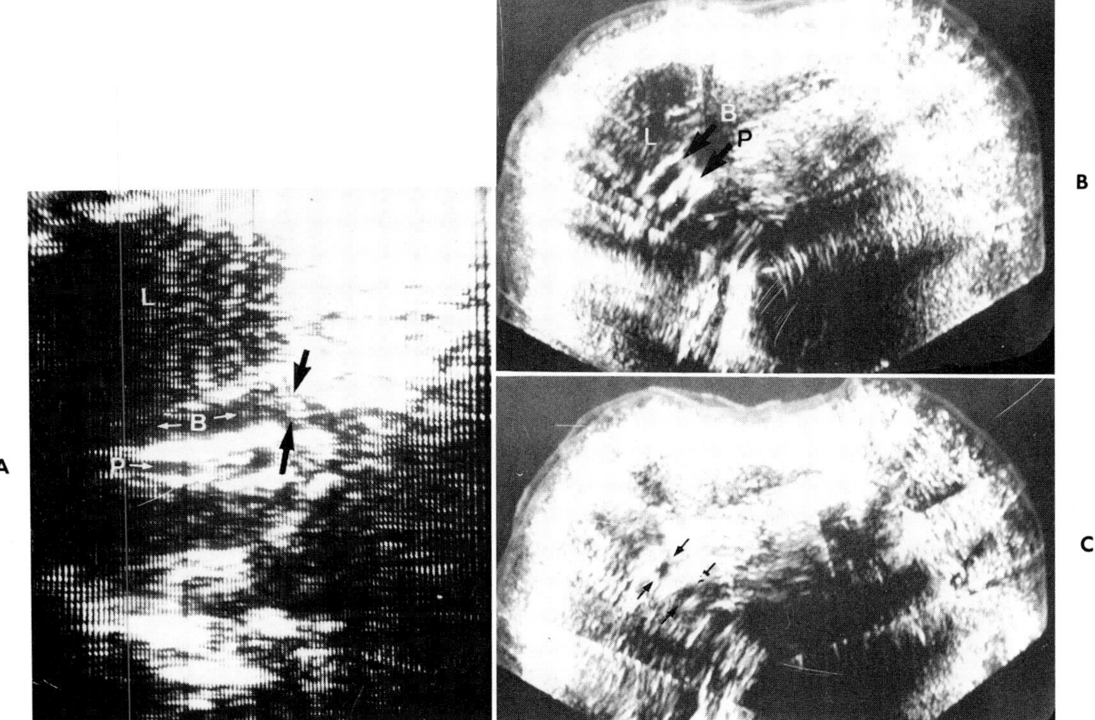

Fig. 26-11. Gun sign. **A,** Oblique scan of right upper quadrant displaying twin parallel, coupled sagittal sections of obstructed main bile duct *(B)* and portal vein *(P)*. Stones *(arrows)* are seen in inferior segment of bile duct. *L,* liver. **B,** Transverse scan of hilar region displaying three parallel lines delineating twin sections of biliary hilar junction *(arrow B)* and portal division *(arrow P)*. **C,** More caudal parallel scan displaying two transverse sections of main bile duct *(arrows)*. Portal vein is deeper-lying element.

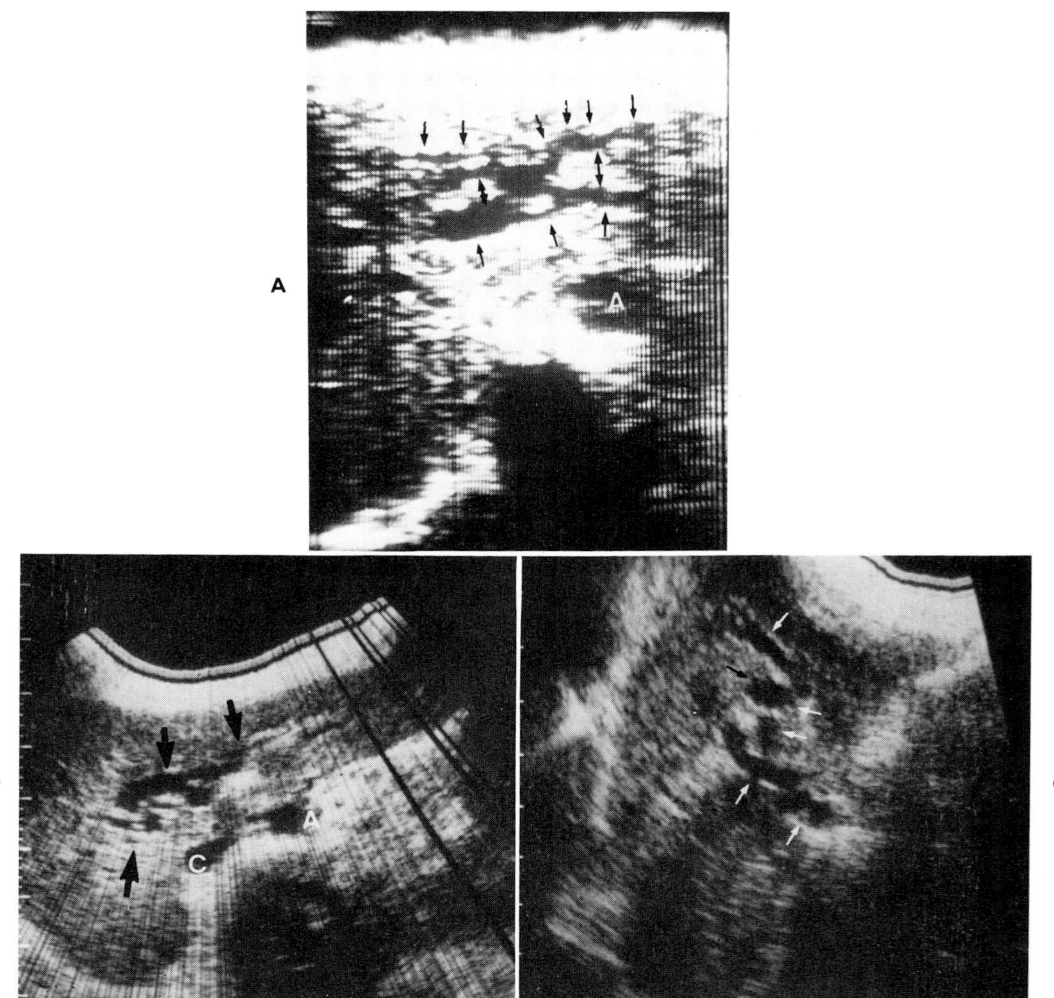

Fig. 26-12. Dilatation of intrahepatic bile ducts. **A,** Oblique recurrent real-time subcostal liver scan displays rich tubular network *(arrows)*. Peripheral location of some enlarged ducts indicates their biliary nature. *A,* aorta. **B** and **C,** Two more examples. *C,* vena cava.

There are pitfalls in the search for a "main" bile duct dilatation. As previously stated, the bile duct is displayed in front of the portal vein, which is often visualized in front of the vena cava. Three distinct tubular elements are then visualized from back to front: the vena cava, the portal vein, and the bile duct. The portal vein may be in close contact with the vena cava, but, in other cases, there is an ultrasonically dead space between the vena cava and portal vein (Figs. 26-18, *B,* and 4-17, *C*). This echo-free space, delineated by the anterior wall of the vena cava and the posterior wall of the portal vein, must not be confused with a tubular element. In that case, the portal vein would be considered the third tubular element from the back and would then be taken for the bile duct and, since the portal

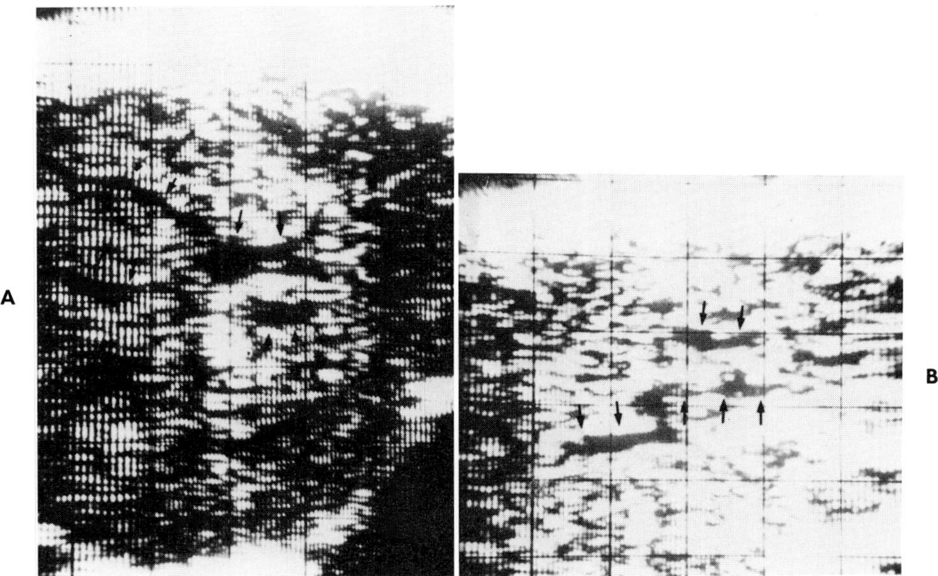

Fig. 26-13. Dilatation of intrahepatic bile ducts. **A,** Real-time oblique recurrent subcostal scan showing dilated tubular network *(arrows).* **B,** More caudal scan displaying peripheral enlarged ducts *(arrows).*

vein is wide, for a dilated bile duct. In the hilar area the adjacent sections of the common hepatic duct and proximal infundibulum present another pitfall on sagittal scans: the use of multiple scanning directions, as well as a real-time study of junctions, is mandatory. Multiple scans also enable one to avoid the pitfall of a false gun sign arising from a dilated cystic duct.

The study of the main bile duct is not limited to the assessment of its diameter. It also includes a careful search for stones. Solitary stones in the common bile duct are reflective and contrast with the surrounding transparent bile (Fig. 16-22, *B*). A main bile duct filled with stones is more difficult to display, since the sharp contrast between stones and bile no longer exists. Choledochal stones will be discussed in more detail a little farther on.

Dilatation of intrahepatic biliary ducts

In a rich, high-gain gray scale display of the liver texture, the dilated intrahepatic radicles are readily apparent (Figs. 26-12, 26-13, 26-15, *A* and *B,* 26-17, 26-27, *B,* and 26-28). As already indicated in Chapter 4, the portal branches become very narrow as they leave the hilum and are displayed only on subcostal recurrent real-time scans. The farther the normal biliary radicles are from the hilum, the more difficult they are to display. On the other hand, a dilated biliary network is displayed even very distally in the periphery of the liver (Figs. 26-12, *A,* 26-13, 26-27, *B,* and 26-28), at which point their diameter may reach several millimeters, whereas portal vessels will almost never attain that caliber peripherally (Fig. 26-14). This is an important feature in differentiating between dilated bile ducts and dilated portal vessels. Multiplicity of branches is also characteristic of

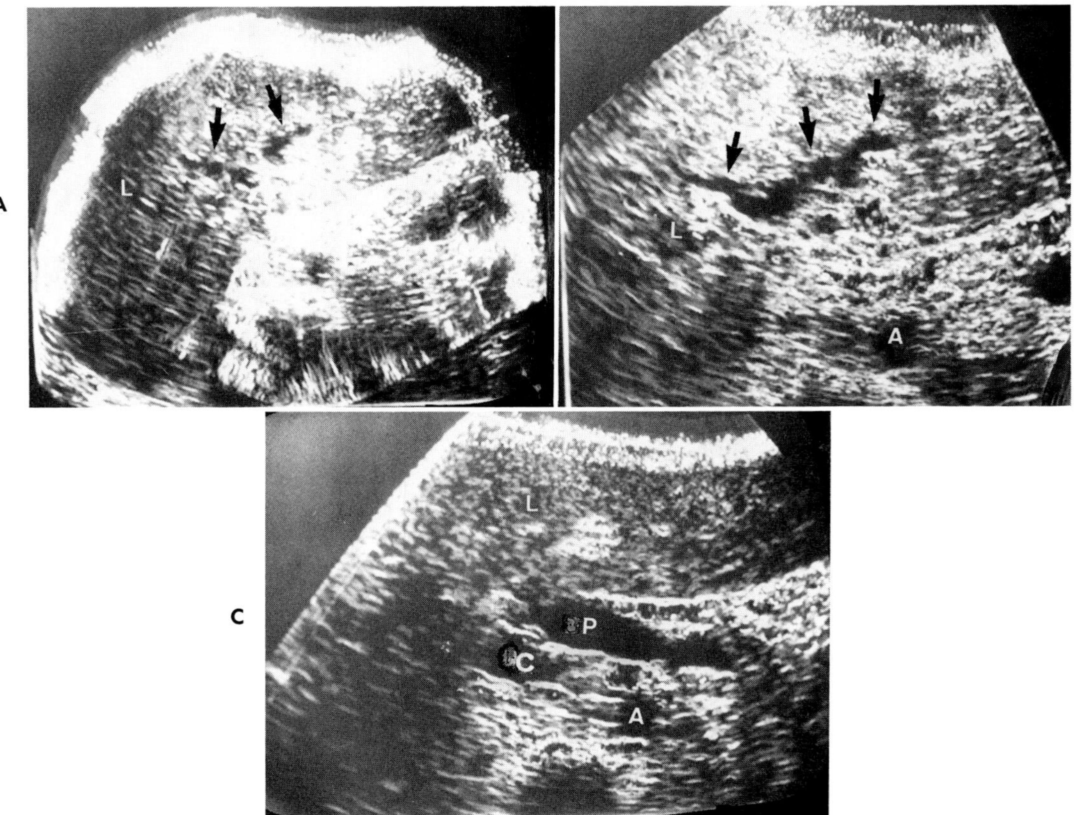

Fig. 26-14. Differential diagnosis. These three scans are of cirrhotic patient with jaundice. **A** and **B,** Transverse scans of enlarged liver *(L)* displaying dilated intrahepatic tubular network *(arrows)*. There are central tubular elements, but no peripheral dilated ones. *A,* aorta. **C,** Oblique scan of right upper quadrant showing portal vein *(P),* identified by its junction with splenic and mesenteric veins. There is no satellite image of dilated bile duct: dilated network belongs to portal system and not to biliary tree. *C,* vena cava.

the biliary ducts: sectional images of a dilated biliary network are often tortuous and many (Figs. 26-12, 26-13, and 26-28), unlike the portal network, which tends to be straight or linear. A helpful sign, recently described by Cosgrove and Dunn (1976), is a tendency to acoustic reinforcement deep to the dilated bile ducts, since bile is even more transparent than blood, but, in my opinion, this sign is not constant and reliable. To these morphological criteria must be added the essential study of the branching of the hilar bile ducts with the main bile duct and the gun sign observed in the hilar region.

CAUSES

Stones

The presence of stones in a dilated (Fig. 26-15, *B*) or normal-sized (Fig. 26-17, *A*) gallbladder or a small gallbladder, due to chronic infection (Fig. 26-18, *B*), is only an accessory sign. A valuable diagnosis is based on the direct display of choledochal stones.

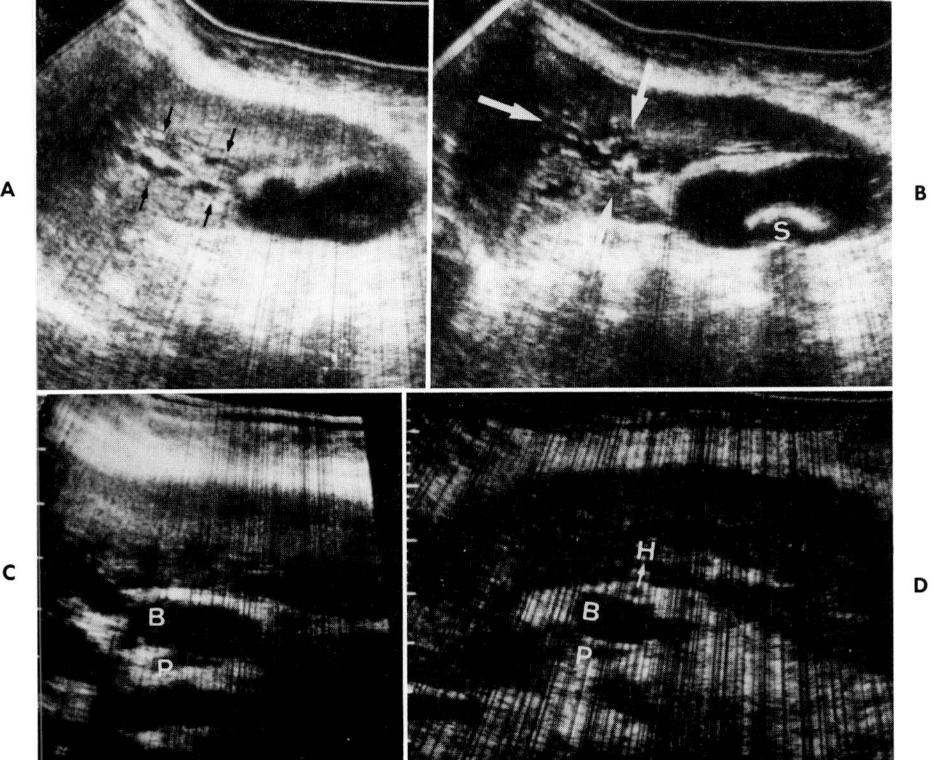

Fig. 26-15. Obstructive jaundice. **A,** Sagittal scan of right hepatic lobe showing dilated biliary network *(arrows).* Gallbladder seems moderately dilated. **B,** Parallel scan again displaying dilated intrahepatic bile ducts *(arrows).* Dilatation of gallbladder appears more clearly, and there is large gallstone with acoustic shadow *(S).* **C,** Oblique scan displaying dilated common bile duct *(B)* and short segment of flattened portal vein *(P).* **D,** Transverse scan of bile duct also showing flattened portal vein and transverse section of hepatic artery *(H)* close to anterior wall of common bile duct. Choledochal stone is not displayed.

When there are only a few or small stones, these are easily displayed, thanks to the sharp contrast between the stones and surrounding bile (Figs. 26-16 to 26-20). Acoustic shadows (Fig. 26-16, *A*) are much rarer than in gallbladder lithiasis and not so sharply marked.

Diagnosis is much more difficult when the bile duct is completely filled with stones, since the contrast between bile and stones has then disappeared (Fig. 26-18, *A*). An acoustic shadow and the presence of a frankly dilated hepatic duct, even though the common bile duct is not visualized, are then valuable signs. A hilar gun sign and dilatation of the intrahepatic network may be the only positive findings, since in a case of lithiasis with chronic infection the gallbladder is usually not dilated (Figs. 26-18, *B,* and 26-19, *C*). Chronic angiocholitis sometimes brings about diffuse tubular stenosis, leading to false-negative diagnoses. This point will be discussed farther on.

A choledochal parasitosis (distomiasis) will, of course, be confused with lithiasis until high-resolution real-time imaging enables one to see the little animal moving—if it moves.

Text continued on p. 426.

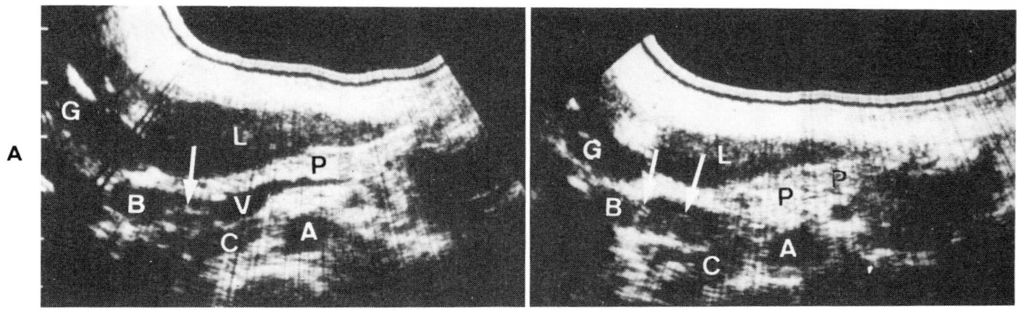

Fig. 26-16. Lithiasis of common bile duct. **A,** Transverse scan of upper abdomen showing reflective area *(arrow)* of stones in enlarged bile duct *(B)*. There is posterior acoustic shadow. *G,* gallbladder; *L,* liver; *V,* splenoportal junction; *P,* pancreas; *C,* vena cava; *A,* aorta. **B,** Oblique scan. Here, bile duct is cut along its sagittal axis. Stones are marked by *arrows.*

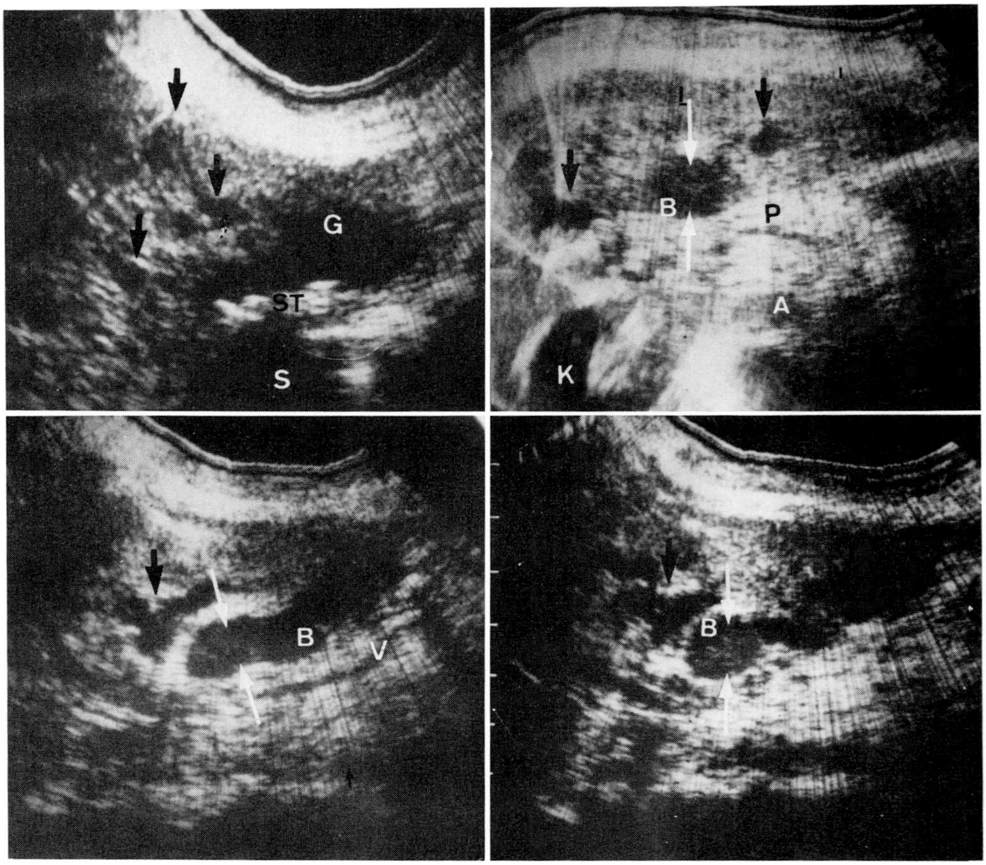

Fig. 26-17. Obstructive jaundice due to common bile duct lithiasis. **A,** Sagittal scan of right upper quadrant showing layer of stones *(ST)* with posterior acoustic shadow *(S)* in lowest part of gallbladder *(G)*. *Black arrows* mark dilated intrahepatic bile ducts. **B,** Transverse scan displaying enlarged hepatic duct *(B),* in which stones are marked by *white arrows. L,* liver; *P,* pancreas; *A,* aorta; *K,* right kidney. **C,** Oblique scan cutting common bile duct *(B),* which is filled with stones *(white arrows),* along its sagittal axis. *V,* portal vein. **D,** Parallel, 1 cm more caudal scan also showing choledochal stones.

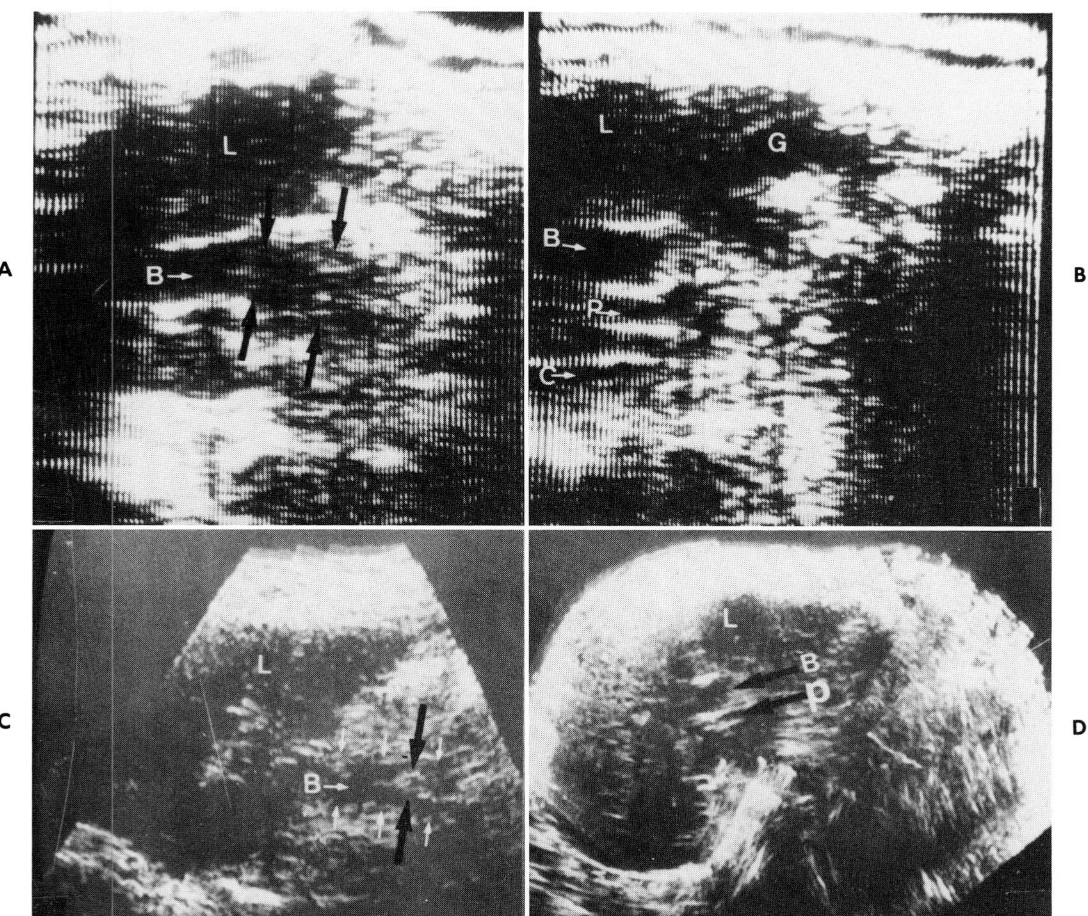

Fig. 26-18. Bile duct filled with stones. **A,** Sagittal scan of right upper quadrant in real time displaying enlarged bile duct *(B)* behind liver *(L)*. Its lower part is occupied by scattered, rather intense echoes *(arrows)*. At level of stones, posterior wall image of biliary duct is poorly delineated because of acoustic shadows. **B,** Parallel, more lateral scan passing through small biloculate gallbladder *(G)* shows, from front to back, liver, enlarged bile duct, portal vein *(P)*, and vena cava *(C)*. Images of bile duct and portal vein give rise to gun sign. Echo-free area between vena cava and portal vein must not be confused with tubular structure. **C,** Sagittal contact scan of right upper quadrant showing main bile duct *(small white arrows)* behind liver. Stones *(black arrows)* are displayed in distal segment of bile duct. **D,** Gun sign in hilar region. Transverse scan shows three parallel lines of wall images belonging to hilar biliary junction *(B)* and portal division *(P)*. As in **B,** biliary dilatation has reversed usual proportion of biliary duct to portal system.

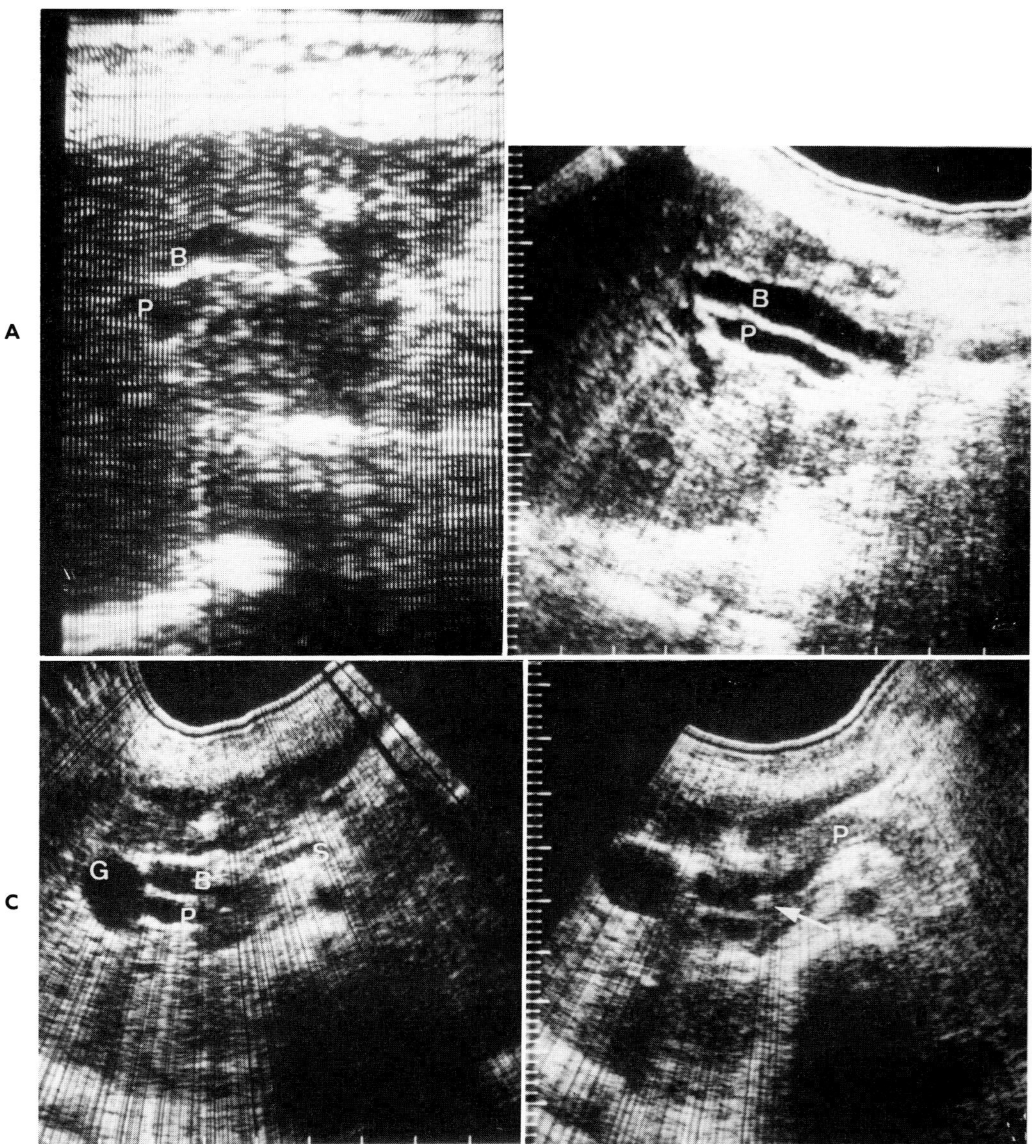

Fig. 26-19. Choledocholithiasis. **A,** Oblique recurrent real-time scan showing dilated biliary junction *(B)* in front of portal division *(P)*. **B,** Oblique scan of right upper quadrant showing twin sagittal sections of dilated bile duct and portal vein. **C,** Here, twin sections appear, on transverse scan, proximal to poorly dilated gallbladder *(G)*. *S,* splenic artery and vein. **D,** More caudal parallel scan displaying normal pancreas *(P)*. Obstacle was choledochal stone *(arrow)*.

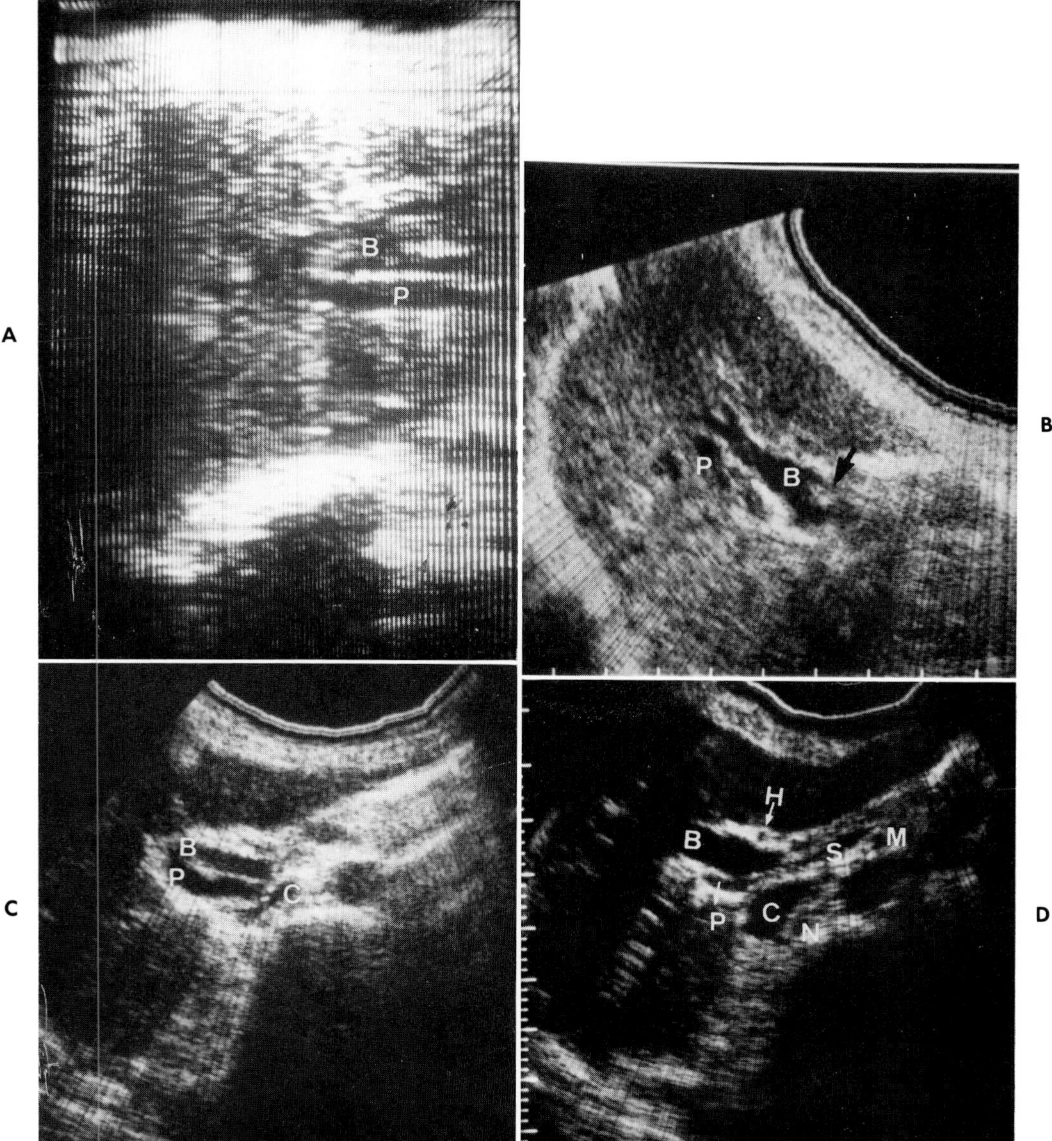

Fig. 26-20. Obstructive jaundice—gun sign at different levels. **A,** Oblique recurrent subcostal scan of liver showing dilated biliary network *(B)* in front of portal division *(P).* **B,** Oblique scan of right upper quadrant displaying sagittal section of dilated bile duct *(B).* Short segment of portal vein *(P)* has also been cut. **C,** Two tubular elements are better displayed on this oblique scan. *C,* vena cava. **D,** Transverse scan also showing dilated common bile duct in front of flattened portal vein. Transverse section of hepatic artery *(H)* is seen just in front of anterior wall of common bile duct. *N,* lymph node; *S,* splenic vein; *M,* SMA. Jaundice was due to choledochal stones, one of which is displayed in **B** *(arrow).*

Pancreatic origin

Inflammatory enlargement of the pancreas can bring about compression of the biliary tree and jaundice (Fig. 26-21). Compression and dilatation are transitory in cases of subacute recurrence. Lithiasis is often associated.

Of course, in most cases it is *tumors* of the pancreas that produce jaundice (Figs. 26-22 to 26-26). As pointed out in Chapter 23, tumors adjacent to the common bile duct are often small at the time they produce tubular obstruction. Their ultrasonic display is nevertheless possible, since their volume is sufficient to enlarge the contour of the head and produce a recognizable tumor image (Figs. 26-23 to 26-25, as well as Fig. 23-4). Adapted scans are often able to outline the tumoral mass and its relation to the dilated bile duct (Figs. 26-23, *C* and *D,* 26-24, *B,* and 26-25, *B*). Obstructions of pancreatic origin give rise to the most typical global dilatations of the biliary tree. They are therefore the easiest to recognize. As already stated in Chapter 23, the echopattern of ampulloma and intrapancreatic cholangiocarcinoma is no different from that of pancreatic carcinoma.

Compression above the pancreas

Lymph nodes can compress the main biliary duct above the pancreas (Fig. 26-27). In such cases, dilatation occurs only in the superior part of the biliary tree. Such masses are easily displayed, but their differentiation from a pancreatic mass may be difficult.

Text continued on p. 433.

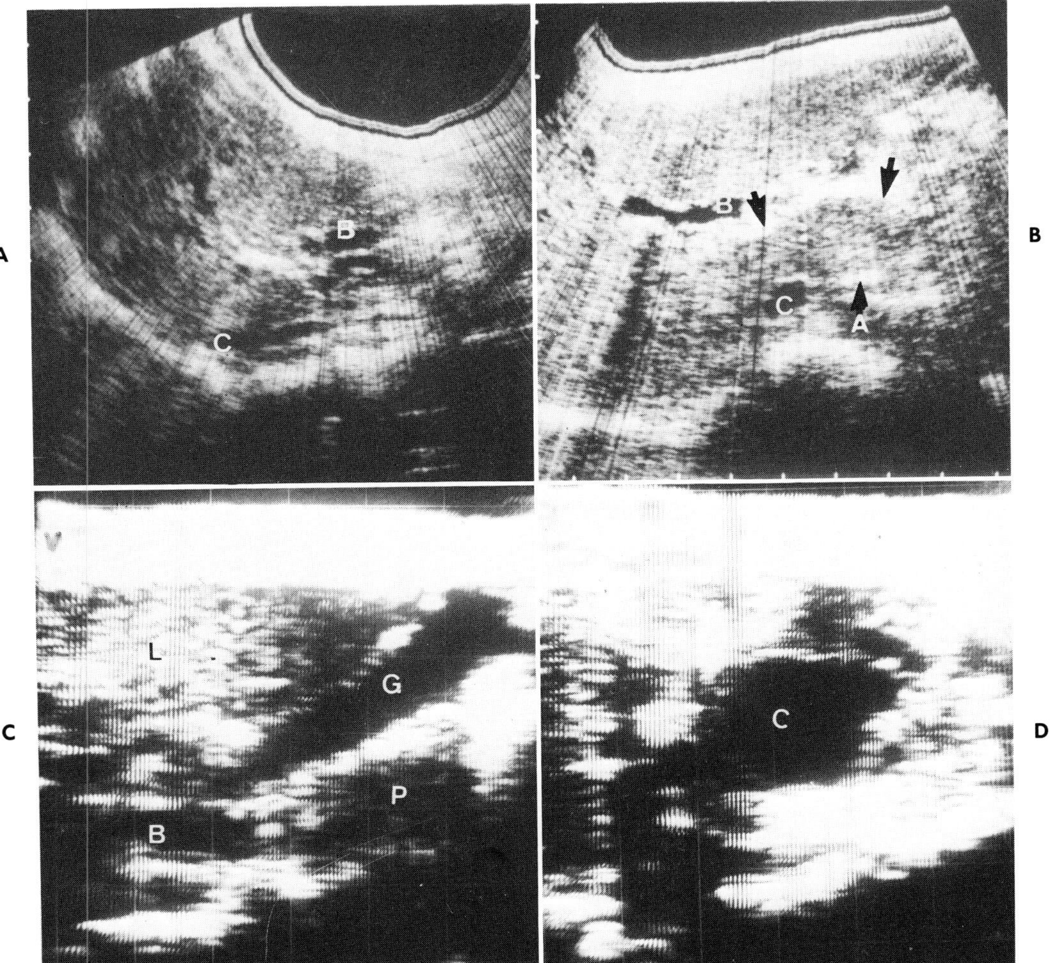

Fig. 26-21. Two examples of jaundice due to chronic pancreatitis. **A,** Sagittal scan of right upper quadrant showing infrahilar gun sign. *B,* bile duct; *C,* vena cava. **B,** Transverse scan showing enlarged, reflective body of pancreas *(arrows)* with micronodulation. At surgery, subacute recurrence superimposed on chronic pancreatitis was found. *A,* aorta. **C,** Sagittal real-time scan of another patient showing enlarged, sonolucent head of pancreas *(P).* Bile duct is dilated, but not gallbladder *(G). L,* liver. **D,** Parallel, more internal cut showing liquid collection *(C)* representing pseudocyst. In this case also, subacute recurrence has developed on chronic pancreatitis.

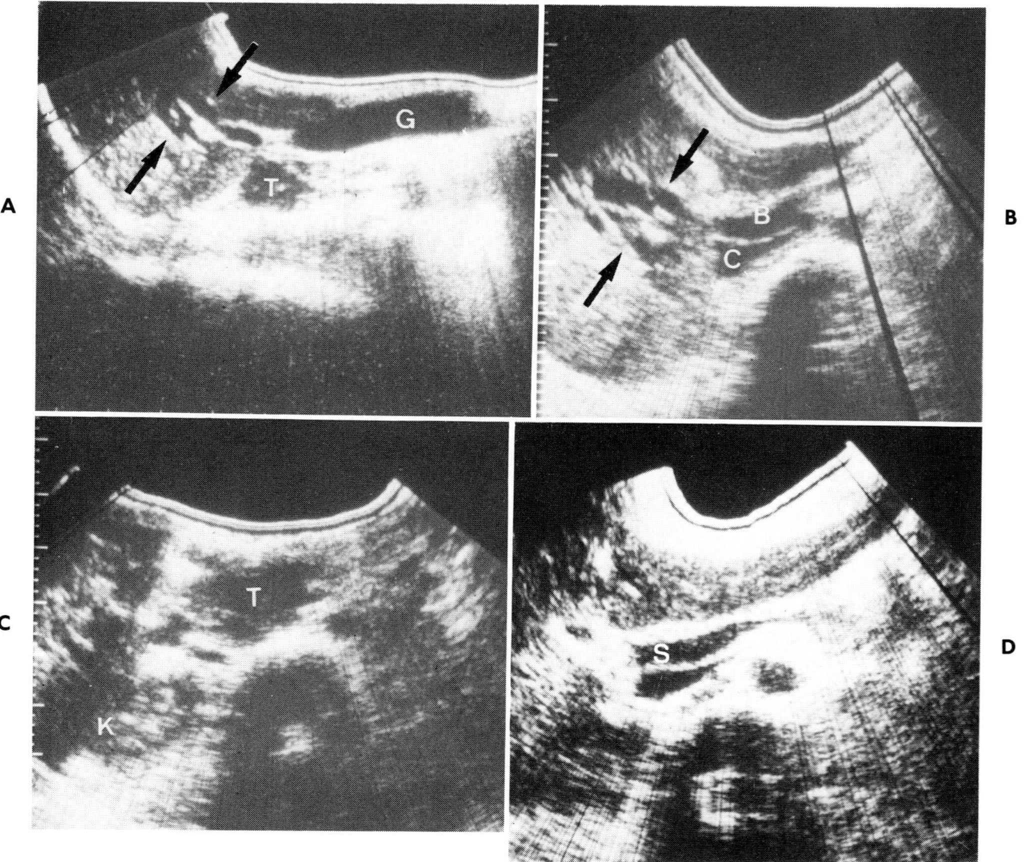

Fig. 26-22. Obstructive jaundice due to pancreatic tumor. **A,** Sagittal scan showing enlarged gallbladder *(G)* and dilated intrahepatic bile ducts *(arrows)*. Section deals with lateral extension of tumor *(T)*. **B,** Transverse scan again displaying dilated intrahepatic biliary network. Enlarged bile duct *(B)* is outlined in front of vena cava *(C)* and origin of left renal vein. Under normal conditions (as in **D**), tubular element outlined in front of origin of left renal vein is splenoportal junction. **C,** More caudal parallel scan passing through pancreatic tumor. *K,* right kidney. **D,** Sagittal scan showing usual pattern of splenoportal junction *(S)*, in front of vena cava in normal patient.

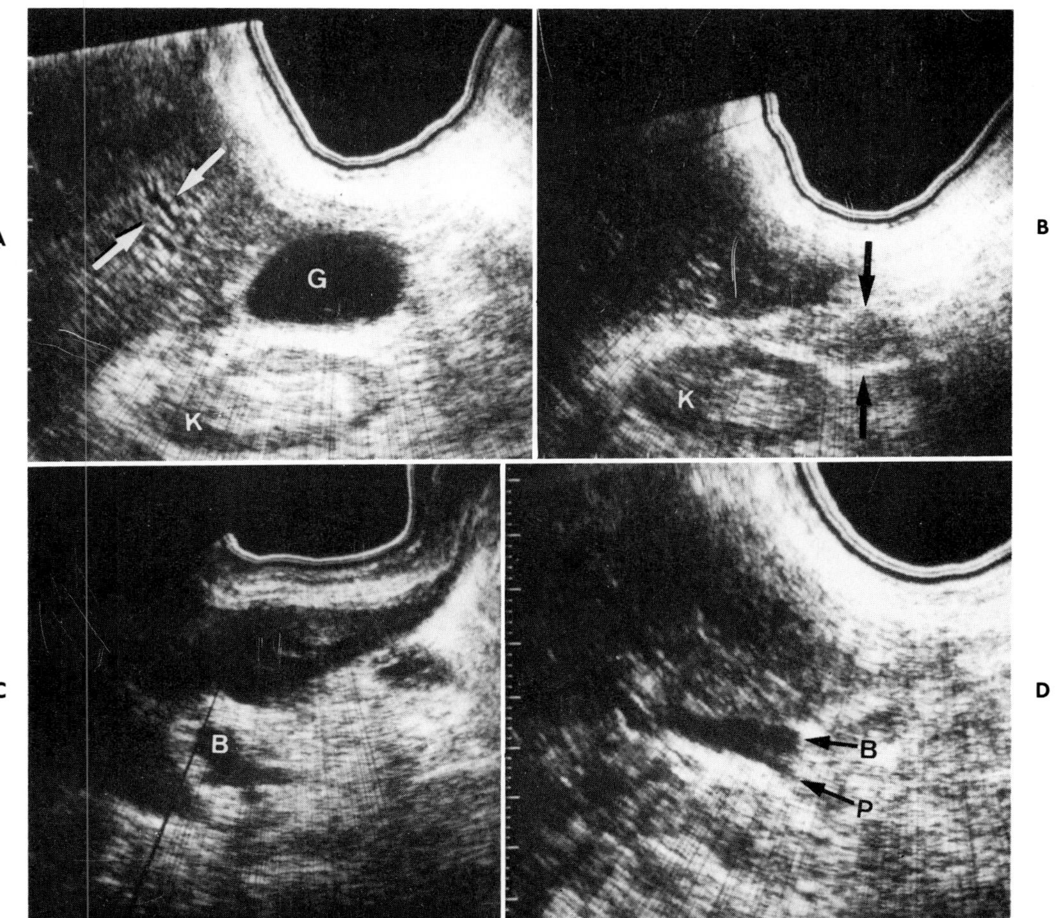

Fig. 26-23. Obstructive jaundice of pancreatic origin. **A,** Sagittal scan showing dilated gallbladder *(G)* and dilated intrahepatic bile ducts *(arrows). K,* kidney. **B,** Parallel, more internal scan passing through lateral extension of pancreatic head tumor *(arrows).* **C,** Oblique scan of right upper quadrant displaying dilated biliary duct *(B)* in hilar area. **D,** Another oblique scan showing dilated "main" bile duct *(B)* in front of flattened portal vein *(P).*

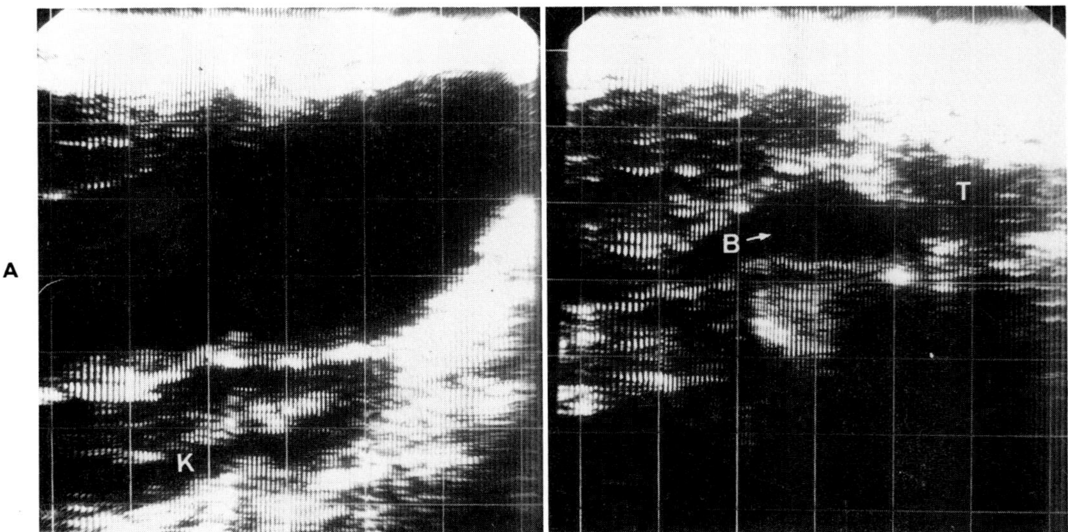

Fig. 26-24. Obstructive jaundice of pancreatic origin. **A,** Sagittal scan of gallbladder with giant dilatation. Gallbladder is so enlarged that it has flattened right kidney *(K).* **B,** Sagittal scan of enlarged bile duct *(B).* Its course is interrupted by small pancreatic tumor *(T).*

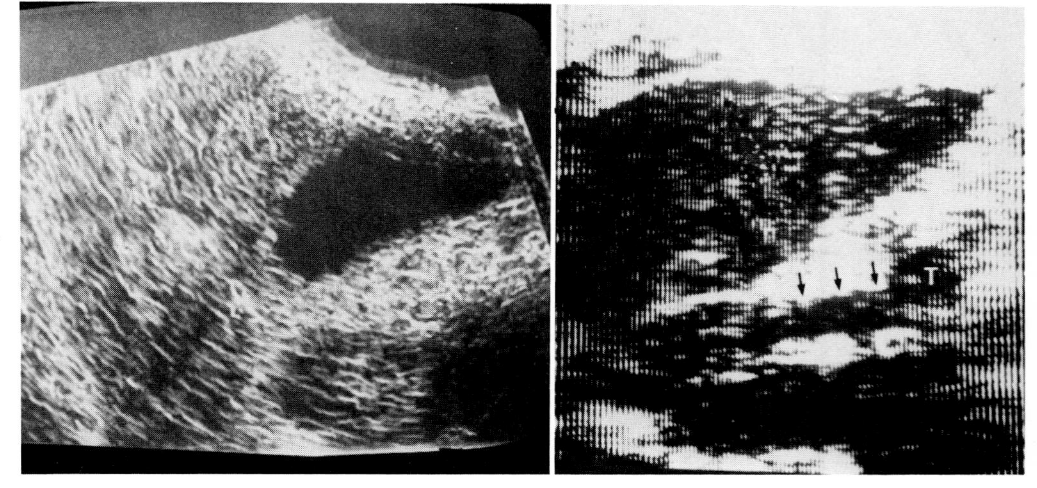

Fig. 26-25. Obstructive jaundice of pancreatic origin. **A,** Sagittal scan of enlarged gallbladder. **B,** Sagittal scan of common bile duct *(arrows).* In this case, as in that illustrated in Fig. 26-24, course of common bile duct is interrupted by small tumoral nodule *(T).*

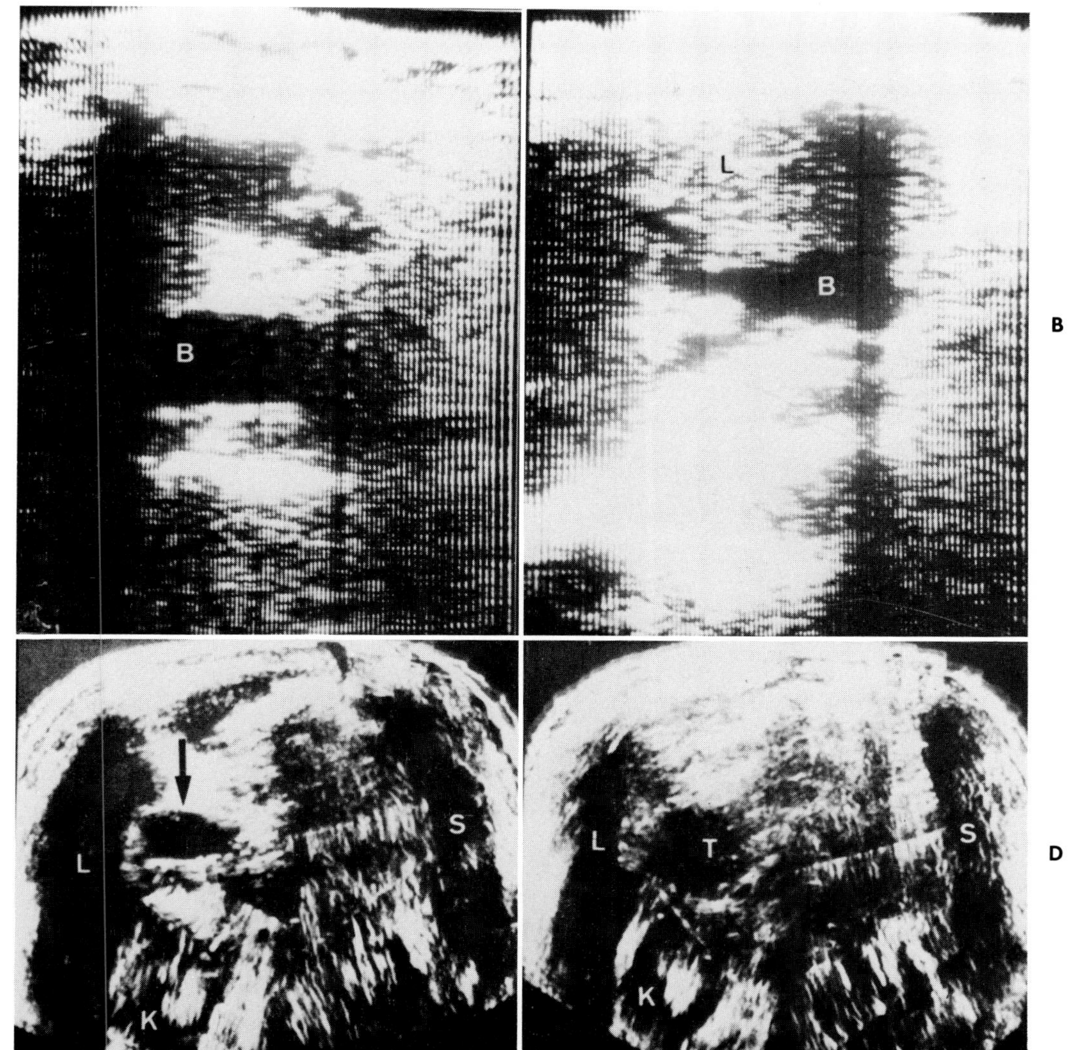

Fig. 26-26. Obstructive jaundice of pancreatic origin. **A,** Sagittal scan of right upper quadrant displaying enlarged bile duct *(B).* **B,** Oblique subcostal recurrent liver scan displaying dilated hilar biliary junction and several biliary branches. *L,* liver. **C,** Transverse scan displaying horizontal section of enlarged bile duct *(arrow)* in front of right kidney *(K). S,* spleen. **D,** Parallel, more caudal scan displaying rounded sonolucent section of tumor of pancreatic head *(T)* in close contact with liver and kidney.

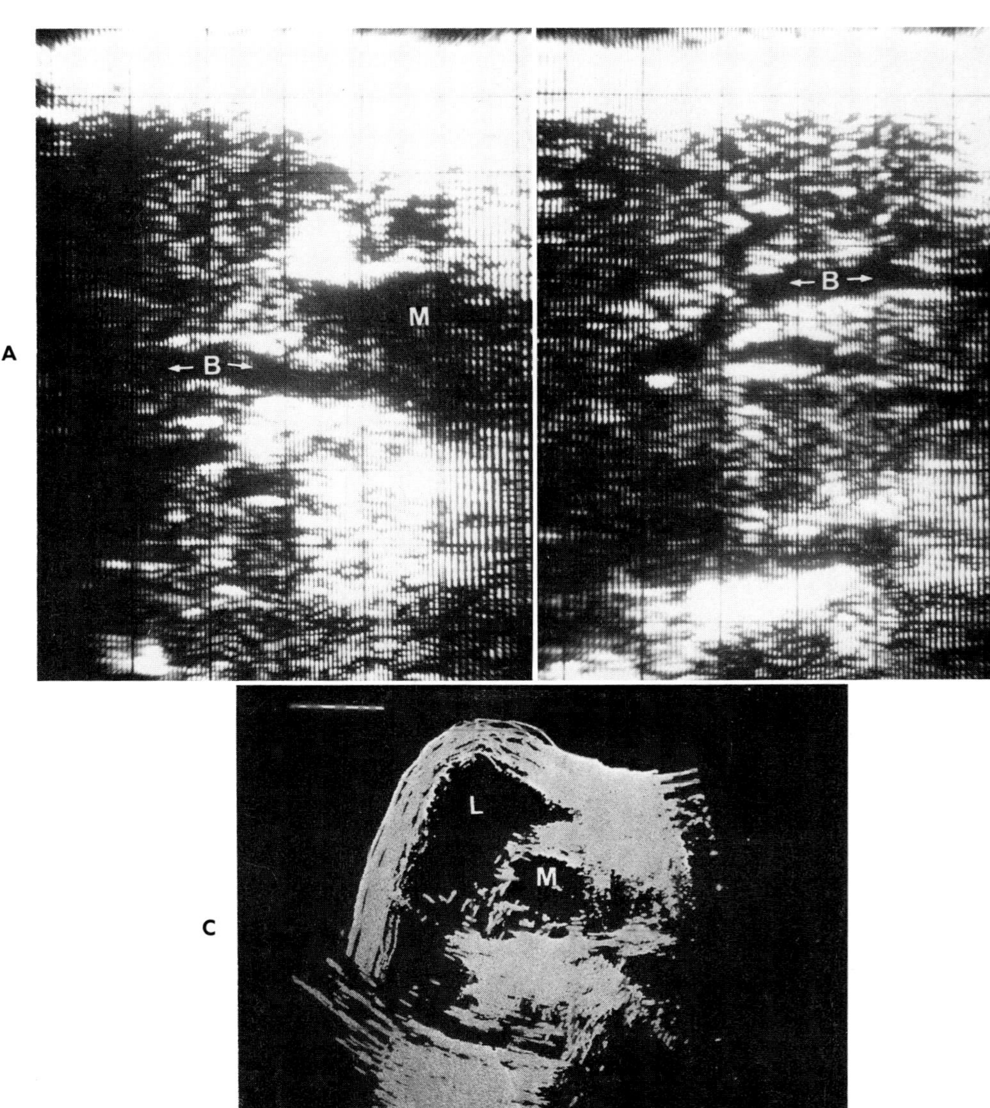

Fig. 26-27. Obstructive jaundice. **A,** Sagittal scan of right upper quadrant showing dilated bile duct *(B),* which is interrupted at rather high level by sonolucent mass *(M).* **B,** Oblique subcostal recurrent scan of liver displaying significant dilatation of biliary network *(B).* **C,** Horizontal scan of upper abdomen displaying mass already disclosed in **A** behind liver *(L).* This mass was metastatic lymph node, secondary to bladder carcinoma.

Obstruction at the level of the hilus

The ultrasonic signs of tumors of the gallbladder and hilus have already been discussed (Chapter 17). These tumors give rise to infrahepatic masses, including stones, characterized by their proper reflections and acoustic shadows. Images of polyps within the gallbladder may also be displayed. Finally, an evident sign is dilatation of the intrahepatic bile ducts (Fig. 26-28).

Postoperative jaundice

After surgery for biliary obstruction, biliary dilatation should decrease within a week. Its persistence indicates accidental bile duct ligature. With luck, it is then possible to display the level of ligature (Fig. 26-29). In other cases the absence of common bile duct dilatation even though the hilar and intrahepatic bile ducts are dilated indicates infrahilar stenosis (Fig. 26-30).

Congenital anomalies

Congenital stenosis or aplasia in infants brings about the same ultrasonic patterns as does surgical infrahilar ligation. The pattern of choledochal cysts has been discussed in Chapter 17.

Intrahepatic cholestasis

The ultrasonic symptomatology of cirrhosis of the liver has already been discussed (Chapter 10), as has that of hepatic metastases (Chapter 8), and hepatic primary tumors (Chapter 9). Intrahepatic cholestasis may also occur in parasitoses (Chapter 11).

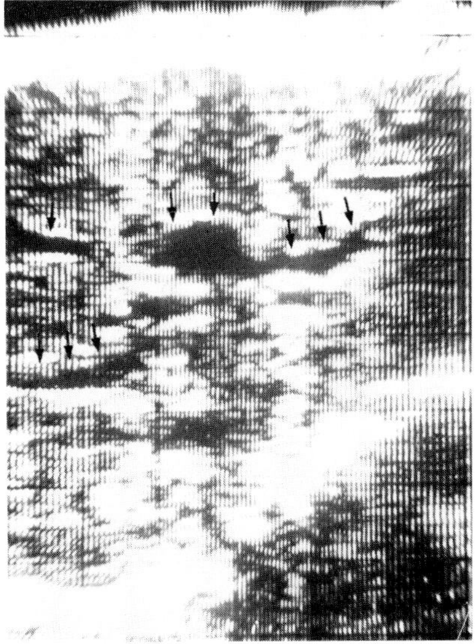

Fig. 26-28. Typical image of dilatation of intrahepatic biliary network *(arrows)*. If such image is solitary, without associated dilatation in another part of biliary tree, obstruction must be proximal. In this case, it was hilar extension from gallbladder tumor.

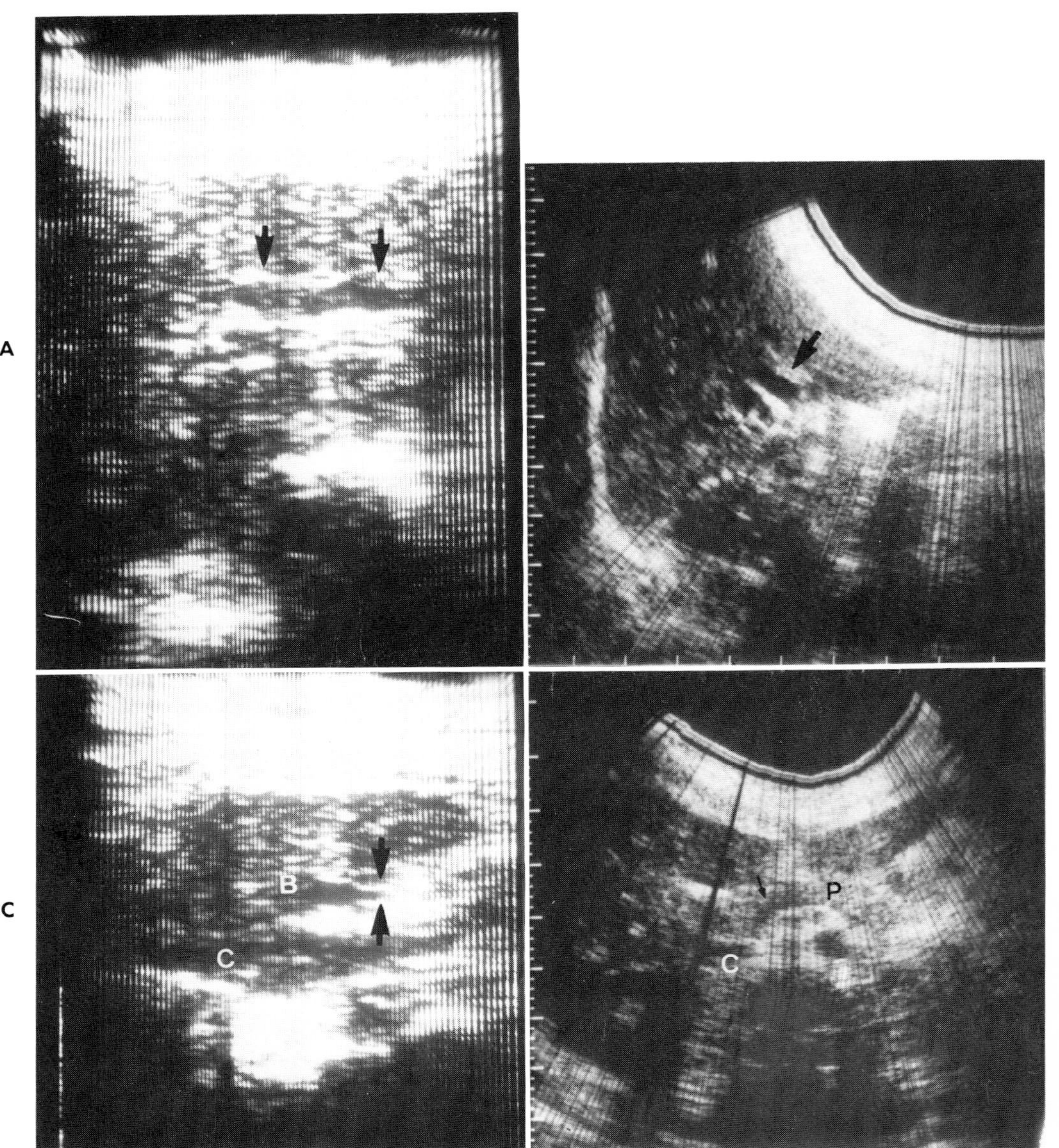

Fig. 26-29. Postoperative jaundice. Examination was carried out 8 days after operation for cholelithiasis. **A,** Oblique recurrent liver scan showing dilatation of intrahepatic bile ducts *(arrows).* **B,** Sagittal scan displaying hilar gun sign *(arrow).* **C,** Another sagittal scan showing narrowing and stop *(arrows)* of bile duct *(B). C,* vena cava. **D,** Transverse scan displaying no dilatation of juxtapancreatic bile duct. *P,* pancreas; *arrow,* splenoportal junction. Second operation showed accidental ligation of common hepatic duct.

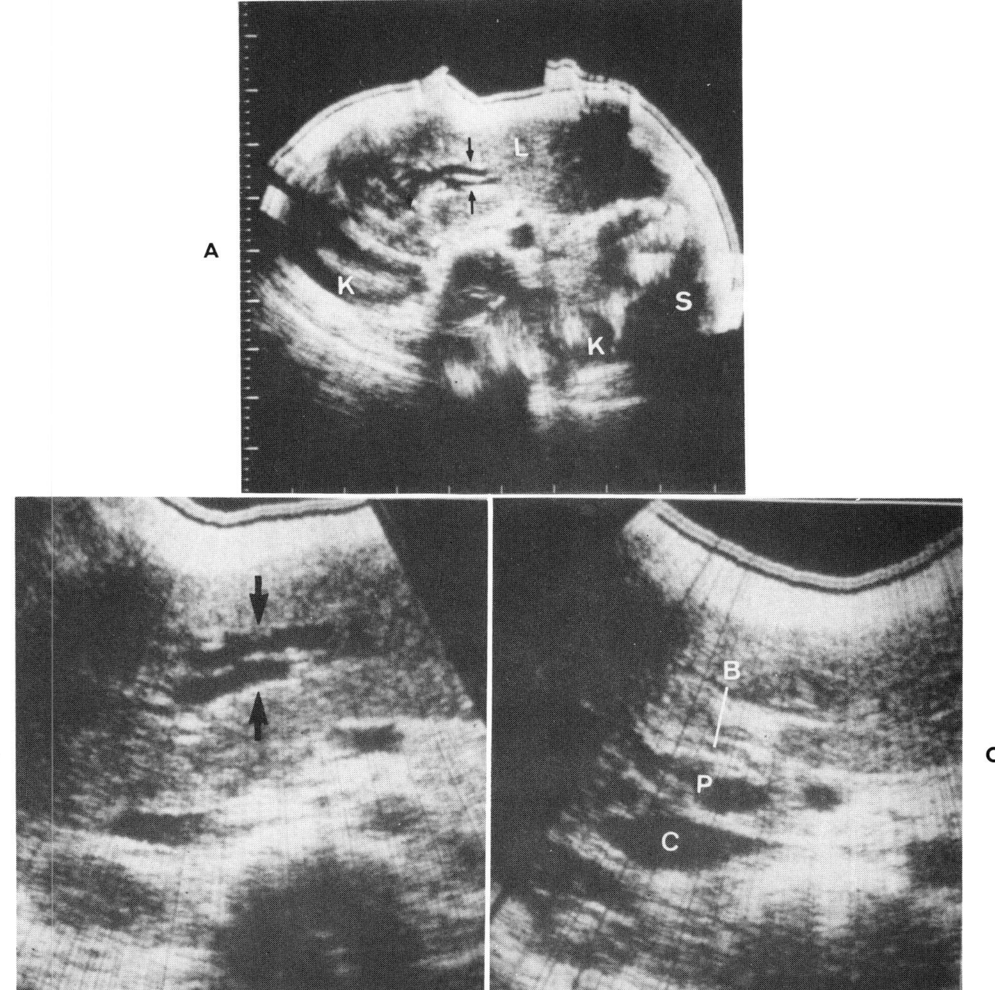

Fig. 26-30. Postoperative jaundice. Patient underwent right hepatectomy because of multilocular echinococcosis. Few months later, transient jaundice with fever appeared. **A,** Transverse scan of remaining hypertrophic left lobe of liver *(L)* showing typical gun sign *(arrows)*. *K,* kidneys; *S,* spleen. **B,** Gun sign *(arrows)* also displayed on more cranial scan. **C,** Oblique scan of right upper quadrant showing, from back to front, vena cava *(C),* portal vein *(P),* and undilated bile duct *(B)*. Stenosis is necessarily infrahilar. This was confirmed by percutaneous cholangiography. Surgery showed hilar stenosis, which was due, not to previous operation, but to parasitic involvement.

Hepatitis

Jaundice due to hepatitis is an exclusion diagnosis, since no dilatation of the biliary network exists. The normal appearance of the biliary tree must be verified by examinations at intervals of a few days. A large gallbladder may be found, but it empties normally. A preexisting large main bile duct, due to chronic necrotizing papillitis, may be found in nonobstructive jaundice, but, in such cases, hepatic scans usually do not display a corresponding dilatation of intrahepatic bile ducts. There is often an associated nonspecific hepatomegaly and occasionally transient pancreatic swelling (Chapter 7).

• • •

These different types of jaundice can be analyzed in a logical fashion. The lower the obstruction, the clearer the dilatation with the exception of some stone-filled common bile ducts, in which the infrahepatic manifestations are difficult to show. The most important sign remains dilatation of the intrahepatic network, which permits one to affirm the obstructive nature of the jaundice and to decide to perfom surgery. From a practical point of view this, of course, is the crucial decision.

RELIABILITY OF ULTRASONOGRAPHY—DIAGNOSTIC POLICY

We studied a group of 240 patients with jaundice (30 nonobstructive and 210 obstructive cases, examined in our department from March 1, 1969, to March 1, 1977). The overall rate of success of differential diagnosis of obstructive and nonobstructive jaundice was 85%. There were two false-positive diagnoses of nonobstructive jaundice (with, in fact, a dilated biliary tree without obstruction). The false-negative diagnoses of obstructive jaundice mainly involved choledochal lithiasis, with diffuse biliary stenosis in eight cases. This study was actually very heterogeneous, since techniques and imaging were vastly improved in those eight years, along with knowledge of abnormal signs. In the thirty-two cases of obstructive jaundice that we examined from March 1 to November 1, 1977, combining real-time and last-generation contact scanning, we made only one false-negative diagnosis, also owing to diffuse narrowing in a case of lithiasis. With the latter exception, we were able to diagnose seven cases of choledochal lithiasis correctly.

Anyway, I must again emphasize the importance of correlative studies, such as radiology of the abdomen, GI series, and hypotonic duodenography. Scintigraphy with newer radionuclide pharmaceuticals can be valuable in the analysis of jaundice. Computerized axial tomography may be useful rarely in the evaluation of a retroperitoneal mass, in case ultrasonography fails. We are far from convinced of the utility of the images of intrahepatic bile duct dilatation provided by computerized axial tomography. In our opinion, since one can display a gun sign in the infrahepatic, as well as the hilar, area, the direct display of a dilated intrahepatic biliary network confers on ultrasonography a much greater value. When positive, a correct ultrasonographic examination is sufficient to decide for surgery. In our opinion, it is only in the event of finding a discrepancy between clinical data, laboratory results, and ultrasonic images that instrumental cholangiography is to be considered. In these cases, we advocate "skinny" needle percutaneous cholangiography, rather than endoscopic retrograde cholangiography. Our equipment for transjugular cholangiography is slowly rusting in its box. By and large, with present imaging, instrumental cholangiography is necessary in less than 5% of cases, and this rate should decrease, since its indications are only sclerosing cholangitis, congenital hepatic fibrosis, or very proximal postoperative stenoses. As for angiography, this has no interest save for a few rare hepatic lesions, especially parasitoses, such as multilocular echinococcosis; but it may be useful as a preoperative step to display the vascular anatomy. In obstructive jaundice, surgery is always the method of treatment, even if only as a palliative. Angiography as an attempt to evaluate the feasibility of operating is therefore not justified. As a matter of fact, our surgical colleagues are now used to operating on the basis of our ultrasonic diagnosis.

REFERENCES

Barnett, E., and Morley, P.: Abdominal echography, Borough Green, England, 1974, Butterworth & Co. (Publishers), Ltd.

Cosgrove, D. O., and Dunn, F.: Ultrasonic differentiation between blood and bile vessels in the liver, World Federation of Ultrasound in Medicine and Biology, San Francisco, 1976, Abstract No. 551.

Goldberg, B. B.: Ultrasonic cholangiography gray scale B-scan evaluation of the common bile duct, Radiology **118:**400-404, 1976.

Hassani, N.: Ultrasonography of the abdomen, Heidelberg, Germany, 1976, Springer-Verlag.

Holm, H. H., Kristensen, J. K., Rasmussen, S. N., Pedersen, J. F., and Hancke, S.: Abdominal ultrasound, Copenhagen, 1976, Munksgaard, International Booksellers & Publishers, Ltd.

Leopold, G. R., and Asher, W. M.: Fundamentals of abdominal and pelvic ultrasonography, Philadelphia, 1975, W. B. Saunders Co.

Perlmutter, G. S., and Goldberg, B. B.: Ultrasonic evaluation of the common bile duct, J. Clin. Ultrasound **4:**107-111, 1975.

Rettenmaier, G.: Personal communication, 1975.

Stone, L. B., Ferruci, J. T., Jr., Warshaw, A. L., Wittenberg, J., and Slutsky, M.: Gray scale ultrasound diagnosis of obstructive biliary disease, Am. J. Roentgenol. Radium Ther. Nucl. Med. **125:**47-50, 1975.

Taylor, K. J. W., Carpenter, D. A., and McCready, V. R.: Ultrasound and scintigraphy in the differential diagnosis of obstructive jaundice, J. Clin. Ultrasound **2:**105-115, 1974.

Weill, F., Becker, J. C., Kraehenbuhl, J. R., Heriot, G., and Walter, J. P.: Clinical atlas of ultrasonic radiography, Paris, 1973, Masson & Cie., Editeurs.

Weill, F., Bourgoin, A., Aucant, D., Eisenscher, A., Faivre, M., and Gillet, M.: L'exploration tomo-échographique des dilatations de la voie biliaire principale. Sa place dans le bilan radiologique d'un ictère, Arch. Fr. Mal. App. Dig. **63:**453-472, 1974.

Weill, F., Gisselbrecht, H., Ricatte, J. P., Kraehenbuhl, J. R., Schraub, S., and Becker, J. C.: Diagnostic tomo-échographique des dilatations vésiculaires, Arch. Fr. Mal. App. Dig. **60:** 49-54, 1971.

PART V

THE SPLEEN

CHAPTER 27

EXAMINATION TECHNIQUE–ECHOANATOMY

Two different situations must be considered: the examination of a nonpalpable spleen and the examination of patients with frank splenomegaly.

THE SPLEEN OF NORMAL SIZE

In children and infants, contact scanning is difficult to use. The infant is constantly moving and breathing. Although children are more cooperative, they are often ticklish. There are few procedures so amusing but also unproductive as to tickle the ribs of a little girl with a transducer. With real-time technique, it is possible to obtain satisfactory intercostal sections of the spleen with the patient in the right lateral decubitus position (Fig. 27-1, *A* to *C*). Rib shadows interfere with the completeness of splenic images (Fig. 27-1, *D*), but the multiplicity of cuts permits one to visualize and analyze the bulk of the splenic tissue. In adults, similar real-time techniques may be used to assess splenic texture, but we prefer contact scanning, particularly to delineate contours. It is easier to evaluate the volume of the spleen, as well as its anatomical relations with neighboring organs, in contact scans than on narrow real-time images. In contact scans of the spleen the patient is first examined supine. Transverse scans are made from the xiphoid process to the umbilicus, centimeter by centimeter (Fig. 27-2). The patient is then positioned in right lateral decubitus. Intercostal scans may then be used, but we prefer sagittal sections parallel to the axillary line (Fig. 27-3). With this technique the problem of acoustic shadowing of the ribs is minimized by compounding. Finally, transverse scans are performed also in the lateral position.

ENLARGED SPLEEN

In the case of an enlarged spleen the different scanning planes are similar, but the spleen extends below the costal margin, so that it is possible to place the RTH in contact with the spleen in a position quite similar to the oblique recurrent subcostal scan used for the hepatic examination (Fig. 27-4). Oblique recurrent splenic scans are invaluable for study of the splenic tissue echopattern, since multiple sections are then possible, without manual interference and acoustic shadowing. One is then able to show small textural abnormalities. Sagittal subcostal contact scans are also performed when the spleen is enlarged.

ECHOANATOMY

Shape and contours

With the very first transverse scans, a global appreciation of the size and shape of the spleen is possible (Figs. 27-5 to 27-10). The external convex aspect of the spleen blends with the thoracoabdominal wall. Its medial aspect is, of course, better defined and is usually somewhat concave or rectilinear. (See Figs. 27-5 to 27-8.)

Text continued on p. 446.

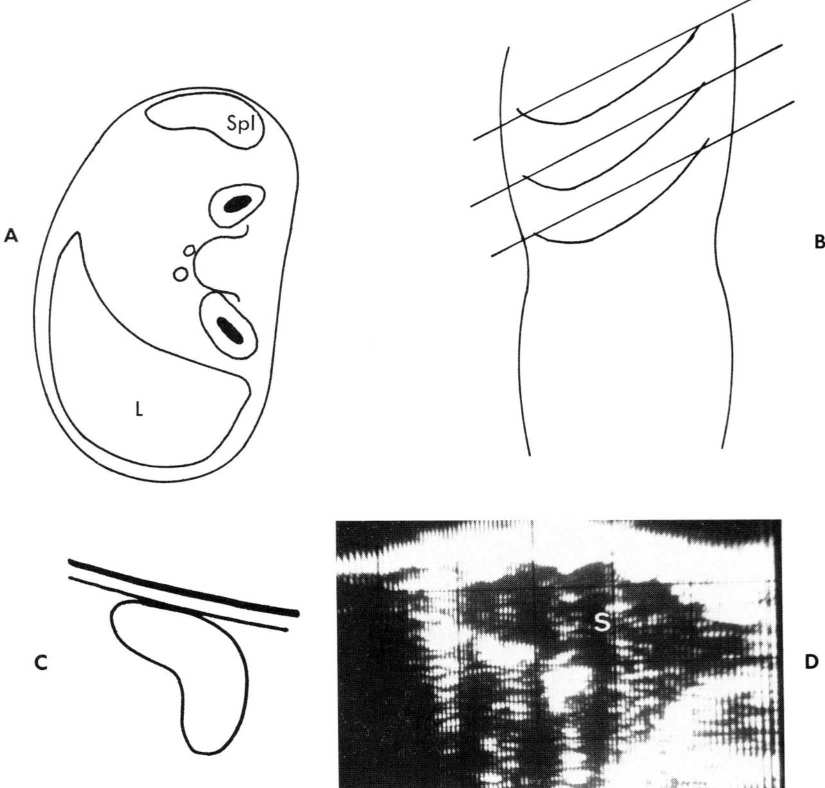

Fig. 27-1. A to **C,** Scanning planes and positions. **A,** Right lateral decubitus positioning. *L,* liver; *Spl,* spleen. **B,** Different scanning planes. **C,** Schematic intercostal section. **D,** Intercostal real-time scan of infant's spleen. Several acoustic shadows of lower ribs are displayed.

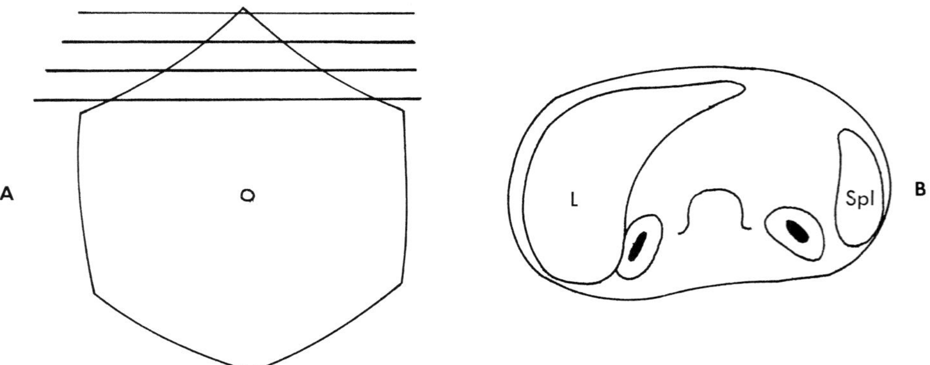

Fig. 27-2. Transverse contact scanning. **A,** Scanning planes. **B,** Schematic drawing of result.

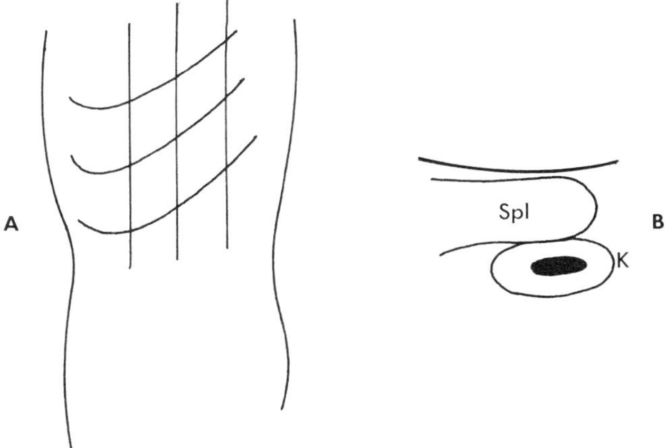

Fig. 27-3. Lateral sagittal axillary scanning. **A,** Scanning planes. **B,** Schematic drawing of result. *Spl,* spleen; *K,* kidney.

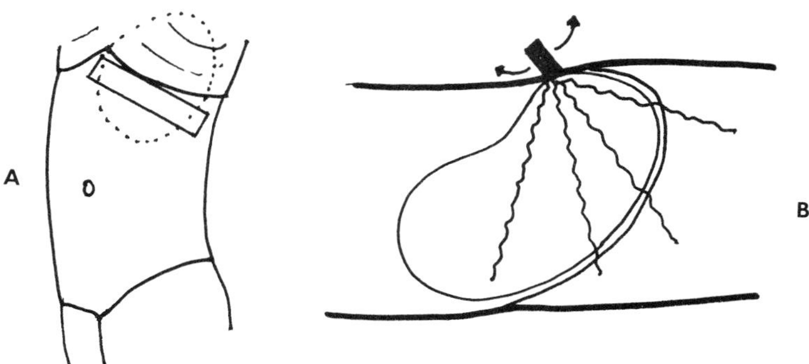

Fig. 27-4. Left subcostal oblique recurrent splenic real-time scanning in a case of splenomegaly. **A** and **B,** Positioning of real-time head.

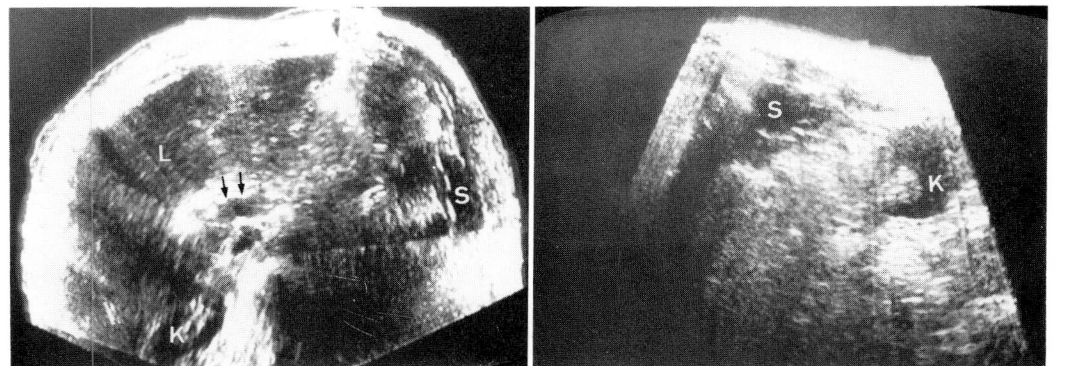

Fig. 27-5. Normal spleen. **A,** Transverse scan of upper abdomen displaying small spleen *(S)*. Splenic tissue is less reflective than liver tissue *(L)*. *Arrows,* portal vein; *K,* kidney. **B,** Sagittal lateral axillary scan in same patient. Spleen is displayed at short distance from left kidney.

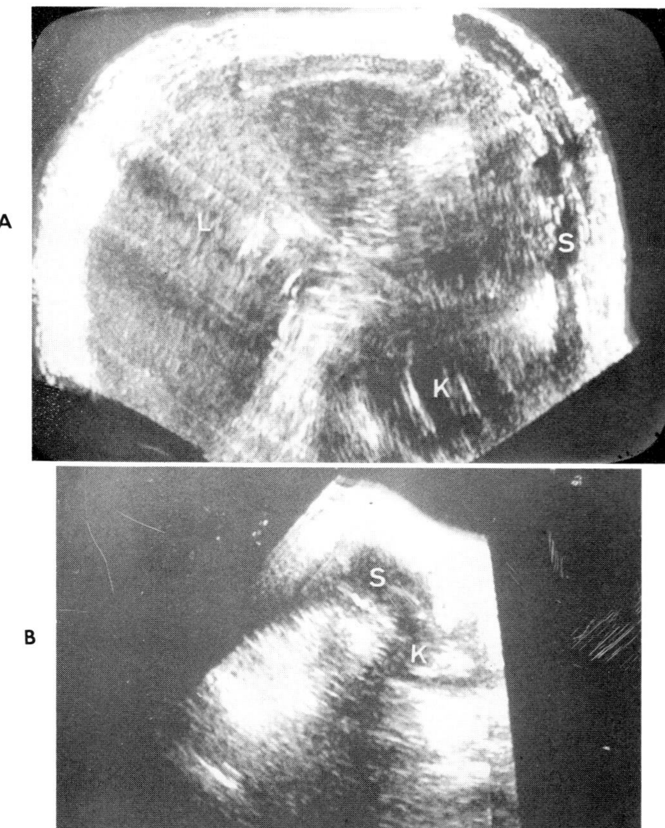

Fig. 27-6. Normal spleen. **A,** Transverse scan of upper abdomen in stout patient showing small spleen *(S)*. *K,* kidney. **B,** Lateral sagittal scan showing relation of spleen to left kidney.

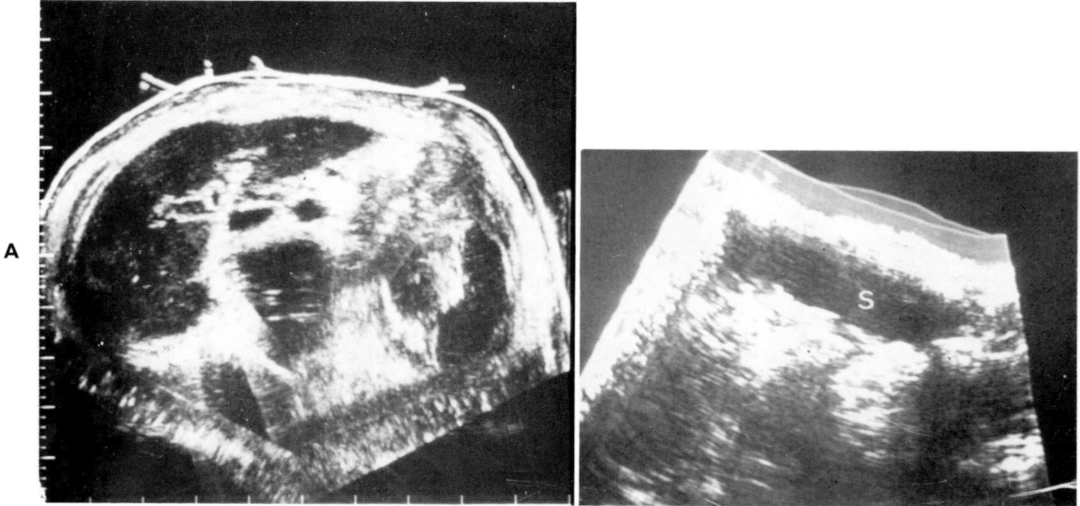

Fig. 27-7. Normal spleen. **A,** Transverse scan of upper abdomen showing larger spleen. Organ is well developed along anteroposterior axis. **B,** Lateral sagittal scan of spleen *(S)* showing normal craniocaudal length.

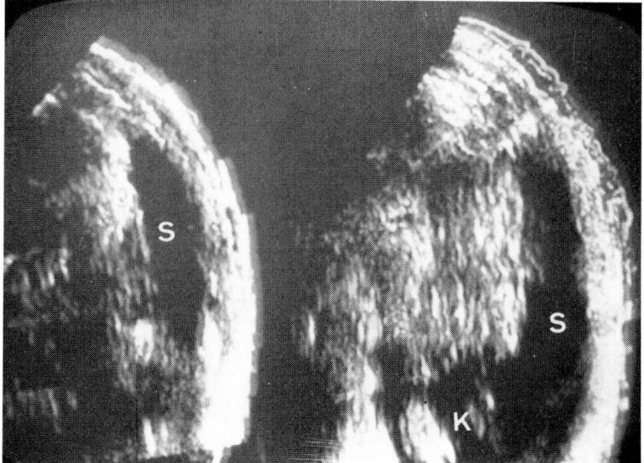

Fig. 27-8. Two parallel scans of left upper quadrant. Size of spleen *(S)* is at upper limit of normal. Relations of spleen and kidney *(K)* are demonstrated on lower scan (right). Internal aspect of spleen is rectilinear.

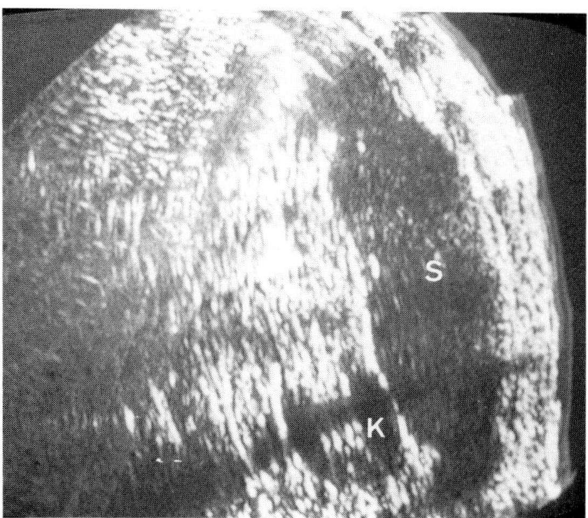

Fig. 27-9. Transverse section of slightly enlarged spleen *(S)*. Medial aspect of organ is slightly convex. It is in close contact with kidney *(K)*.

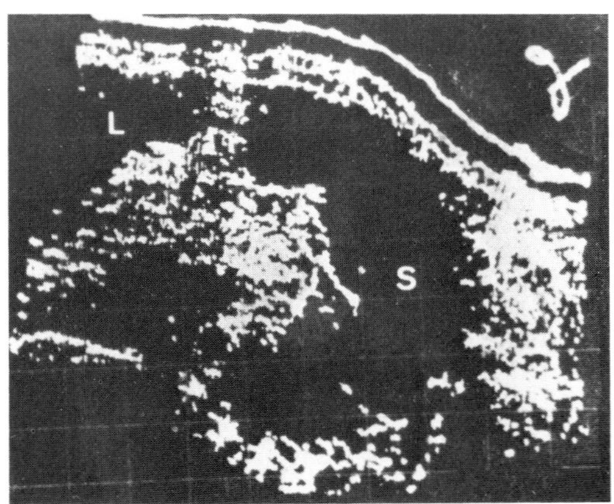

Fig. 27-10. Oblique subcostal recurrent section of enlarged spleen *(S)*. Medial aspect of spleen is undulated. *L,* liver.

Although the medial aspect may be minimally convex, it is never frankly convex. This is an important feature in the differentiation of some left upper quadrant tumors of large volume, such as those which will be seen in the next chapter. Frank concavity of the medial border of the spleen is not abnormal (Fig. 27-10). In sagittal axillary cuts performed with the patient in the right lateral decubitus position, the splenic section is ovoid. Unfortunately, the upper pole is not well seen, since the left lower lobe of the lung lies between the transducer and the spleen (Fig. 27-11). Therefore the upper limit of the spleen as it appears on ultrasonic sagittal sections is usually not the real upper limit of the organ. On the other hand, with an anterior approach, the interposition of colonic gas also compromises the display of the upper pole. The possibility that one has missed a lesion of the upper pole of the spleen because of physical inaccessibility must be kept in mind except for the very enlarged spleen, in which the entire organ is visible.

Echopattern

The splenic tissue echopattern is particularly sonolucent, sometimes almost of liquid type—in fact, it is the echopattern of the splenic blood. It is, however, always possible with sufficient gain or high frequency, to build a solid or at least semisolid tissue echopattern, which should be perfectly homogeneous (Figs. 27-7 to 27-9 and 27-12). Areas of abnormal reflectivity are always due to splenic lesions. Splenic reflectivity is always less in normal conditions than that of the liver. The hepatic image is saturated before the tissue echopattern of the spleen is displayed. (See Figs. 27-5 to 27-7.)

Anatomical relations

The spleen is usually located posteriorly enough to be adjacent to the left kidney, as shown by transverse scans (Figs. 27-7, *A,* 27-8, *B,* and 27-9) and by lateral sagittal scans (Figs. 27-5, *B,* 27-6, *B,* and 27-12). The relations between the lower pole of the spleen, the upper pole of the left kidney, and the tail of the

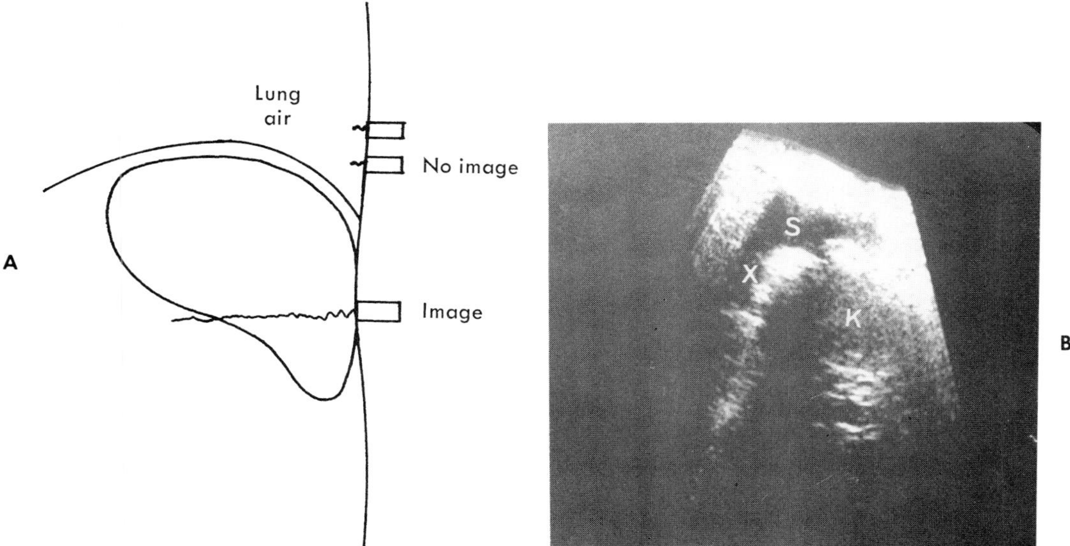

Fig. 27-11. Pulmonary air interposition in examination of upper pole of spleen. **A,** Schematic representation. **B,** Example of lateral sagittal scan. Upper pole of spleen *(S)* is masked by acoustic shadow *(X)*. *K,* kidney.

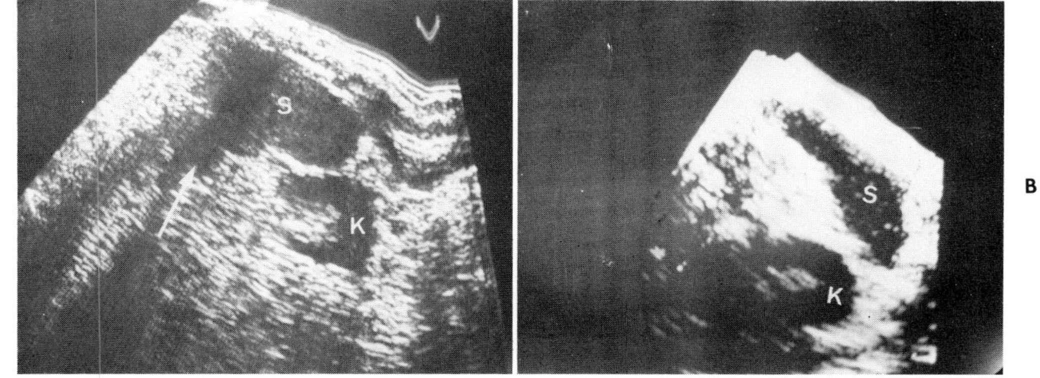

Fig. 27-12. Splenic upper pole. **A,** Another example of poor display of splenic upper pole, this time due to rib shadow *(arrow)*. On this lateral sagittal scan, note close contact of spleen *(S)* with left kidney *(K)*. **B,** Here, lateral sagittal scan seems to display quite completely upper pole of spleen. Actually, even such images as these are deceiving. There is always loss of at least 2 cm in display of upper pole. In this case, relation of spleen to kidney is less close.

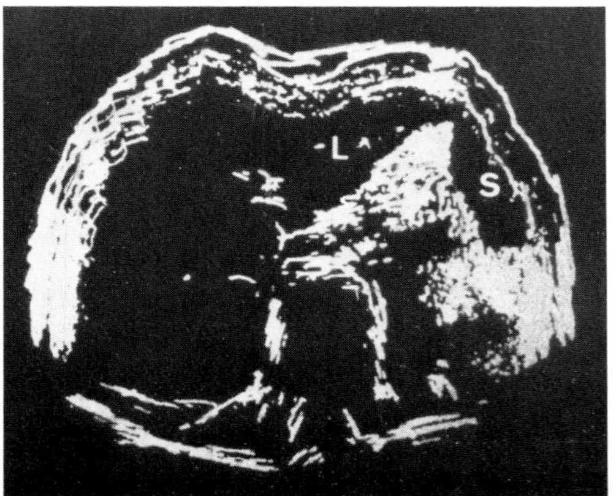

Fig. 27-13. Anteriorly located spleen *(S)*. Despite fact that splenic size is normal, anterior limit of organ is in close relation with margin of left hepatic lobe *(L)*.

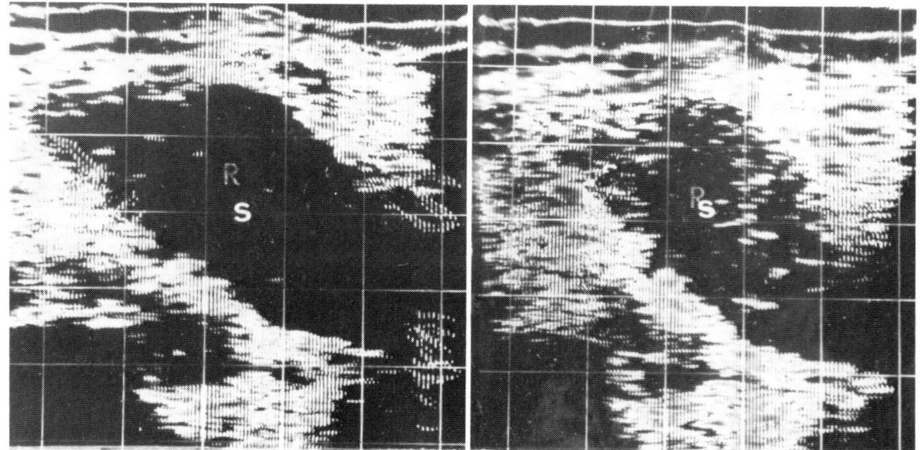

Fig. 27-14. Transverse real-time scan of epigastrium. Sonolucent mass corresponding to epigastric spleen *(S)* is displayed. (From Weill, F., Becker, J. C., Kraehenbuhl, J. R., Heriot, G., and Walter, J. P.: Clinical atlas of ultrasonic radiography, Paris, 1973, Masson & Cie., Editeurs.)

pancreas have already been discussed in Chapter 19 (Fig. 19-12, *A* and *B*). Rarely the spleen is located more anteriorly and is then in contact with the left lobe of the liver, rather than the left kidney (Fig. 27-13). Usually, direct contact between the left hepatic lobe and the spleen is observed only in the case of splenomegaly (or hepatomegaly). In a few patients with a hypoplastic left lobe of the liver, a mobile and anteriorly located spleen can be found in the epigastrium. The mobility of the mass, which is palpable, and the absence of a normal splenic image in the left upper quadrant enable one to identify such an epigastric spleen (Fig. 27-14) and to differentiate it from a pathological mass.

When there is ascites, transverse scans display a sonolucent band between the

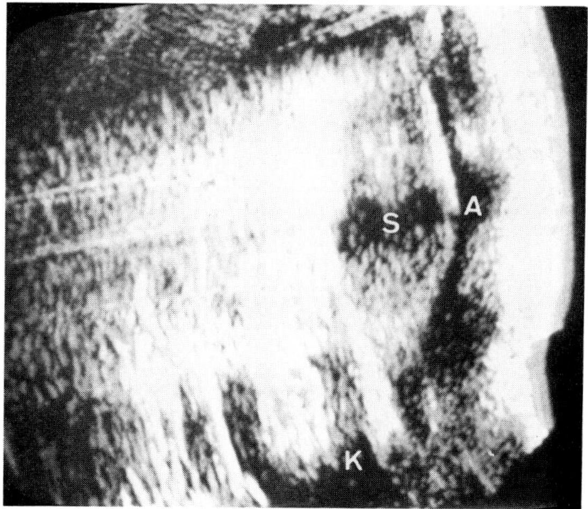

Fig. 27-15. Ascites. Transverse scan of left upper quadrant showing sonolucent band of ascites *(A)* between spleen *(S)* and abdominal wall. *K,* left kidney.

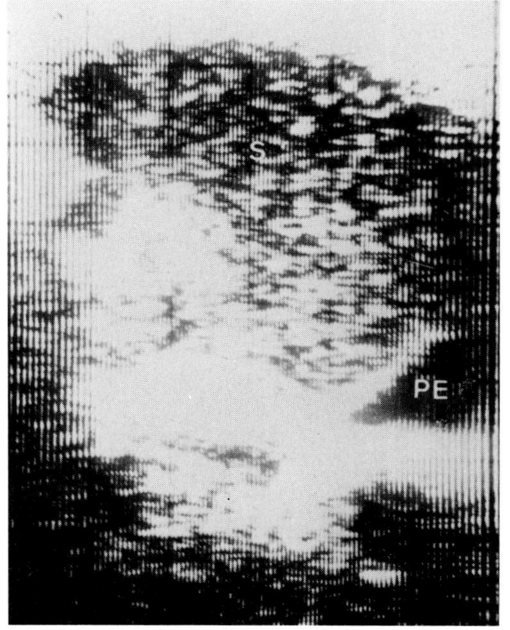

Fig. 27-16. Another abnormal juxtasplenic image. *PE,* pleural effusion; *S,* spleen.

spleen and the abdominal wall (Fig. 27-15). The thickness of this liquid band changes with the position of the patient. This is an important element in the differential diagnosis of a splenic hematoma. A left pleural effusion may also appear as a posterolateral sonolucent crescent (Fig. 27-16) or above the upper pole of the organ on sagittal axillary scans (Fig. 27-17).

Is the spleen normal? Is it enlarged? A few characteristics of the normal spleen

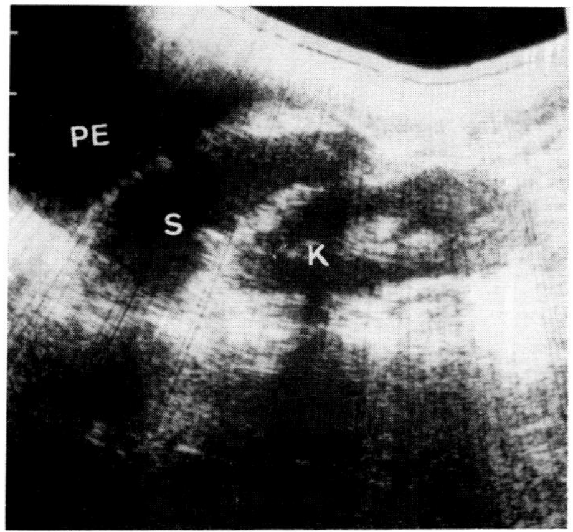

Fig. 27-17. Left pleural effusion *(PE)* displayed on sagittal lateral scan. Presence of liquid in pleural space enables one to better outline upper pole of spleen *(S)*. *K,* left kidney.

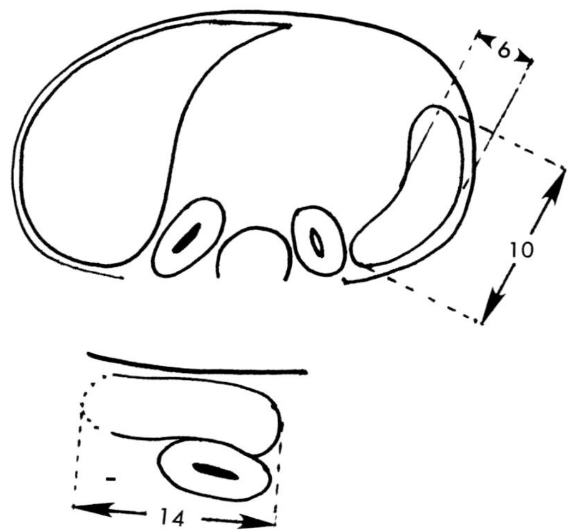

Fig. 27-18. Splenic size criteria.

have already been described. The first was the concave, rectilinear, or only slightly convex outline of the medial aspect of the spleen. The sonolucent, homogeneous echopattern of the spleen and its low refractivity are other normal features. There are also ultrasonic criteria for splenomegaly. A normal, nonmobile spleen does not clear the costal margin. In addition, the different organ dimensions may be measured on splenic sections. We consider that the anteroposterior diameter of the spleen must not exceed 10 cm; the transverse diameter must be less than 6 cm and the craniocaudal length under 14 cm (Fig. 27-18). The lack of precision in the display of the upper splenic pole must, however, be borne in mind when evaluating the craniocaudal diameter. At least two diameters must exceed their normal values before the spleen is considered enlarged. (See Chapter 28.)

CHAPTER 28

THE PATHOLOGICAL SPLEEN

NONSPECIFIC SPLENOMEGALY

When the spleen is enlarged, it becomes particularly accessible to ultrasonic scans, even if it does not clear the costal margin. I have indicated (Chapter 27) my *criteria of splenomegaly.* The spleen enlarges along its anteroposterior diameter, extending then from the left kidney up to the margin of the left lobe of the liver (Figs. 28-1 to 28-5). The extension of the spleen to the midline and even toward the right side of the abdomen may be such that the left hepatic lobe is displaced posteriorly (Figs. 28-5 and 28-15). The spleen also enlarges transversely. Its medial aspect becomes slightly convex (Figs. 28-3 and 28-4) but does not bulge. With sufficient transverse swelling the left kidney is flattened (Figs. 28-6, 28-7, and 28-11). Finally, the spleen grows along its craniocaudal axis, which is displayed through lateral sagittal scans in right lateral decubitus (Figs. 28-6 and 28-7). As in the case of the liver, in nonspecific splenomegaly the *tissue echopattern* is perfectly homogeneous. However, the spleen may be less sonolucent than normal, approaching the reflectivity of the liver (Fig. 28-3, *B*). This increased reflectivity may be caused by fibrosis. When the spleen is both enlarged and increased in reflectivity, it is difficult to distinguish from the left lobe of the liver, whereas, when the splenic tissue has its normal low reflectivity, the differentiation between two neighboring organs is obvious at first glance (Figs. 28-1, 28-5, and 28-8, *B*).

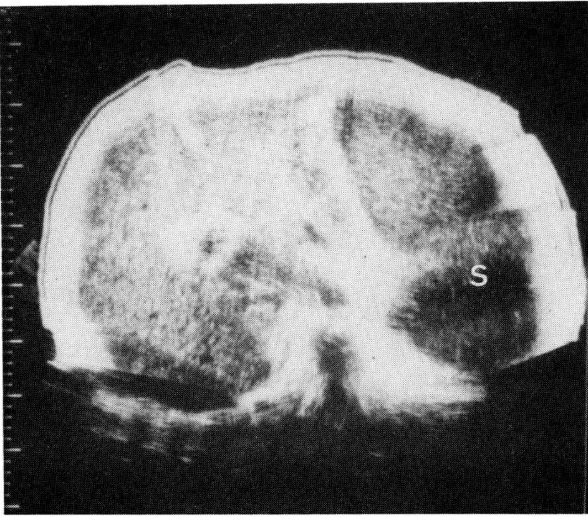

Fig. 28-1. Transverse scan of upper abdomen in case of lymphoma. Medial aspect of enlarged spleen *(S)* remains concave. Note lesser reflectivity of splenic tissue compared to liver.

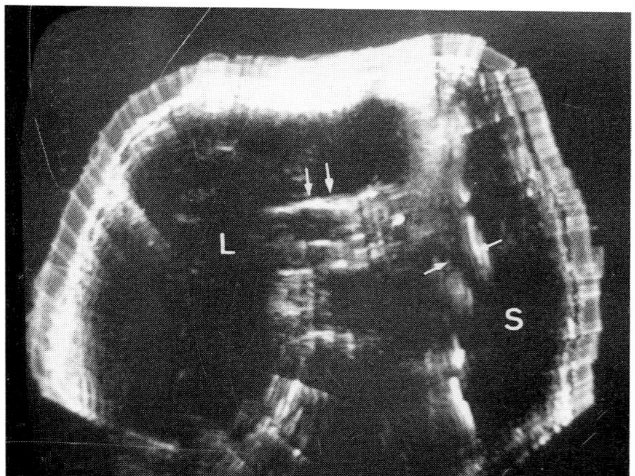

Fig. 28-2. Moderate enlargement of spleen *(S)* in case of cirrhosis. Internal aspect of organ is concave. In close contact with this aspect, enlarged splenic vein *(opposed arrows)* is displayed. Rounded margin of left hepatic lobe *(L)* is due to artifact. In close contact with this lobe, portal vein is obliquely cut *(parallel arrows).*

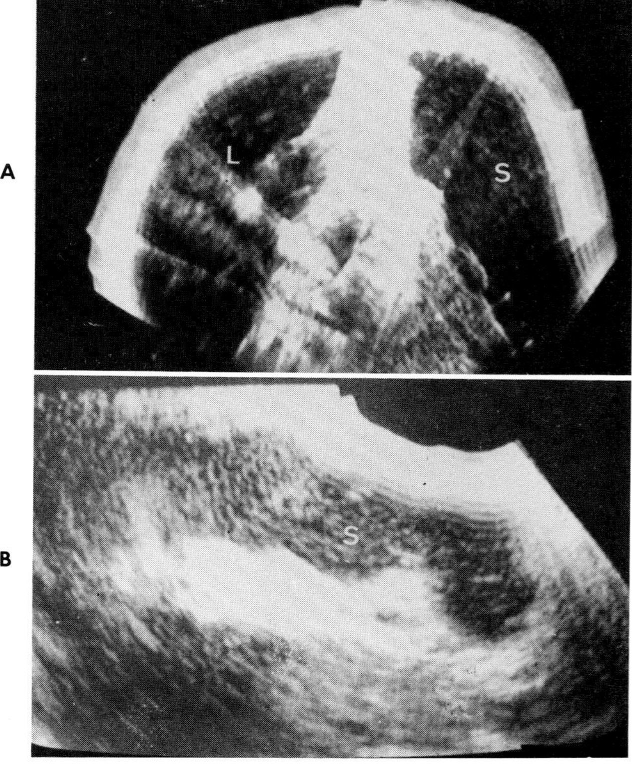

Fig. 28-3. Splenomegaly in case of lymphoma. **A,** Transverse scan. Liver *(L)* is of normal size. Spleen *(S)* is increased in size along all its diameters; medial aspect is undulated. **B,** Sagittal scan. Undulated shape of internal aspect is again displayed. Tissue echopattern remains homogeneous, but level of reflectivity is increased.

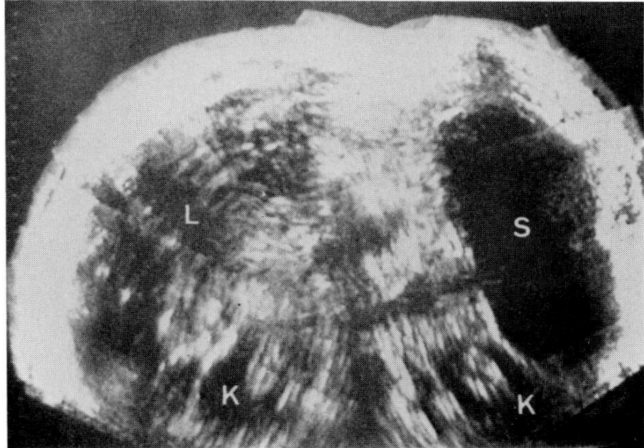

Fig. 28-4. Splenomegaly. Internal aspect of spleen *(S)* is rectilinear. General shape of section is oval, but not rounded. Left kidney *(K)* is slightly flattened. Echopattern remains less reflective than that of the liver *(L)*. This splenomegaly is caused by chronic lymphoid leukemia.

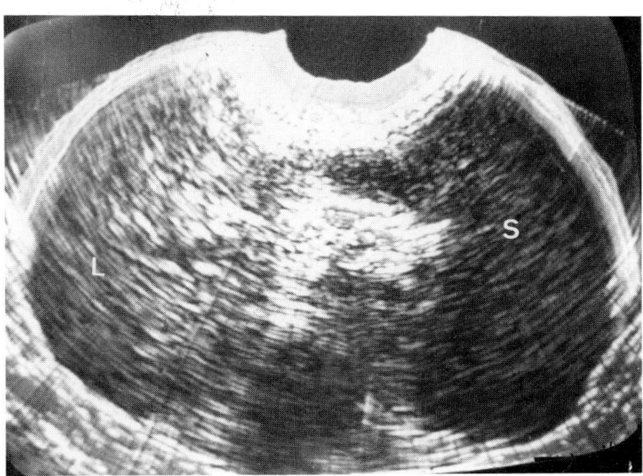

Fig. 28-5. Large spleen in hemolytic anemia. Transverse section of spleen *(S)* has area at least equal to that of liver *(L)*. Spleen extends to right beyond midline and comes in contact with small left hepatic lobe, but echopattern of spleen remains homogeneous and less reflective than liver.

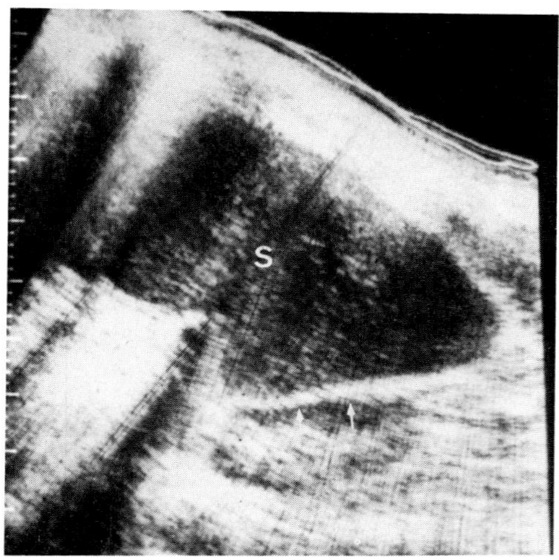

Fig. 28-6. Splenomegaly displayed on lateral sagittal scan. Note moderate flattening of external renal contour *(arrows). S,* spleen.

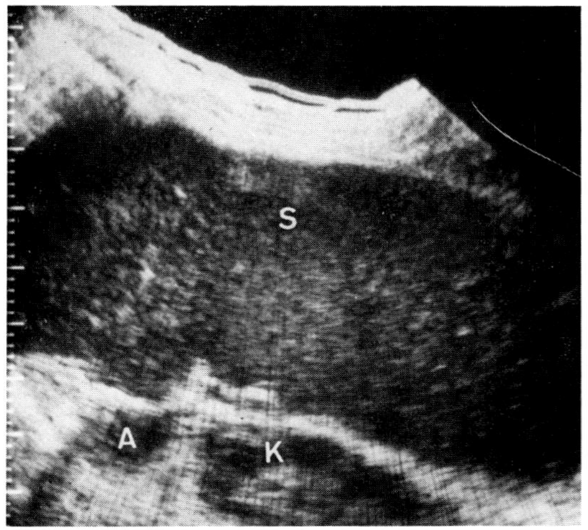

Fig. 28-7. Extreme enlargement of spleen *(S)* with moderate flattening of renal lower pole *(K). A,* adrenal gland.

One of the main causes of nonspecific splenomegalies is cirrhosis. The cirrhotic splenomegaly does not usually attain the volume of the spleen in lymphoma. An important associated sign is the dilatation of the portal venous network, as described in Chapter 10 and illustrated again in Fig. 28-8. In the presence of a nonspecific splenomegaly, another *associated sign* to search for is the presence of *lymph nodes* (Figs. 28-9 and 28-10), such an association being significant for *lymphoma.* Lymphomas will be dealt with again in the discussion of splenomegalies with focal involvement. Multiple *other pathological processes,* unfortunately without any associated ultrasonographic signs, may also give rise to images of non-

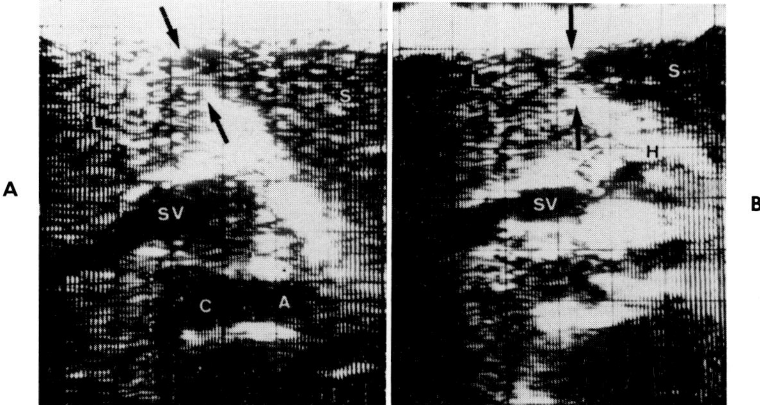

Fig. 28-8. Associated signs of splenomegaly—portal hypertension. **A,** Transverse real-time scan displaying left hepatic lobe *(L)* and medial aspect of spleen *(S),* which are in close contact. Reflectivity of spleen is much less than that of liver. *Arrows* point to limit between two organs. Posterior to area of contact and left hepatic lobe, enlarged splenic vein *(SV),* sagittally cut, is shown. *C,* vena cava; *A,* aorta. **B,** Another scan, slightly oblique, showing splenic vein from splenic hilus *(H).* Since sensitivity is lower than in **A,** difference in reflectivity between splenic and liver tissue is more obvious.

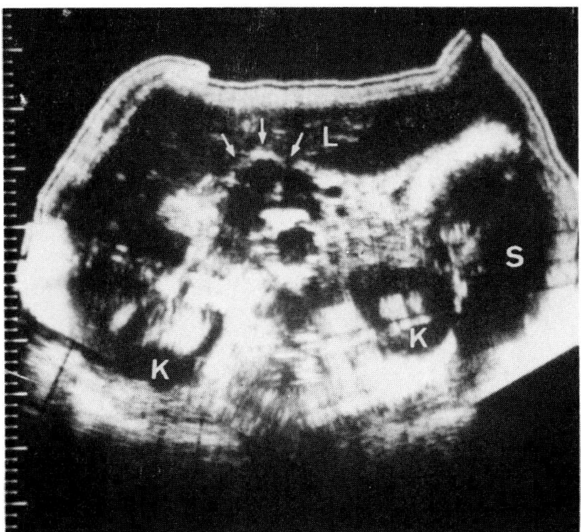

Fig. 28-9. Associated signs of splenomegaly—lymph nodes. This transverse scan of upper abdomen shows enlarged spleen *(S).* Sonolucent mass *(arrows)* is displayed between aorta and liver *(L).* This image belongs to lymphoma. *K,* right and left kidneys.

specific splenomegaly. As a resident or former resident, you know them all, of course, by heart.

LYMPHOMAS

In lymphomas, there are often echopattern anomalies. The level of reflectivity may increase. Reflective areas that are more or less nodular with more or less regular margins may appear (Figs. 28-11 to 28-14). This has also been reported by Vicary and Souhami (1977). By and large, any heterogeneity of the splenic tis-

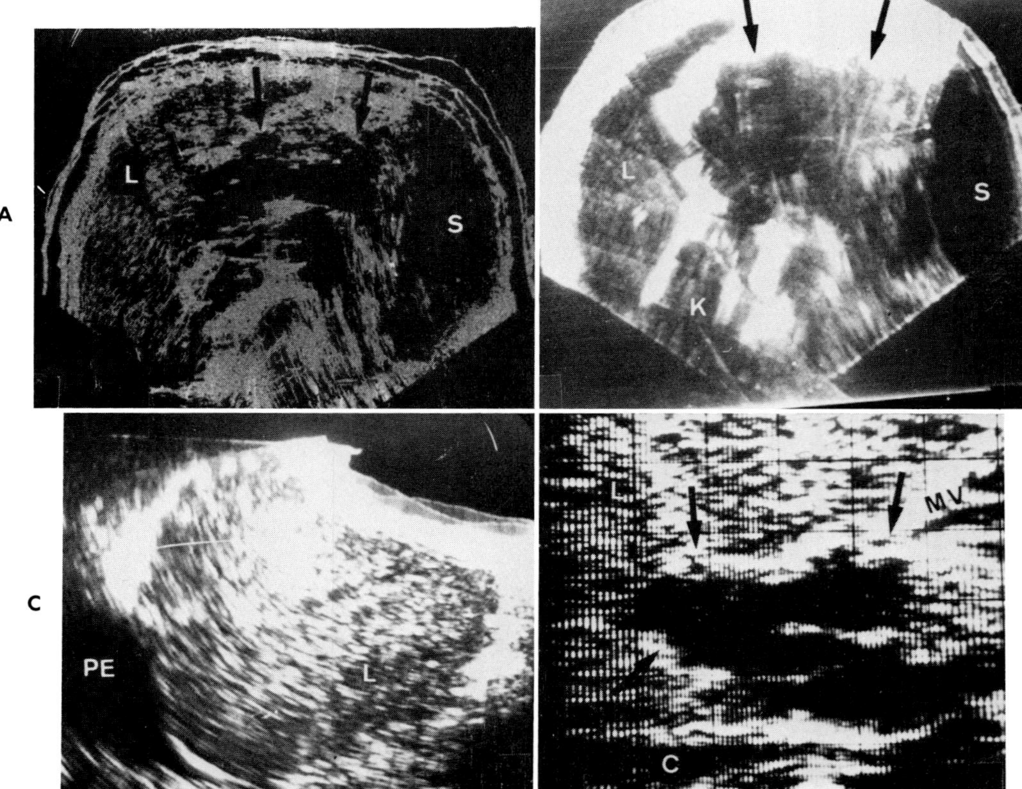

Fig. 28-10. Associated signs of splenomegaly—lymph nodes. **A,** Transverse scan of upper abdomen showing enlarged spleen *(S).* Between liver *(L)* and great vessels, polycyclic sonolucent mass is displayed *(arrows).* **B,** More caudal scan displaying extension of sonolucent mass. *K,* kidney. **C,** Sagittal scan of right upper quadrant showing hepatomegaly with angle sign and with areas of abnormal reflectivity. Above diaphragm is transparent area of pleural effusion *(PE).* **D,** Sagittal real-time scan passing through vena cava *(C)* again shows sonolucent mass with polycyclic margin *(arrows).* Mesenteric vein *(MV)* is displaced forward. This combination of signs is typical of lymphoma.

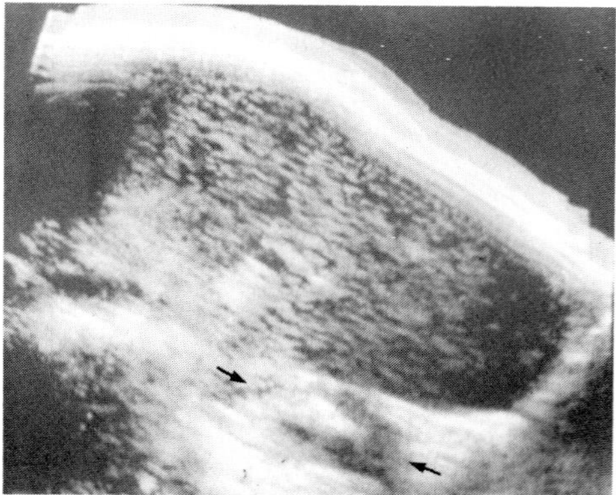

Fig. 28-11. Splenomegaly with abnormal tissue echopattern displayed on lateral sagittal scan. Level of reflectivity is abnormally high. This is Hodgkin's disease. Note flattened kidney *(arrows).*

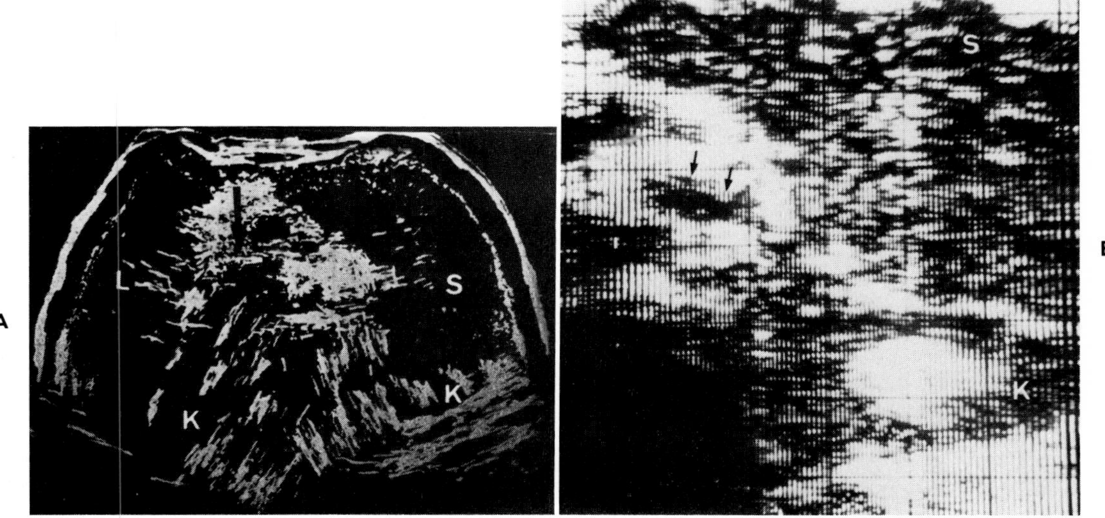

Fig. 28-12. Splenomegaly with abnormal tissue echopattern. **A,** Transverse scan of upper abdomen displaying enlarged spleen *(S)* extending to right beyond midline. There are a few lymph nodes *(arrow)* in relation with liver *(L)* and right kidney *(K)*. **B,** Splenic left oblique subcostal recurrent scan showing heterogeneous tissue echopattern. There are different areas of abnormal reflectivity, delineating a few sonolucent nodules. Note splenic vein *(arrows)* in hilar area. This abnormal echopattern is due to Hodgkin's disease. *K,* kidney.

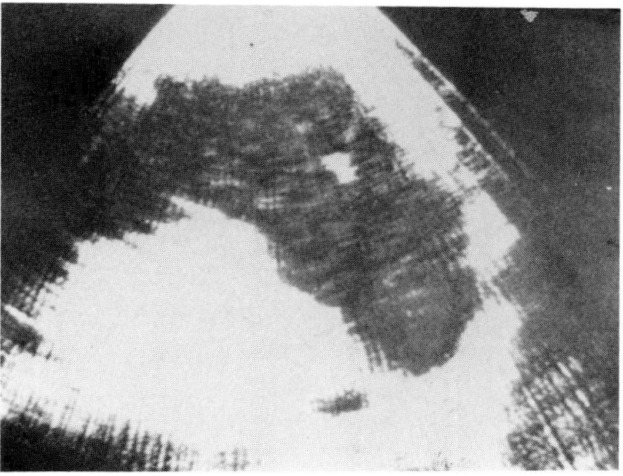

Fig. 28-13. Splenomegaly with abnormal echopattern in case of lymphatic leukemia. Oblique recurrent scan of spleen displays area of abnormally high reflectivity. There is one frank reflective nodule.

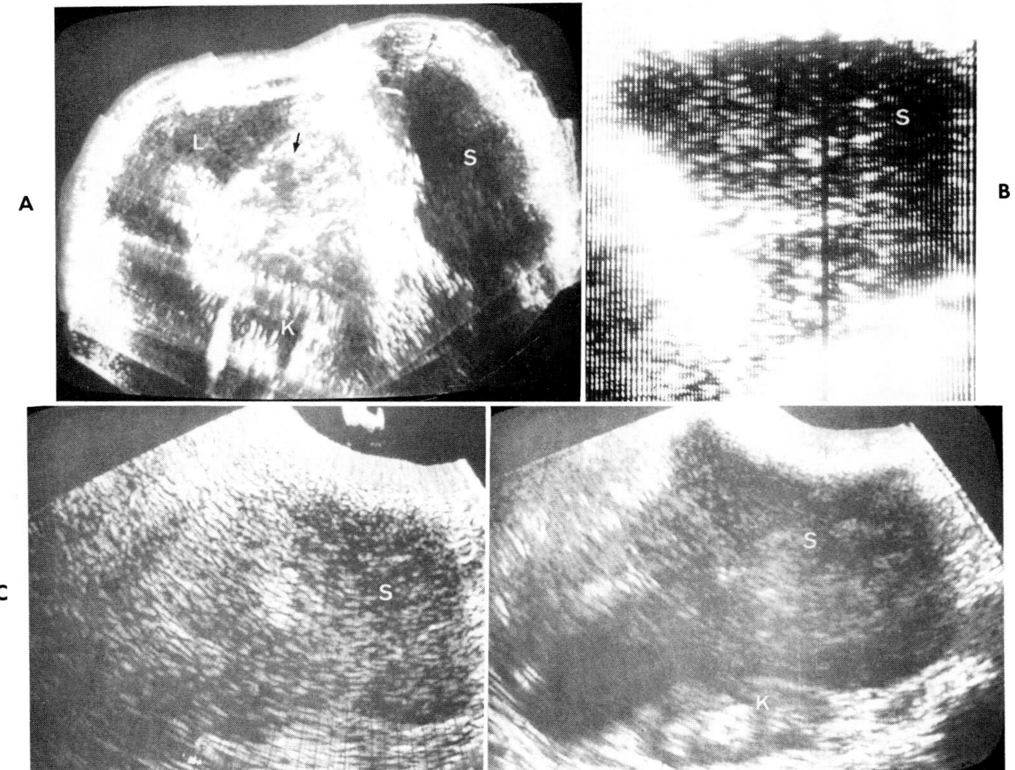

Fig. 28-14. Splenomegaly with abnormal echopattern (lymphoma). **A,** Transverse scan of upper abdomen displaying splenic contours. Splenic echopattern is slightly heterogeneous. There are a few lymph nodes *(arrow)* behind left hepatic lobe *(L)*. *S,* spleen; *K,* right kidney. **B,** Subcostal oblique recurrent real-time scan of spleen better displaying heterogeneous tissue pattern with areas of high reflectivity. **C** and **D,** More oblique recurrent scans, in gray scale contact scanning, also displaying heterogeneous echopattern with areas of abnormal reflectivity. *K,* left kidney.

sular echopattern is to be considered pathological. With gray scale imaging, whether with a real-time machine or a scan converter, it is now possible to diagnose the splenic involvement in lymphomas with good reliability. Successive examinations, in the course of chemotherapy, enables one to follow up objectively the course of improvement or, on the contrary, a recurrence.

SPLENIC TUMORS

In a splenic tumor, ultrasonography displays splenic enlargement, with important heterogeneity of the tissular echopattern (Fig. 28-15). Marginal humps may bulge out. At this moment, there is no specific ultrasonographic symptomatology leading to differentiation between either the different kinds of splenic sarcoma or a splenic sarcoma and metastatic deposits. A common complication of splenic sarcoma is infarct, which may produce marginal hematoma (Fig. 28-16).

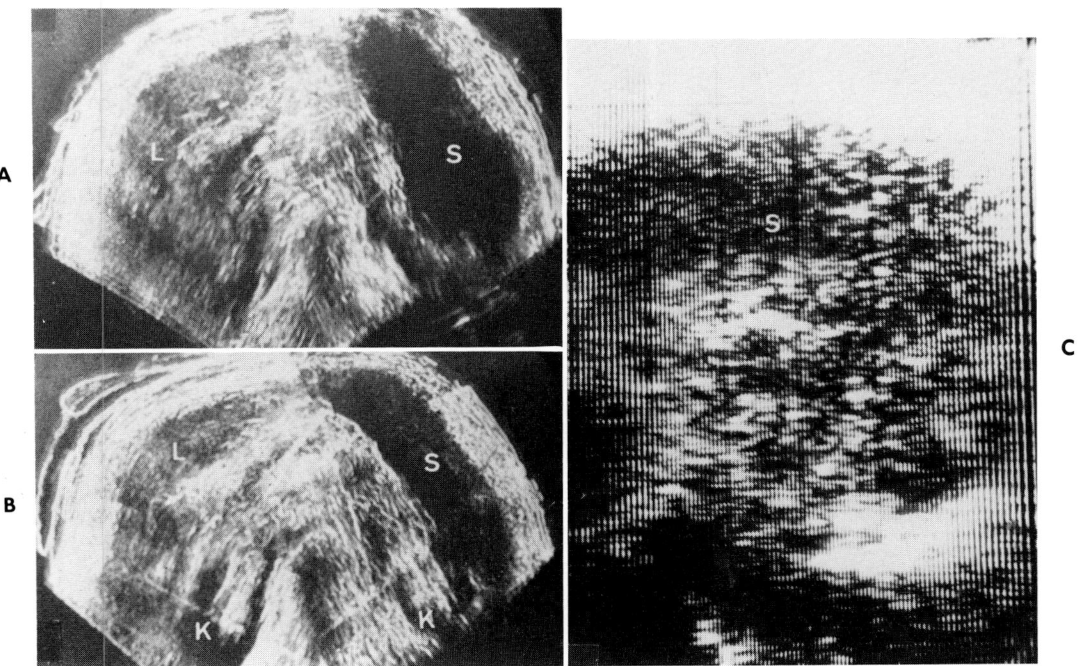

Fig. 28-15. Splenomegaly with tumoral echopattern. **A** and **B,** Two parallel transverse scans of upper abdomen showing splenomegaly *(S).* Internal aspect of spleen appears slightly convex in **A** and slightly concave in **B.** *L,* liver; *K,* kidney. **C,** Intercostal real-time scan displaying multiple areas of heterogeneity, similar to mottled pattern of metastatic deposits in liver. This is splenic lymphosarcoma.

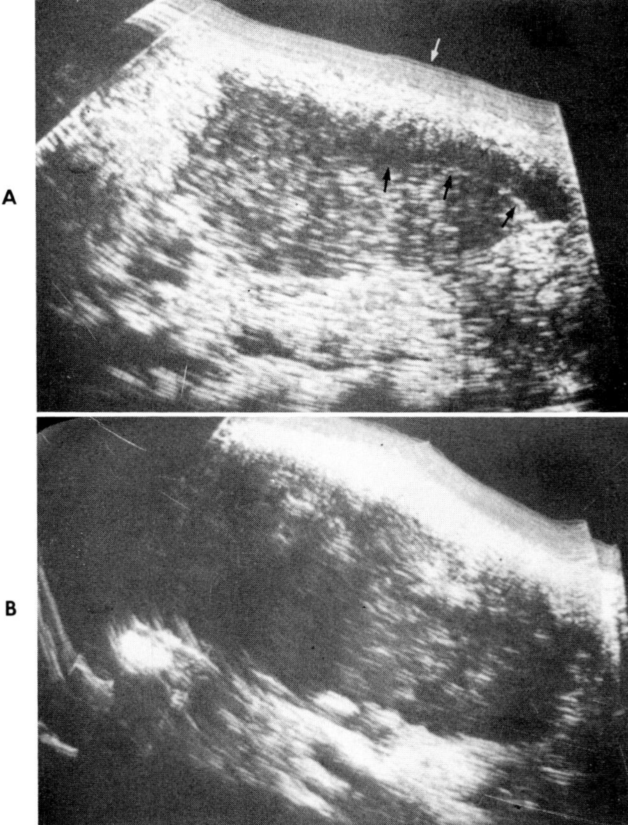

Fig. 28-16. Splenomegaly in tumor with hematoma. **A,** Lateral sagittal scan. Spleen is enlarged and clears costal margin *(white arrow).* Along superficial aspect of organ, sonolucent band *(black arrows)* is displayed; it belongs to hematoma. Tissue echopattern of spleen is heterogeneous, of mottled type. **B,** Oblique subcostal recurrent scan again displaying heterogeneous tissue echopattern. This splenomegaly with hematoma was caused by lymphosarcoma.

SPLENIC CYSTS

Parasitic cysts of the spleen (Fig. 28-17) are similar to parasitic hepatic cysts. Because the spleen is normally so lucent, one might be puzzled as to whether there is a cyst or only a rounded spleen. In fact, however, since splenic cysts possess well-delineated walls with posterior reinforcement, their pattern can be distinguished. A mature hydatid cyst, filled with daughter vesicles, is easier to recognize in the spleen than in the liver, since the solid pattern of such a cyst contrasts sharply with the sonolucent pattern of the splenic tissue. An immature hydatid cyst is, however, indistinguishable from a nonparasitic cyst (Fig. 28-18).

SPLENIC HEMATOMAS

A subcapsular hematoma gives rise to a double splenic contour delineating a marginal band of different echopattern, usually sonolucent (Fig. 28-16, *A*). The

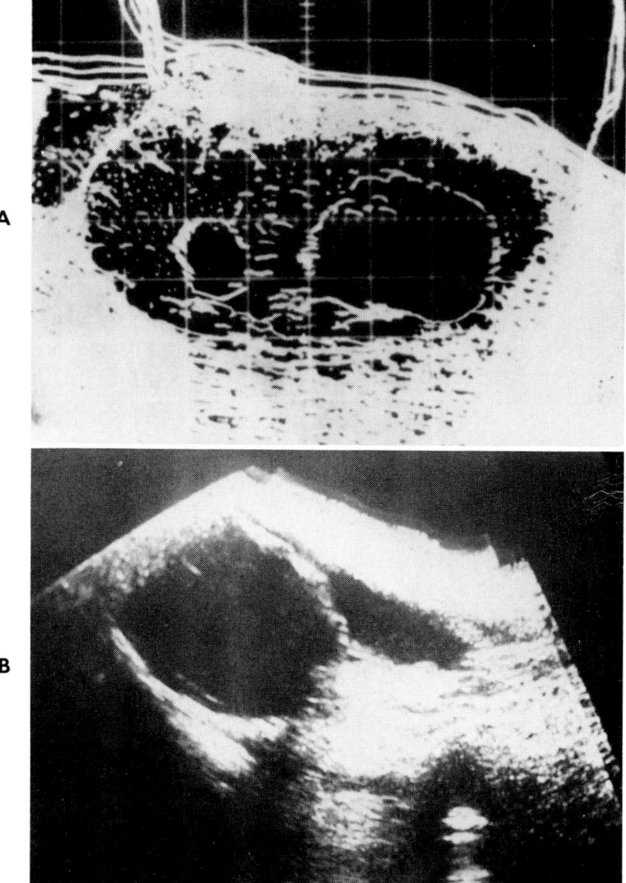

Fig. 28-17. Splenic cysts. A, Oblique subcostal recurrent scan. Spleen is enlarged. Two well-delineated cystic areas are displayed. They represent immature echinococcal cysts. B, Old, mature, calcified splenic echinococcal cyst in upper pole displayed on lateral sagittal scan. (A courtesy Dr. Roussille and Dr. Duquesnel, Lyons, France.)

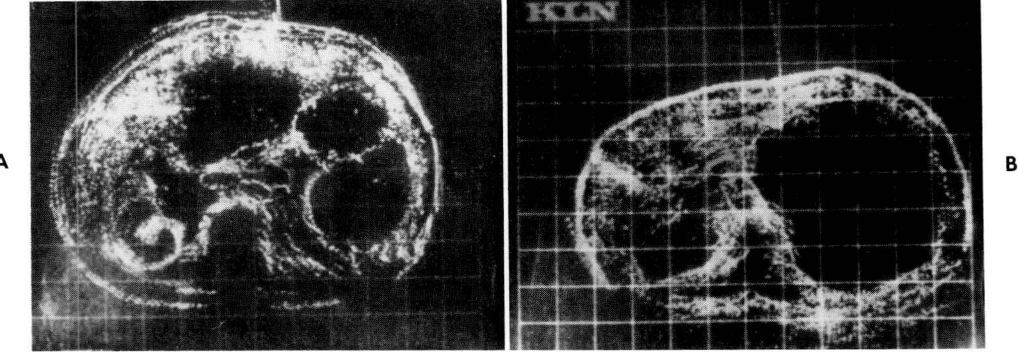

Fig. 28-18. Splenic cysts. A, First transverse scan of pregnant woman (7 months) showing two cystic elements. B, Two months later (i.e., 10 days after delivery), patient was examined again, in emergency condition. Splenic image was replaced by large sonolucent collection corresponding to spontaneous hematoma, which had developed on nonparasitic splenic cyst. (Courtesy Dr. Roussille and Dr. Duquesnel, Lyons, France.)

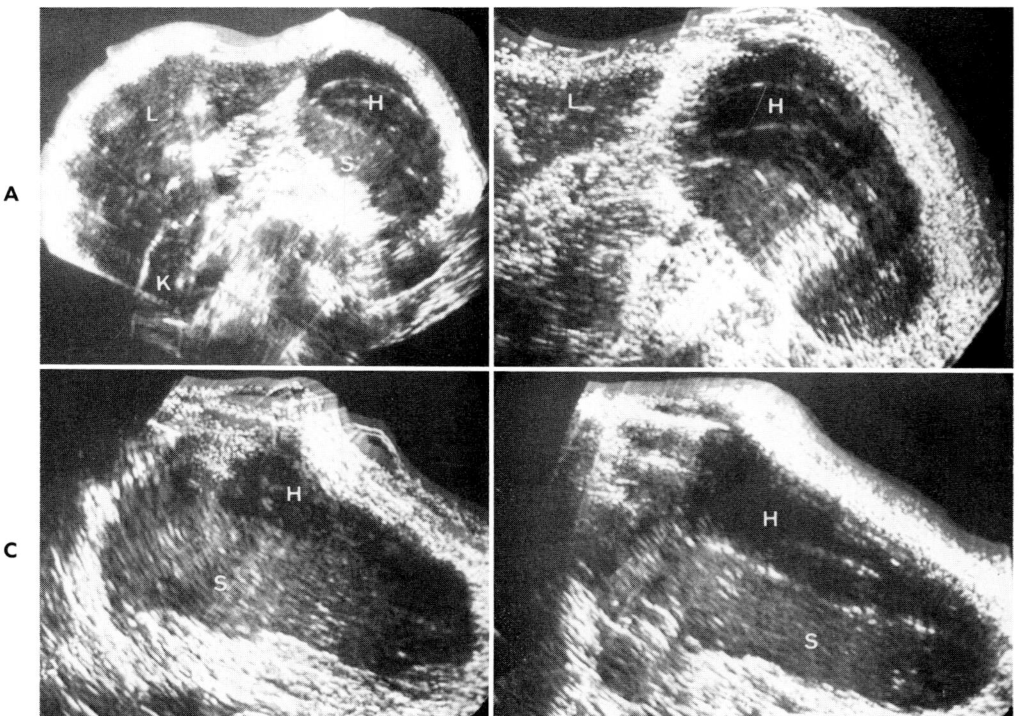

Fig. 28-19. Spontaneous hematoma. Young man with anemia complained of pain in left upper quadrant. His spleen was large, and sonolucent band was displayed between splenic tissue and abdominal wall. This was case of myelogenous leukemia. **A,** Transverse scan. *S,* spleen; *H,* hematoma; *L,* liver; *K,* kidney. **B,** Larger scale transverse scan. **C** and **D,** Oblique recurrent subcostal scans.

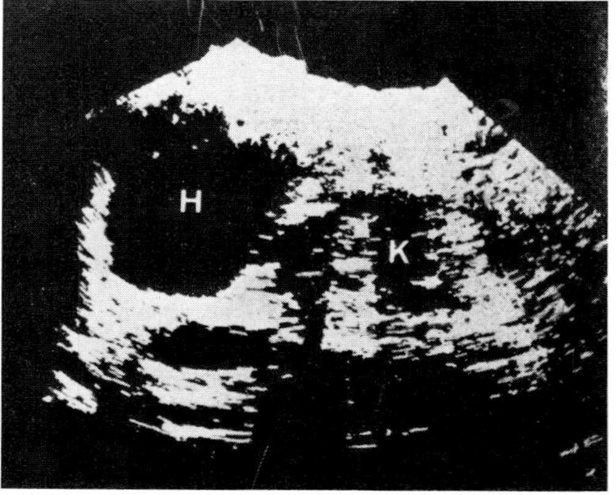

Fig. 28-20. Posttraumatic hematoma displayed on lateral sagittal axillary scan. Hematoma *(H)* is displayed as well-marginated sonolucent collection in relation to kidney *(K)*.

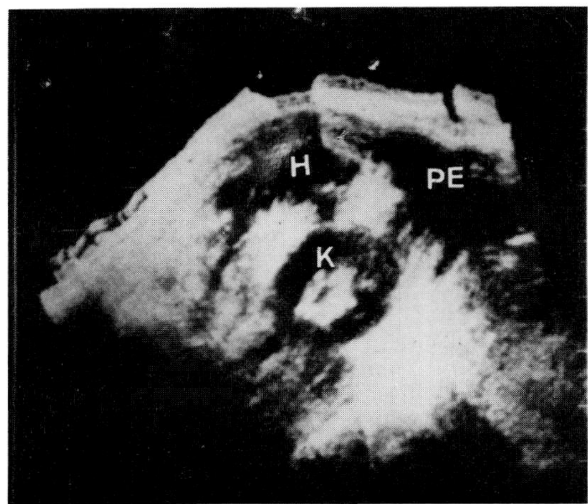

Fig. 28-21. Hematoma. Patient underwent splenectomy for traumatic rupture. In days after operation, recurrent anemia developed to slight degree. Examination was performed with patient in right lateral decubitus. Transverse scan shows, between kidney *(K)* and lateral wall, sonolucent collection *(H)* representing postoperative hematoma. *PE,* pleural effusion.

pattern of a hematoma is absolutely similar whatever its origin—spontaneous (e.g., infarcts, blood diseases, and altered blood coagulation) or traumatic (Figs. 28-16, *A*, and 28-19 to 28-21). The greater the splenic enlargement, the more easily the splenic hematoma is displayed; if a hematoma arises from a spleen of normal size, as is usually the case with trauma, it is much more difficult to show a small hematoma, especially if it is located in the upper pole. Therefore only a positive ultrasonic diagnosis of hematoma is reliable. In case of trauma, if unable to display a traumatic hematoma, we always perform splenic angiography.

DIFFERENTIAL DIAGNOSIS

A moderately enlarged spleen is easily identified between the left kidney and the lateral thoracic wall; but, in the case of a *large mass* occupying the whole left upper quadrant, the mass may be an enlarged spleen or another organ. In the latter case, the spleen is pushed away and flattened and may be impossible to show. As a rule, even a greatly enlarged spleen retains its shape. Its medial aspect remains concave, rectilinear, or slightly convex; but a splenic mass never shows a frankly rounded shape in transverse scan, whereas a renal or adrenal tumor has just that shape. (See Fig. 28-22.) This shape has also been observed in several sarcomas arising from the posterior abdominal wall (Fig. 28-23). Tumors of the pancreatic tail are smaller, so that no problem of differentiation from an enlarged spleen arises except for cystadenomas, which, as seen in Chapter 23, may become very large. I have seen several tumors arising from the gastric wall, extending to the left upper quadrant, and suggesting splenomegaly (Figs. 25-36 and 28-24). I once interpreted a huge hepatic tumor, arising from the margin of the left hepatic lobe and occupying the whole left upper quadrant, as an enlarged spleen. These different considerations indicate that, if there is doubt as to the splenic nature of a mass in the left upper quadrant, the best answer is to find the spleen, even if it is compressed by

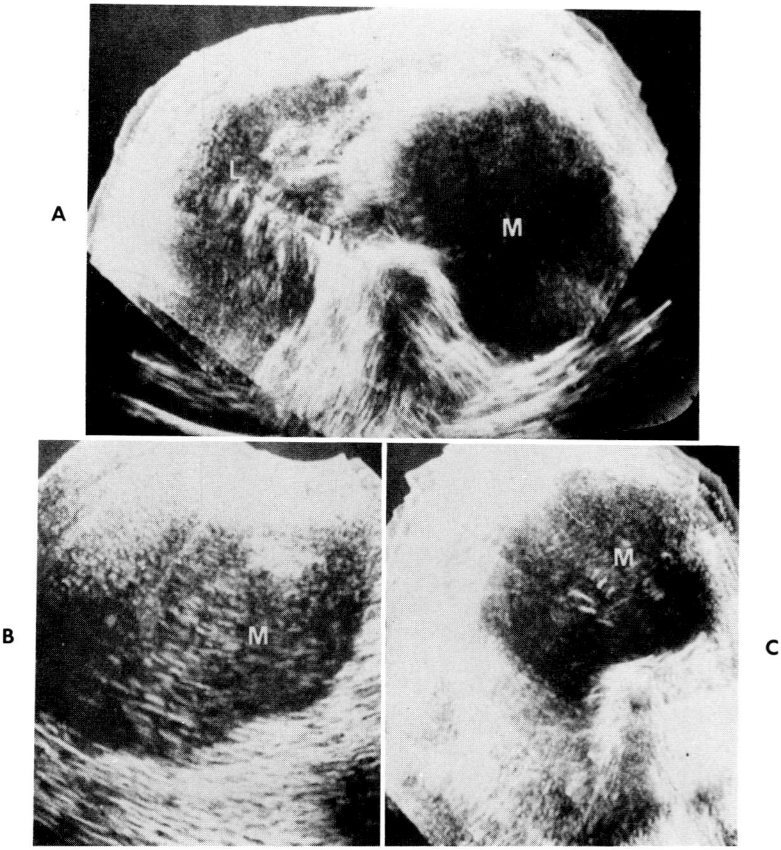

Fig. 28-22. Differential diagnosis—renal mass. Patient was referred for splenomegaly. **A,** Transverse scan of upper abdomen displaying sonolucent mass *(M)* occupying left upper quadrant. There is no renal image. Internal aspect of mass is frankly convex. *L,* liver. **B,** Intercostal scan. **C,** Lateral transverse scan made with patient in right lateral decubitus. Rounded shape of tumoral section enables one to rule out splenomegaly. Once again, radiological information must be gathered in comprehensive way and IV urography performed.

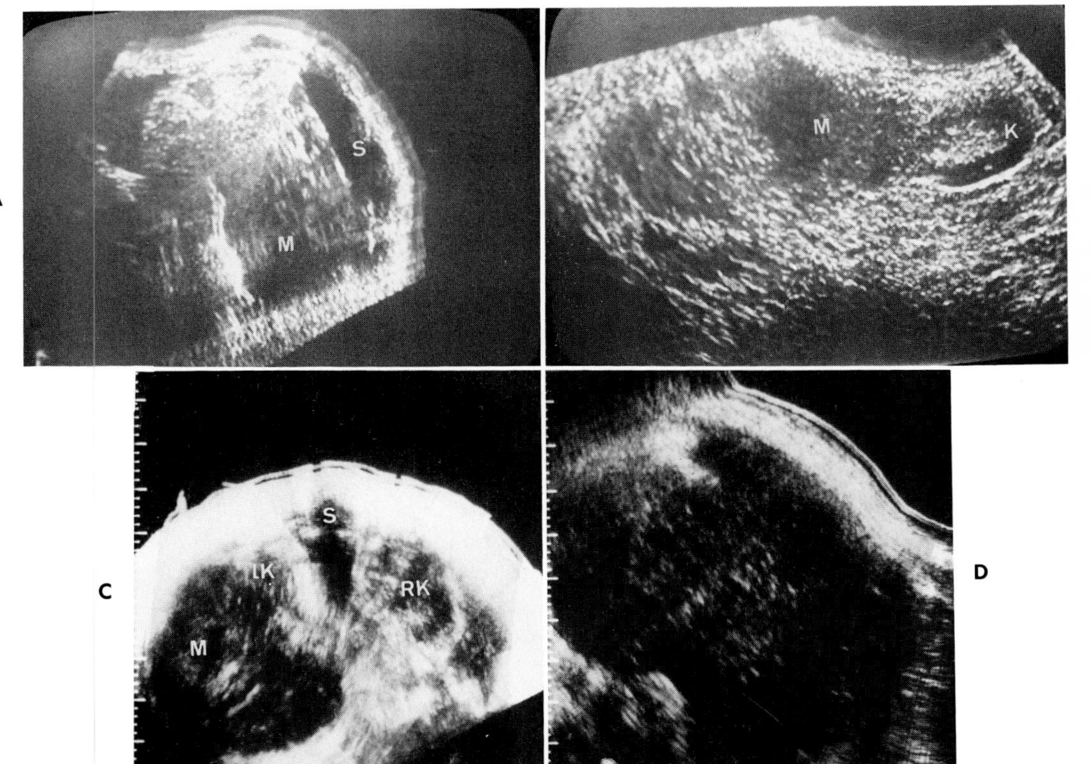

Fig. 28-23. Differential diagnosis of left upper quadrant masses. **A** and **B,** Correct diagnosis of nonsplenic mass. Patient was referred for splenic investigation because of polycythemia. "Enlarged spleen" had been palpated. **A,** Transverse scan showing normal spleen *(S)*. There is large, solid mass *(M)*, which could be renal tumor. **B,** Lateral sagittal scan displaying normal kidney *(K)* displaced downward by mass. Mass, neither renal nor splenic, was retroperitoneal rhabdomyosarcoma. Even if spleen had not been displayed, rounded shape of mass with convex contours would not be consistent with diagnosis of splenic mass. **C** and **D,** Incorrect diagnosis of splenomegaly. **C,** Transverse scan of patient in prone position shows large heterogeneous mass *(M)* on left side, flattening left kidney *(LK)*. *S,* spine; *RK,* right kidney. **D,** Intercostal scan. Mass was diagnosed as tumoral spleen. Final diagnosis was rhabdomyosarcoma arising from posterior muscles.

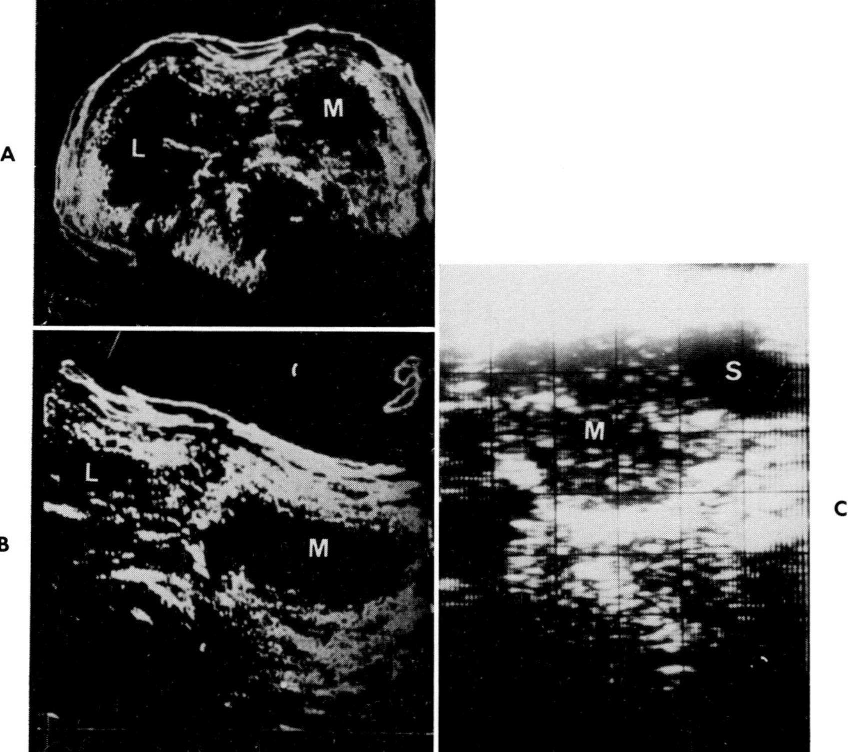

Fig. 28-24. Differential diagnosis—gastric tumor. Barium study, as well as endoscopic examination, indicated presence of extragastric mass. **A,** Transverse scan showing mass *(M)* occupying left upper quadrant. *L,* liver. **B,** Left recurrent subcostal scan displaying oval shape of mass, which could be splenic. **C**, Intercostal real-time scan showing normal spleen *(S)* in relation to mass, which was finally found to be schwannoma with extragastric development.

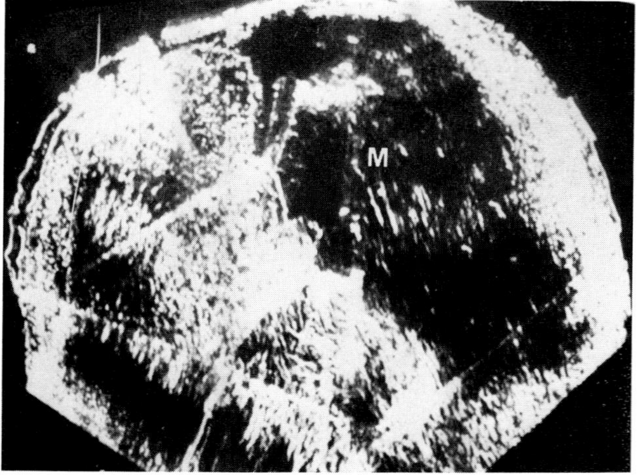

Fig. 28-25. Differential diagnosis—mass in left upper quadrant. On this transverse section, mass is seen to have undulated and slightly convex internal aspect; its anterointernal margin is angular. Echopattern is heterogeneous, of mottled type. Our diagnosis was tumoral splenomegaly. Actually, mass was renal carcinoma.

the tumor. If no specific splenic image is displayed, it is usually possible to rely on the fact that an honest spleen and an honest nonsplenic tumor are different in shape on transverse sections, but enlarged spleens and other masses, like all of us, are not always absolutely honest. A mass in the left upper quadrant may have a typical splenic shape but turn out to be a renal tumor (Fig. 28-25). As a rule, the left kidney, flattened as it may become, is always easily displayed behind an enlarged spleen; but the spleen is much more difficult to display next to a large nonsplenic mass. Large masses in the left upper quadrant, however, must also be evaluated by intravenous urography.

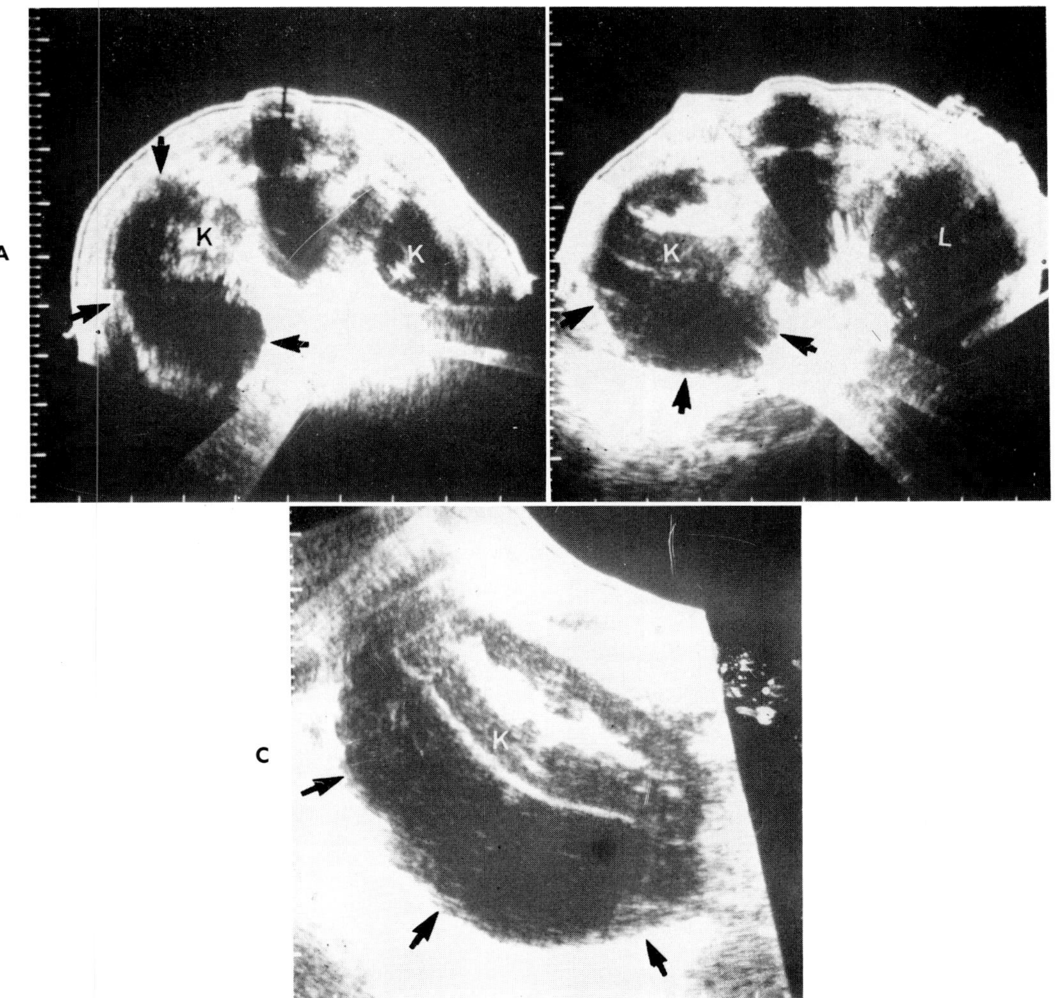

Fig. 28-26. Differential diagnosis—hematoma of left upper quadrant. Patient was referred after blunt trauma. **A,** Transverse scan made with patient in prone position showing fluid collection *(arrows)* around left kidney. It could be splenic or renal hematoma. *K,* kidney. **B,** More cephalic parallel scan again showing hematoma. *L,* liver. **C,** Sagittal scan showing close relation of hematoma to anterior aspect of kidney without cephalad extension. Splenic image was normal: hematoma was of renal origin.

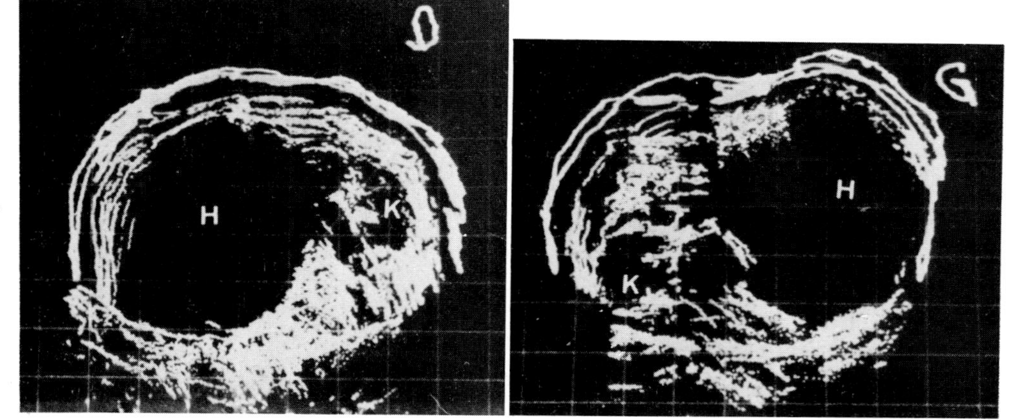

Fig. 28-27. Differential diagnosis—hematoma of left upper quadrant. **A,** Transverse scan, made with patient in prone position, of child who had undergone trauma, showing huge hematoma *(H)* occupying left upper quadrant. *K,* normal right kidney. **B,** Transverse scan made with patient in supine position again displaying collection. It is too large to be splenic hematoma. Besides, left renal image is not displayed. As a matter of fact, it was collection of blood and urine due to renal rupture.

In cases of *hematoma,* other possibilities may be considered. As is the case for the liver, the presence of a sonolucent marginal band may be due to ascites. (See Fig. 27-15.) The differentiation is possible through positional changes, with which an ascitic band disappears or changes in shape, whereas a sonolucent band belonging to a hematoma remains unchanged in location and shape. When a hematoma is large, it can occupy the whole splenic area (Figs. 28-18, *B,* 28-20, and 28-21). After trauma, a large hematoma may also belong to the kidney. It is necessary to display the proper image of the kidney in case of a splenic hematoma or, conversely, the splenic image in case of a renal hematoma. (See Fig. 28-26.) This is not always easy if the hematoma is really large enough to occupy the whole left upper quadrant (Fig. 28-27); but such a giant hematoma is not likely to be of splenic origin, since the splenic capsule is too fragile to extend that far without rupture and intraperitoneal hemorrhage. In any case, the discovery of a giant hematoma in the left upper quadrant requires emergency surgery, often without even the delay of angiography.

Once the diagnosis of a pathological splenic process has been made, one has to take a second diagnostic step, which is the *differential diagnosis of the possible splenic lesions.*

I have already emphasized the importance of associated signs, such as portal hypertension or the presence of lymph nodes. The presence of an abnormal echo-pattern leads, according to the clinical and ultrasonic features, either to lymphography, to splenic angiography, or to both examinations successively. Ultrasonically guided biopsy would, of course, be the only procedure leading to a definite diagnosis; but the spleen is much more fragile than the liver, and this is likely to lead to hemorrhage, especially since in many cases of splenomegaly there are clotting problems.

RELIABILITY AND DIAGNOSTIC POLICY

The reliability of splenic ultrasonography is excellent except for lesions in the upper pole. Its sensitivity, with regard to tissue echopattern abnormalities, in my opinion, is better than that of scintigraphy, as demonstrated, for instance, by the display of hematomas; but, owing to the problem of a possible failure in displaying the upper pole, a seemingly normal ultrasonographic result may prove insufficient. Occasionally, scout films of the abdomen may show a calcified mass in the upper pole. When this is not the case and the upper pole has not been displayed by ultrasonography, other procedures may prove useful. Since scintigraphy is able to show this upper pole and to display small, superiorly located spleens, hidden under the diaphragm and inaccessible to ultrasonography, this procedure retains a great value in splenic examinations. Another contribution of scintigraphy is easy identification of a normal spleen in cases involving a large mass in the left upper quadrant, large masses always being a difficult diagnostic problem. Scintigraphy displays the splenic nature of the mass or, on the contrary, shows that the spleen is displaced and compressed—a result that is not always achieved by the combination of ultrasonography with IV urography. A retroperitoneal sarcoma can also be differentiated from simple splenomegaly by CT scanning. I advocate the following sequence of procedures if ultrasonography is not definitive: IV urography, scintigraphy, and then, if necessary, CT scanning.

In the most difficult cases, selective angiography is helpful in showing the exact origin of a left upper quadrant mass, especially with exceptional large adrenal masses.

REFERENCES

Barnett, E., and Morley, P.: Abdominal echography, Borough Green, England, 1974, Butterworth & Co. (Publishers), Ltd.

Goldberg, B. B., Kotler, M. N., Ziskin, M. C., and Waxham, R. D.: Diagnostic uses of ultrasound, New York, 1975, Grune & Stratton, Inc.

Hassani, N.: Ultrasonography of the abdomen, Heidelberg, Germany, 1976, Springer-Verlag.

Holm, H. H., Kristensen, J. K., Rasmussen, S. N., Pedersen, J. F., and Hancke, S.: Abdominal ultrasound, Copenhagen, 1976, Munksgaard International Booksellers & Publishers, Ltd.

Kristensen, J. K., Buemann, B., and Kuhl, E.: Ultrasonic scanning in the diagnosis of splenic hematomas, Acta Chir. Scand. **137:**653-657, 1971.

Leopold, G. R., and Asher, W. M.: Fundamentals of abdominal and pelvic ultrasonography, Philadelphia, 1975, W. B. Saunders Co.

Vicary, F. R., and Souhami, R. L.: Ultrasound and Hodgkin's disease of the spleen, Br. J. Radiol. **50:**521-522, 1977.

Weill, F., Becker, J. C., Kraehenbuhl, J. R., Heriot, G., and Walter, J. P.: Clinical atlas of ultrasonic radiography, Paris, 1973, Masson & Cie., Editeurs.

CHAPTER 29

PRACTICAL ADVICE, OR HOW TO DO BETTER THAN WE DID

DIAGNOSTIC POLICY

At the end of this ultrasonic study of pathology of the digestive organs, some practical advice may perhaps be useful. No procedure, including ultrasonography, is error-free; but most errors are due to faulty interpretation, rather than the physical limitations of the imaging procedure. Often errors are produced by arriving at a diagnosis too rapidly with an inadequate number of scanning planes. Since one is dealing with tomographic sections, an inadequate number may fail to reveal important pathological elements. It is thus necessary to emphasize the point that multiple scans, performed in each of the views that constitute the logical procedure of the examination, are compulsory. As in any radiological procedure, clinical intuition must be used, but it must be within the framework of a strict examination protocol. One view or direction of scan may disclose a lesion or prove that a finding previously considered to represent a lesion was merely an artifact. Each step of the examination procedure must be followed in every patient. The most typical liquid collection must be assessed thoroughly with multiple cuts and different levels of sensitivity. After such thorough analysis, it may finally appear to be solid or to contain solid elements.

If one has succeeded in displaying an abnormal image in real time and then in contact scanning, the reliability of the diagnosis is enhanced. Similarly, repeating an examination after a few hours or a day, first without preparation and then on a fasting patient, helps to rule out pseudopathological images of gastric or intestinal origin. This is particularly true for images in the left prerenal area.

Fluoroscopy, radiography, and high- and low-contrast films, are all employed in conventional radiologic procedures. Similarly, real-time imaging and contact scanning with high and low contrast must also be used in a comprehensive way. No technique, sophisticated though it may be, is able to display all the anatomical and pathological features of interest. This is a general concept in medicine and applies equally to ultrasound imaging. I have frequently emphasized the need to relate the ultrasonic findings to those of other radiological procedures. This is the reason that I dealt with gastric and colonic tumors only with differential diagnosis and not in an individual chapter: the diagnosis of this type of tumor is a function of conventional radiology, not ultrasonography. Ultrasound imaging must not be considered competitive with other types of radiological examinations, but rather complementary.

Ultrasonography permits one to make the best selection of various radiological techniques. For example, it is totally irrational to begin the workup of a patient suspected of harboring a pancreatic carcinoma or having jaundice with angiography

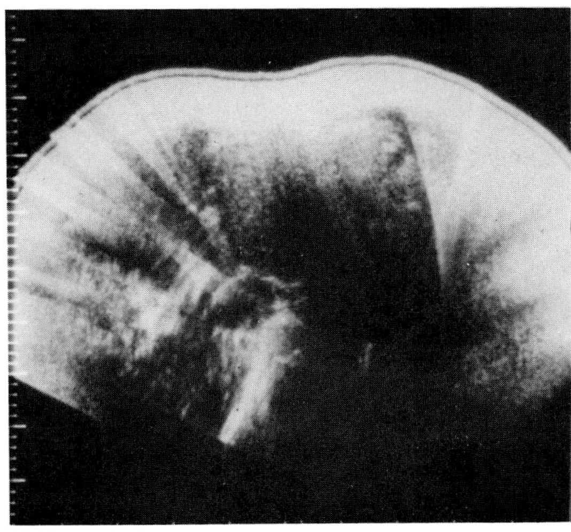

Fig. 29-1. Complete failure of ultrasonic examination, due to small size of left lobe of liver and presence of gas in bowel. Such failure occurs with 5% of patients.

or retrograde pancreatography. Unfortunately, in many hospitals, such procedures are, in fact, followed.

The era of direct visceral radiology has now been entered. Ultrasonography, as well as computerized tomography, is able to display direct images of soft tissue organs. Indirect procedures, such as contrast angiography, remain useful but should be used in selected cases, such as the search for a pancreatic islet cell tumor or the hemodynamic study of a case of portal hypertension. Within the area of direct visceral radiology, one is now confronted with a choice between ultrasonography and computerized tomography. These modalities offer different advantages and disadvantages and examine different physical aspects of the tissues. Whereas computerized tomography reveals the electron density of the tissues, ultrasound gives information primarily about the elastic properties of the tissues. Whereas computerized tomography is useful for visualizing and distinguishing a wide variety of densities, including air, fat, bone, and contrast material, ultrasound is primarily useful in the tissues that are close to water density. Computerized tomography is chiefly indicated, for instance, in evaluation of the abdominal-thoracic extensions of lymphoma (Kreel, 1977); but, since ultrasonography is a simple and flexible method, it should generally be used first, so that a more rational use of computerized tomography, which is costly both in terms of money and radiation, can subsequently be made. Keep in mind how easy and important it is to cut along the sagittal axis of the gallbladder, the common bile duct, or the portal vein and how valuable it is to evaluate the motion pattern of the vena cava. Obviously, none of these things can be done with computerized tomography, which can also be the only effective procedure, as illustrated in Fig. 29-1.

SELECTION OF AN ULTRASONIC MACHINE

The choice of an ultrasonic machine is a difficult matter. If the manufacturer knows better than the radiologist how the machine has been built, the radiologist knows better than the maker what one is entitled to expect from it. There is no doubt that the radiologist requires the combination of real-time and contact scanning techniques. At the present time, both types of machines must be purchased separately, and this is expensive. Complementary real-time machines must be made available at a reasonable price and be used to take advantage of the sophisticated electronic devices, such as the scan converter, that are already incorporated in the contact scanners. This seems to be at hand with digitized scan converters.

No radiologist would seriously consider purchase of a radiographic unit for GI radiology without an image amplifier and television monitor. Anyone who purchases only a contact scanning machine is deliberately preparing to lose at least half the available ultrasonic information. At the present time, two ultrasonic devices, one contact and one real time, cost less than sophisticated radiological equipment and enable one to obtain at least as many diagnoses, even if they are different ones. Technology is changing so fast that it is almost impossible to forecast what ultrasonographic processes will be used in the future (e.g., transmission ultrasonography, Doppler imaging, or image computer processing). However, in the near future, I personally see more promise in flexible, high-resolution real-time machines than in fully automatic "slicers"—provided real-time imaging really attains high resolution. Anyway, at present, as previously stated, real-time and contact scanning are necessarily used as complementary techniques.

Now that the principle of simultaneous purchase of a real-time and contact scanning machine has been established, I should like to emphasize the *criteria of technical quality*. This quality is to be assessed by the detail of the hepatic tissue echopattern and display of the tubular structures within the liver, such as portal and hepatic veins. The tissue echopattern must appear as a rich group of small, sharp echoes. On proper scans, with a frequency of 3.5 MHz, tubular elements 2 mm in diameter are to be outlined. At the present time, real-time machines of the first generation, that is, those with a mechanical displacement of the transducer, seem to display a better tissue echopattern than do the multiarray transducers. Another point is the size and flexibility of the RTH. It should be light and capable of displacement in a variety of positions—a quality announced for last-generation real-time machines, in addition to high resolution.

In contact scanning, two kinds of qualities must be assessed—mechanical and electronic. The first mechanical quality is the rigidity of the articulated scanning arm, which assures reproducibility of the scanning plane. One must be able to change the direction of the scanning arm easily, so as to perform transverse oblique and sagittal scans. It is also important for one to be able to angle the scanning plane cranially or caudally. These different movements must be controlled through individual, reliable, and handy electromagnetic brakes. The movements, if possible, should be able to be managed with only one hand and without effort.

There are also various indispensable electronic qualities. One of these is a good balance of the TGC. The TGC curve must be prominently displayed and easy to adjust. It is useful to know the level of the initial gain, the number of decimals per centimeter of gain compensation, and the maximum amplification in depth. Although with a good machine it is possible with the majority of patients and in most examinations to obtain good images with a standard TGC curve, fine adjustments must be available. It is also necessary to be able to adjust the sensitivity in a direct way. In constructing total-body sections, one may wish to change the sensitivity as the transducer moves from one part of the body to the other, for example, when passing from the ribs to the epigastrium. For this reason the control must be manageable and within reach of the left hand while the right is performing the scan. The level of intensity in decibels must be displayed, so that quantitative comparisons can be made. For gray scale imaging the monitor screen must be large enough, and the image must appear without significant flickering. Its inscription must be rapid, to avoid artifacts due to slowing of the transducer movement. The more rapidly the image is produced, the less likely important vascular images are to blur. It is essential that one be able to obtain high-quality tissue images without filling the images of the vessel lumina. This occurs when there is a high noise level in the machine, and one then sees an apparent filling of vascular and cystic structures, due to background noise. At high sensitivity levels, noise may produce a falsely semisolid echopattern in a liquid structure.

I would suggest the use of films of wider dynamic range than Polaroid. Such systems are now available. Polaroid film should be reserved for emergency examinations.

The quality of the transducer and the way it is focused have important effects on the quality of the image. The acoustical dynamic range of the machine and the dynamic range of the gray scale display interact with the fundamental image quality of the transducer to determine the reliability of the registration and the final image quality. These technical qualities contribute to meeting two clinical criteria in contact scanning: display of the normal Wirsung's duct and easy differentiation between the pancreas and stomach or duodenum.

A final point that must be considered in selecting a machine is reliability and rapidity of service and maintenance. In small communities this may be a crucial element in deciding which machine to purchase.

PRACTICAL TRAINING

The best method of training, of course, is to read this book and give a copy of it to all your friends, so that they can recite it to you at every occasion. If you have never practiced ultrasonography, a good introduction would be to restudy your anatomy books. It is, of course, useful to attend courses and seminars. However, despite all these guides, practical training is compulsory. An experienced radiologist requires at least 2 months of practical training to learn the basic elements of abdominal ultrasonography. This is not in excess of what is required for other procedures such as angiography. A reasonable way to proceed is to take a first training course of about 6 weeks followed by independent practice and then return for a second training period to clear up remaining problems. It is, however, possible to reduce the necessary training period by practicing scanning on your husband or wife, colleagues, secretary, technicians, or lovers. The American Institute of Ultrasound in Medicine has recommended that one avoid using ultrasound for demonstration or training to prevent any presently unknown biological effects on human guinea pigs. However, at a seminar organized in London by the World Health Organization (October, 1977), Hill summarized the data of multiple experiments and concluded that, at the levels of energy used for diagnostic imaging, there is no evidence at all of any harmful biological effects.

When enough experience has been obtained, one must keep a constant eye on the quality of the images. Hepatic tissue architecture must look alike from one scan to another, from one examination to another, and from one patient to another. There must be a similar balance of gray shades. Such reliability is now easy with the machines of the newest type. Reproducibility of image quality is essential for the communication of ultrasonic data and discussions among colleagues. Regular conferences among ultrasonographers in the same hospital or community provide another source of stimulation; but, if one participant brings high-contrast images, the second saturated ones, and the third artifacts, no discussion is possible.

These different forms of training should help avoid the delays, the errors, and the approximations of truth through trial and error that were the lot of those who had to learn by themselves.

Good luck and go ahead!

REFERENCES

Hill, C. R.: Personal communication, 1976.

Kreel, L.: Computerized tomography using the EMI general purpose scanner, Br. J. Radiol. **50:**2-14, 1977.

Index